X-RAY CT FOR GEOMATERIALS

PROCEEDINGS OF THE INTERNATIONAL WORKSHOP ON X-RAY CT FOR GEOMATERIALS, GEOX2003, 6–7 NOVEMBER 2003, KUMAMOTO, JAPAN

X-ray CT for Geomaterials

Soils, Concrete, Rocks

Edited by

Jun Otani & Yuzo Obara
Department of Civil and Environmental Engineering, Kumamoto University, Kumamoto, Japan

A.A. BALKEMA PUBLISHERS LISSE / ABINGDON / EXTON (PA) / TOKYO

Published by: A.A. Balkema, a member of Swets & Zeitlinger Publishers
www.balkema.nl and www.szp.swets.nl

ISBN 90 5809 666 1

X-ray CT for Geomaterials; Soils, Concrete, Rocks – Otani & Obara (eds.)
© 2004 Swets & Zeitlinger. Lisse, ISBN 90 5809 666 1

Table of Contents

Preface

X-ray Computed Tomography (CT) scanning has been widely used for years as a medical diagnosis technique. To date, this technique is attracting increasing interest for its applicability as a tool in non-destructive testing in engineering. Particularly the testing of *geomaterials*, materials comprising any kind of matter composed of geological substance, such as soils, rocks, concrete and pavement, proved to be very fruitful. The current book forms one of the first reports about the application of X-ray CT in the non-destructive testing of the mechanical properties of geomaterials such as deformation and failure.

This work comprises one special lecture, three keynote lectures and 35 technical papers that were presented at the International Workshop on X-ray CT for Geomaterials (GeoX 2003) in Kumamoto, Japan that was held from 6 to 7 November, 2003.

The four major themes during this gathering are:

- Recent advances of X-ray CT technology in hardware and software
- State-of-the-art of the application of X-ray CT scanning in the testing of geomaterials
- Current world-wide research activities
- Future prospects of X-ray CT applications

This book is intended for researchers and professionals working in the field of geotechnical engineering, soil, rock and concrete engineering and geology.

The topics which are discussed in this book are:

1. Mechanical properties such as deformation and failure of geomaterials
2. Hydraulic properties such as seepage and diffusion of liquids in geomaterials
3. Interaction between geomaterials and other materials
4. Geo-environmental applications
5. New applications
6. Miscellaneous

This workshop was held under the supports of the Faculty of Engineering, Kumamoto University, ISSMGE/TC9, ISSMGE/TC34, ISSMGE/TC35, the Society of Rock Engineering in West Japan, the Japan Society of Civil Engineers, the MMIJ Kyushu Branch, Japan and the Kyushu Branch of Japanese Geotechnical Society. We would like to express our sincere gratitude to all the societies and groups for their strong support to this workshop.

It is our hope that this workshop will be the beginning of a new horizon in the progress of new technologies in geomaterials testing.

Jun Otani
Chairman of GeoX 2003

X-ray CT for Geomaterials; Soils, Concrete, Rocks – Otani & Obara (eds.)
© 2004 Swets & Zeitlinger. Lisse, ISBN 90 5809 666 1

Organization

Organizing Committee:
Prof. Jun Otani (Chairman, Kumamoto University, Japan)
Prof. Yuzo Obara (Co-Chairman, Kumamoto University, Japan)
Dr. Toshifumi Mukunoki (Secretary General, Queen's University, Canada)

Advisory Group:
Prof. H. Akiyama (Kumamoto University, Japan)
Prof. A. Asaoka (Nagoya University, Japan)
Prof. M.D. Bolton (Cambridge University, U.K.) Chairman of ISSMGE/TC35
Prof. J. Desrues (Laboratoire 3S, France)
Prof. A. Hirata (Sojo University, Japan)
Prof. M. Hori (University of Tokyo, Japan)
Prof. A. Iizuka (Kobe University, Japan)
Prof. K. Ikeda (Tohoku University, Japan)
Prof. T. Ishida (Yamaguchi University, Japan)
Prof. K. Kaneko (Hokkaido University, Japan)
Dr. Y. Kikuchi (Port and Airport Research Institute, Japan)
Prof. M. Kimura (Kyoto University, Japan)
Prof. K. Konagai (University of Tokyo, Japan)
Prof. O. Kusakabe (Tokyo Institute of Technology, Japan)
Mr. G.A.M. Kruse (GeoDelft, Netherlands)
Prof. K. Matsui (Kyushu University, Japan)
Prof. K. Matsuki (Tohoku University, Japan) Chairman of Rock Mechanics Division of MMIJ
Prof. A. Murakami (Okayama University, Japan)
Prof. H. Ochiai (Kyushu University, Japan) Chairman of ISSMGE/TC9
Prof. M. Ohtsu (Kumamoto University, Japan)
Prof. F. Oka (Kyoto University, Japan) Chairman of ISSMGE/TC34
Prof. R.K. Rowe (Queen's University, Canada)
Prof. S. Sture (University of Colorado, U.S.A.)
Prof. K. Sugawara (Kumamoto University, Japan) Chairman of ISRM National Group
Dr. M. Takahashi (National Institute of Advanced Industrial Science and Technology, Japan)
Prof. A. Vervoort (K.U. Leuven, Belgium)
Prof. G. Viggiani (Laboratoire 3S, France)
Prof. R.C.K. Wong (University of Calgary, Canada)
Prof. A. Yashima (Gifu University, Japan)

Special lecture

X-ray CT for Geomaterials; Soils, Concrete, Rocks – Otani & Obara (eds.)
© 2004 Swets & Zeitlinger. Lisse, ISBN 90 5809 666 1

Recent advances on X-ray CT

M. Fujii & K. Uyama
Toshiba IT & control systems corporation, Inspection Equipment Division, Tokyo, Japan

ABSTRACT: X-ray CT has been being developed to meet each requirement in medical and industrial field respectively. Medical CT, aiming high speed and high spatial resolution, has achieved 3D (3 dimension) isotropic spatial resolution and quick scan by multi-slice CT. The latest multi-slice CT can take 16 slices (min. 0.5 mm × 16 slices) simultaneously in 1 rotation in 0.5 s. Industrial CT is separated into 2 extremes of aiming high penetrating ability and aiming of high spatial resolution. For high resolution, micro-CT with μm-order resolution has been developed. Besides, the application of 3D shape extracted from CT data to DE (digital engineering) is being schemed actively. Starting from prior application, i.e. quality management, development and analysis, the application of CT to DE is progressing to a new method of engineering.

1 INTRODUCTION

X-ray CT (Computed Tomography) is applied in many industrial fields, as CT has ability of making accurate Images and 3D (3 dimension) data, which could not obtain by usual non destructive testing.

X-ray CT for medical use was invented in 1970s, and was popularized quickly. Stimulated by that, industrial application was started to investigate in 1980s. Medical X-ray CT was started in a system with scanning method of translate-rotate (TR here after) with only 1 channel detector. These early CT has best Images in principle, in spite of many methods of CT later were developed and used practically. CT continued to aim high speed scanning and high resolution, has been progressed to multi-slice CT with scanning method of rotate-rotate (RR here after), with 2 dimensional array detector, obtaining 10 and several slices along Z (body axis) direction in 1 rotation.

CT for industrial use was started in an attempt of scanning of wood or coal etc., which can be scan at X-ray tube voltage of 120 kV, which is applied for human body. Medical CT aims high speed scanning, while, industrial CT is going to be separated into 2 extremes of aiming high penetrating ability and of aiming high spatial resolution. Particularly for high resolution, micro-CT with spatial resolution of μm-order has been developed.

Industrial CT is being used in quality management, development and analysis of trouble for material and products using it's accurate Images. Moreover, it is being attempted actively to apply CT to digital engineering, extracting 3 dimensional shape of object.

2 X-RAY CT

There are 2 types of CT of penetration-type and emission-type. Between these, penetration-type is mainly used, in which X-ray is radiated to object from outside. X-ray CT uses X-ray tube of acceleration-voltage of 100 to 400 kV-class, and further uses 1 to 12 MV linear accelerator for more penetrating ability (Tonner & Stanley 1992).

There are examples of CT for trial using synchrotron radiation of X-ray, extracting monochromatic ray, making image of specified element (Nagata et al. 1993).

On the other hand, X-ray scatter imaging, in which X-ray scattered in the object by Compton scattering is measured, is used in the field of security to detect narcotic or explosive, as whose image is sensitive to materials of low atomic number. This method enables the imaging from one side only, irradiating X-ray to the object and detecting the backward scattering. Examples of CT using the X-ray scatter imaging are reported (Gupta et al. 1987).

3 PROGRESS OF X-RAY CT

The principle of CT is "An image on a closed plane can be reconstructed if projections in all directions through any points on the plane are given". Scanning method of CT systems which satisfies this condition and gives aimed image-quality and is as quick as possible, has been being groped. At present the scanning method is converging to TR and RR, from balancing between ability and cost.

Figure 1 shows scanning methods of CT. RR method, shown in Figure 1a, in which X-ray fan beam covers object, is able to scan only by rotation of X-ray tube and X-ray detector around the object. In RR, data pitch at object is fixed by channel pitch of the detector. Notable characteristic of RR is high speed scanning.

Figure 1b is rotate-only (RO here after) method of micro-CT, which is RR basically. RO rotates object taking magnified projections with micro-focus X-ray tube, whose focal size is from sub-μm to 10 μm, and with X-ray I.I. (Image Intensifier).

Figure 1c is TR method, which is used for middle energy industrial CT. Characteristic of this method is high dimensional accuracy in comparison with medical CT and micro-CT. TR has more advantage to be able to construct CT system flexibly to meet demands on objects, i.e. size and required image quality (Fujii 1999).

4 MEDICAL CT

Medical CT was developed increasing detector channels, aiming high speed and high spatial resolution. Initial TR CT, in which X-ray tube and detector translate and rotate around human body, has limitation in speed, so is replaced by RR. Initial RR system has 320 ch detector with fan angle of about 30° and needs about 10 s for 1 scan. Although the matrix of the image was about 320 × 320, image quality and speed was epoch-making as compared with 2D image of other X-ray inspection system.

At present, main current is continuous rotating multi-slice CT, achieved by various technical innovations. The progress is shown in Figure 2 directly. Figure 2a is an image which is converted to vertical cross-section from axial slices taken with standard condition by single slice CT, which was popular in 1990s. Figure 2b is an image which is taken by latest multi-slice CT. The technical advance is seen at a glance.

The concept of the multi-slice CT is to realize isotropic high resolution and high speed scanning. Isotropic means directionally homogeneous, i.e. data of 3D image is obtained by Voxel of equal size in 3 direction x, y, z. According to the isotropy, more

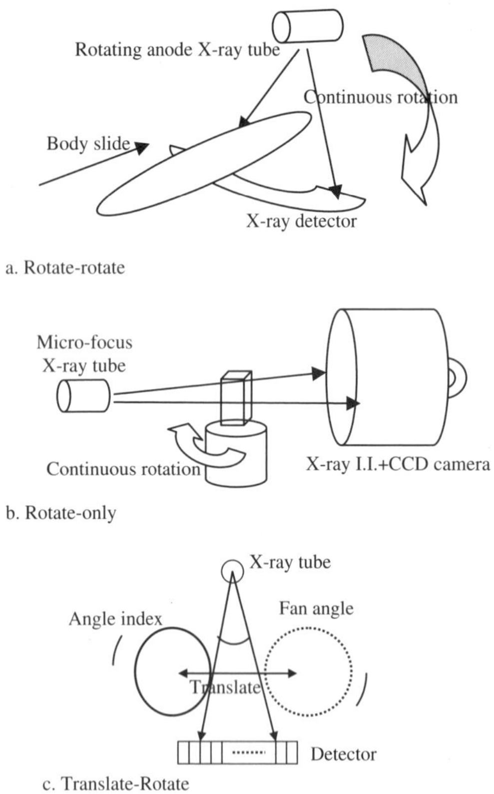

Figure 1. Scanning methods of CT.

a. prior (7mm slice-width)

b. latest (1mm slice-width)

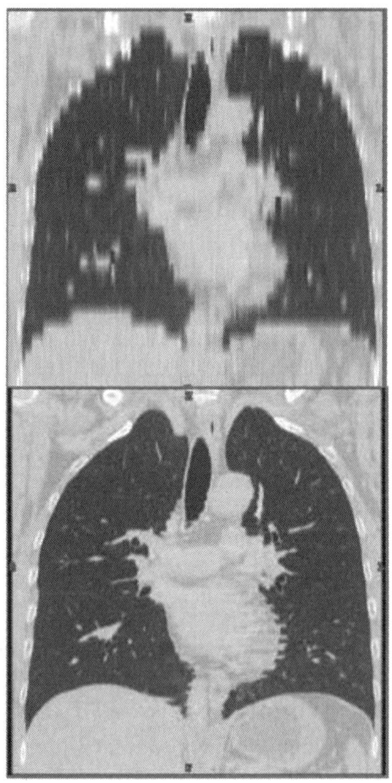

Figure 2. Advance in resolution by multi-slice CT.

precise 3D image or MPR (Multi-Planer Reconstruction) image is possible.

Figure 3 is an appearance of latest multi-slice CT. This CT can take fine 16 slices (minimum slice width 0.5 mm × 16 slices) simultaneously in 1 rotation in 0.5 s (Ozaki 2003). This system has achieved by various technical innovations. Starting from single slice CT, the followings were developed in 1985 to 1993, i.e. continuously rotating high speed CT with slip ring (Mori et al. 1987), helical scan technology (Mori 1986), which moves object in scanning, and technology of real time reconstruction. Scanning time was realized 0.5 s for 1 rotation in 1998. On the base of these technologies, the multi-slice CT was developed, in which X-ray detector, DAS (Data Acquisition System), image reconstruction algorithm and reconstruction system were newly developed.

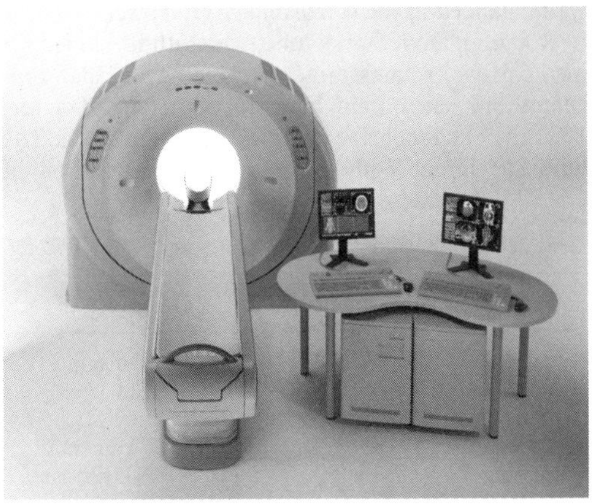

Figure 3. 16 row Multi-slice CT Aquilion™.

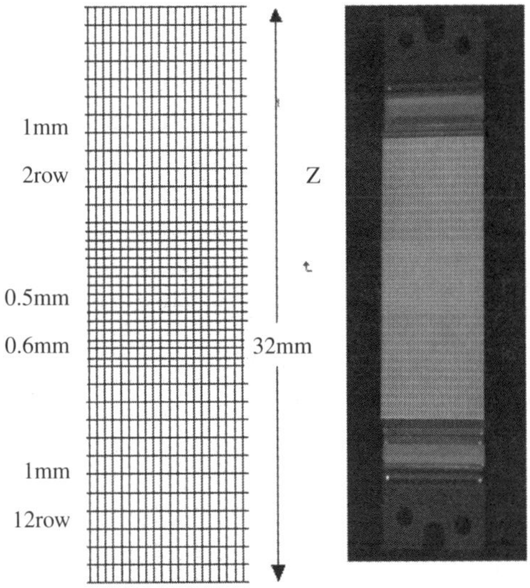

Figure 4. Construction and appearance of the SSMD detector.

The detector, SSMD (Selectable-Slice thickness Multi-row Detector) was developed to realize 16 slices in 1 rotation in 0.5 s. This is a SDD (Solid State Detector), which is constructed by array of scintillator and photodiode, 896 ch in channel direction, 40 cells in direction of body axis, making 2D array of total about 36,000 cells. Figure 4 is 20 ch of SSMD detector. The 40 cells in body axis direction is selected by switch to 16 outputs to the 16 DAS channel, here the cells are combined flexibly making slice width variable. The slice width is selectable from 0.5 mm to 8 mm.

Prior algorithm of image reconstruction is fanbeam backprojection which is limited to 2 dimensional plane. If this algorithm is applied to helical scan CT, strong helical artifact appears, which originate from cone angle error, i.e. inclination of X-ray pass from scanning plane. Backprojection should be correct along projection-pass, so that Feldkamp method (Feldkamp 1984) of algorithm is adaptable to solve cone angle problem. Feldkamp method is an 3D backprojection for circular scanning not for helical. So, the TCOT (True Cone beam Tomograpy Reconstruction Algorithm) method is developed, which is a 3D backprojection applicable to helical scan. The data to be backprojected on to the reconstruction plane, is the data of nearest detector row, which varies as view angle (i.e. rotation angle) varies. The row also varies depending on the position on the plane, in a view. Further, to eliminate helical artifact, helical weight is applied to the data according to the distance of the row from the plane. Helical weight which covers (not 0) over 360° rotation is used for small helical pitch. Helical weight which covers 180° + fan angle + α is used for large helical pitch, that makes half reconstruction.

The exclusive reconstruction system was developed, which is adapted to cone angle exactly, easily applicable to the CT with high throughput. The recon. system has powerful backprojection, which has a rate of minimum 0.4 s for 1 slice reconstruction in spite of 3D backprojection. In the case applied to real time fluoroscopy with 2D cross-sectional image, quick reconstruction of 12 images/s in 512 matrix is possible. The recon. system adopts basic construction of multiple microprocessor with pipe line processing.

Figure 5 is a sample of image which is obtained for large area in short time. Area of 640 mm is taken in about 20 s, here the image from the breast to the abdomen is obtained.

5 INDUSTRIAL CT

Table 1 shows transition of industrial X-ray CT in Japan. In this table main models of medical CT are included in bracket for reference. Initially industrial CTs were constructed using technology and hardware of medical CT. Now on industrial CT, developments are advancing with original technology in middle energy TR CT with 400 kV-class X-ray tube and in micro-CT with micro-focus X-ray tube.

Table 2 shows combinations of X-ray source and X-ray detector for CT based on actual use. Possible X-ray sources are almost 4 kinds of micro-focus X-ray tube, mini-focus X-ray tube, rotating anode X-ray tube and linear accelerator (linac). For CT the balance on X-ray source between focal size and X-ray power is important to obtain aimed spatial resolution and penetrating ability.

Micro-focus X-ray tube, whose X-ray focus is from sub-μm to 10 μm, mainly has acceleration-voltage from 100 kV to 225 kV. Using this tube largely magnified projection-data of object without degradation in sharpness is obtained.

Mini-focus X-ray tube, whose X-ray focus is from 0.1 mm to a few mm, has acceleration-voltage from several 10s kV to 450 kV. X-ray tube emits bremsstrahlung of X-ray when electron beams hits target in the tube of high vacuum. The target is cooled by flowing water or oil to keep temperature below melting point, as about 100% of input electric power is dissipated to heat. Tungsten, which has high melting point, is used for the target, as X-ray maximum output is limited by melting of target. Besides, as focal size is smaller, X-ray maximum output is limited lower, because concentration of heat on the target is larger. From this view, mini-focus X-ray tube is well balanced in focal size and X-ray power.

Rotating anode X-ray tube, which is developed for medical use, rotates target preventing thermal concentration, can obtain large tube current of a few 100 mA. The focal size is same as the mini-focus. The tube has large X-ray power, however, duration of

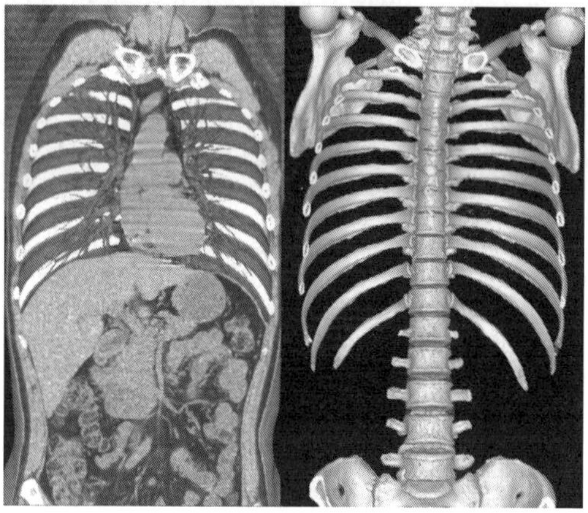

Figure 5. An inspection of breast and abdomen.

Table 2. Combinations of X-ray source and X-ray Detector.

Source	Combination	Detector
• Micro-focus	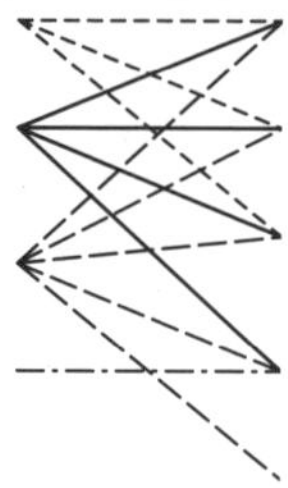	• IP: imaging plate
• Mini-focus		• X-ray I.I. + TV camera
• Rotating anode		• FPD: flat panel detector
• Linear accelerator (linac)		• X-ray line sensor
		• multi-track X-ray line sensor

Table 1. Transition of industrial X-ray CT in Japan.

Year	Method	Source	Detector (channel)	Time (s)	Matrix
1970s	(TR, RR)	(RA120 kV)	(gas 320)	(4.5/9)	(256/320/512)
1980s	• TR	420 kV	solid 8	60	256
	• RR	RA130 kV	gas 320/512	12	320/512
	(RR)	(RA130 kV)	(gas 512)	(3)	(512)
1990s	• TR	450 kV	solid 88/176	60/120	512/1024/2048
	• RO	micro-focus	CCD camera 1300 equiva.	30	do.
	(RR)	(RA130 kV)	(solid 512/900)	(1)	(512)
2000s	• TR	450 kV	solid 176	20	512/1024/2048
	• RO	micro-focus	CCD camera 1300 equivalent	20	do.
	• Cone beam	do.	FPD 1200/2400	40	do.
	(RR multi-slice)	(RA135 kV)	(solid 512/900, 900 × 16 rows)	(0.5)	(512/1024)

RA: rotating anode

X-ray emission is limited in short time, as the whole target is hard to cool down owing to the structure, which has bearings for rotation in vacuum.

Linear accelerator is used for large object, over 100 mm in case of steel. The acceleration of electron is done by high frequency electric field, differently from other X-ray source, and gives high energy X-ray over 1 MeV to about 12 MeV of acceleration energy is ordinarily used. The X-ray detector is designed to keep detection efficiency notwithstanding it is difficult to catch the X-ray with high penetrating ability.

Various CTs are possible with various scanning methods and with various combinations of source and detector, which are shown in Table 2. Although, the main current of industrial CT goes to two directions. One is the middle energy TR CT whose objects are aluminum casting of car engine and so on. This CT uses 400 kV-class mini-focus X-ray tube aiming high penetrating ability. Another is the micro-CT, whose main objects are semiconductor, secondary battery and printed circuit board. This CT obtains cross-sectional image of small structure by taking magnified projections with the micro-focus X-ray tube. The micro-CT uses RO method, which has high X-ray detection efficiency, because X-ray power is not large.

6 MIDDLE ENERGY INDUSTRIAL CT

Figure 6 is an appearance of middle energy industrial CT with TR method. Figure 7 is its system construction. The X-ray tube, detector, scan mechanism etc. are enclosed in X-ray shield box with interlock for safety, so that, the system can be set up easily. TR scan is done by moving object differing from medical CT. The X-ray measuring part comprises X-ray tube of 450 kV, which has the highest energy among X-ray tube, X-ray detector which has high catch up ability of X-ray with scintillator and photo diode.

In industrial CT, image quality is required for various objects in material and in shape, differing from medical use, such as plastics, ceramics, metals and complexes of these. TR method acquires data in translate motion, so that, it can select size of scan area, data pitch, which concerns spatial resolution directly, and data quantity flexibly making it possible to apply for various application.

In TR, the data is acquired by trigger of translate pitch, and the data of fan angle α is acquired in 1 translation. Rotation of α and 1 translation is alternatively repeated, and scan is completed when $180°/\alpha$ times of translations are done. The data pitch (X-ray pass pitch) is as finer as the trigger is finer, so that, channel number of the detector is not dominant to the spatial resolution differing from RR. So, the detector can be constructed with enough space between channels preventing crosstalk and preventing scattered X-ray to enter the detector cell.

The detector developed has tungsten separators of enough thickness between cells against crosstalk,and

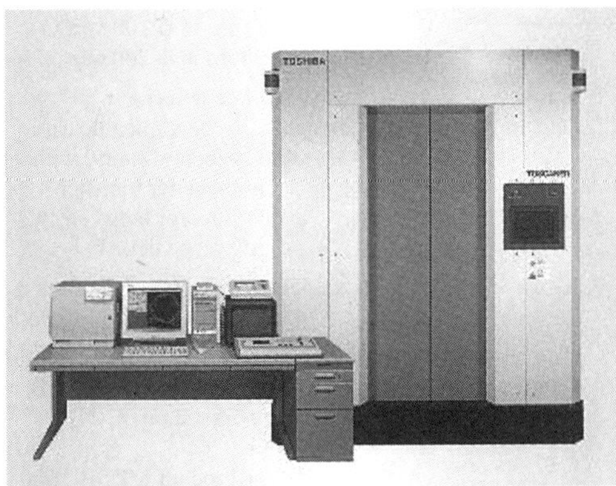

Figure 6. Appearance of middle energy industrial CT.

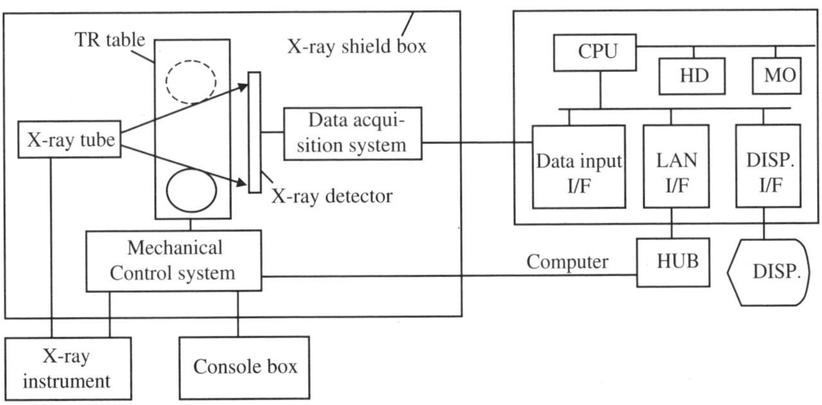

Figure 7. System construction of the middle energy industrial CT.

Table 3. Specification of the middle energy industrial CT.

Item	TOSCANER-24500AV
1. Scan method and mode	translate-rotate (fan angle 30°) mode: half/full/double-full, normal/fine
2. Max. object thickness	aluminum: 300 mm, Fe: 110 mm, Achril:600 mm (condition: double-full, s.w. = 4 mm, 430 kV)
3. Scan area and available objects	scan area: ϕ 300/ϕ 600 changeable object max.size: ϕ 600 × H600 mm object max. weight: 100 kg
4. Slice width	1/2/3/4 mm changeable
5. Scan time (include recon.)	30 s ~ 600 s (option 20 s) by mode change
6. Dimensional accuracy	±0.1 mm at ϕ 300 mm
7. Detectability of defect in AL	drill hole: ϕ 0.4 mm in ϕ 100 mm ϕ 0.8 mm in ϕ 200 mm crack (length10 mm, thickness 4 mm): 0.03 mm in ϕ 100 mm 0.09 mm in ϕ 200 mm
8. X-ray detector	type: solid state detector main det.: 176 ch, applicable to s.w. below 4 mm, with anti-scatter tungsten-collimator between ch.s reference det.: 1 ch
9. X-ray	max.: 450 kV, 5 mA (1.5 mmfocus) 450 kV, 2 mA (0.8 mmfocus) scan: 430 kV, 2 mA (0.8 mmfocus)
10. Data processing	• CPU: Xeon 2.8 GHz × 2, 1 GB • MD: PC workstation 36 GB • DVD, MO • display: 21 type ultra VGA 1600 • OS: Windows 2000 professional

also has tungsten collimators between channels against scattering. This structure is as more important as energy is higher to obtain image of good contrast and high dimensional accuracy, which is important to digital engineering described later.

Table 3 is the main specification of the middle energy industrial CT. The scan area is selectable of 600 mm and 300 mm. The minimum scan time is 20 s including data acquisition, reconstruction and display. Maximum object thickness is 110 mm for steel, 300 mm for aluminum.

This CT is aimed to scan bodies from high-z materials like metals to low-z materials like plastics. For this purpose, the scan time is widely selectable shown in Table 3. But, if scan time is elongated simply, detector overflows, so that, here scan mode is changed. In addition to the prior half-scan, full-scan and (double) full-scan were developed. Data of 360° is acquired at full-scan, and 720° at (double) full-scan. In these scans, data of same pass is combined to data equivalent to long integration time.

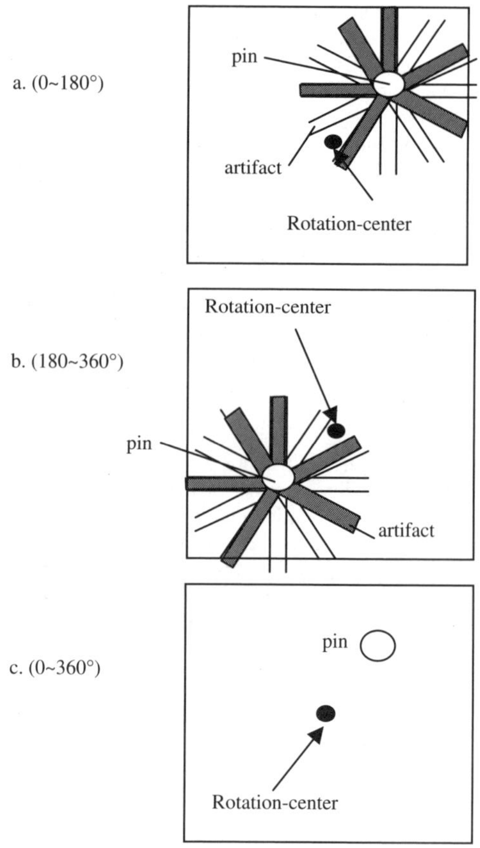

Figure 8. An illustration of cross-sectional image of a pin with artifact.

Another merit of the (double) full-scan is to be able to eliminate residual spoke artifact. The spoke artifact originates from discrepancy of translation-center from rotation-center. Although the translation is adjusted carefully, there remains possibly small residual discrepancy. Figure 8 is an illustration of cross-sectional image of a pin. Figure 8a is a first image obtained by scan of 0° to 180°. Figure 8b is a second image obtained by scan of 180° to 360°. Figure 8c is the final image of the full-scan, i.e. is the added image of the first image and the second image, here the second image is turned 180° before addition as its start location is 180°. Figure 8a has residual spoke artifact around the pin, which appears by angular step of fan angle (here 30°) and whose brightness is opposite at opposite direction. Figure 8b has quite same artifact around the pin as Figure 8a, so that, in Figure 8c spoke

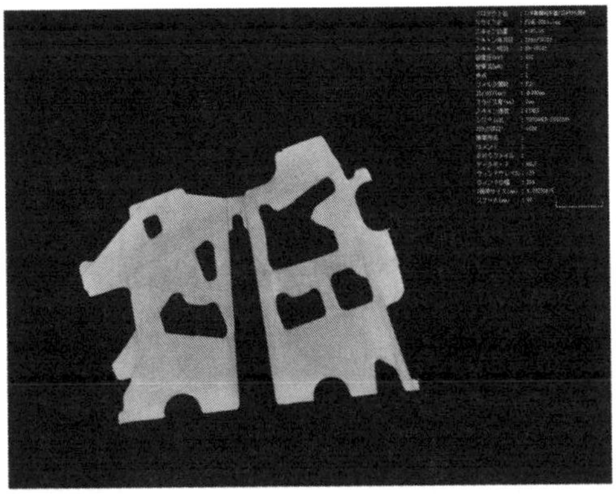

a. half-scan

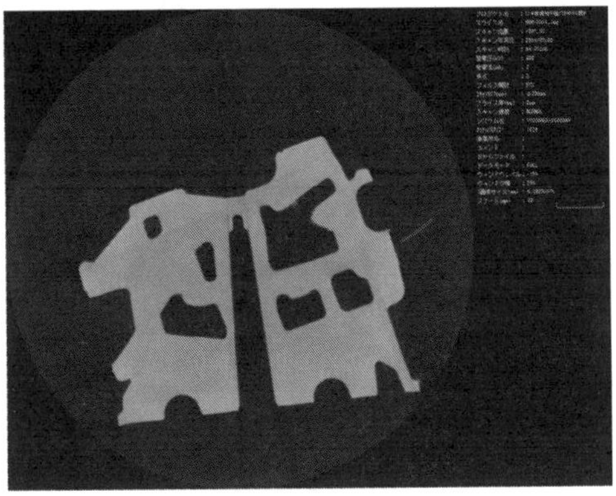

b. full-scan

Figure 9. An example of images by half-scan and full-scan of a cylinder head of a car.

artifact is eliminated. So, image quality is improved in (double) full-scan. Besides, said addition in image is almost same as addition in raw data.

Figure 9 is an example of images by half-scan and full-scan of a cylinder head of a car. Figure 9a is half-scan. Figure 9b is full-scan. The difference of the image quality is recognized obviously.

7 MICRO-CT

There is X-ray fluoroscopic system with the micro-focus X-ray tube and X-ray I.I., which convert X-ray image to visible, yields a few 100 times of magnification of X-ray projection-image. This system is applied mainly to inspect semiconductor and secondary battery. The micro-CT was developed from this X-ray fluoroscopic system.

Figure 10 is an appearance of the micro-CT. Figure 11 is system construction of the micro-CT. With the

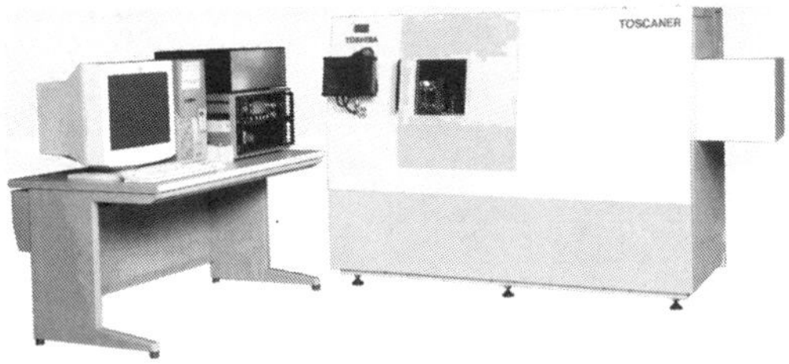

Figure 10. Appearance of the micro-CT.

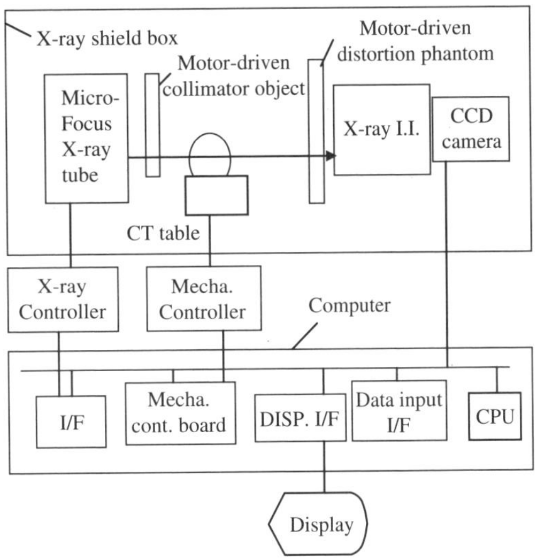

Figure 11. System construction of the micro-CT.

X-ray shield box the system can be set up easily. Projection-images are obtained taking the output of the X-ray I.I. by TV camera, in rotating the object, which is set on the CT table between the tube and the X-ray I.I. From the projection-images, the data on the slice line which is parallel to the rotation surface is extracted for projection-data of CT. As in general the slice line does not coincide to horizontal direction of TV camera, the projection-data is obtained by interpolation, which is processed as data of ordinary RR CT.

The micro-CT has "continuously variable geometry", in which the position of the CT table and the X-ray I.I. can be set continuously toward the X-ray tube direction, and has electric zooming of the X-ray I.I., which changes the detection field of the X-ray I.I., so that, the magnification of X-ray projection-image is continuously variable in wide range. So, for example from a few mm of an electric device to about 200 mm of a structure can be scanned. In general the spatial resolution is higher as the magnification is larger. The spatial resolution of about 5 μm is achieved for maximum magnification.

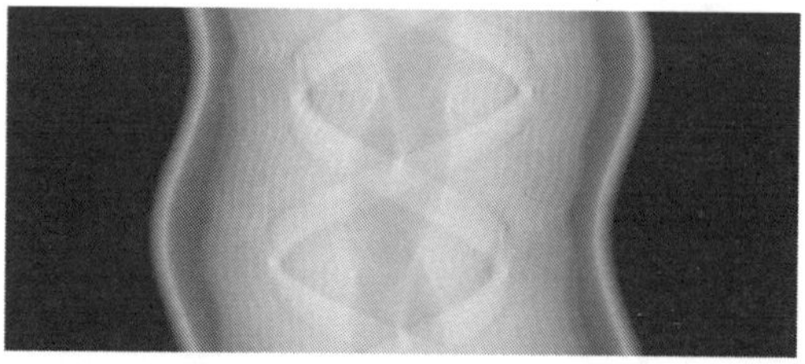

Figure 12. CT projection-data of an object.

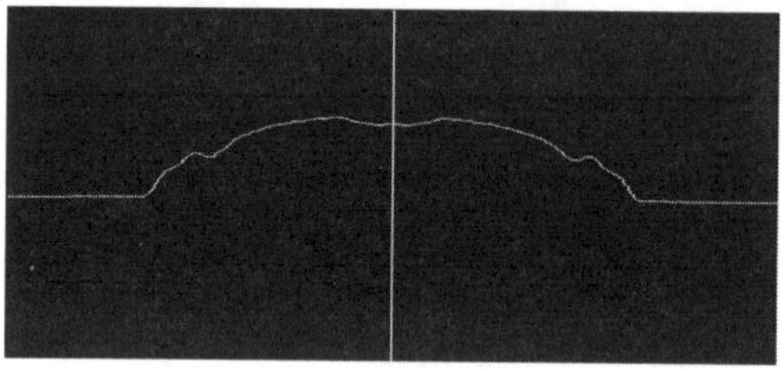

Figure 13. The added projection-data in rotation direction.

The micro-CT also has functions of multi-slice, which gets 5 slices in 1 rotation, cone-beam-scan, which gets 3D data in 1 rotation.

Geometry of micro-CT is continuously variable, in contrast fixed or step-changed of others. Because of this variable geometry, micro-CT is required to do setting of scan condition and calibrations before scan. Calibrations are for image distortion, for rotation-center on image, for focus to rotation-center distance, etc., and for those same as ordinary CT. These calibrations are somewhat troublesome as it is needed whenever geometry changed. So, automatic calibration was developed. When scan condition is changed and that needs a calibration, the system displays the calibration needed and execute automatically.

Most important calibration is for rotation-center on image, which is called centering. The position of rotation-center on image moves when the CT table or the I.I. moves or the zooming is changed. If centering is incomplete, the passes of backprojections shift leading incorrect image.

A software named "auto-centering" is described below which is an automatic calibration of centering, in which rotation-center is obtained from the projection-data of CT scan of the object itself not pin phantom. Figure 12 is CT projection-data of an object, channel in horizontal, rotation in vertical. Figure 13 is the added projection-data in rotation direction. The added projection-data should be symmetrical with respect to rotation-center, as addition is in 360°. The rotation-center is obtained finding symmetrical center by use of correlation method. If there is not "auto-centering", operator must exchange object and pin phantom every time when geometry varies.

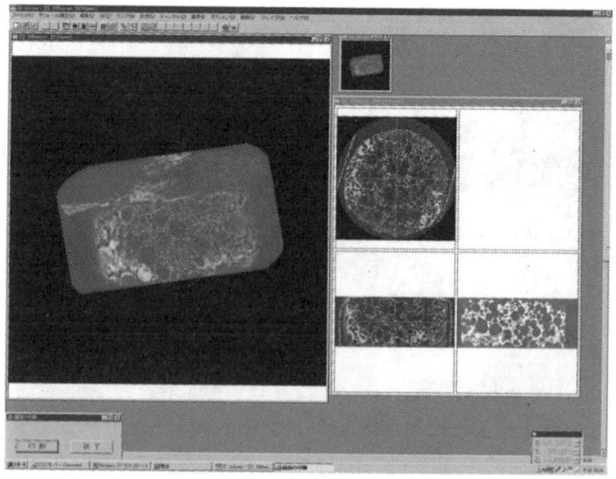

Figure 14. 3D image (left) and MPR image (right) of an artificial bone on which live bone is grown up.

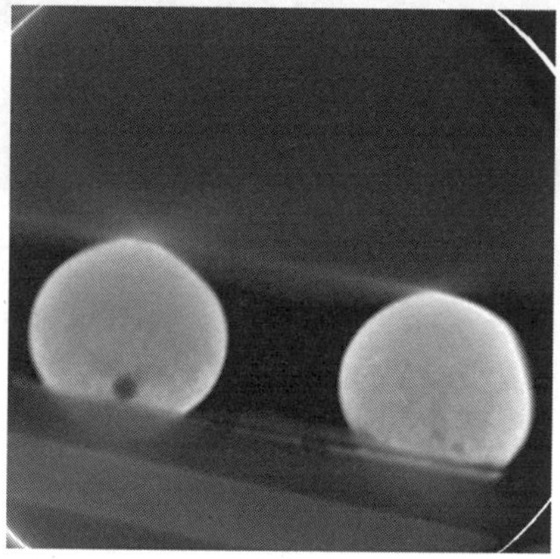

Figure 15. An example image of BGA (Ball Grid Array).

Figure 14 (left) is a 3D image of an artificial bone on which live bone is grown up, whose depth in Z direction is 2 mm, whose slice width and slice pitch is both 30 μm, whose pixel size is 5.3 μm. Figure 14 (right) is MPR image, a circle is standard cross-section, bottom 2 is vertical cross-section whose location is indicated on the standard. Here, arbitrarily inclined cross-section also can be displayed. Changing the cursor line on the standard, the bottom 2 can be changed in real time.

Figure 15 is an example image of BGA (Ball Grid Array), whose diameter is about 500 μm, left ball with a void, right ball with small separation in jointed part.

8 TREND OF CT

Medical CT achieved volume data by helical scan, isotropic spatial resolution by multi-slice CT. At present important approach is "Time". If data in area over

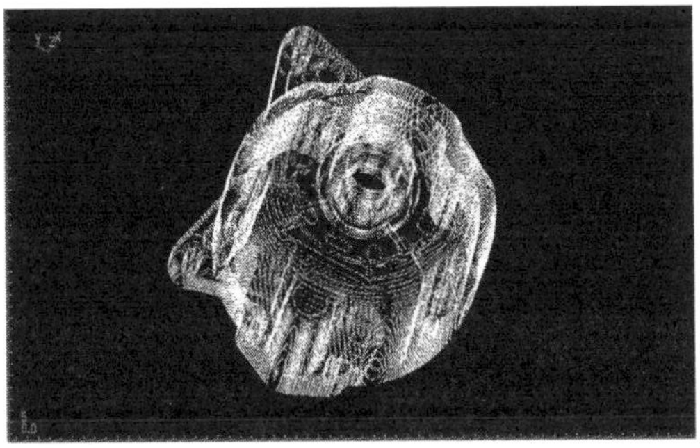

a. the image of cloud of points

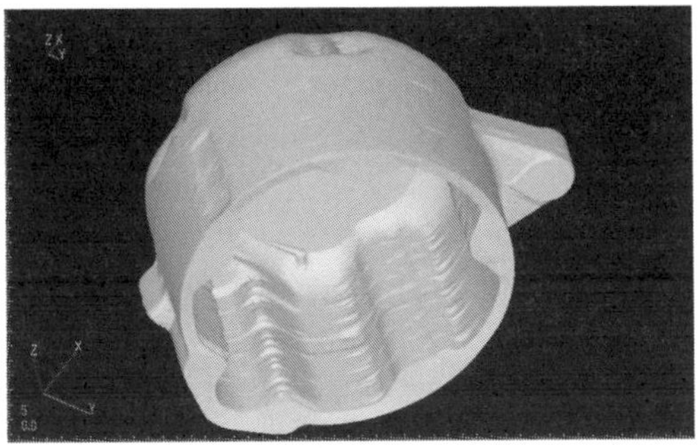

b. the shaded image of STL data

Figure 16. 3D data of aluminum-casting by CT modeler.

100 mm is acquired in a same time, heart motion can be taken to images, though now only suspected motion is visualized by extracting phase data from obtained data in about 30 s. If CT acquires the ability of "Time", heart motion is visible in real time, that is one of future-images of medical CT.

On the other hand, micro-CT is being accelerated in advance. X-ray detector will move from X-ray I.I. and CCD camera to FPD (Flat Panel Detector), which has not image distortion, so, calibration with grid is not necessary. Especially FPD has advantage for cone-beam-scan which is sensitive to image distortion.

Besides, digital engineering (DE), for new application of CT is noticed. DE is a method using 3D data taken by CT and using computer, to do inspection, to make drawing, to do analysis of product manufactured for trial, to make copy from existing body, and so on. Not only outer surface but complicated surface structure and internal structure also should be described accurately in DE. The data of mechanical or optical 3D coordinate measuring machine can not satisfy this requirement. The continuous cross-sectional information obtained by X-ray CT is accurate and complete 3D information, practically useful for DE.

Software, "CT modeler" is developed for extracting 3D shape from CT data. Figure 16 shows images

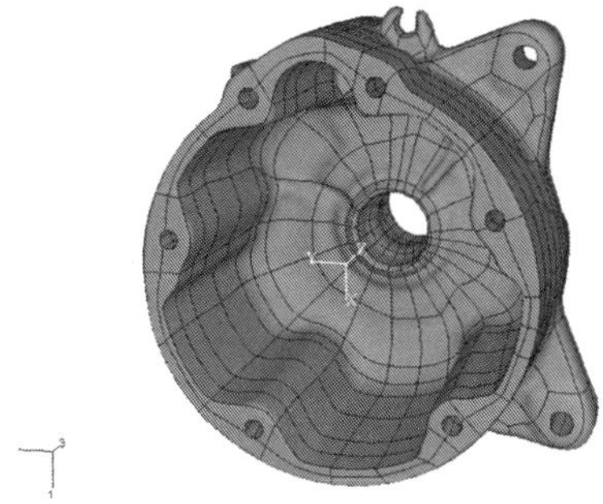

Figure 17. 3D CAD data.

processed by CT modeler of aluminum-casting. Figure 16a is the image of cloud of points, in which outline of body is indicated by points in 3D coordinate. Figure 16b is the shaded image of STL (Standard Triangulation Language) data, in which body shape is indicated by triangular surfaces. The STL data can be used to make copy of the body using rapid prototyping machine.

Figure 17 shows a 3D CAD data, which is obtained by converting the data of cloud of points. The application to DE possibly can make new progress of CT.

9 CONCLUSION

Medical CT, aiming high speed and high spatial resolution, has achieved 3D isotropic spatial resolution and quick scan by multi-slice CT.

Industrial CT is separated to 2 extremes of aiming high penetrating ability and of aiming high spatial resolution. For high resolution, micro-CT with μm-order resolution has been developed. Besides, the application of 3D shape extracted from CT data to DE is being schemed actively. Starting from prior application, i.e. quality management, development and analysis, the application of CT to DE is progressing to a new method of engineering. It is desired that CT technology is useful in various fields and developments go well.

The authors thank Mr. M. Ozaki for his offer of information about the development of medical CT.

REFERENCES

Feldkamp, L.A., Davis, L.C. & Kress, J.W. 1984. Practical cone-beam algorithm. *J. Opt. Soc. Am. A* 1(6): 612–619.

Fujii, M. 1999. Progress of industrial computed tomography and reverse engineering. *Journal of the Japanese Society for Non-destructive Inspection* 48(9): 566–573.

Gupta, N.K., Rodenbaugh, R.F., Silver, M.D. & Silvers, E.A. 1987. Back scatter imaging tomography with high efficiency detectors. *Work in progress, in review of progress in quantitative NDE, June, Williamsburg, VA.*

Mori, I. 1986. Computerized tomographic apparatus utilizing a radiation source. USP4, 630, 202.
Mori, I. et al. 1987. Whole-Body X-ray CT scanner, TCT-900S. *TOSHIBA review* 42(2): 80–82.
Nagata, Y. et al. 1993. Imaging of specified element by monochromatic X-ray using Synchrotron Radiation. *4th Symposium on new Materials and Nondestructive Evaluation of these Products* 3–1: 79–84.
Ozaki, M. 2003. Key technologies of multislice CT scanner, *Journal of the Japanese Society for Non-destructive Inspection* 52(6): 276–279.
Tonner, P.D. & Stanley, J.H. 1992. Supervoltage Computed tomography for large aerospace structures. *Materials Evaluation*, December: 1434–1438.

Keynote lectures

X-ray CT for Geomaterials; Soils, Concrete, Rocks – Otani & Obara (eds.)
© 2004 Swets & Zeitlinger. Lisse, ISBN 90 5809 666 1

Tracking strain localization in geomaterials using computerized tomography

Jacques Desrues
CNRS – Université de Grenoble – Laboratoire 3S

ABSTRACT: Shear banding is a very common phenomenon in Geomaterials. The process which gives rise to shear bands is known as "Strain localization", according to the experimental observation that the deformation process is diffuse at first, and then tends to concentrate in narrow zones called shear bands, one or several. Computerized Tomography has proven to be a very powerful tools to track strain localization in geomaterial specimens. Indeed, localized patterns consisting of several sets of complex shear band mechanisms have been revealed by experiments made on different kind of sands, clay, and clayey rocks. Moreover, quantitative density measurements allowed by Computerized Tomography, provided appropriate calibration is performed, have brought a new insight on so-called "critical state" supposed to be reached in large strains in granular materials: it has been shown that in case of strain localized specimens, this theoretical concept can be matched inside, and only inside, the shear bands. An overview of the techniques developed and the results obtained so far using computerized tomography in the context of strain localization in Geomaterials is given, including the recent advances; encouraging perspectives are drawn for the future use of this powerful technique.

1 INTRODUCTION

Essentially known at first for its medical applications, **Computerized Tomography** (CT) has become nowadays a common tool in the engineering field. Specific devices have become available for industrial and research applications involving specimens or structures made of different kinds of materials, for different purposes including geometrical characterization, defect detection, phase transition, pore fluid flow, and others. Microtomography has developed, taking advantage of the constant improvement of image capture and processing techniques. On the other hand, newly available large equipments offering synchrotron radiation facilities, like the European Synchrotron facility (ESRF) in Grenoble, France, have made possible to develop experiments using high energy X-ray beams as sources for high-resolution Computerized Tomography.

In the 20 past years, using computerized tomography has changed from a pioneering high-tech exotic experimental approach to a still high-tech but well-recognized powerful experimental method.

In the context of Geomechanics, Computerized Tomography was especially appealing for characterizing the heterogeneous deformation structures develop in the specimens when approaching rupture. Indeed, it has been realized in the past 20 years that **Strain Localization** affects most laboratory tests performed on soil specimens. In specially designed laboratory experiments, as for example *plane strain* or *biaxial tests*, direct observation can be sufficient to characterize the geometry of the shear bands. However, in the most common laboratory tests in Geomechanics, namely the axisymmetric *triaxial test*, localization patterns are more difficult to detect and describe. The homogeneity of the void ratio distribution over the specimen during the test, especially when approaching the limit strength, is an essential point to consider for a correct interpretation of the overall volume change measurements. A stabilization of the global volume change for sufficiently large deformation is often considered as the indication of having reached a limit or critical state. But is it a correct interpretation ? If it is recognized that deformation becomes not homogeneous, what is the local evolution of the void ratio as strain localization takes place in the specimen? 55 years ago, Casagrande and Watson (1938) were already asking these questions: "*Whenever distinct failure occurs, then the expansion in volume of the sample as indicated by the standpipe readings takes place in the shearing zones only and the actual void ratio in the shearing zone after failure cannot be determined, except that we can conclude that the increase must be very substantial. This increase* *continues until a void ratio is reached at which continuous movement takes place. Theoretically, this void ratio should be the same regardless whether the test is started in very loose state and the void ratio decreases during the test, or whether the test is started in a dense state and the sample expands in the shearing zone until the void ratio is reached which allow continuous movement without further change in void ratio. It is this void ratio which I originally defined as the "critical value" (critical density).*" Nowadays, constitutive modeling has made significant progresses, strain localization has become an important research field in geomechanics and the experimental tools available have improved quite a lot. After the experimental studies devoted to strain localization in rheological (or "element") tests for soils and granular materials since the late 70's by Vardoulakis *et al.* (1979, 1980, 1982), Arthur *et al.* (1977, 1982), Tatsuoka *et al.* (1990), Desrues *et al.* (1984, 1985, 1989, 1991), and others, it is clear that strain localization affects most of the laboratory tests, even if refined axisymmetric triaxial tests seem to show a special resistance to localization. Hence several authors posed the question of the physical relevance of global volumetric strain measurements, and raised some doubt on the validity of the critical void ratio measurements based on global volume change measurements. In 1977, Vardoulakis stated in his Dissertation that "*for an overcritically dense sand the critical state cannot be reached following an overall homogeneous deformation. The critical state can only be reached inside the shear bands*". At the end, the concept of critical void ratio itself can be questioned. Is there really a unique void ratio attained after large deviatoric strain independently of the initial density, at a given mean pressure? This challenging question was one of those which motivated the author for trying to develop quantitative field measurements methods in bulk materials: strain field with *stereophotogrammetry*, density field with *tomography*.

Computed Tomography (CT) is a valuable tool to study strain localization in granular materials. It allows to observe quantitatively the evolution of the density field inside 3D sand specimens subjected to a mechanical loading. A better knowledge of the inception and development of the localization in shear bands (SB) can be obtained with such investigations. Both the local behavior (inside the SB) and the global one (SB patterning at the scale of the specimen or structure) are quantitatively described. The present paper reports on different studies performed by the author and his co-workers in Laboratoire 3S "*Sols, Solides, Structures*" since the years 1980 on sand, clay and rock specimens, using CT method to characterize the onset of strain localization under loading up to failure.

2 X-RAY IMAGING TECHNIQUES USED IN GEOMATERIAL TESTING

Different authors have used X-ray imaging in experimental studies on geomaterials. In most cases, these studies revealed strain localization taking place in the test. Indeed, during the process of strain localization, not only the shear strain but also the volumetric strain are locally increased. In dense sands sheared under moderate confining pressure, conventional triaxial tests show dilatancy. The response to a purely deviatoric stress loading is a deviatoric strain combined with a significant volume increase of the specimen. When strain localization appears, shear bands can be the locus of very significant density changes due to localized dilatancy. Roscoe *et al.* (1970) in the 60's performed experimental studies on plane strain models of different geotechnical structures such as retaining walls. They used an X-ray technique to follow the displacement of small lead shot distributed in the sand mass. They observed dark bands on the radiographs, and stated that, "*this dark band represents the rupture surface, in which the sand has dilated to the critical state*". Figure 1

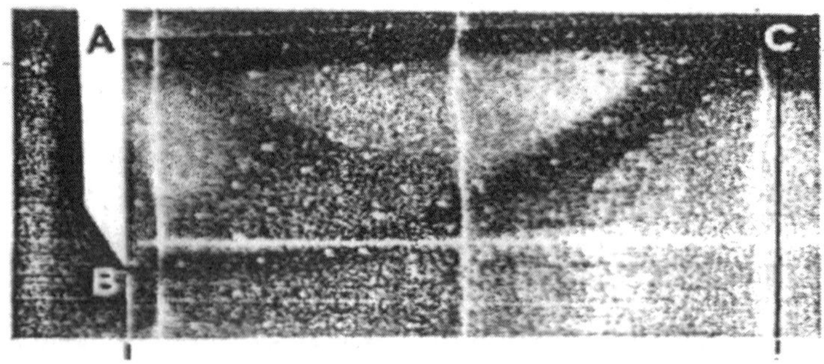

Figure 1. X-ray photography used on plane strain models allowed Roscoe *et al.* his collaborators to show the large dilatancy taking place in shear zones in retaining wall models. After Roscoe *et al.* (1970).

shows a typical example of the pictures presented in the review paper by Roscoe (1970). The same observation was made using the same X-ray technique by other authors – in triaxial tests by Kirkpatrik *et al.* (1968); in flowing sand masses in hoppers by Bransby *et al.* (1975), and later by Michalowsky (1990); in a simple shear apparatus by Scarpelli *et al.* (1982); in the Directional Shear Cell by Arthur *et al.* (1977,1982); in a plane strain biaxial test by Vardoulakis *et al.* (1982); in a thick-walled hollow cylinder test by Alsini *et al.* (1992), and others. Although using X-ray, these studies were not tomographic X-ray methods: in tomographic methods, the density maps are measured in specific planes (in fact, slices) in the specimen or model, while the X-ray methods referenced above were providing averaged attenuation maps through the complete soil mass in the direction perpendicular to the plane of the picture. These X-ray measurements have given most valuable qualitative information on localization patterning in sand specimens and sand box models. However, they generally suffer two limitations: the lack of quantitative data on the observed density changes, and the limitation to plane strain experiments – except for Kirkpatrick (1968). In a number of cases, an attempt to obtain quantitative data was concentrated on the displacement of lead shot disposed in the soil mass, but not on the density field of the soil itself.

As far as tomography applied in soil mechanics is concerned, a pioneering paper was published by Arthur in 1970. At that date Computerized Tomography was not available, but tomographic images were already obtained, using a special arrangement of moving source and photographic plate. The technique was shown to be able to provide pictures of the internal organization of 3D gravel specimens (Fig. 3.36 in the paper cited). Tomography was presented as a promising tool for soils mechanics, due among other qualities to its capacity to provide quantitative measurements. Personal discussions with Dr. J.R.F. Arthur may have influenced the interest of the author of the present paper for tomography.

3 FIRST ATTEMPTS TO MEASURE DENSITIES IN THE SHEAR BANDS

3.1 *Stereophotogrammetry gives some first local volumetric strain incremental measurements*

3.1.1 *Stereophotogrammetric method*

In the early years1980, knowing the already mentioned experimental work performed by Vardoulakis *et al.* (1979, 1980, 1982) in Karlsruhe, the author started to study experimentally strain localization. The need of a strain field measurement method, both accurate and easy to process, was clearly identified as a key point. Following other authors – Butterfield *et al.* (1970), Benefice *et al.* (1979), it was decided to develop so-called *false relief stereophotogrammetry*. High resolution photographic shots on glass plates were taken, a professional stereo comparator apparatus made by Leica was used for data acquisition and a specific data processing software was developed. The author has developed and extensively used this method. In Desrues *et al.* (1984), it is explained how stereophotogrammetry can be used to determine the displacement field of plane strain specimens, then to compute the strain field from these measurements, and finally to characterize quantitatively the volumetric strain, especially in shear bands – see also Desrues *et al.* (1985).

The tools developed and the experience acquired are still used in our current research projects in 2003, although numerical image correlation software becomes nowadays a valuable alternative. Indeed, numerical image correlation is easier to use, faster and hence give richer images in a number of cases. However there is still cases in which stereophotogrammetry is better, especially when strong discontinuities like cracks and sliding planes are concerned.

3.1.2 *A stimulating result*

In a large testing program devoted to strain localization in dense sand (Hostun RF) under low confining pressure (50–100 kPa), it was observed as expected that dilatancy effect was very strong in the incipient shear bands, but decreased and eventually vanished after some relative displacement on the adjacent blocks. A clear illustration of this observation is given in Figure 2. On this figure, deviatoric and volumetric incremental strain components are presented as maps of symbols which are sized proportionally to the local value of the component. In the test considered, a first shear band appears at the increment 6–7; both shear strain (on left upper picture) and volumetric dilating strain (left lower) occur in the band. The unique shear band remains the localized deformation mode for a while. It can be seen in the figure (middle) that during the increment 10–11, almost no volumetric strain is observed inside the band (lower), although large shear occurs (upper). Eventually, after large overall and localized deformation, a second shear band appears. Increment 11–12 shows that both the old and new shear bands are active (shear strain in right upper picture) but only the new one undergoes dilation (volumetric strain in right lower picture). It can be concluded from this observation that the density inside the band tends to a limit value, reached for large localized strains but for short overall equivalent strains (in an element test).

3.2 *Gammametry used for local measurements of density in plane strain sand specimens*

Gamma-ray absorption is an alternative technique for density measurements. It has been used by several

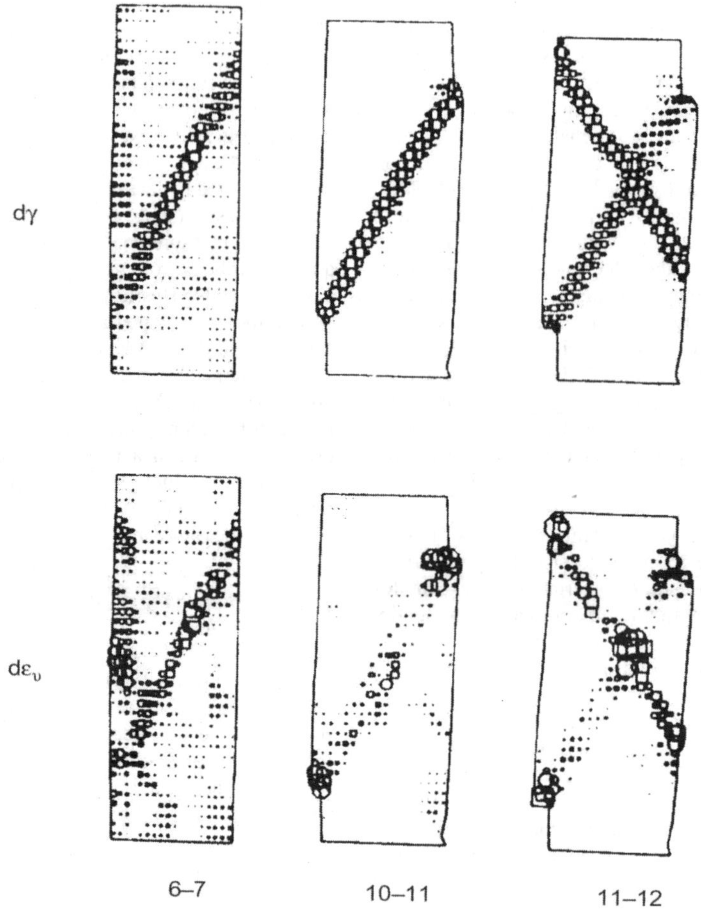

Figure 2. Dilatancy in recent versus old shear band: *towards a limiting void ratio?* After Desrues (1991) p. 139.

authors in the past. Some references can be found in a paper by Tan & Fwa (1991). In the context of strain localization studies, this technique was used in Grenoble by Desrues (1984), and Desrues *et al.* (1985) to perform quantitative measurements of mass density changes in the localized shear zones of sand specimens subjected to plane strain loading. These two studies were made respectively on plane strain test specimens, and on true Triaxial specimens. In both cases, the specimen was loaded up to failure in the testing apparatus, then unloaded and kept pressurized by vacuum applied inside the specimen. Then it was transferred on a special measuring device allowing to enlighten the specimen with a collimated gamma-ray beam. The intensity of the attenuated beam was measured by a detector. Figure 3 illustrates the Principe of the measure. The specimen was placed with its plane strain face perpendicular to the beam; mass density profiles could be obtained, as illustrated in Figure 4 which shows the profile recorded across a shear band. Figure 5 presents a profile for a complete section of the specimen shf18, with comparison of the profile before and after the test.

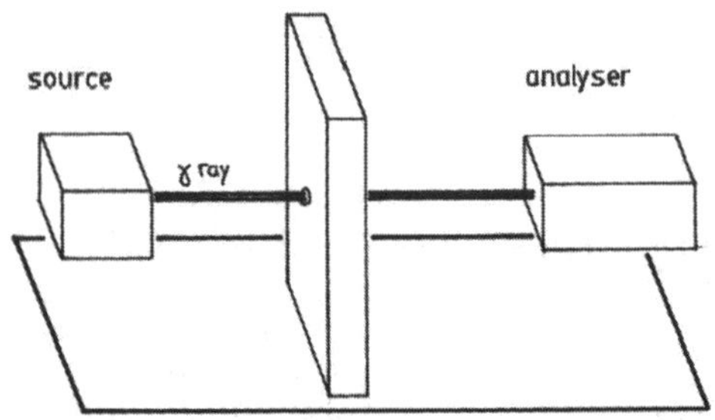

Figure 3. Gamma-ray device used to measure the local density in Shear Bands in plane strain specimens. After Desrues (1984).

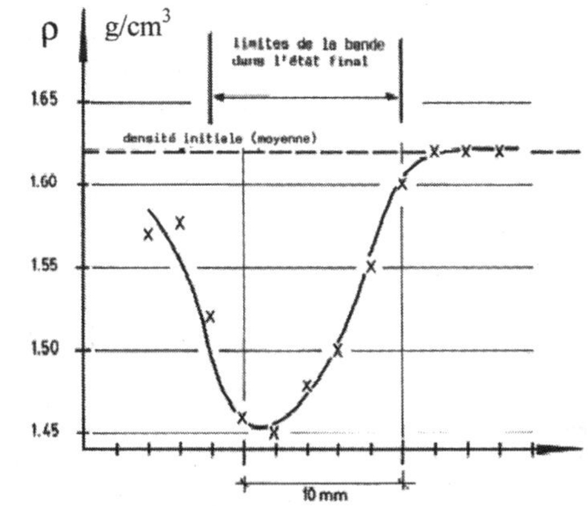

Figure 4. Density profile across a shear band in plane strain test SHF06, recorded by gamma-ray absorpion. Units g/cm^3, mm. (dense specimen, low confining pressure). After Desrues (1984).

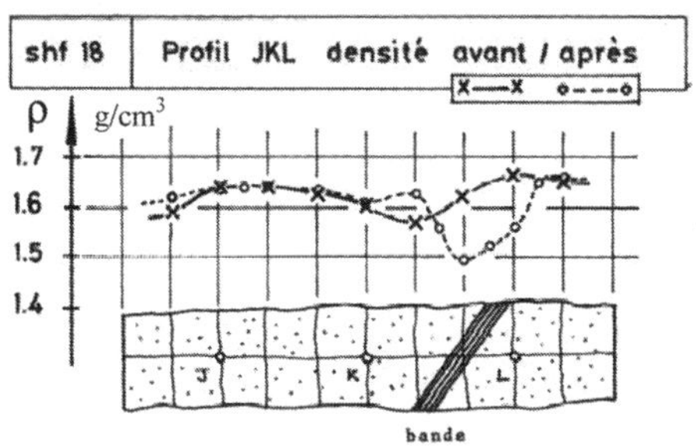

Figure 5. Density profile before and after loading in test shf18 (dense specimen, low confining pressure). After Desrues (1984).

In both cases, significant dilation has taken place in the shear bands, much more than in the rest of the specimen. An estimation of the mass density inside the shear bands at large strain was given by these experiments, which was in the range [1.45–1.50] g/cm^3. Figure 6 shows two profiles obtained using the same technique in a loose specimen, test shf20. All the specimens were tested in plane strain, with the same low confining pressure (about 80 kPa). In Figure 6, the profiles before and after do not differ significantly, the mass density remains about 1.45 g/cm^3 both in the shear bands and outside.

Figure 7 presents another plane strain test, but this one has been performed in the True Triaxial apparatus of Laboratoire 3S-Grenoble. In this apparatus, six rigid platens can be moved to deform the initially cubical specimen into a right-angled prism, with three different principal strain and stresses in the three orthogonal directions parallel to the edges of the specimen. Hence, the test is displacement-controlled and many authors asserted – at least by that time – that in such conditions strain localization is not possible. An experimental technique, consisting in painting the rubber membrane surrounding the sand specimen, allowed us to show that this assertion was false. We were able to see after the test the shear band which had taken place while the specimen was hidden into the closed box of the apparatus: indeed, during the deformation, the intensity of the deformation was so high locally that the paint was taken off from the membrane, keeping memory of the traces of the shear bands on the faces of the specimen (see Figure 7). The specimen is thicker, and its initial geometry is such that the shear band had to be reflected several times on the rigid platens to develop. The profile shows very clearly again that the density inside the shear bands is completely different from the density outside,

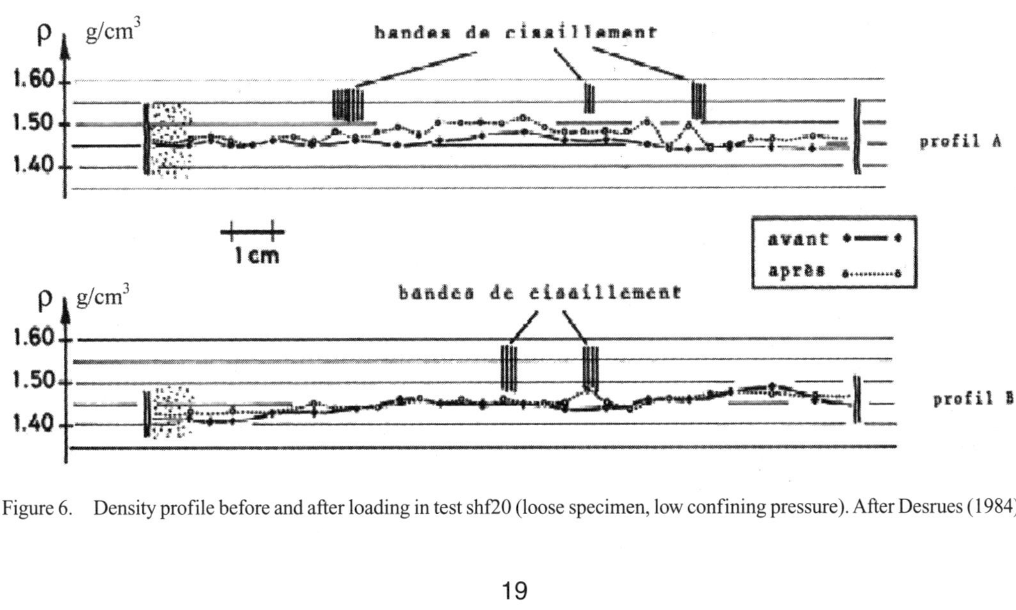

Figure 6. Density profile before and after loading in test shf20 (loose specimen, low confining pressure). After Desrues (1984).

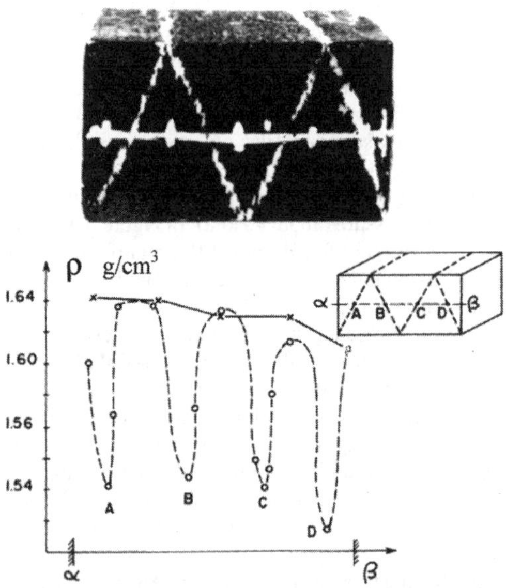

Figure 7. Density profile before (solid line) and after (dashed line) loading in a True Triaxial test (dense specimen, confining pressure 300 kPa. After Desrues *et al.* (1985).

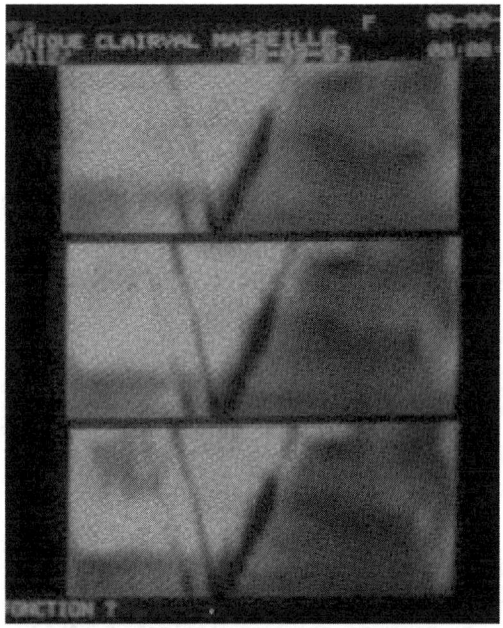

Figure 8. CT scan of three slices parallel to the plane strain plane in resin-injected specimen shf01 loaded to failure under biaxial test conditions. After Desrues (1984).

which does not differ much of the density before the test. The average mass density inside the shear bands is about 1.52 g/cm^3. More details on the latter test can be found in reference Desrues *et al.* (1985).

From these different results it could be stated (consistently with the discussion in paragraph 3.1.2 above) that for a given confining pressure, the density or void ratio inside the shear bands tends to a limit value, the same for dense and loose specimens. More tests, with repetition and verifications would have been necessary to establish firmly the result, but the technique was rather difficult and hence not well-suited for extensive investigation. In addition, like X-ray studies mentioned above, it was still limited to plane strain. However, these studies were preparing the next step, namely Computerized Tomography.

3.3 *First studies using CT*

3.3.1 *CT imaging "frozen" plane strain sand specimens*

A first study by the author using CT was made in 1982, and gave promising results on quantitative local measurements of mass density in the shear bands. This study was reported only in the Doctor of Science Thesis of the author, Desrues (1984) (in French, available for free download on internet at the URL http://A1phnum/hps1/etagere.htm).

After performing the test shf01, the specimen was injected by an epoxy resin. Some time later, on an invitation by Professor Sawczuk in Marseille, France, the author had an opportunity to access to a medical X-ray scanner in a medical center *Clinique Clairval*. Figure 8 was obtained, confirming that the shear bans patterns observed on the face of the specimen were identically developed inside, and that they were places of large dilation. Some attempts were made to calibrate the scanner to get quantitative results, but it was difficult to insure the complete saturation of the pores by the resin. Hence, we had three phases to deal with, namely grains, resin and air. Calibration was not possible. It was decided to try other approaches, not using resin injection (or insuring full saturation by resin).

3.3.2 *CT imaging a first series of axisymmetric triaxial specimens made of different sands*

Another series of preliminary tests with CT control was undertaken in 1984 (Colliat *et al.* 1988). The study was performed using the X-ray scanner facilities of LETI laboratory in Grenoble, thanks to Dr. Ing. Pleyber and Martin who operated the scanner. The mechanical tests were performed on a special apparatus, designed specifically to allow the tomodensitometric survey of the specimens during Triaxial tests performed in the LETI laboratory, an electronic laboratory, not a soil mechanics one. The device consisted of a rather rustic, manually operated mechanical press. The confining pressure was produced by atmospheric pressure acting on the membrane of a dry sand specimen under inner vacuum. After a given loading step, the specimen was unloaded and, still under vacuum, removed from the loading device and placed in the scanner. It was then possible to control the homogeneity of the density over the specimen at several stages of the test. Another limitation of the study was the lack of calibration of the scanner for our material, due to limited access time available. Hence, only qualitative (or quantitative but relative) results could be obtained.

The study was dealing with the improvement of test conditions in axisymmetric Triaxial test, using end platens lubrication and reduced slenderness. Strain localization was searched, considering that the objective of Triaxial tests on soils is to characterize the homogeneous response of the material. Once localized, the response of the tests should not be used as input data for calibrating constitutive models.

All the figure presented were directly photographed on a cathode ray tube (CRT) display. They can be interpreted as classic X-ray pictures. In the pictures, the darker a zone is, the looser the material inside that zone is. When profiles are shown, they concern the attenuation along the zone indicated by dotted in the picture. Differences in lightness and darkness are to be interpreted in relative terms, because the system was not calibrated.

Figures 9 (top) and 9 (bottom) show the density inside the conventionally tested specimen, rough ends and slenderness ratio L/D = 2, at 10% axial strain. At this stage, a typical failure surface was evident to direct observation on the surface of the specimen. In Figure 9 (top), a cross-section is shown at the middle height of the specimen (Z = 10 cm); the failure surface appears clearly as a dark straight line on the picture. Darker means looser, so this figure confirms the strong dilatancy observed inside the shear bands under low mean pressure, reported above and in a number of other works. In Figure 9 (bottom) another cross-section is shown, a few centimeters below the upper platen (Z = 15 cm). The brighter central zone, surrounded by a gray ring, is the section of the less deformed central cone, induced by end restraints (less dilatancy). Moreover, the trace of the failure surface on this cross section appears distorted; this indicates that, during its development, the surface could not penetrate the relatively rigid zone of the central cone, but had to pass around it. This observation was original to the author's knowledge. Although indicating only relative values, the density profiles deserve comment: the lower density, recorded inside the failure surface, is quite the same in both sections (1670 units); the mean value outside the surface, in the central section shown in Figure 9 (top), is about 1730, while the value in the rigid cone, in Figure 9 (bottom), is markedly denser (1880). (These units are uncalibrated, but in monotonic increase with density).

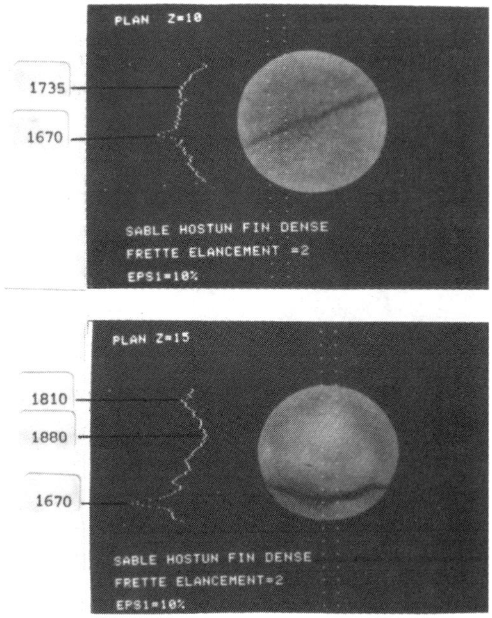

Figure 9. Conventional axisymmetric Triaxial test JLCD37: (top) Z = 10 cm, (bottom) Z = 15 cm.

For the improved tests (lubricated ends, reduced slenderness L/D = 1), a question arises: does a specimen that remains cylindrical after deformation conceal some strong internal heterogeneities? Figure 10 (top) shows a section from just beneath the upper lubricated platen; this rather surprising picture reveals that a very small rigid cone is generated by the small porous stone placed for drainage at the center of the lubricated platen. In Figure 11, a schematic of the actual arrangement, the cone is bordered by a small shear surface, clearly identified by the high void ratio (dark circle in Figure 10-top). The density measure is, again, about 1650 units. The half angle of this small cone can be estimated at 25° from another cross-section, 1 cm beneath, as shown in the figure. This cone, being only a local perturbation, cannot affect significantly the overall measurements neither of axial load, nor of total volumetric change.

Figure 10 (bottom) shows the central cross-section (Z = 5 cm) of the specimen tested with improved conditions, once sheared at 20% axial strain. Conversely to the previous case (conventional test conditions), no failure surface appears clearly inside the specimen, despite the large axial strain. However, the homogeneity is not perfect, as a diffuse heterogeneity can be observed. A denser (white) small zone is located located in the middle of the cross-section, with density count about 1800, surrounded by a darker large zone, with irregular shape, non symmetrically distributed with respect to the center of the cross-section; then a whiter crown around, along the border of the cross-section. In the darker zone, the density count is about 1700, only slightly denser than in the density measured in the failure surfaces. From these observations, we could only state at that time that "this supports the idea of a critical void ratio, which can be reached immediately after localization inside the shear bands, or at large strains in the homogeneous specimens" – Colliat-Dangus *et al.* (1986). Further experiments were announced, to clarify the generality of these preliminary results; they are reported here in section 4.

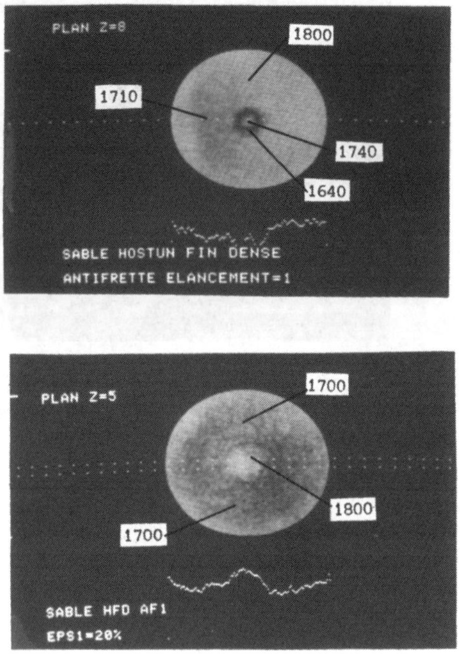

Figure 10. Improved axisymmetric Triaxial test JLCD38: (top) Z = 8 cm, (bottom) Z = 5 cm.

In the same study, a large program of high pressure triaxial tests (up to 15 MPa in confining pressure) were performed, on Hostun sand and on a calcareous sand so-called SC-sand. The latter is made of very small pieces of shells, which are easily broken by the stress concentrations arising in the grains at the contact points between them. Hence, it is very contractive especially at high mean effective stress. Figure 12 shows that the less distorted cones near the top and bottom ends of the specimen, induced by the friction on the platens, undergo less contraction than the rest of the specimen: indeed, darker means looser so the material in the cones is less dense than elsewhere. Figure 13 shows the evidence of a contractive shear band taking place in a sand specimen in large strain: the oblique white band on the right side of the picture is denser than the rest of the specimen. Although purely qualitative, this observation is interesting and it was probably the first one to be described when published in Colliat-Dangus (1986).

3.3.3 *Other studies using CT imaging system in Geomechanics*

To the author's knowledge, before the middle of the 1990's, very few comprehensive studies using CT in the context of soil testing have been reported in the geotechnical literature. As far as rocks are concerned, Raynaud *et al.* in 1989, Fabre *et al.* in 1989 and Vinegard *et al.* in 1991 have published studies on specimens subjected to axisymmetric triaxial loading, and showed that both initial heterogeneity and local density changes induced by the internal failure mechanisms in rock specimens can be accurately described with this technique. Hicher *et al.* (1994) have used tomography to study strain localization in clay

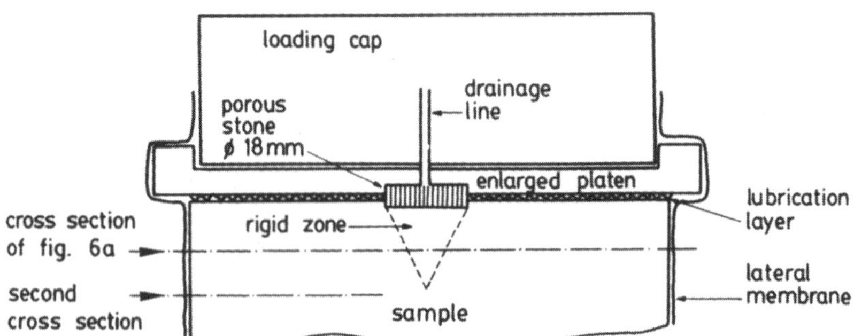

Figure 11. Lubricated end, porous stone and tomographic cross-sections locations in improved axisymmetric triaxial test JLCD38. After Colliat-Dangus *et al.* (1986).

specimens; their study shows that shear bands take place in the tests, and the density change in the shear band is increased with respect to the rest of the specimens, whatever it is dilating (over consolidated specimens) or contracting (normally consolidated specimens). In Undrained tests, no density change is observed in shear bands, although direct observation confirms the presence of localized deformation in these tests.

Later with respect to the studies discussed here, Sture and his collaborators have obtained very similar results to those reported here in section 4. The tests were made on a sand – see Alshibli *et al.* (2000) and (2003). This work is remarkable, because the tests had

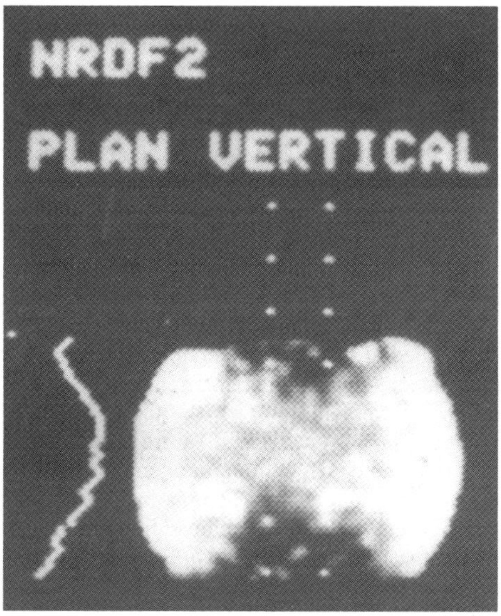

Figure 12. Vertical section of a calcareous sand specimen SC-sand tested under 10 MPa effective confining pressure. The « rigid » cones induced by friction on the top and bottom platens show less contractancy than the rest of the specimen.

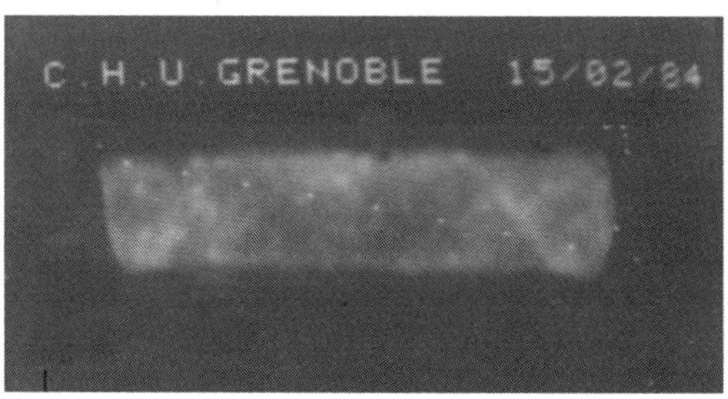

Figure 13. Vertical section of a calcareous sand specimen SC-sand tested under 500 kPa effective confining pressure up to very large axial strain (60%). Initial slenderness ratio was 1. A contactant shear band is observed (oblique white band on the right side of the picture).

been performed at very low effective mean stress in micro-gravity in the space shuttle, then the specimens were scanned using CT after coming back to the earth. However, the comparison of the results with ours essentially shows that what happens in virtually zero gravity is not different from what had been already observed in 1 g gravity.

4 A COMPREHENSIVE STUDY OF STRAIN LOCALIZATION IN AXISYMMETRIC TESTS ON *HOSTUN RF SAND* USING CT

The study reported in the present section started in 1990. It was devoted to strain localization in triaxial tests on sand, and was undertaken by Mokni (1992). A first preliminary set of results from this study was presented by Desrues and Mokni (1991). This section is an expanded version of a paper by Desrues *et al.* (1996); the major additions (subsection 4.3) relate to a complementary study performed some years after the first set of tests, using a higher mean effective stress range and an improved scanner-triaxial configuration. A parallel study done by Tillard-Ngan (1992) in her thesis on marls, has been published in the reference Tillard *et al.* (1993).

The experimental program discussed here involved two series of CT controlled triaxial tests: the first study was performed on loose and dense Hostun RF sand under constant low confining pressure of 60 kPa, and the second on the same sand at three different initial densities (dense-medium-loose) under a higher confining pressure of 400 kPa.

4.1.1 *Material: Hostun RF sand*

Hostun RF sand is a fine granular siliceous sand, uniformly graded, with D50 = 0.32 mm, uniformity coefficient = 1.7, minimum and maximum volumetric weight of 13.24 and 15.99 kN/m^3, respectively (in terms of mass density: 1.35 and 1.63 g/cm^3; in terms of void ratio, 1.00 and 0.65). The grain specific density is 2.65. It is the sand used as a reference material in the studies performed in Grenoble Laboratory 3S/IMG since 1978 by Desrues (1984), Hammad (1991), Mokni (1992) and others. A detailed description of Hostun RF sand can be found in Flavigny *et al.* (1990).

4.1.2 *X-ray computed tomography*

Only a brief description of X-ray computed tomography is given here. More details on the apparatus used in the present study can be found in Latière *et al.* (1987), Colliat *et al.* (1988), Raynaud *et al.* (1989), and general information on Computed Tomography in Bossi *et al.* (1990) and Blumenfeld and Glover (1981). Computed Tomography uses an apparatus commonly known by its medical name as an "X-ray scanner".

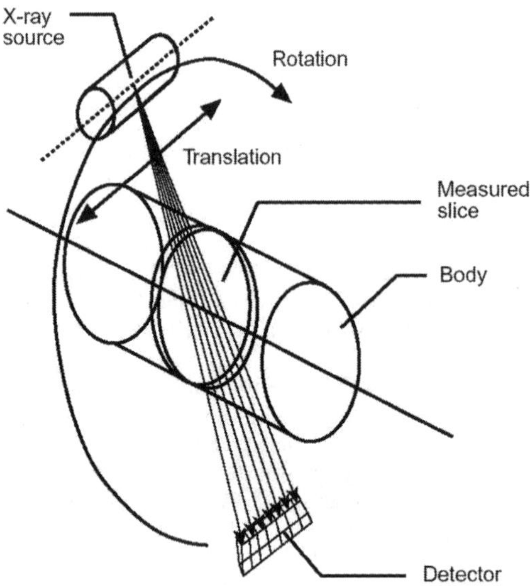

Figure 14. Computed tomography is based on the recording of a set of attenuation profiles of a collimated X-ray beam through a body: each profile is obtained by translation of the beam, and the set of profiles, by rotation of the beam direction in a plane perpendicular to the axis of the measurement field, and the procedure results in a radiographic density map of a slice of the body, whose thickness depends on the width of the beam.

This non-destructive testing method provides cross-sectional images of the attenuation of a X-ray beam through a body. Looking at the physics of the phenomenon, it can be shown (Bossi *et al.* 1990) that the measurement of attenuation which results from CT is predominantly proportional to the electron (mass density of the material under inspection. If the material is made up of a uniform chemical composition, the measurement is proportional to the local mass density of the object. The technique is illustrated in Figure 14: a collimated X-ray beam is moved rotationally and translationally across the body, together with a detector which records a few attenuation profiles for each incidence. The width of the collimated beam determines the thickness of the plane measured slice. The cross-sectional image is constructed numerically from the set of profiles recorded. By placing a triaxial specimen with its axis coincident with the axis of the scanner, and moving the specimen along the axis, a complete set of cross sections is obtained. Using appropriate image software, the slices can be placed next to each other to construct a complete 3-D image of the specimen.

The scanner ND8000 used in the experiments is a medical apparatus, installed in the CNRS Laboratory LMA, Marseille, France. The experimental set-up is presented in Figure 15. The scanner itself is represented in this sketch only by the source and detector, and the volume called measurement field. In this field can be placed a triaxial cell, aluminium made in order to be transparent to X-rays. The axial displacement is applied by a screw jack, at constant speed. The reaction frame is made of strong steel beams; they have to encircle the full scanner since no metallic element can be put inside the measurement field, except the aluminium cell vessel. However, the tests presented in the paper Desrues *et al.* (1996) were performed in a less elaborated configuration, in which the confining pressure was applied by vacuum inside the specimens; hence no cell was used; in addition, the loading stage of the test was done outside the measurement field, in a separate loading frame.

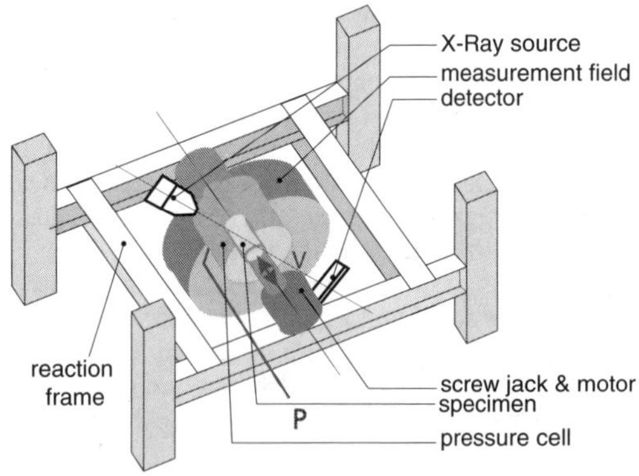

Figure 15. Experimental set-up: specimen, triaxial cell, scanner field measurement and reaction frame.

The resolution of a CT scanner at the object is determined by the source and detector dimensions and the position of the object under test with respect to them (Bossi *et al.* 1990). The spatial resolution, and the density resolution, are two different things – but related together in a complex way. When measuring, for example, the density of water in a bottle, the homogeneity of the specimen is almost perfect and the only cause of local error is the noise of the apparatus (dominated by the quantic noise of the source). In the scanner used, the standard deviation of the density in a water bottle, over a square zone including about 2000 pixels, is currently recorded as 0.2%. This is a measure of the density resolution. However, when measuring heterogeneous specimens, the spatial resolution plays a role in the local measurement. In an ideal apparatus, an infinitesimal point in the object should affect only an equivalent point in the image. In real apparatuses, the imaging system creates an image of an infinitesimal point as a blurred or broadened intensity distribution that overlaps and inteferes with the images of neighbouring points (Blumenfeld and

Glover 1981). The spatial resolution of an imaging system is the parameter that specifies how far apart two very small high-contrast objects must be to be detected as separate in the displayed image. Following the constructor' information, in the scanner used, the spatial resolution can be up to seven pairs of lines per centimeter, which means that the minimum distance between discernable small objects is about 0.7 mm. In the tests presented, the scanner tuning was optimized for density resolution, rather than spatial; in that case, using the practical rules given by Bossi *et al.* (1990), the spatial resolution can be estimated as 2.5 pair of lines per centimeter, i.e. 2 mm. Practically however, there is other reasons why the boundaries of the heterogeneities in the specimens can be blurred and broadened: the partial volume effects, which occur for example when the boundaries (of the specimen, of heterogeneities) are not perpendicular to the slice. Hence, the local measurements must be considered with caution, especially when the heterogeneities are small or narrow with respect to the apparatus spatial resolution. In the tests presented, the thickness of the slice was set to 4 mm. Hence, the density maps recorded represent the averaged density over a 4 mm thick slice of the body, perpendicular to the axis of the apparatus. After reconstruction from the profiles recorded, the density map is obtained as a discrete set of numbers supposed to represent the average density over small elements of the picture, the pixels. In the ND8000, each pixel represents a $0.7 \times 0.7\,mm^2$ square of the medium plane of the slice.

In a granular material, with a grain size finer than the scanner resolution, the local attenuation can be directly linked to the local density of the material. As indicated before, the underlying physics show that in a material with homogeneous chemical composition the relation between the radiological attenuation and the mass density is linear. A calibration has been carried out, using several sand specimens deposited carefully to produce well-defined loose, medium and dense densities. After checking the homogeneity of the deposit , averaged measures of the radiological attenuation over the specimen were recorded and compared to the mass density (g/cm^3) of the deposit. The measured data points were fitted using the following linear calibration relation, illustrated in Figure 16:

$$W = 0.00132 \times H + 1.222$$

where W is the mass density in g/cm^3, and H the radiographic absorption. The mean deviation from the linear approximation is about $7 \times 10^{-3} g/cm^3$, i.e. a relative error of approximately 0.5% in mass density. Using the ND8000 scanner in its standard (medical) configuration, the output data H is expressed in the so-called Hounsfield scale, in which the absorption is -1000 units in air and 0 in water. When testing materials, it can be convenient to shift the density window

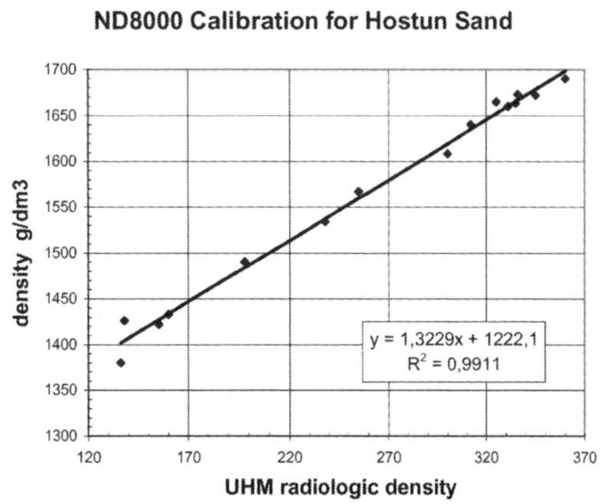

Figure 16. ND8000 Calibration of CT measurements for Hostun sand in term of mass density: mass density is defined by global measurement of the specimen mass divided by its volume; radiographic density is given by the average over of the specimen.

of the apparatus in order to improve the sensibility in the relevant range. In the test program reported, the water absorption was set to -300 units (the abbreviation MHU is used in the present paper, for Modified Hounsfield Units).

During the triaxial tests, the scanning program was conducted as follows: complete scanning with a full set of slices placed next to each other in the initial and final states; partial scanning: 3 slices – bottom, middle, top – in the intermediate states. The images were recorded numerically on computer hard disc.

After the tests, the density images were explored using image processing software's. There were two basic operations: reconstruction of axial or parallel to axis views on the basis of full scanning states, and measurement of density averages over well defined regions such as shear band or part of shear band, and full section of the specimen.

The density measurements were done using specific devices available from the workstation, allowing us to define interactively a region of interest (ROI) and to get the mean value and standard deviation over the region. Profiles along lines could be obtained too, and local point measurements including maximum and minimum over a zone. Averages over zones were preferred to eliminate possibly less significant local measurements. To estimate the accuracy of the evaluation of the averaged local density over a shear zone, some measurements on a zone were repeated, each time including the definition of the region of interest; the scatter of the void ratio was found to be about 0.02.

However, the possible effect of the spatial resolution on the local measurement deserves some comments. The spatial resolution of the apparatus, estimated to

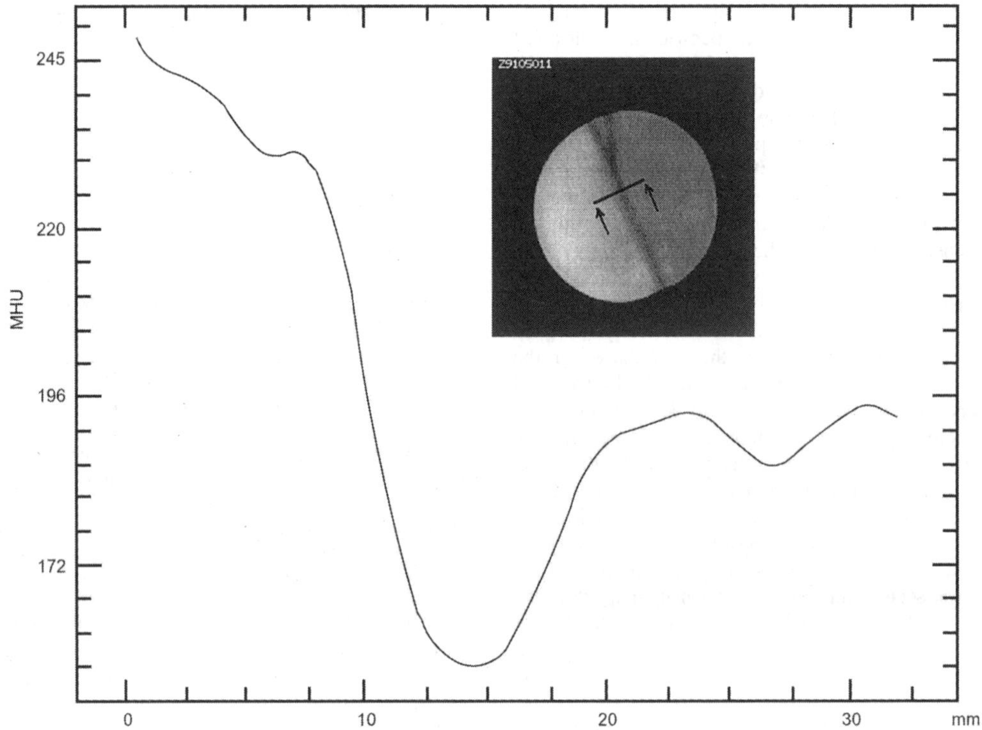

Figure 17. Density profile recorded in a shear band: the trace of the profile is indicated on the density map.

2 mm in the configuration used, is smaller than the shear band thickness (estimated in the range 20 to 30 mean grain size, namely 6–9 mm). A typical density profile across a shear band in a dense specimen is presented in Figure 17. This profile appears more as a round-shaped trench with a smooth transition with the neighboring soil mass than a sharp cut with homogeneous density inside. Such a profile can be interpreted as the indication of an influence of the spatial resolution; in fact, it looks like a typical PSF (point spread function), which quantifies the broadening of the intensity distribution of a small contrasted object by an imaging system.

On the other hand, the actual density profile in shear bands can be a smooth curve. It is possible too that, being so close to the grain scale, only an average measure over the band has a physical meaning at the continuum level. The spatial resolution of the scanner used was not sufficient to address these questions in the present study. Practically, for each local measurement, several samples were taken in order to control that the measure obtained was representative.

4.1.3 *Triaxial test procedure*

The tests performed in this study were axisymmetric triaxial tests, i.e. had an axisymmetric geometry (specimen shape) and loading conditions (constant lateral pressure, and increasing axial load). The material was deposited by pluviation from a large funnel through a nozzle at a constant drop height. For the loose specimens, the nozzle diameter was 40 mm and the drop height null, which gave approximately 20% relative density. For the dense specimens, relative density was about 90%. These techniques ensure homogeneity and reproducibility. The material was tested dry. The latex membrane, wrapping the lateral sides of the specimen, was approximately 0.35 mm thick. The diameter of the specimens was 100 mm, the its height was 100 mm (except RFDT4, whose height was 200 mm). Axial load and axial displacement were measured.

The specific features were:

- An anti friction device was used to reduce the perturbations due to friction between the specimen and the platens. It consisted of polished steel platens (larger than the specimen) and two rubber discs, 0.4 mm.
- thick, coated with silicon grease. Drainage (air) was ensured by a 18-mm central porous stone on each platen. For comparison, a single test was performed in "conventional" test conditions, i.e. no anti friction device and slenderness ratio 2.
- The confining pressure was obtained by applying an internal vacuum inside the specimen, without a

Table 1. Triaxial tests on Hostun RF sand ($\sigma_3 = 60$ kPa).

Test name	Height h_0 (mm)	Diameter d_0 (mm)	Slenderness h_0/d_0	ρ_0 at $\sigma_c = 60$ kPa (g/cm^3)	Test conditions
rfdt3	101.0	100.3	1.0	1.663	Dense, lubricated
rfdt6	100.0	100.0	1.0	1.665	Dense, lubricated
rfdt7	100.0	100.0	1.0	1.660	Dense, lubricated
rfdt4	196.0	101.0	1.94	1.640	Dense, non lubricated
rfdt8	100.0	100.0	1.0	1.673	Dense, soft inclusion
rflt1	100.0	100.6	1.0	1.380	Loose, lubricated
rflt2	192.0	100.9	1.90	1.426	Loose, non lubricated
hfdt1	100.0	100.0	1.0	1.64	Dense, short, NL

confining cell. The difference between the atmospheric pressure and the lower internal pressure was fixed at 60 kPa.

- In this study, the test was not performed directly inside the scanner measuring field. The test procedure consisted in the following successive steps – the pressurized specimen was submitted to a small strain increment in a loading frame, then unloaded, dismounted from the frame, and placed in the scanner for tomography. This sequence was repeated 8 to 12 times, depending on the amount of final deformation.

During the swap between the tester and the scanner, the specimen was kept under its nominal confining pressure by a continuously active vacuum line. Handled carefully, it was not subjected to other disturbance than the effect of the repeated loading–unloading cycles. It is well known that specimens tested under cyclic loading accumulate volumetric strains as the number of cycles increases; however, the effect of ten cycles is not significant with respect to the question addressed in this paper, namely the large density changes undergone in shear bands. In fact, a comparison was made between a typical test under scanner and a test performed in the classical way on a triaxial apparatus. In the latter, the sand was tested dry, without unloading sequences, and the volumetric change was measured by recording the expelled cell fluid. It was found that the scanner density averaged over the specimen and the volumetric strain curve measured using the classical soil mechanics procedures on a monotonic loaded specimen of the same dry sand under the same test conditions were very close (Figure 13 in reference Desrues and Mokni, 1991).

4.2 *Results and analysis*

4.2.1 *Test program*

The series of tests performed on Hostun RF sand is listed in Table 1. Both dense and loose, lubricated and non lubricated, long and short, homogeneous and slightly perturbed specimens were prepared and tested in order to observe the effects of these different test conditions on the onset of localization, and the subsequent localization patterns.

4.2.2 *Localization patterns observed*

The onset of localization and the development of a complete localization structure inside the specimens were very clearly revealed by the density maps in the dense case. Conversely, in the loose specimens, it was difficult to observe localization structures, because the density in the localized strain zones did not change significantly.

In the dense specimens, localization was observed to depend very much on the test conditions. Hereafter a few tests showing different typical localization patterns are described.

In Test rfdt4, performed on a long and non lubricated specimen, a single shear plane appeared at a global axial strain $\varepsilon_a = 7\%$, and remained the unique localization structure for larger strain. This is a common observation in conventional triaxial testing. Figure 18 shows two tomograms of the specimen at $\varepsilon_a = 13\%$. The left picture is taken perpendicular to the axis of the specimen approximately at middle height, while the right one is parallel to the axis and contains it. The dark band is the trace of the shear plane. It can be noted that the trace is not perfectly straight, which means that the localization zone is not a perfect plane.

The stress ratio versus axial strain curve for this test is presented in Figure 19. It shows a very marked peak, arising as soon as $\varepsilon_a = 3$–4% while the mean void ratio increase is abruptly stopped, but not before $\varepsilon_a = 7\%$. In contrast to that rather simple localization pattern, test hfdt1, which was performed on a short but non lubricated specimen gave a quite different localization pattern as revealed by the CT images of Figure 20. In that figure, the upper picture is a tomogram perpendicular to the axis of the specimen, taken near the upper platen. A rigid cone, attached to the end platen, can be observed in that picture. This cone

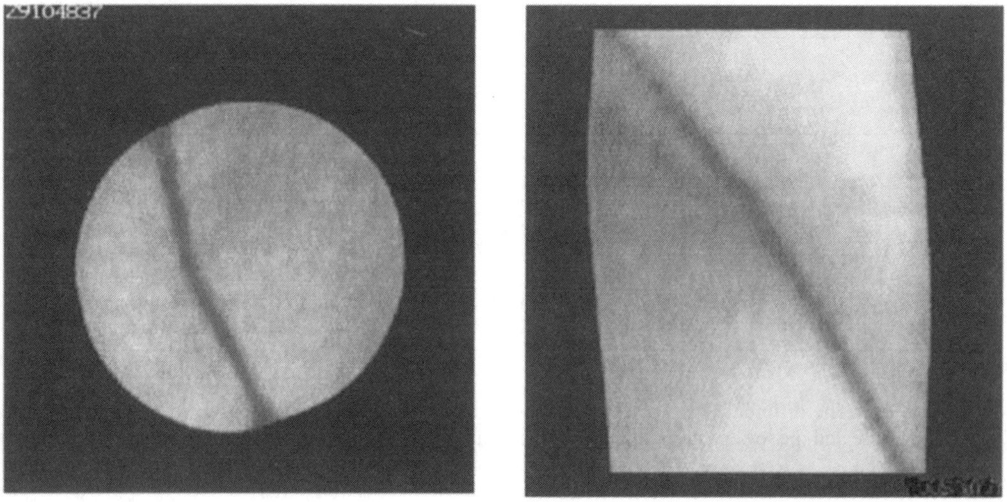

Figure 18. Trace of the single shear plane in Specimen rfdt4 (ε_a = 13%): (left) trace of the shear zone in a section perpendicular to the axis in a cross-section 72 mm above the bottom platen in the initial state; (right) containing the axis of the specimen.

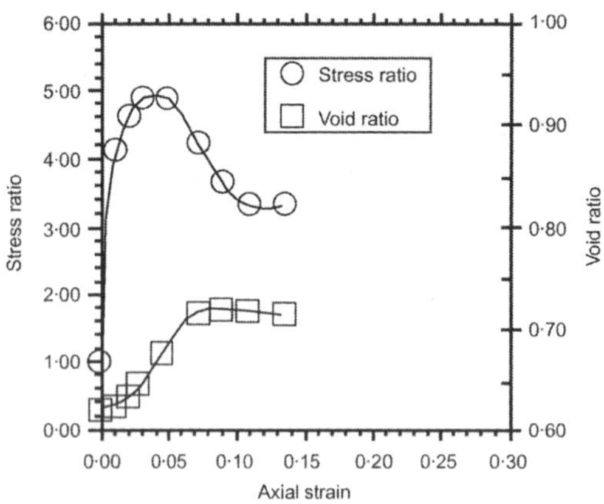

Figure 19. Stress ratio and void ratio plotted against axial strain recorded during test rfdt4.

is delimited by a circular shear surface which is the locus of a large dilatancy. The lower picture is taken approximately at the middle of the specimen. It reveals that the rest of the specimen outside the rigid cone is severely affected by strain localization along surfaces with approximately straight traces in the planes perpendicular to the axis. This surprising figure is discussed in detail later on.

When short lubricated specimens were tested – which is the standard of advanced triaxial testing on granular materials since the 80's – the onset of localization was significantly delayed. For example, in Test rfdt6, the density field at ε_a = 16% showed only the very beginning of a localized structure, which became really clear only at 20%. In rfdt7, the localization started at 16%, but in rfdt8 the density field at 19% was still non localized.

The variation of stress ratio versus axial strain presented in Figures 21, 22, 23 show that the peak in the stress curves in these tests was much softer than in Test rfdt4 (Fig. 19) performed under regular (non-lubricated) conditions. In addition, the peak occurred at larger axial strain. The three void ratio versus axial strain curves look similar and seem to tend towards the same constant value. On the other hand, there is no apparent correlation between the occurrence of the plateau in volume change and the peak stress. The global volume change evolution is observed not to stop before an axial strain in the range from two to three times the strain at stress peak. The question of the physical relevance of the global volume curves is discussed later on.

The localization patterns observed in these specimens were different from one test to the other, and showed complex geometry as illustrated in Figures 24 and 25. In both these specimens, the localized deformation is organized with a single rigid cone attached to one of the platens, while the other platen does not generate any cone. Outside the cone, complex patterns are observed. In Figure 24, the localized strains are developed mainly on one side of the specimen. Indeed, this test was marked by a severe rotation of the upper platen in the NW direction (direction of the upper left corner of the cross-section pictures). In Figure 25, the rigid cone is clearly seen on the bottom

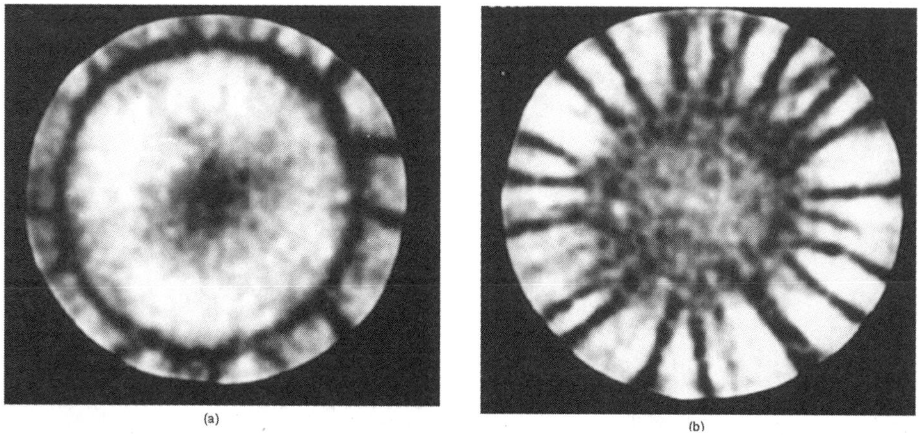

Figure 20. Two cross-sections recorded in specimen hfdt1, revealing complex localization patterns (a) near the upper platen and (b) at middle height of the specimen for $\varepsilon_a = 13\%$ (positions of the cross-sections in the initial state: (a) 80 mm and (b) 50 mm from the bottom platen).

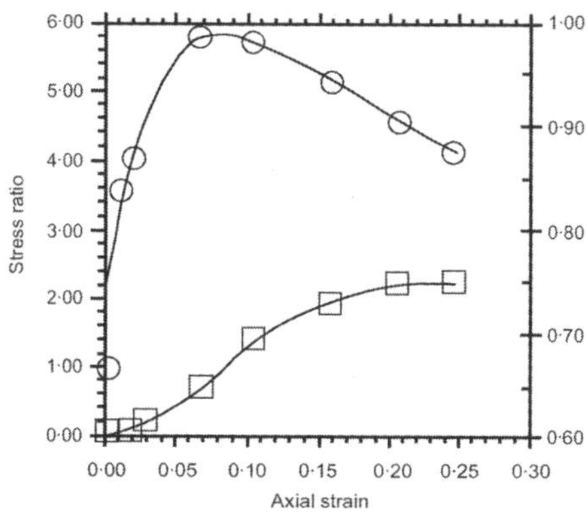

Figure 21. Stress ratio and void ratio plotted against axial strain recorded during test rfdt6.

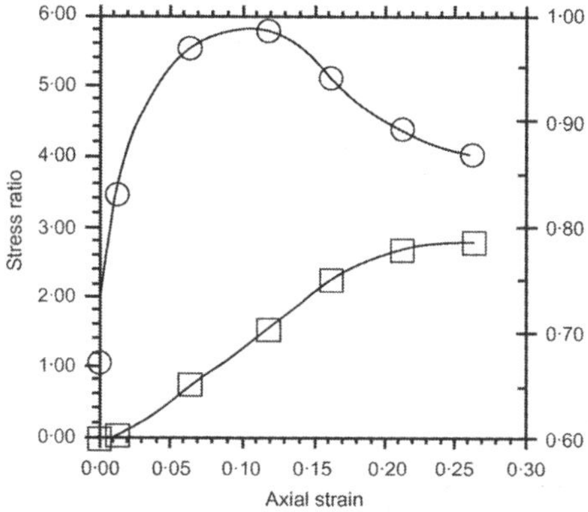

Figure 22. Stress ratio and void ratio plotted against axial strain recorded during test rfdt7.

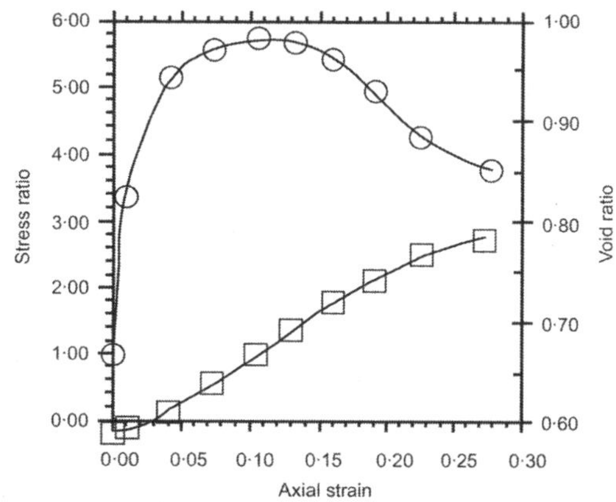

Figure 23. Stress ratio and void ratio plotted against axial strain recorded during test rfdt8.

cross section, and complex patterns can be observed in the top cross section. There are two apparently undistorted zones (white on the picture) separated by a more disturbed zone, and sliced again by dark lines which are intense shear zones. At first, it seems difficult to extract some general information from such pictures. However, a detailed image analysis of the density maps obtained during Test rfdt8 revealed a pattern which may be somewhat generic. Figure 26 shows the six upper tomograms in the specimen strained at 27%. The distance of the mean plane of each slice from the upper platen is 4, 8, 12, 16, 20, and 24 mm.

As shown in Figure 26, a black central circle appears on the top picture, and gets bigger in diameter as the tomograms are taken further from the top. Besides this approximate circle, one can notice a set of pairs

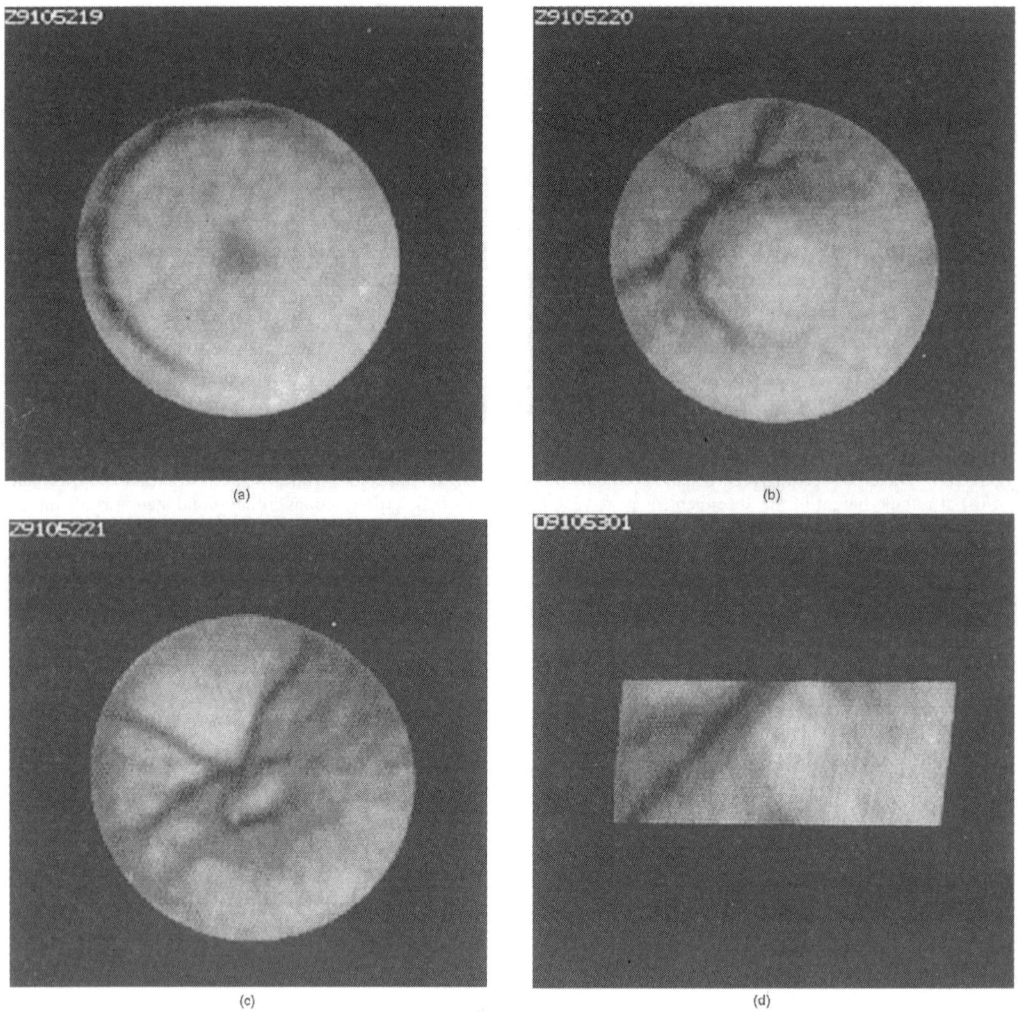

Figure 24. Localization patterns in specimen rfdt6 (ε_a = 20%): (a) bottom, (b) middle and (c) top cross-sections and (d) one axial reconstruction (positions of the cross-sections in the initial state: (a) 20, (b) 50, (c) 80 mm from the bottom platen).

of approximately straight and parallel black lines. The direction of each pair passes through the specimen axis and is approximately radial. The spacing between the twin lines in each pair increases from one tomogram to the lower one, as does the diameter of the circle. On the sixth tomogram, the spacing is quite large but the lines remains approximately parallel by pairs. Each individual line is clearly not passing through the specimen axis.

As shown in Figure 27, the trace of an inverted V appears on a profile reconstructed from the set of slices placed next to each other. The inverted V can be seen on the bottom picture, which was reconstructed in a plane perpendicular to the mean direction of one of the pairs observed on the tomograms. The upper pictures present the adjacent slices, aligned along the direction of the medium line of the considered pair. The reconstruction was performed on three different parallel planes perpendicular to the same pair (only one is shown on the figure). It was found that the V shapes were superposable, while the trace of the specimen contour was not, since it was cut at different distances from the central axis. Figure 28 illustrates the geometrical interpretation of these observations. Localization pattern in this specimen involves two kinds of structures; first a cone centered on the axis of the specimen, with its tip outside the specimen, and its contour matching exactly the specimen's bottom section; secondly,

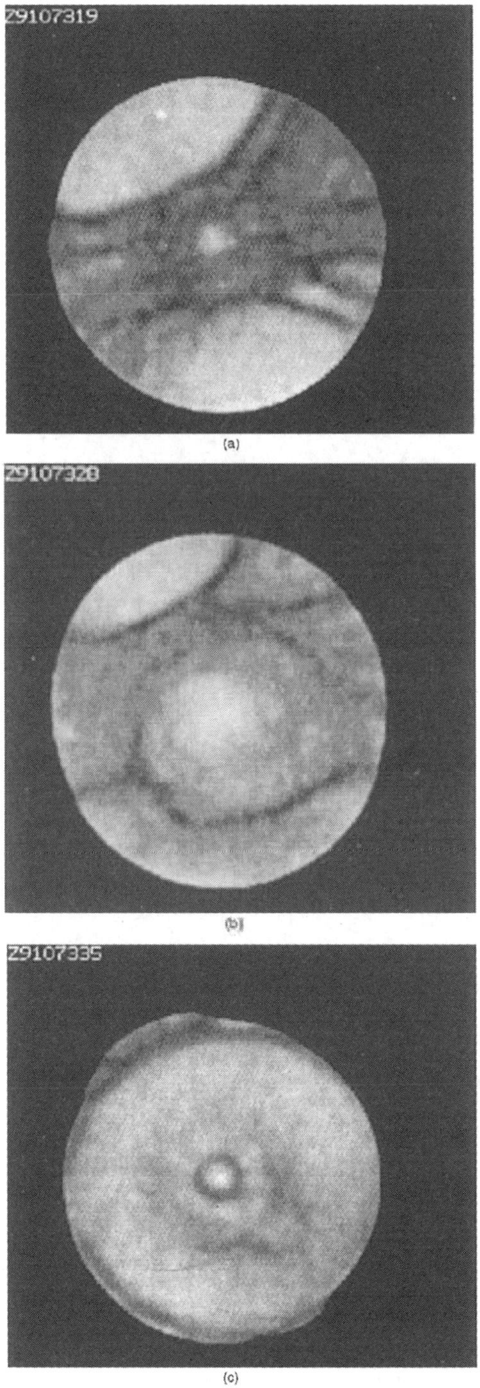

Figure 25. Localization patterns in specimen rfdt7 (ε_a = 26%): (a) top, (b) middle and (c) bottom cross-sections (positions of the cross-sections in the initial state: (a) 80, (b) 50, (c) 20 mm from the bottom platen).

a set of plane strain mechanisms associated in pairs, each pair of plane crossing on a line which is a diameter of the top section. In the figure are presented schematically the traces of the shear zones on one cross-section close to the top platen, and on one reconstruction parallel to the axis. The comparison of these traces with the experimental observations shown in Figure 27 shows the consistency of the geometrical interpretation. From measurements made on different reconstructed sections parallel to the axis, or including the axis, the angle of the cone and the angles between the planes associated in pairs is approximately the same, in that case $60° \pm 5°$. There is not a symmetric cone with its tip at the bottom, neither a symmetric set of crossing planes with their edges at the bottom.

Although these findings were not observed as clearly in every specimen tested, they can be recognized in Figure 20. Furthermore, refined observation of the patterns obtained in the loose specimens in this study, although rendered more difficult due to the low contrast between the localization zones and the rest of the material, suggests that the same kind of organization can be present. This is illustrated by Figure 29 which presents a cross section of a loose specimen strained axially at 42%. So it is proposed that this organization is not fortuitous but somewhat general in axisymmetric specimens, at least when there is no major heterogeneity in geometry, initial state or loading condition. Indeed, any major heterogeneity breaking the symmetry will induce the selection of one direction as the preferred plane strain direction. On the other hand, Test rfdt8 showed that a strong local heterogeneity can play no role if it does not break the symmetry of the specimen. In that specific test, a soft perturbation, namely a cotton sphere 1 cm in diameter was placed on the axis of the specimen. Figure 30 shows that the localization pattern was not influenced by this imperfection.

Conversely, we present in Figure 31 a set of tomographic sections realized on a specimen of calcareous sand under high confining pressure, in a study performed in our Laboratory in Grenoble, and reported in reference Colliat-Dangus (1986). The specimen was loose, non lubricated, with aspect ratio 1. Due to the breakage of the brittle calcareous grains, the material exhibited very large contractancy during the test. Only the final state of the deformation is observed, but the figure shows clearly that the strain localization, organized on a cone like in dilating specimens, has induced localized contractancy indicated by the white circle on the sections (the black disc on the top section is the hole let by the drainage porous stone). In fact, the specimen is the same as the one illustrated in Figure 13, examined in Laboratory LETI in 1986; but the images in Figure 32 result from a second CT examination, several years later, using a different CT scanner, namely the scanner ND8000 used in the experiments described in the present section. This second

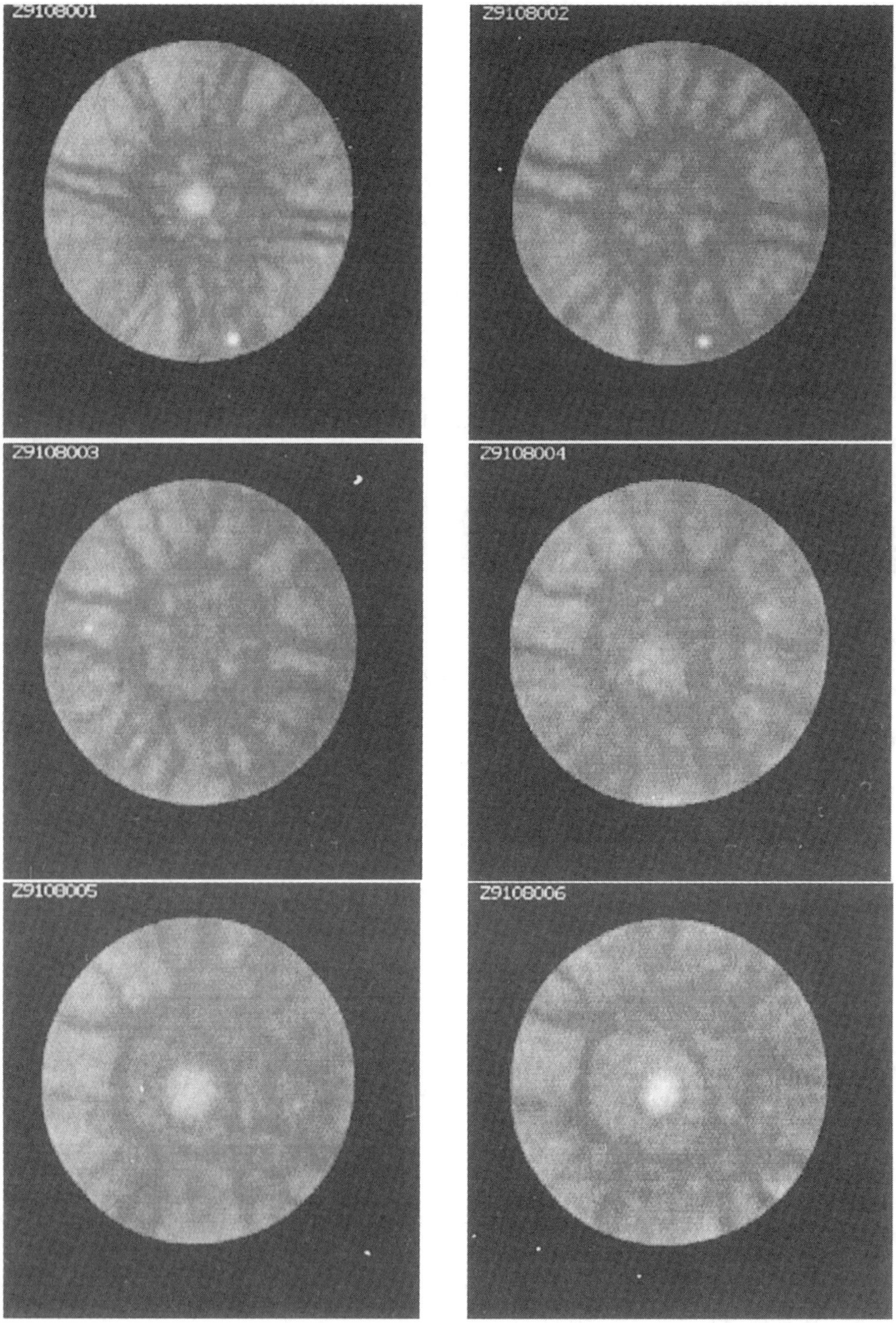

Figure 26. Six adjacent tomograms across the upper part of specimen rfdt8 (ε_a = 27%) (positions of the cross-sections in the initial state: (a) 4, (b) 8, (c) 12, (d) 16, (e) 20, (f) 24 mm from the top platen).

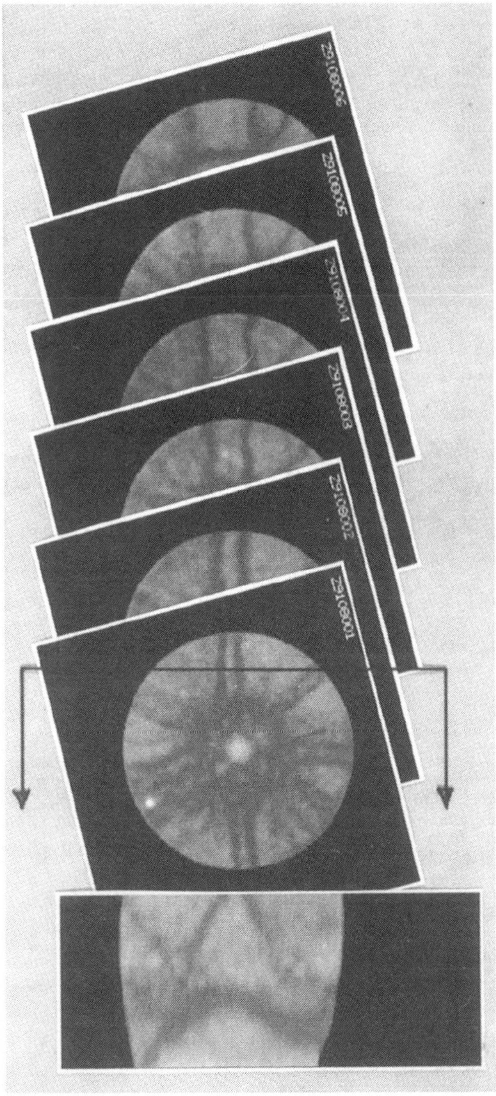

Figure 27. Localization patterns in specimen rfdt8: reconstruction of the density of the specimen on a plane parallel to the axis, and perpendicular to a pair of localization planes (bottom picture shows the inverted V produced by the two associated planes intersecting on the top platen; the trace of the cone appears as a parabola oriented towards the lower platen).

examination is more precise than the first one, it shows that what was interpreted as a plane in Figure 13, due to the limited number of tomographic sections, was in fact a cone. Conversely to the observations made on dense Hostun Sand, no shear plane was observed in addition to the localized shear cone in that specific case of very contractant material.

4.2.3 *Void ratio evolution recorded locally and globally*

The numerical images of the cross sections recorded along the tests by CT give not only qualitative but also quantitative information. Using this information, it has been possible to monitor the evolution of the global and local densities during the tests (cf. section 4.1.2). For convenience, the results are presented in terms of void ratio, using the classical relation: $e = \gamma_s/\gamma_d - 1$ with γ_s the grain specific gravity and γ_d the dry volumetric weight of the material. Figure 32 presents the comparison between global and local evolution of the void ratio for the set of loose and dense specimens tested in this study. "Global" means averaged over a cross section of the specimen (open symbols), while "local" stands for averaged over a zone identified as a localized shear zone (closed symbols). The data are plotted in a void ratio versus global axial strain graph.

4.2.3.1 Global measurements

Global curves appear similar for the 4 tests rfdt3, rfdt6, rfdt7 and rfdt8. After a rather long dilatant stage (from 0 to 20%), these curves show a more or less smooth transition to something which could be interpreted as a common plateau. The curve for rfdt4, however, is significantly different: the evolution leads abruptly to a plateau which is lower than the latter, and comes before.

4.2.3.2 Local measurements

Local curves depart from the global ones as soon as a localized zone is detected for the specimen considered. The slope of the curve is higher, indicating that the void ratio averaged over the localized zone changes faster than the global one, at least when both are plotted versus the global axial strain. The major result however is that *all these local curves tend to reach a same plateau*, the level of which is significantly higher than the final level of the global curves. The void ratio corresponding to the ultimate part (plateau) of the local curves is approximately 0.85 ± 0.02. This value has been confirmed by numerous measures on the different dense specimens.

4.2.3.3 Loose specimens

For the loose specimens rflt1 and rflt2, the global and local evolution of the void ratio do not differ much, when they are discernible. Both tend to a plateau again, which is found to coincide with the plateau of the local curves for the dense specimens.

4.3 *A complementary study at $\sigma_3 = 400\,kPa$*

A complementary study was undertaken on the same sand, Hostun RF, in 1995 by the author and P. Bésuelle, and remained unpublished until the present paper, except a short paper Bésuelle *et al.* (1995) in French. The study was organized as a continuation of the

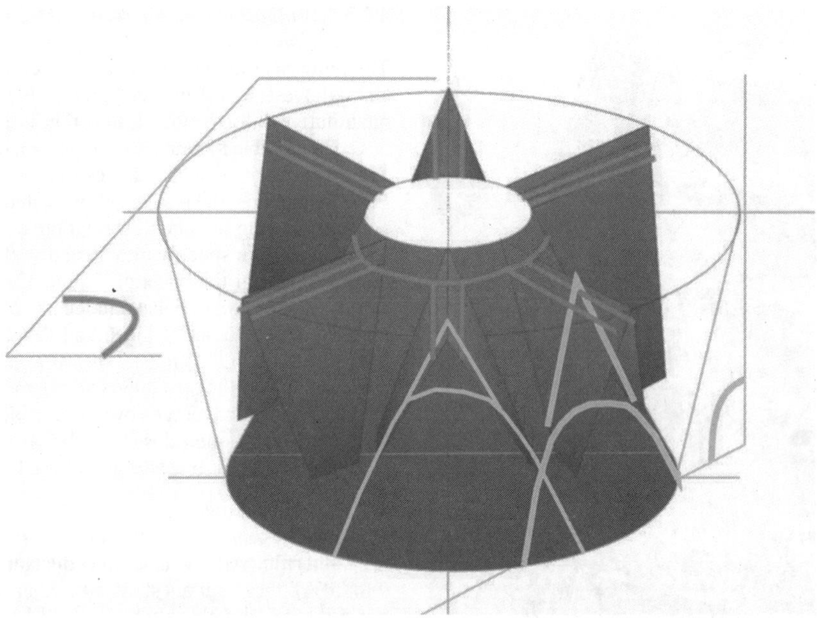

Figure 28. Idealized representation of the patterning in test rfdt8.

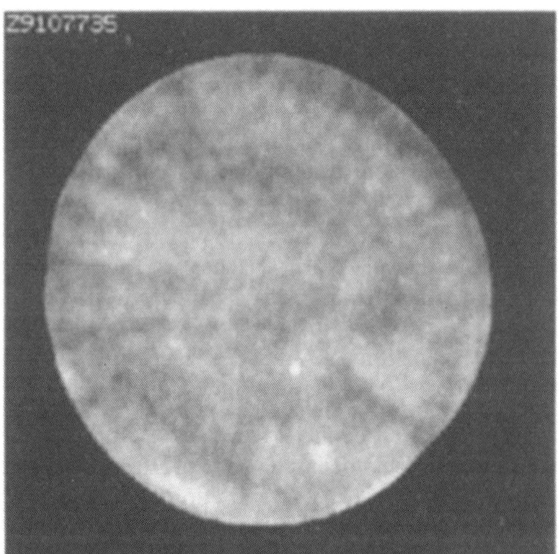

Figure 29. Localization patterns in loose specimen rflt2 ($\varepsilon_a = 42\%$).

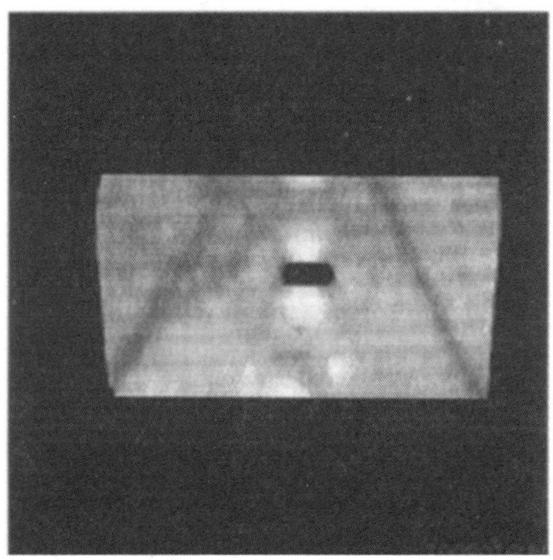

Figure 30. Reconstruction of void tomogram of specimen rfdt8: dark disc in the middle of the picture is a soft imperfection placed on the axis of the specimen; localization zones did not pass through the imperfection Void ratio (global or local).

previous one, with improved test conditions and higher mean effective stress. By that time the manuscript of the paper Desrues *et al.* (1996) was already submitted, and the present data could not be incorporated.

4.3.1 *Improved test conditions*
The major change in test conditions is that the tests were performed *in-situ*, i.e. directly inside the CT scanner, using a specially designed Triaxial cell together with

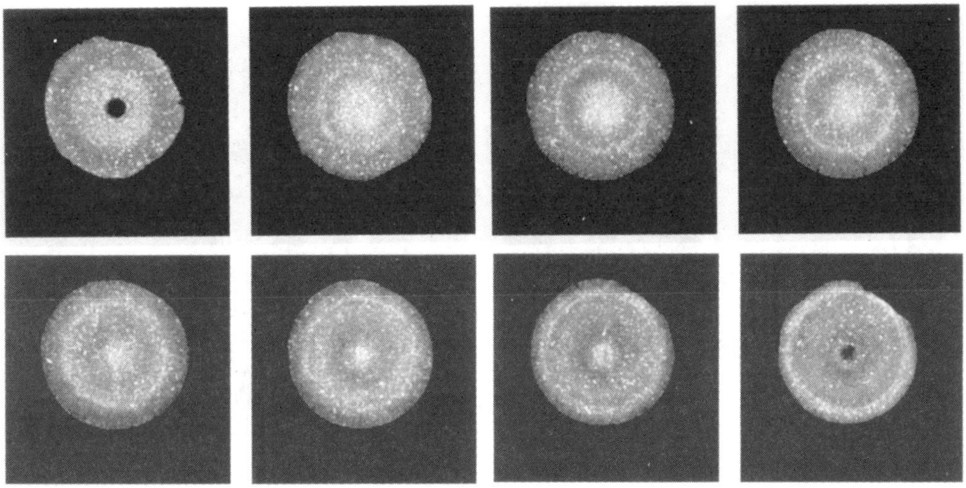

Figure 31. Demonstration of contractant localized shear zones in sand: from upper left to low right, eight adjacent tomograms across a calcareous sand specimen tested under high confining pressure. The white circle is the trace of a shear zone organized along a cone.

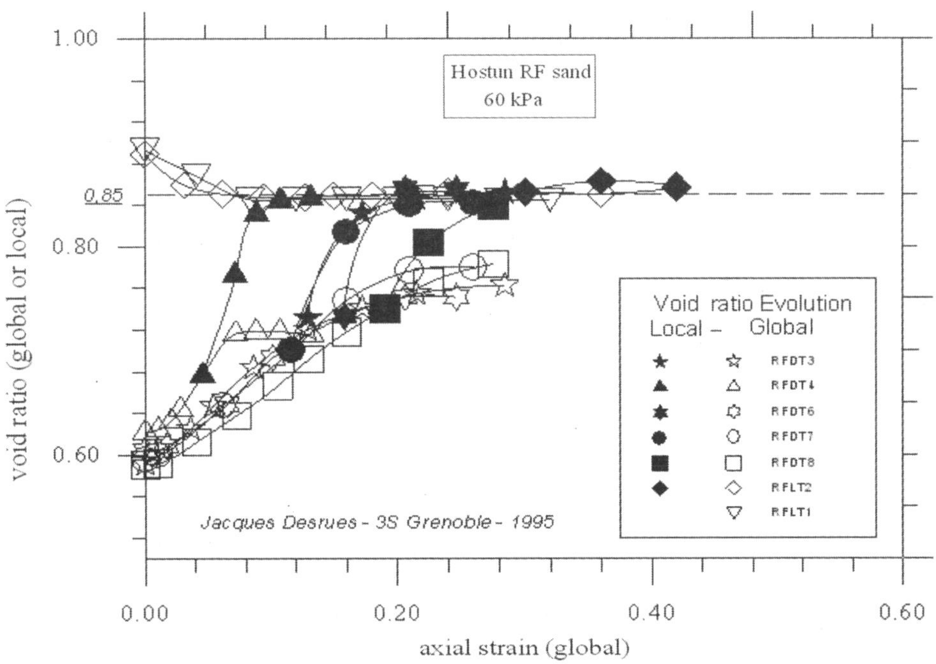

Figure 32. Global and local evolution of the void ratio in loose and dense Hostun RF sand specimens submitted to axisymmetric triaxial test under 60 kPa effective confining pressure.

the loading frame described in Figure 15 above. The cell (shown in Fig. 33) is made of aluminium, a material chosen for its low X-ray absorption. It is equipped with drainage lines, loading piston, and cell pressure regulation facilities. The specimen was prepared at a given initial density (dense, medium, loose), then put inside the cell while kept under vacuum; the vacuum was released after pressurization of the cell. Then the

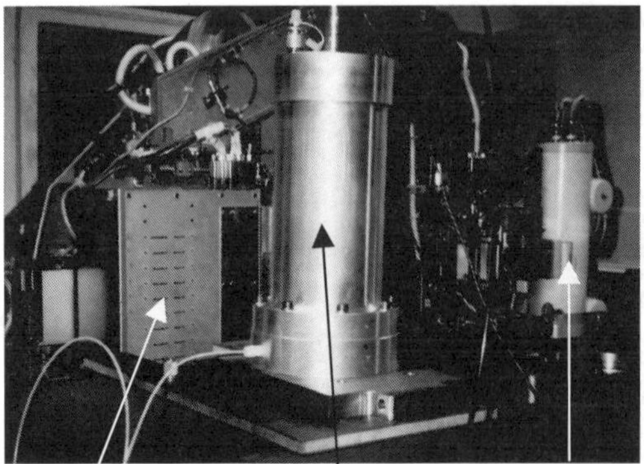

Figure 33. The aluminium triaxial cell used for *in-situ* tests in the CT scanner in LMA, Marseille.

dense unlubricated

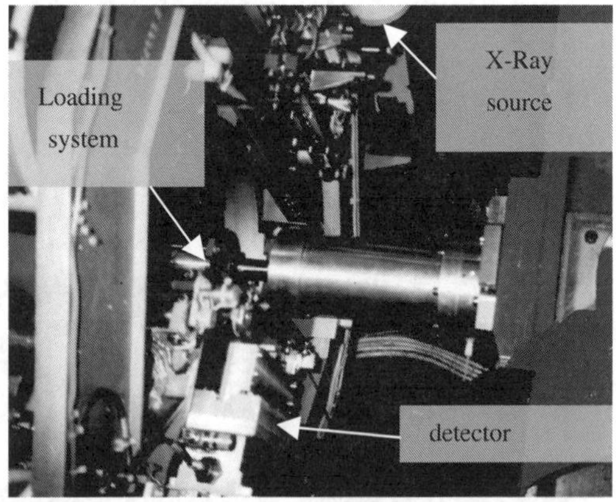

Figure 34. The triaxial cell ready for insertion in the measuring field of the scanner. The cell is fixed in horizontal position on the red beam which is part of the loading frame described in Figure 15.

Table 2. Complementary triaxial tests set on Hostun RF sand (σ_3 = 400 kPa).

Test name	Height h_0 (mm)	Diameter d_0 (mm)	Slenderness h_0/d_0	ρ_0 at σ_c = 400 kPa (g/cm^3)	Test conditions
RF04FD	140	70	2.0	1.700	Dense, unlubricated
RF04FM	140	70	2.0	1.568	Medium, unlubricated
RF04FL	140	70	2.0	1.445	Loose, unlubricated

cell was fixed in horizontal position on the loading frame (Fig. 34). The axial loading was applied using a screw jack fixed on the loading frame on the other side (labeled "loading system" in the figure). Horizontal displacement of the loading frame together with the triaxial cell fixed on it, with respect to the CT scanner apparatus, allowed to scan sets of cross-sections through the specimen. The scanning could be done without unloading the specimen.

As for possible perturbations of the stress state, due to the bending moment induced by gravity acting in the perpendicular direction to the axis of the specimen, their effect was minimized by using a rather high cell pressure: 400 kPa.

4.3.2 *Results*

Table 2 present the characteristics of the different tests. Three densities were tested. The slenderness ration was equal to 2. No anti-friction device was used. We know from the previous study that such a slenderness ratio and end friction conditions will favour single shear band mechanisms with respect to more smeared patterns as shown before (Fig. 26). However, in this complementary study we are interested more in characterizing the void ratio evolution inside the shear band. Figures 35 and 36 show the comparison between three tests performed under CT scan control on dense, medium and loose specimens of Hostun RF sand. In Figure 35, the stress ratio versus axial strain curve show the typical evolution from dense to loose specimens: the peak is lower, it comes later, and the softening is slower, as the initial density decreases (or initial void ratio increases). The open symbols indicate the first CT scan on which shear bands can be observed; it can be said that the first observation of shear with the CT is always after the peak, and the non-localized post-peak portion of the test seems to be longer as the specimen is less dense. The local void ratio curves confirm the observations made at low mean stress level: a ultimate void ratio in large strain, so-called "critical void ratio" in the framework of critical state theory, can only be reached inside the shear bands since strain localization stops the evolution of the deformation process in the major part of the specimen, as soon as it takes place. See for example the void ratio value at the plateau of the global curve for the dense specimen in Figure 36, compared

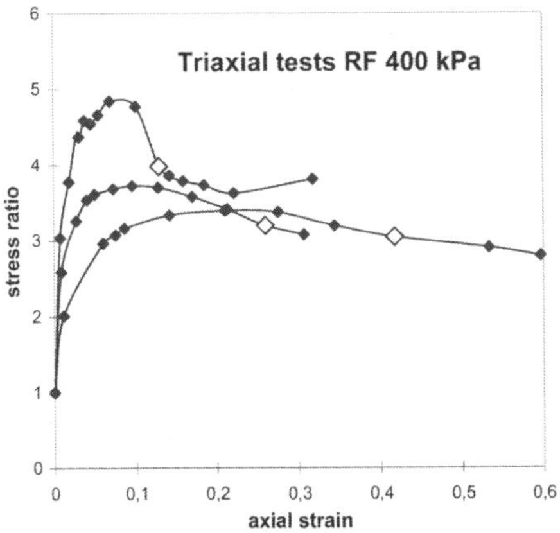

Figure 35. Comparison of the stress-ratio versus axial strain curves for three tests performed under CT scan control on dense, medium and loose specimens of Hostun RF sand. The open symbols indicate the first CT scan showing localization.

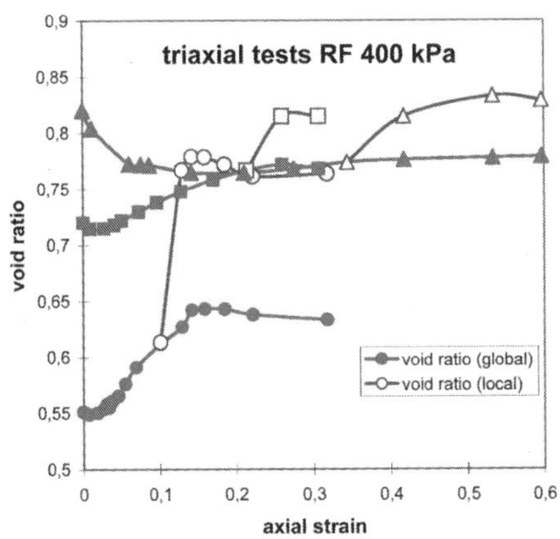

Figure 36 Comparison of void ratio versus axial strain curves for three tests performed under CT scan control on dense, medium and loose specimens of Hostun RF sand. The curves with full symbols are global (average) measurements, while the curves with open symbol are local measurements within the shear bands.

to the same quantity for the medium and loose tests: the first is less than 0.65, while the others are higher than 0.75, which makes a very significative difference.

As for the critical void ratio observed within the bands is concerned, it can be estimated at 0.83 ± 0.02 from the tests presented. It should be noticed that the measures taken within the band in the case of the dense specimen is somewhat lower. This remains to be confirmed by other tests. If it was confirmed, it could be due to the fact that the mean effective stress inside the specimens after localization is no more homogeneous, and could be significantly different in dense and loose specimens.

Figures 37 and 38 illustrate the deformation observed in the three tests. Although strain localization is clearly observed in all cases, with one or several shear planes, the observed density variations in sets of cross sections in each specimen do not allow to detect clearly volumetric strain localization in the medium and loose cases. Density is a good marker for strain localization only if localized shear strain induces significant volumetric strain, which is linked to dilatancy.

4.4 *Discussion and conclusion*

4.4.1 *Patterning*

This study reveals that the more or less cylindrical or barrel-like shape of the axisymmetric specimens strained in laboratory tests may conceal internal complex structures involving strain localization. To the authors' knowledge, the localization patterns revealed in this tomographic study had not been described previously. However, they can be seen as a generalization of the figure described by Desrues *et al.* (1985) on cubical specimens tested in a true triaxial apparatus. Figure 39 reproduced from this reference shows the final deformation state of a cubical specimen tested under axisymmetric stress conditions. It can be seen that two plane strain mechanisms take place simultaneously in the specimen, in such a way that the "axisymmetric" test condition can be met, at least with respect to the two orthogonal directions of the apparatus. The two mechanisms are selected by the geometry of the specimen and the apparatus. In cylindrical specimens, under ideal test conditions, there is no constraint which could select a particular mechanism. Only imperfections can induce such a selection, but they have to be rather strong to succeed in that process. Indeed, the full development of a given mechanism is a matter of global organization of the deformation over the specimen, not only local. If the conditions for strain localization are met somewhere in the specimen, for a given shear direction, it is not sure at all that this will give rise to a developed shear band.

Even if a shear band starts propagating, it can be arrested by some stronger, or less stressed zone in the specimen and then let another incipient shear band become the major one. It has been observed in plane strain experiments that near the peak load, several incipient shear bands can appear simultaneously, but only one will become a fully developed one. Examples of this are given in Desrues (1991), pages 132–134 or in Desrues *et al.* (1985).

Hence, the further development of an incipient shear plane can be possible or not depending on the behavior of other regions of the specimen, at some distance from the initiation point.

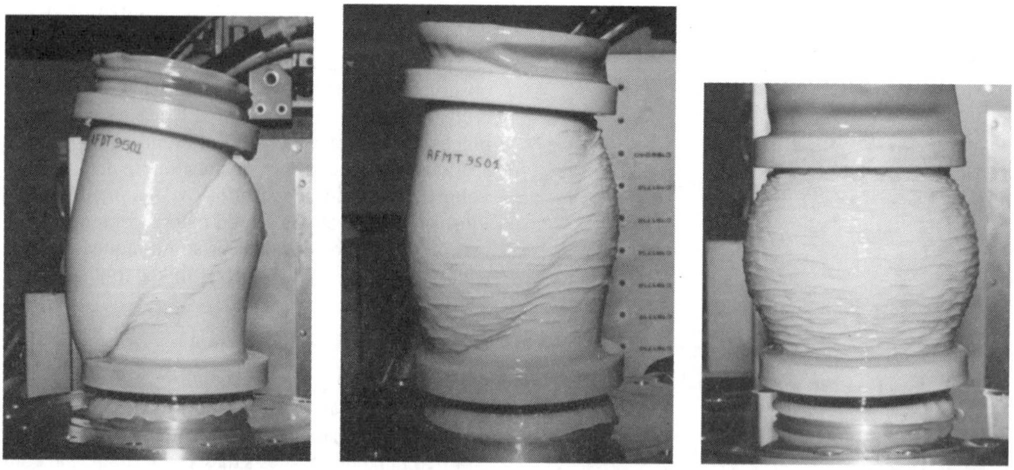

Figure 37. Three specimens of Hostun RF sand loaded to failure under CT control at $\sigma_3 = 400\,\text{kPa}$. From left to right: dense, medium dense, loose. One localized shear plane is clearly visible in dense and loose cases, while in the loose specimen a set of shear mechanisms could be observed on the membrane.

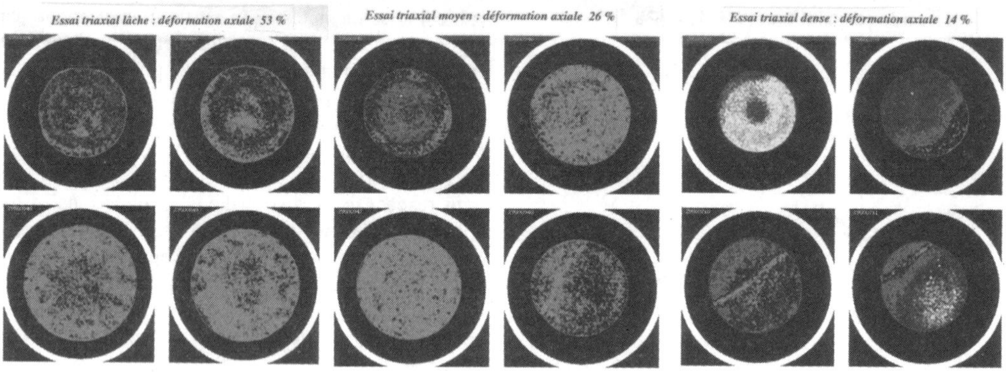

Figure 38. For the three specimens shown above, four cross sections were taken by CT, equally distributed along the z-axis in each specimen. The dilating shear band in the dense specimen is clearly shown, while the localized structure is not clearly revealed in the two other tests. This illustrates that density is not always a good marker of shear strain, depending on the dilating behavior of the material.

Given the orientation of the shear bands with respect to the axial stress direction, an axisymmetric specimen has more degree of freedom in the selection of an active mechanism than a plane strain test. In the latter, the degrees of freedom for shear bands is limited to (i) the initiation point, and (ii) a binary choice between left and right orientation; while in ideally axisymmetric specimens, the direction of the steepest line in the localization plane is another degree of freedom. It has been shown incidentally in this study (Fig. 30) that an imperfection, even strong, which does not break the symmetry does not act as an attractor for the localization. In the authors' opinion, the results presented in this section suggest that symmetry of the specimen state (geometry, density, stresses) is a stabilizing factor with respect to localization. The stabilization is relative, it does not suppress definitely localization but it leads to smoother global response characteristics, and complex localization patterns involving multiple mechanisms, taking place at large axial strain. Conversely, symmetry breaking imperfections, either diffuse or local, are more likely to induce single mechanism localization like the shear plane shown in Figure 18. Globally biased initial density distribution, even slight as the one observed in specimen rfdt4, bad centering of the specimen, and non parallel platens are other examples of such global imperfections which may induce marked localization. On the other hand, end-restraint

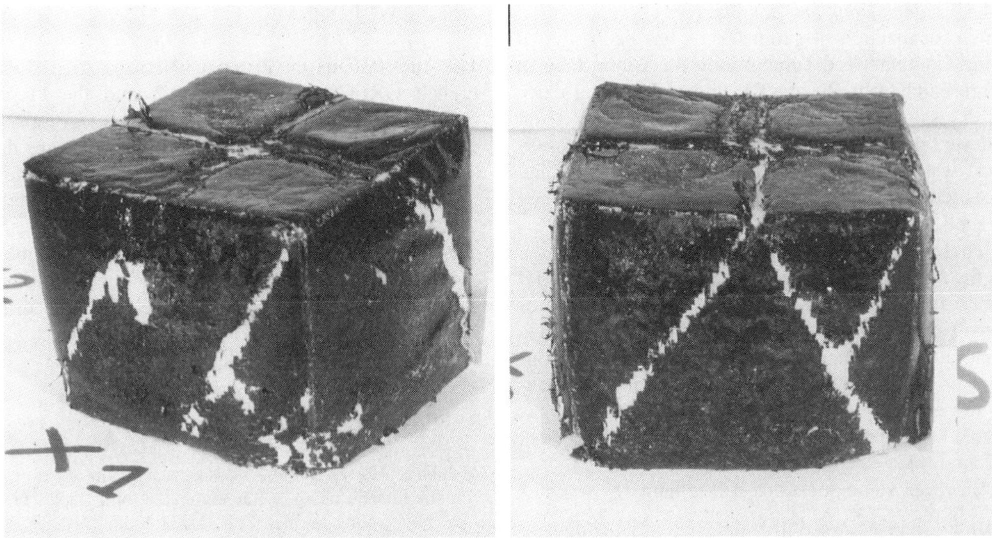

Figure 39. Localization pattern in a true triaxial specimen tested in axisymmetrical stress conditions (after Desrues *et al.*, 1985).

effects due to imperfect end lubrication may play a stabilizing role with respect to the development of a single mechanism over the sample, because they reinforce the axisymmetric constraint, favoring the distribution of the localized deformation over a large number of mechanisms. It is the case of Test rfdt1(Figure 20) which was tested under severe end restraint: non-lubricated ends and reduced slenderness (aspect ratio 1). Of course, such extreme test conditions are not good practice, because they induce a very heterogeneous stress field in the specimen, and artificially increase the strength.

In conclusion, it can be stated that more or less complex localization patterns can develop in laboratory specimens, depending on test conditions. Constraints favoring symmetry, like end platen friction, and small aspect ratio, induce multiple localization modes, while circumstances favoring symmetry breakage, like biased density profile, bad centering of the specimen , tilted platen, local weakness of the material, are likely to produce unique and severe localization modes. In any case however, soon or late localization will come.

4.4.2 *Towards a limit void ratio*

The following conclusions can be drawn from the comparison of the global and local measurements using CT during this series of tests, and from the observation of localization patterns within the specimen:

(i) the final plateau observed in the volumetric strain versus axial strain curves for dense dilating specimens is not physically relevant; it cannot be interpreted as the manifestation of a limit void ratio, but as an effect of the strain localization process inside the specimen.

(ii) a limit void ratio is measured however, but inside the shear bands. Figure 32 shows a strong tendency of the local void ratio to stabilise after a large jump during the first stage of the localization development, and a remarkably good agreement between the final void ratio of the different tests.

Moreover, the local curves for the loose contracting specimens tend to the same plateau. For Hostun RF sand under the confining pressure considered, $\sigma_3 = 60\,\text{kPa}$, the limit void ratio is estimated to 0.85 ± 0.02. The corresponding dry volumetric mass is $1.43 \pm 0.03\,\text{g/cm}^3$. At $\sigma_3 = 400\,\text{kPa}$, we found again a tendency toward a same plateau, at about 0.83 ± 0.02, which is not much different from the previous case. In the second study, the number of tests was not large enough and some discrepancy was observed between the dense case and the other cases (loose and medium).

Due to the limited spatial resolution of the scanner, the numerical values inside the shear bands must be considered as estimated. A specific study of the influence of the spatial resolution of the scanner on local measurements in fine structures like shear bands is still to be undertaken. In fact, a micromechanical approach of the grain movements in the shear bands could help assessing if a local density in the sense of continuum mechanics can be defined by some homogenization procedure; but this is another study.

4.4.3 *Conclusions and perspectives*

Strain localization in geomaterials has been studied using Computerized Tomography for a long time in our research team. Besides the studies described above on dry sand, other studies have been performed on different geomaterials: Beaucaire Marl, a soft clayey rock, was studied by Tillard-Ngan *et al.* (1993), and more recently a sandstone (Red Vosges Sandstone) by Bésuelle *et al.* (2003).

These studies have brought significant information on the structure of strain localization in complex 3D patterns, and allowed quantitative measurements of density in a zone of localization. The patterns have been later confirmed by other research teams. Contractant shear bands have been exhibited. The capacity to perform *in-situ* test, i.e. under CT control, has been a key improvement with respect to post-mortem CT analysis.

However, some questions still remain:

- How can be assessed the relevance of local density measurements in narrow bands, in the limit of the voxel size ?
- How can we discriminate between narrow shear zones and cracks?
- Can we explore multi-scale localization, with shear strain concentration at different scales ?

Moreover, new questions arise as one moves from continuum to discrete Geomechanics: can we expect CT to help us exploring the deformation processes in granular assemblies, by looking at the behavior of grains as individuals particles ?

For most of these questions, *resolution* is a key point … but not the only one! Advanced mechanical test facilities must be used for tests under CT control, including drainage, pore pressure equilibration in the specimen, and whatever test refinement relevant for the problem under study.

In both these directions, namely increased resolution and advanced geomechanical testing under CT control, new studies have been undertaken by our team in Grenoble, using Synchrotron Radiation at the European Synchrotron Facility *ESRF:*

- *Post-mortem* analysis of small cores taken from plane strain specimens of Beaucaire Marl, perpendicularly to the plane strain plane, in shear bands and outside (see Marello *et al.* in the present book)
- *In-situ* saturated tests with drainage control on Beaucaire Marl (see Lenoir *et al. ibidem*).

However, using Synchrotron Radiation is not the only way to develop high-resolution CT; micro-CT studies using industrial (as opposed to medical) CTs have been presented by a number of teams during the workshop, with convincing results. The use and benefit of Computerized Tomography in scientific studies of geomaterials is probably only at its beginning.

ACKNOWLEDGEMENT

The Author thank the European Network ALERT, the French GRECO "Géomatériaux", and the French GdR "Géomécanique des Roches Profondes" for supporting the present research. Many thanks are due also to Clinique Clairval in Marseille, Laboratoire LETI in Grenoble, and Laboratoire LMA in Marseille for having provided us access to their X-ray CT scanners at different times in the 20 past years. A number of co-workers have been associated to the works summarized here; among them are Frederic Mazerolle, Xavier Reynaud, Moncef Mokni, Dominique Tillard-Ngan, Pierre Bésuelle, Jack Lanier and others.

REFERENCES

Alshibli K.A. *et al.*, 2000. Assessment of localized deformations in sand using X-Ray computed tomography, Geotechnic testing Journal GTJODJ, 23:3, pp. 274–299

Alshibli K.A., Batiste S.N. and Sture S, 2003. Experimental Observations of Instability Phenomena in Sands: Plane Strain Versus Triaxial Compression Conditions, ASCE, J. Geotechnical and Geoenvironmental Engineering, Volume 129, Issue 6, pp. 483–494

Alsini A.,Vardoulakis I., and Drescher A., 1992. Deformation localization in the thick- walled hollow cylinder inflation experiment on dry sand . Géotechnique, 42(1): 395–410.

Arthur J.R.F., 1971. New Techniques to Measure New Parameters. Proc. of the Roscoe Memorial Symposium, Cambridge University on Stress-Strain Behaviour of Soils, Ed. R.H.G. Parry, G.T. Foulis and Co.: 340–346.

Arthur J.R.F., Dunstan T., Al-Ani Q.A.J.L., and Assadi A., 1977. Plastic deformation and failure in granular media. Géotechnique, 27: 53–74

Arthur J.R.F. and Dunstan T., 1982. Rupture layers in granular media. Proc. IUTAM Conf. Def. Fail. Gran. Media, Balkema: 453–459

Benefice P. and Boehler J.P., 1979. The application of stereophotogrametry to the analysis of displacement fields in solid mechanics . Proc. IUTAM conf. on Optical Methods in Mechanics of Solids

Bésuelle P., Desrues J. and Mazerolle F., 1995. Etude tomographique de la localisation dans un sable, Actes du colloque GEO'95, 11–15 décembre 1995 Aussois (France)

Bésuelle P., Baud P. and Wong T. 2003. Failure mode and spatial distribution of damage in Rothbach sandstone in the brittle-ductile transition, Pageoph vol.160 No 5–6, pp. 851–868

Blumenfeld S.M. and Glover G., 1981. Spatial Resolution in Computed Tomography. Radiology of the skull and brain – Technical aspects of computed tomography, Ed. Thomas H. Newton and D. Gordon Potts Ed., The C.V. Mosby Company, 5: 3918–3940

Bossi R.H., Friddell K.D. and Lowrey A.R., 1990. Computed Tomography. Non-Destructive Testing Of Fiber-Reinforced Plastic Composites, Ed John Summerscales Ed., Elsevier Applied Science, 2: 201–252

Bransby P.J. and Blair-Fish P.M., 1975. Deformation Near Rupture Surfaces In Flowing Sand. Géotechnique, 25(2): 384–389

Butterfield R., Harkness R. and Andrawes K.Z., 1970. A Stereophotogrammetric Method For Measuring Displacement Fields. Géotechnique, 20(3): 308–314

Casagrande A. and Watson J.D., 1938. Compaction Tests And Critical Density Investigations Of Cohesionless Materials For Franklin Falls Dam, Merrimack Valley Flood Control. Corps Of Engineers, U.S. Army, U.S. Engineering Office, Appendix Bii: Bii-7

Colliat-Dangus J.L., 1986. Comportement des matériaux granulaires sous fortes contraintes, *Thèse de doctorat* – Université de Grenoble (in french, PDF version available)

Colliat-Dangus J.L., Desrues J. and Foray P., 1988. Triaxial Testing Of Granular Soil Under Elevated Cell Pressure. Advanced Triaxial Testing For Soil And Rocks – Astm Stp 977, Ed. R.T. Donaghe- R.C. Chaney And M.L. Silver, Astm: 290–310

Desrues J., 1984. La localisation de la déformation dans les matériaux granulaires. thèse de Doctorat es Sciences, USMG – INPG Grenoble (in french, PDF version available)

Desrues J. and Duthilleul B., 1984. Mesure du champ de déformation d'un objet plan par la méthode stéréophotogrammétrique de faux relief. Journal de Mécanique Théorique et Appliquée, 3(1): 79–103

Desrues J., Lanier J. and Stutz P., 1985. Localization Of The Deformation In Tests On Sand Sample. Engineering fracture mechanics, 21: 909–921

Desrues J. and Hammad W., 1989. Experimental study of the localisation of deformation on sand: influence of mean stress. In Proc. XIIth ICSMFE – Rio de Janeiro (1): 31–32

Desrues J., 1991. An Introduction to Strain Localisation in Granular Media. Physics of Granular Media – proc. Winter School Les Houches Feb. 90, Ed DODDS J.A. and BIDEAU D., Nova Sciences Publ.: 127–142

Desrues J., Mokni M. and Mazerolle F., 1991. Tomodensitom, trie et localisation dans les sables. Deformation of soils and displacement of structures – X ECSMFE, Ed. Associazione Geotechnica Italiana, Balkema: 61–64

Desrues J., Chambon R., Mokni M. and Mazerolle F., 1996. Void ratio evolution inside shear bands in triaxial sand specimens studied by computed tomography, Géotechnique 46(3): 529–546

Fabre D., Mazerolle F. and Et Raynaud S., 1989. Caractérisation tomodensitométrique de la porosité et de la fissuration de roches sédimentaires. Rocks at great depth, Ed. Maury V. and Fourmaintraux D., Balkema: 297–304

Flavigny E., Desrues J. and Palayer B., 1990. Le Sable d'Hostun "RF" – note technique. Revue Française de Géotechnique (53): 67–69

Hammad W., 1991. Modélisation non linéaire et étude expérimentale de la localisation dans les sables. Thèse de doctorat, UJF – INPG Grenoble

Hettler A. and Vardoulakis I., 1984. Behaviour of dry sand tested in a large triaxial apparatus. G, otechnique, 34(2): 183–198

Kirkpatrick W.M. and Belshaw D.J., 1968. On the interpretation of the triaxial test. G, otechnique, 18(3): 336–350

Latiere H.J. and Mazerolle F., 1987. The X-ray scanner. A tool for the examination of the intravoluminal crystalline state of aluminium. Engineering Fracture Mechanics, 27(4): 413–463

Michalowski R.L., 1990. Strain localization and periodic fluctuations in granular flow processes from hoppers. Géotechnique, 40(3): 389–403

Mokni M., 1992. Relations entre déformations en masse et déformations localisées dans les matériaux granulaires. Thèse de doctorat, UJF – INPG Grenoble

Raynaud S., Fabre D., Mazerolle F., *et al.*, 1989. Analysis of the internal structure of rocks and characterization of mechanical deformation by a non-destructive method: X-ray tomodensitometry. Tectonophysics, 159: 149–159

Roscoe K.H., 1970. The influence of strains in soil mechanics. Géotechnique, 20: 129–170

Scarpelli G. and Wood D.M., 1982. Experimental observations of shear band patterns in direct shear tests. Proc. IUTAM Conf. Def. Fail. Gran. Media, Balkema: 473–484

Tan S. and Fwa T., 1991. Influence of voids on density measurements of granular materials using gamma radiation techniques. Geotechnical testing journal GTJODJ, 14(3): 257–265

Tatsuoka F., Sakamoto M., Kawamura T., Fukushima S., 1986. Strength and deformation characteristics of sand in plane strain compression at extremely low pressures. Soils and Foundations, 26(1): 65–84

Tillard D., 1992. Etude de la rupture dans les geomat, riaux cohesifs. Application à la marne de Beaucaire. Thèse de doctorat, Université Joseph Fourier – Grenoble I

Tillard-Ngan D., Desrues J., Raynaud S. and Mazerolle F., 1993. Strain localisation in the Beaucaire marl. Geotechnical Engineering of Hard Soils – Soft Rocks, Balkema: 1679–1686

Vardoulakis I., 1979. Bifurcation analysis of the triaxial test on sand samples. Acta Mechanica, 32: 35–54

Vardoulakis I., 1980. Shear Band inclination and shear modulus of sand in biaxial tests. Int. J. Num. Anal. Meth. Geom., 4: 103–119

Vardoulakis I. and Graf B., 1982. Imperfection sensitivity of the biaxial test on sand. IUTAM Conf. Def. Fail. Gran. Media, Balkema: 485–491

Vinegar H.J., De Waal J.A. and Wellington S.L., 1991. CT Studies of Brittle Failure in Castlegate Sandstone. Int. Rock Mech. Min. Sci. and Geomech. Abstr., 28(5): 441–448

X-ray CT for Geomaterials; Soils, Concrete, Rocks – Otani & Obara (eds.)
© 2004 Swets & Zeitlinger. Lisse, ISBN 90 5809 666 1

State of the art report on geotechnical X-ray CT research at Kumamoto University

J. Otani
Department of Civil and Environmental Engineering, Kumamoto University, Kumamoto, Japan

ABSTRACT: Industrial X-ray CT scanner was installed at the Department of Civil and Environmental Engineering, Kumamoto University, Japan in the year of 1996. In this keynote paper, the research activities, which we have done so far from that year, are introduced, precisely. First of all, the background and motivation of this topic are introduced and an X-ray CT apparatus, which we have at Kumamoto University, is precisely introduced with its theoretical background. Then, the contents of our researches up to now are reviewed with the order from fundamental study to boundary value problem. These are: (1) Characterization of soil behavior; (2) Developments of new triaxial compression test apparatus; (3) More positive usage of X-ray CT data; and (4) Bearing capacity mechanism under vertical pile loading. Based on these studies, the effectiveness of X-ray CT scanner for geomaterials or geotechnical engineering is confirmed.

1 INTRODUCTION

A nondestructive method, such as geophysical prospecting or electric prospecting, became a useful tool for investigating the characteristic of soils in geotechnical engineering. An X-ray computed tomography (CT) method which is one of the nondestructive testing method has also been used with the name of an apparatus commonly well-known by the medical diagnostic method which provides the cross sectional images based on the absorption of the X-ray beam through the materials. This X-ray CT scanner was originally invented by Hounsfield (1972) who received Nobel Prize in 1979 shared with Allan Cormack. Because of its relatively new testing apparatus, not many researches on the application to geotechnical engineering have been done. But some of the studies have been done on the topic of soil science (cf. Special Publication editors by Anderson and Hopmans (1994)). For the application to mechanical behavior such as deformation and failure of geomaterials, the studies on rock materials by Verhelst et al. (1995) and those for sand by Desrues et al. (1996) and Tani (1997) have been done at relatively early stage of this application. Kruse et al. (1998) have also applied X-ray CT scanner to centrifuge soil model. But all those researches have used the medical X-ray CT scanner, so that the power of the X-ray is relatively low and as a result, the images which are obtained from scanning may not be clear and thus, the quantitative discussion can not be expected.

Recently, an industrial X-ray CT scanner (TOSCANER-23200 min:TOSHIBA Corp.) has been installed at the group of Rock Engineering in Kumamoto University, Japan. Although not many researches on the application of this industrial CT scanner has been done in geotechnical engineering so far, Hagiwara and Nanba (1990), Sugawara et al. (1997) and Sugawara et al. (1998) have discussed on the possibility of the use of this industrial X-ray CT scanner to rock engineering. Otani et al. (1997) applied this technique to the soil material for the first time in Japan. As far as the applications for soils are concerned, the papers by Alshibili et al. (2000), Wong (2000), and Pralle et al. (2001) have introduced their interesting results concerning the application of X-ray CT for any soils.

In this keynote paper, the research activities, which we have done so far, are introduced, precisely. First of all, the system of X-ray CT scanner, which we have at Kumamoto University, is introduced. Then, the contents of our up-to-dated research topics are introduced with the order as follows:

(1) Characterization of soil behavior;
   1.1 Failure of undisturbed overconsolidated clay
   1.2 Failure of mixed soil with dredged slurry, cement and air foam
   1.3 Soil-structure interaction
   1.4 Seepage and drying
(2) Development of new triaxial compression test apparatus;

(3) More positive usage of X-ray CT data; and
    3.1 Application to numerical analysis
    3.2 Evaluation of particle crushing in soils
(4) Bearing capacity mechanism under vertical pile loading.

Based on these studies, the effectiveness of X-ray CT scanner for geomaterials or geotechnical engineering is confirmed.

2 SYSTEM OF INDUSTRIAL X-RAY CT AT KUMAMOTO UNIVERSITY

2.1 *Theoretical background*

In ideal situations, projections are a set of measurements of the integrated values of some parameter of the specimen which is the integration being along straight lines through the specimen. When X-ray beam propagates through the one-dimensional homogeneous specimen, the intensity of the X-ray, I_0 in terms of the number of photons that enter the specimen changes to that value of I after the attenuation of X-ray in the specimen. This process is expressed by the following equation for the width of the specimen, W with the linear coefficient of absorption, f:

$$I = I_0 \exp\{-fW\}. \tag{1}$$

Then, the projection, p is defined by

$$p = fW = \ln\{I_0/I\}. \tag{2}$$

When the specimen is nonhomogeneous in two dimension, Eq.(2) is rewritten by following line integral form for the case shown in Fig.1:

$$p(r,\theta) = \ln(I_0/I) = \int_{-\infty}^{\infty} f(x,y)dt. \tag{3}$$

in which $f(x, y)$ is the spatial distribution of the coefficient of absorption in two dimension and each line integral by the (r, θ) parameters which are shown in Fig.1. In the X-ray CT scanner, a large number of independent projections are measured by tomographic technique and finally the spatial distribution of the coefficient of absorption, $f(x, y)$ is obtained by the Filtered Back-Projection Method (Kak and Slaney (1987)). In the image processing analysis, following so called "CT-value" is used:

$$\text{CT-value} = (\mu_t - \mu_w)\,\kappa / \mu_w \tag{4}$$

where μ_t: coefficient of absorption at scanning point; μ_w: coefficient of absorption for water; and κ: constant. Here, it is noted that this constant is fixed to a value of 1000. Thus, the CT-value of air should be −1000 because the coefficient of absorption for air is zero. Likewise, this value for the water is 0 from the definition of Eq.(4). The CT images are presented with shaded gray or black color for low CT-value and light gray or white color for high CT-value as all the subsequent black and white images. The total number of levels on these colors is 256. Figure 2 shows the relationship between CT-value and density of the materials. The results of different materials are plotted in this figure and those results show a linear relation among all the results, so that the CT-value can be a parameter for evaluating the change of the density. Therefore, it is promised that the CT-value can be a parameter for evaluating the density change due to the compression of the soils, and the distribution of the density change in soils could be evaluated quantitatively using X-ray CT scanner.

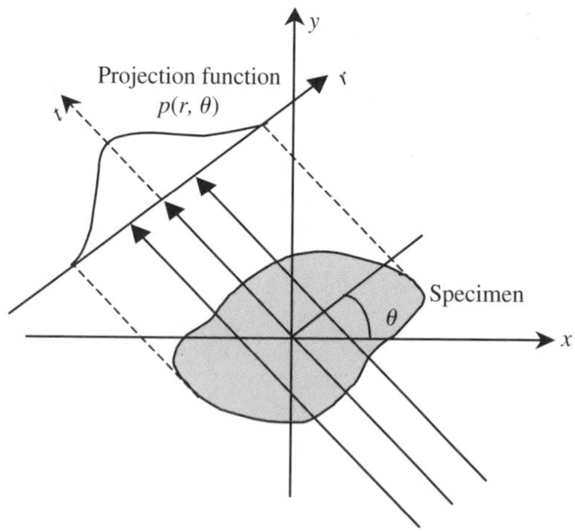

Figure 1. Principle of X-ray CT scanner.

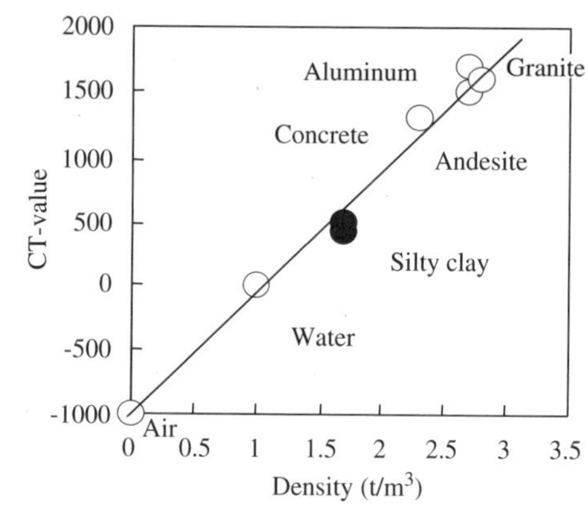

Figure 2. CT-value–Density relationship for several materials.

Figure 3 shows the concept of the X-ray CT image. In general, a digital image is composed of "Pixel" in two dimension, which shows the unit of any kind of images such as photograph and other digital data. But so called

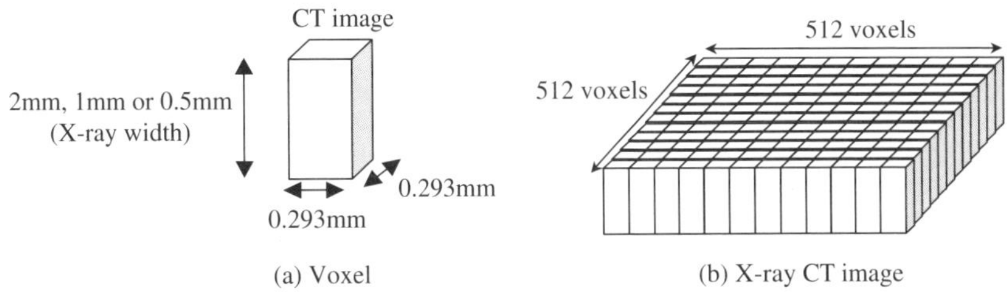

Figure 3. Voxel and the concept of X-ray CT image.

"Voxel" is used for X-ray CT image because the CT image is constructed not only in two dimension but also three dimension. Therefore, the value of X-ray absorption can be defined as the density in each voxel. In our X-ray CT apparatus, the size of this voxel is 0.293 mm × 0.293 mm × the width of X-ray attenuation (1 mm) as shown in Fig.3. In addition, the X-ray CT image can be constructed by the total number of 512 × 512 voxels for the image size of 150 mm diameter in one cross section.

Figure 4 shows the constructing process of the CT image. Fig.4(a) shows the frequency of the CT-values for total of 5 cross sections of a soil sample and Fig.4(b) shows two different cross sectional images for this sample in which the range of CT-value for the case (1) is $-1000 <$ CT-value < 500 while that of case (2) is $0 <$ CT-valuc < 500 as shown in Fig.4(a). As easily realized from those images, different images are obtained although the material is the same. Thus, the image should be constructed along the target range of the density and it is important to note that the CT-image have to be obtained after statistical analysis as shown in Fig.4(a). In our study, all the original images are constructed by the way of case (2) in Fig.4, in which the range of existing CT values is checked for each material and testing. Figure 5 shows the concept of resolution for the X-ray CT scanner used in this study. If one of the soil particle in the soil is larger than the size of single voxel as shown in Fig.5(a), the obtained CT-value can be realized as the density of this soil particle. But if the size of the soil particle is smaller than that of single voxel which is the case of Fig.5(b), the resulted CT-value shows the average sense of the density including both soil particles and voids in one voxel. The case shown in Fig.5(c) is the same situation as Fig.5(b) but some of the soil particles are out of one voxel. And the density of the air foam is more reflected on the average density than the case of Fig.5(b). Those properties are very important for both qualitative and quantitative discussion on the CT images.

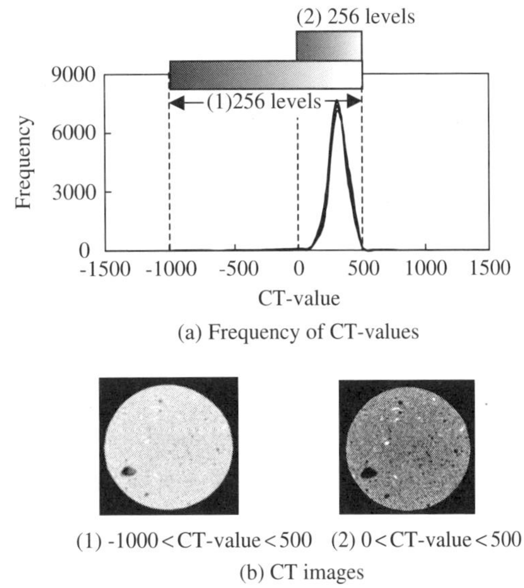

Figure 4. Voxel and the concept of X-ray CT image.

2.2 *System of X-ray CT scanner*

There are several types of X-ray CT scanner systems differentiated by factors such as the scanning time or the number of detectors as shown in Fig.6. The items in Fig.6 are classified as 1st generation (Translate-Rotate 1: T-R1), 2nd generation (Translate-Rotate 2: T-R2), 3rd generation (Rotate-Rotate: R-R) and 4th generation (Stationary-Rotate: S-R). The T-R1 is a rather old system that operates on the principle of a pencil beam. All the others operate on the principle of a fan beam and have been widely used in the medical industry. The system used in this study was the T-R2, which is known for giving the most accurate results but has a longer scanning time equipment than all others of the fan beam type. The S-R system has the shortest scanning time owing to its large number of detectors.

The system of the X-ray CT scanner used here is the same type as that used by Hagiwara and Nanba (1990) and this is shown in Photo 1 and the precise contents in the shield room is shown in Fig.7. In this apparatus, the collimated X-ray is penetrated from all around the circumference of the specimen by rotating and translating the specimen table as shown in Fig.7. The detected data are assembled and the cross sectional images are reconstructed using image data processing

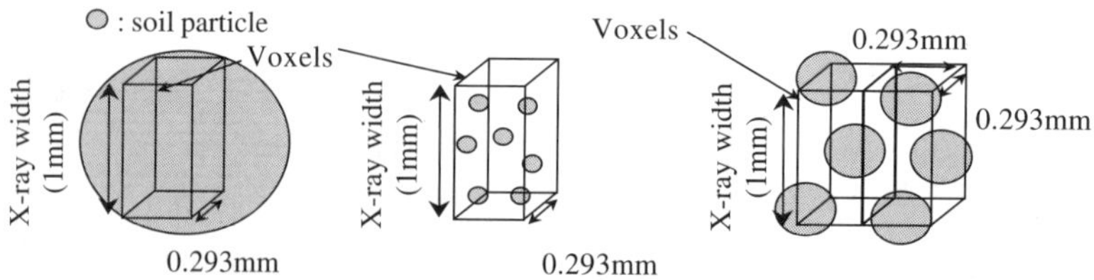

(a) Case of soil particle bigger than voxel (b) Case of soil particle much smaller than voxel (c) Case of soil particle smaller than voxel

Figure 5. Relationship of size between voxel and soil particle.

Scan type	1st generation (Translate-Rotate)	2nd generation (Translate-Rotate)	3rd generation (Rotate-Rotate)	4th generation (Stationary-Rotate)
Source of X-ray X-ray beam detector specimen scan area	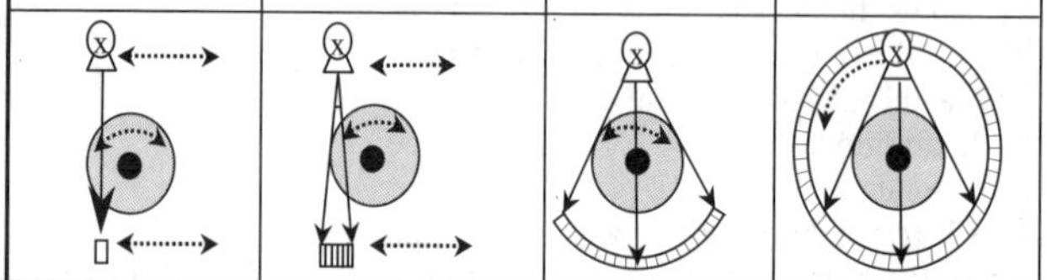			
X-ray beam Angular aperture	0° Parallel beam	3°~30° Narrow fan beam	30°~40° Wide fan beam	30°~40° Wide fan beam
Number of detectors	1	3~60	500~600	1000~2000
Scanning time	4~5 min.	20~120 sec.	3~10 sec.	1~10 sec.

Figure 6. Several types of X-ray CT scanners.

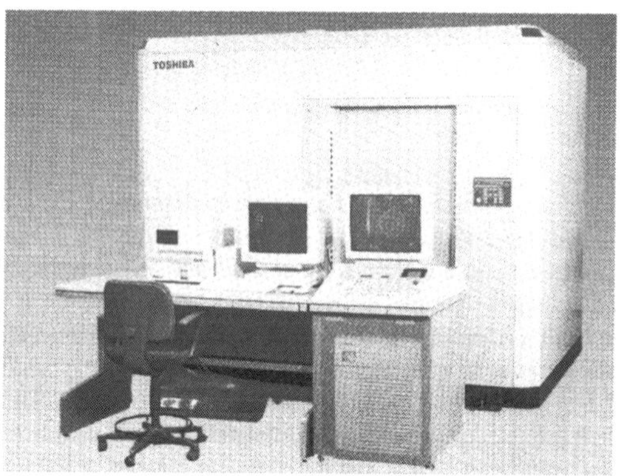

Photo 1. System of X-ray CT scanner at Kumamoto University.

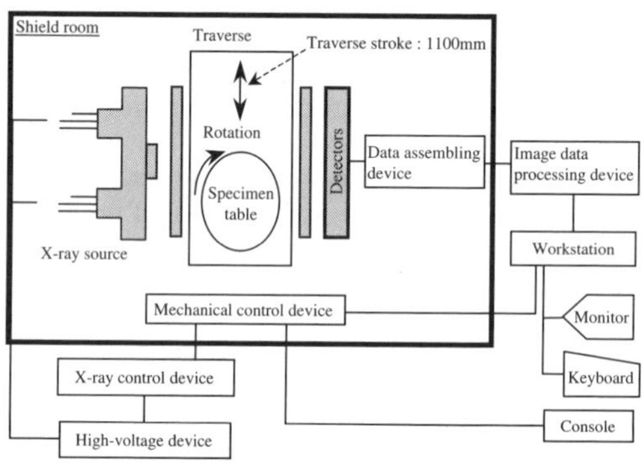

Figure 7. System of industrial X-ray CT scanner.

device by means of the filtered back-projection method. Then, the image is expressed on the monitor of engineering workstation. By using all these cross sectional images around the circumference of the specimen, the three-dimensional (3-D) images can be reconstructed. The contents of the specification on this X-ray CT scanner are shown in Table 1. The medical CT scanners are most commonly equipped with 140 kV X-ray tubes

Table 1. Specification of industrial X-ray CT scanner (TOSCANER-23200 min: TOSHIBA Corp.).

Scan Type	Traverse/Rotation
Power of X-ray	300 kV/200 kV
Number of detectors	176 channels
Maximum size of specimen	D:400 mm × H:600 mm
X-ray beam	0.5 mm, 1 mm, 2 mm
Spatial resolution	0.2 mm (diameter of hole) for 20 mm thickness of steel

while the industrial ones used here is equipped with 300 kV X-ray tubes. Thus, it is easily realized that the capacity of scanning for the industrial use is much higher than that of medical one, so that the possibility of quantitative discussion may be expected.

3 CHARACTERIZATION OF SOIL BEHAVIOR

3.1 *Failure of undisturbed overconsolidated clay*

It has been discussed recently that the failure mechanism of the ground or soil is related to its local deformation or so called "strain localization" of the soil. And it has been also realized that the failure of the soils is caused by the result of the progress of this localization in the soil. Most of the experimental researches on this topic so far are based on direct observation from the membrane or the soil box under plane strain assumption, so that it is very difficult to discuss the mechanical behavior in the soil especially under loading conditions.

The purpose of this research is to characterize the failure in soils using X-ray CT scanner. In this study, an unconfined compression test was conducted on undisturbed silty clay and then, the soil specimen is scanned at every 2 mm thickness along its axis during the test. Here, the two different stress levels which are at the peak and the post-peak conditions, respectively are chosen for scanning stages.

3.1.1 *Test procedure*

The soil specimen used in this study is undisturbed Ariake clay which has been known as a soft clay in Japan. The classification of this specimen is silty overconsolidated clay. A series of unconfined compression test and nondestructive testing using X-ray CT scanner were carried out under following steps:

(1) Unconfined compression test was conducted in the laboratory, in which the size of the specimen was at the diameter of 70.0 mm with the height of 140.0 mm and the density of the specimen is $1.68\ t/m^3$.
(2) When the value of applied stress was around the peak which is the highest value during the test, the loading was stopped and the specimen was moved to the scanning room of the CT scanner shown in Fig.7. The specimen was wrapped up by vinyl sheet during scanning in order to keep the water content unchanged.
(3) Then, the specimen was scanned with every 2.0 mm thickness along the height of the specimen.
(4) After resetting the specimen to the compression test apparatus, the test was restarted until the strain level reaches to fairly a large strain level (post-peak).

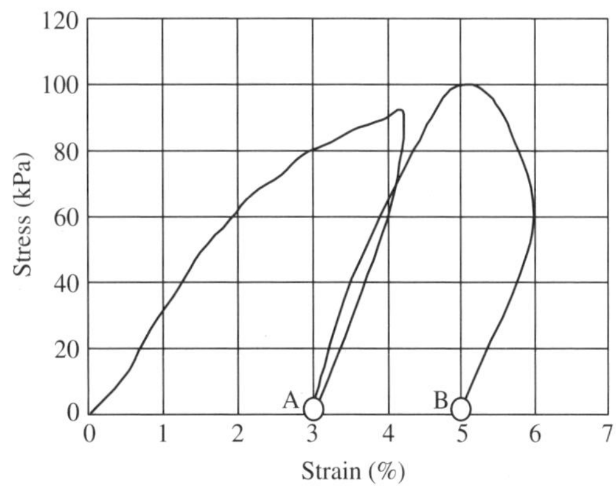

Figure 8. Stress–strain relationship of undisturbed overconsolidated clay under unconfined compression test.

(5) Then, the soil specimen was scanned again with the same procedure as described in (3).
(6) The high frequency noise was filtered from resulted CT-values using the method of Edge-Preserving Smoothing (Nagao and Matuyama (1978)).
(7) These filtered data were used for not only making cross sectional image but also obtaining 3-D image using computer software on workstation in the system.

3.1.2 *Results and discussion*

Figure 8 shows a typical stress–strain relationship for unconfined compression test. A nondestructive testing using X-ray CT scanner was conducted at the strain levels of A and B in the figure, which are related to peak and post-peak conditions, respectively. It is noted that both scanning stages are the conditions of zero stress because the specimen was released from the unconfined compression apparatus in order to scan the specimen.

The CT image in each cross section was obtained based on the distribution of CT-values after scanning the soil specimen. Figure 9 shows some of the cross sectional images for both peak (Fig.9(2)) and post-peak (Fig.9(3)) conditions, in which the locations of the cross sections along the height of the specimen are indicated in Fig.9(1) for both conditions. As described before, the dark region in the image shows low density area while the region of relatively light color shows that of high density. Here, it is easily realized that the area of low density appears around the top part for the peak condition and it also appears for all the heights for the post-peak condition. It is considered that all the dark areas should be the area of strain localization or shear zone. Especially, more complicated localization patterns are observed at the post-peak condition. The change of the density in the specimen can be also realized from the change of colors between two cross sectional images at the same

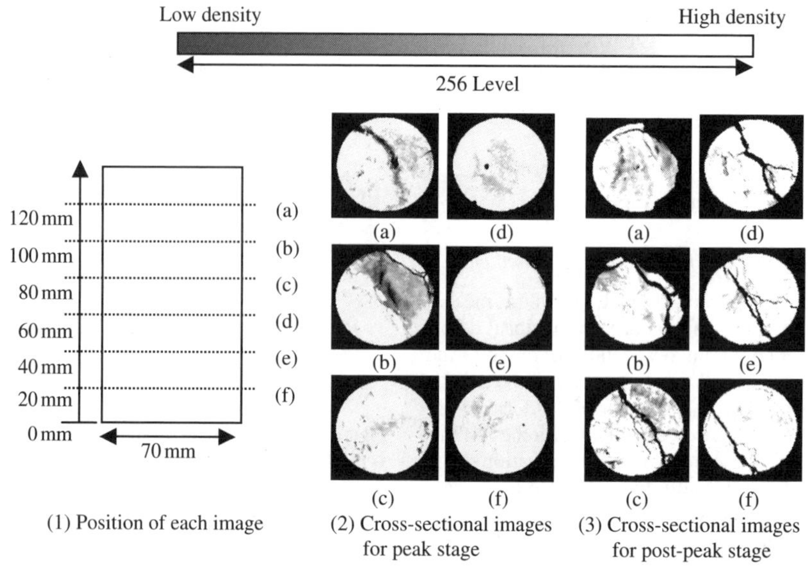

Figure 9. Cross-sectional images.

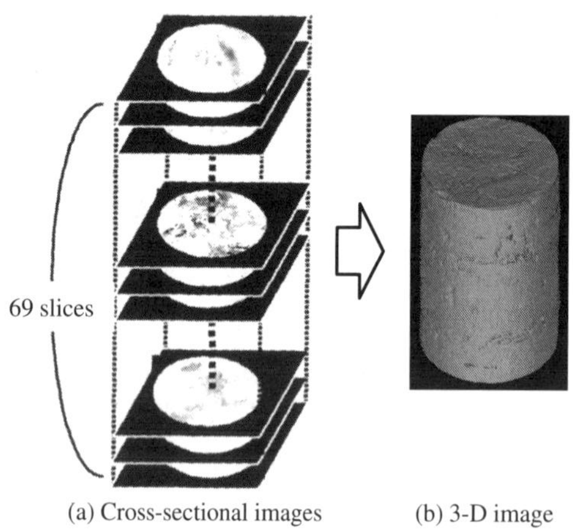

Figure 10. Reconstruction of 3-D image.

location. These cross sectional images which are the total number of 69 images in each condition are used for reconstruction of 3-D image as shown in Fig.10 which is the case of 3-D image at the peak condition. Figure 11 shows the results of 3-D images of the specimen for both peak and post-peak conditions, respectively. In each condition, both outside and inside images are reconstructed. For the images of inside view shown in Fig.11(2), it is assumed that the region of progressive failure is obtained after extracting the right range of CT-value which indicates the area of strain localization. Here, this localization area is presented with the area of white color in the image, in which this definition is

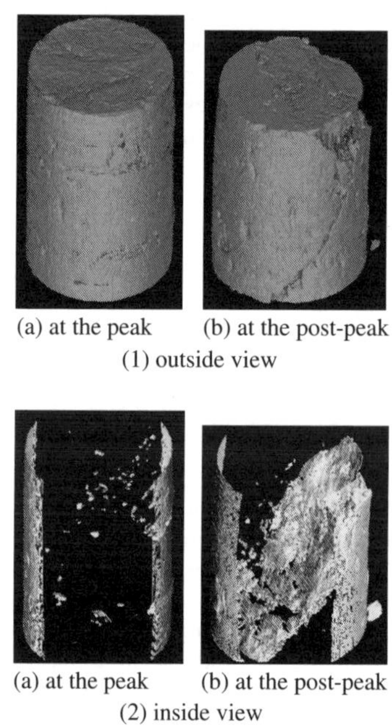

Figure 11. 3-D images in the soil.

the opposite compared to the original definition for CT images. Both the images of outside and inside views show the clear pictures of failure surface in the soil and besides, the progressive failure can be observed in the soil even at the peak condition. This can not be observed from outside view shown in Fig.11(1)(a).

Therefore, it is concluded that the initiation of the failure surface appears around the top of the specimen even at the peak condition, and the failure surface in the soil is clearly shown at the post-peak stage as a result of progressing these local low density areas as shown in Fig.11(2)(b). Figure 12 shows a graphical presentation of failure surface for post-peak condition. The shape and complicated surface condition on the failure surface can be reconstructed and thus the effect of this graphical presentation is confirmed for the results of the X-ray CT scanner. Figure 13 shows the vertical cross sectional images for both conditions. Ten images of equally spaced slice are presented for each condition, in which the location of each vertical cross section is indicated in the horizontal cross sectional image shown at the top of the figure. The soil specimen used here is the undisturbed clayey sample, so that many horizontal weak seams are clearly observed around the top half of the specimen. The shear zone appears around these weak seams at the peak condition as shown in Fig.13(a) and this zone progresses into the soil as shown in Fig.13(b). Thus, it is considered that those weak seams are the origin of the progressive failure for this specimen. Therefore, these results make the discussion of failure mechanism in the soil possible without any destruction of the specimen and this should be a valuable data in order to characterize the failure mechanism of soils.

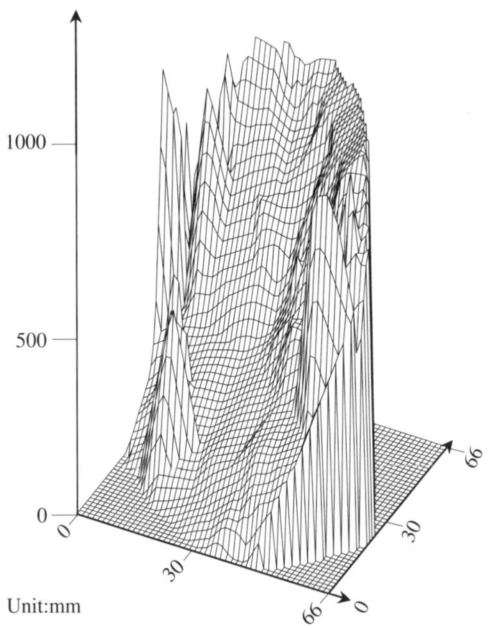

Figure 12. Graphical presentation of failure surface.

3.1.3 *Summary*

Using industrial X-ray CT scanner, the 3-D image of the specimen can be well reconstructed and even the inside view of the soil can be observed without any destruction of the soil.

In order to complete this study, following researches have to be done:

(1) The resolution of the X-ray CT scanner for composite materials such as soils has to be determined.
(2) A thresholding value for void in the soil has to be defined in order to discuss the failure in the soil, quantitatively. This depends on the classification of soil such as sand, clay, and other composite grounds.

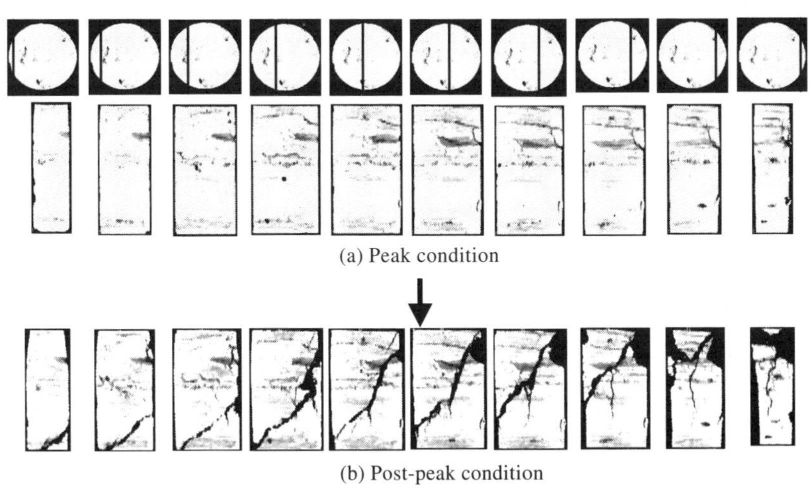

Figure 13. Visualization of vertical cross-sectional images.

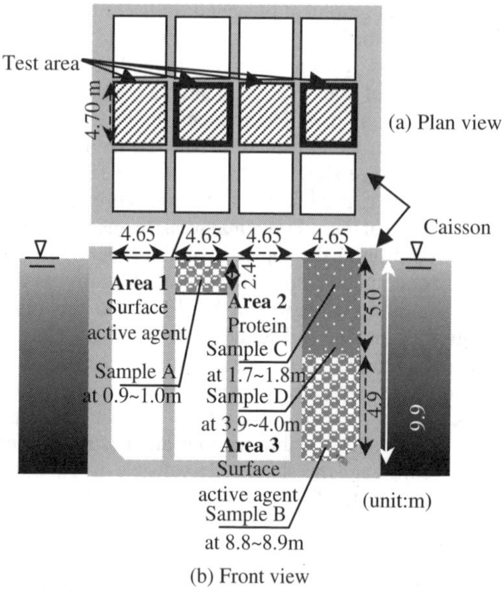

Figure 14. Schematic view of in-situ construction site.

(3) The loading system should be developed in the shield room of the system of X-ray CT scanner, so that the soil specimen can be scanned without any possibilities of stress relaxation.

3.2 *Failure of mixed soil with dredged slurry, cement and air foam*

Recently, so called "mixed soils" or "composite soils" has been widely used around the world. This type of soil can be realized as composite materials mixing with other materials in the soil, such as cement and air foam, so that its mechanical behavior should be complicated compared with just simple soils such as sand and clay.

The purpose of this study is to visualize the engineering property of in-situ mixed soil using industrial X-ray CT scanner. The specimen used in this study is in-situ SGM (Super Geo-Material) which is a light weight soil by mixing dredged slurry with cement and air foam. Those were sampled at the trial construction site of new Kumamoto seaport, Japan. Here, both physical and mechanical properties of in-situ SGM with different air foams are discussed precisely as the three dimensional feature of the soil and the effect of the air foam in the SGM is evaluated quantitatively. First of all, the physical properties of the in-situ SGM are investigated such as non-homogeneity of the soil due to the effect of different air foam. Then, the density evolution and the failure mechanism due to unconfined compression are discussed for the purpose of evaluating the mechanical properties of SGM based on the results of CT scanning with the image processing analysis.

Table 2. Mixing conditions.

	Mass (kg/m^3)	Volumetric fraction (L)
Dry mass	367.0	136.0
Water	624.0	606.0
Cement	100.0	32.8
Air Foam	9.3	225.0
Total	1100.3	999.8

Table 3. In-situ SGM samples.

Agent type	Name of sample	Wet density (t/m^3)	Sampling depth (m)
Surface active	Sample A	1.16	0.9~1.0
	Sample B	1.22	8.8~8.9
Protein	Sample C	1.34	1.7~1.8
	Sample D	1.35	3.9~4.0

3.2.1 *Material of SGM*

Figure 14 shows the schematic view of the site of underwater casting test, in which Fig.14(a) shows the plan view at the site while Fig.14(b) shows its front view. The light weight soils by means of different type of air orientation were constructed in the caisson below the sea level. Here, the air foams consist of the orientation by surface active agent and protein were used. The specimens used in this study were sampled at Area 1, Area 2 and Area 3 as shown in Fig.14 after curing of 28 days. Total number of the specimens was four, which were Sample A, Sample B, Sample C and Sample D and each of those samples was constructed at those areas as shown in Fig.14, respectively. Table 2 shows the mixing condition of those in-situ light weight soils. The dredged slurry used for this light weight soil was Ariake clay which is known as a soft clayey soil deposited around the Kumamoto seaport located in Ariake Bay of Kyushu Island in Japan. The target of the density after curing process of 28 days was expected to be the values between 1.1 and 1.2 t/m^3. The sampling depths were 0.9–1.0 m for Sample A, 8.8–8.9 m for Sample B, 1.7–1.8 m for Sample C, and 3.9–4.0 m for Sample D as shown in Table 3, respectively. Here, the air foam made by surface active agent was used for Sample A and Sample B, while that of protein was used for Sample C and Sample D. As easily realized from Table 3, the densities after curing process were increased comparing with its target value and the effect of curing process on the density change was obvious. The size of the specimen was fixed to be a diameter of 50 mm with the height of 100 mm in this study. It is noted that mixing those materials such as dredged slurry, cement and air forms was done by

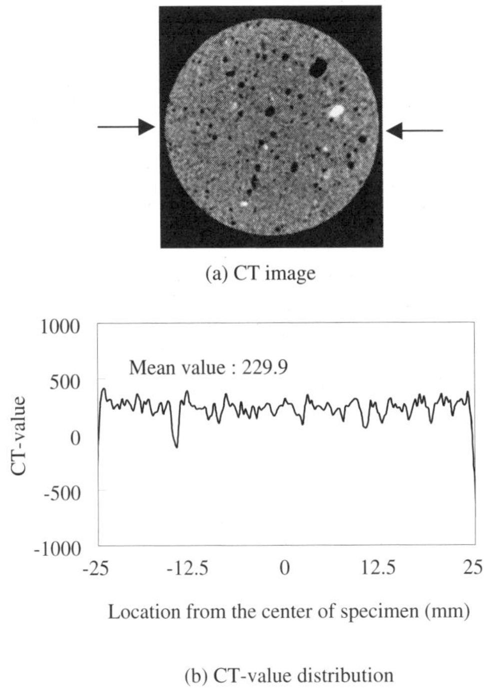

(a) CT image

(b) CT-value distribution

Figure 15. CT image and CT-value distribution for Sample A.

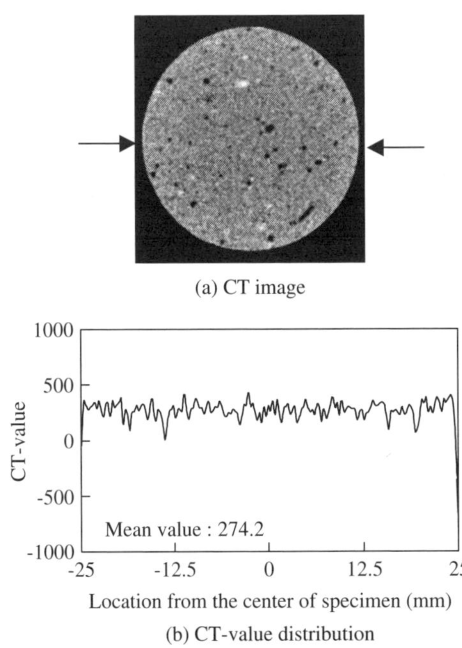

(a) CT image

(b) CT-value distribution

Figure 16. CT image and CT-value distribution for Sample B.

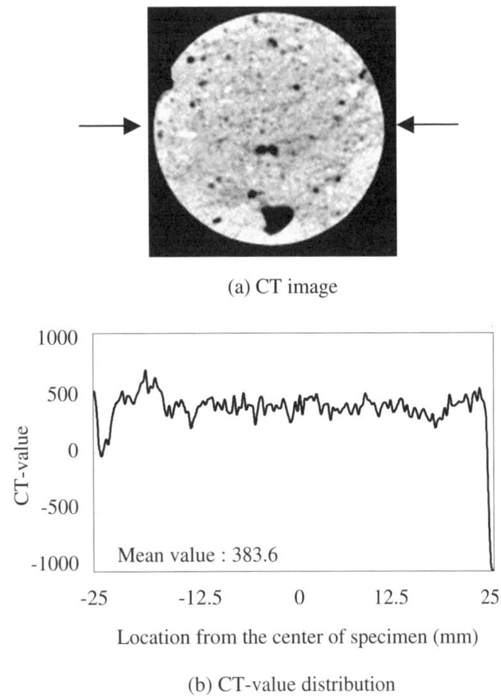

(a) CT image

(b) CT-value distribution

Figure 17. CT image and CT-value distribution for Sample C.

special mixing plant at the construction site. It is also noted that this material becomes hard normally after curing of within one day.

3.2.2 *Physical property*

Figures 15 and 16 show some of the cross sectional images at the central height of the specimen for Sample A and Sample B, which are the cases of the air foam made by surface active agent. Those figures also include the distribution of CT-values along the intersection between two arrows shown in the figure. It is realized that the area of black color shows single air foam or the group of tiny air foams depending upon its size as discussed before while the clear white color in the image means relatively high density area such as the lump of cement. And the color of the image of Sample A is rather dark compared with that of Sample B and this means that the density of Sample A is lower than that of Sample B. Those results convince the effect of sampling depth below the sea level at the construction site and this is obvious when the mean value of CT-values is compared between those two cases, which are shown in Figs 15(b) and 16(b). Figures 17 and 18 show the same results as Figs 15 and 16 for different type of air foam which is protein. It is easily realized that those images for the use of protein are

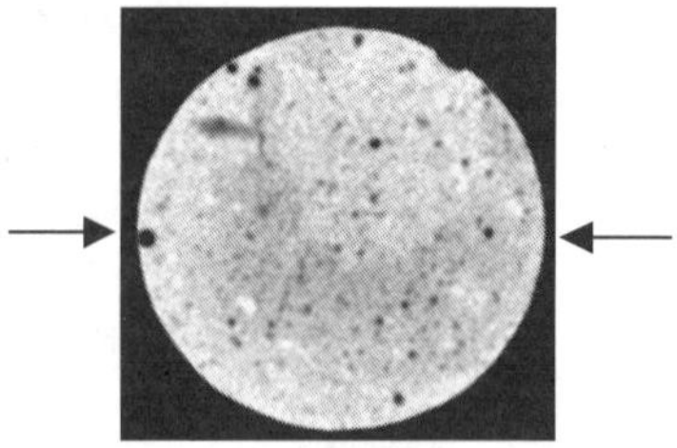

(a) CT image

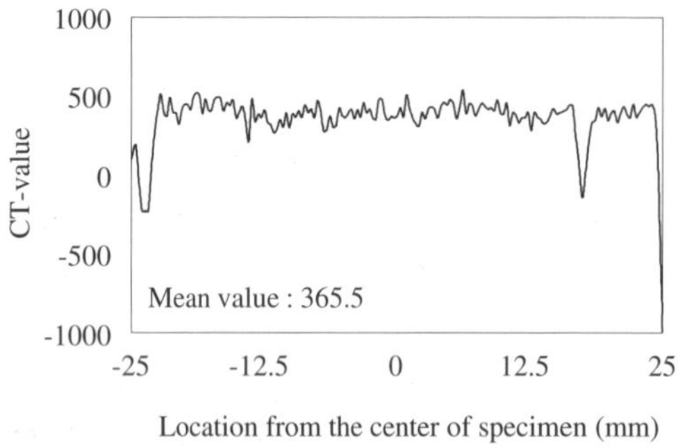

(b) CT-value distribution

Figure 18. CT image and CT-value distribution for Sample D.

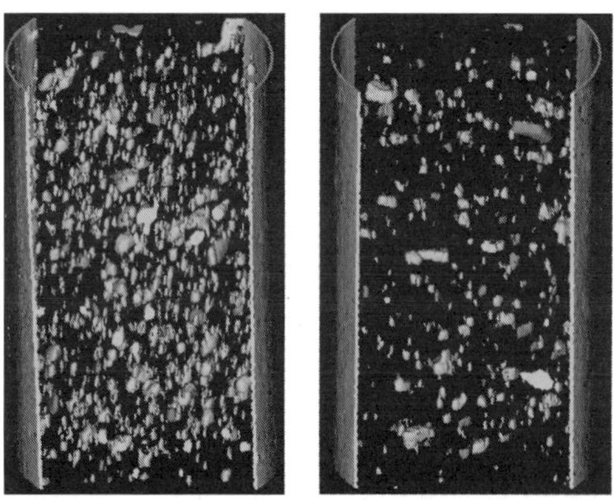

(a) Sample A (b) Sample B

Figure 19. 3-D binary image for air foams for Sample A and Sample B.

much lighter than those for the use of surface active agent as a whole and it is obvious that the density for the samples of protein is much larger than those of surface active agent. Therefore, the density of the SGM with air foams by protein is easily increased even for the low water pressure due to the effect of construction depth in the ocean. When the image of Sample C is compared with that of Sample D, there is not much change and this is obvious for the comparison of the mean CT-value as shown in Figs.17(b) and 18(b). This is because those specimens were sampled at the same area of in-situ site and the sampling depth is not much different between those two samples.

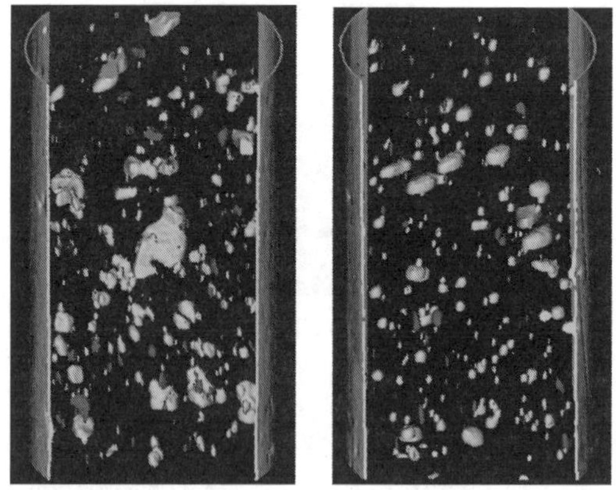

(a) Sample C (b) Sample D

Figure 20. 3-D binary image for air foams for Sample C and Sample D.

An X-ray CT image is a digital image based on CT-values as described before and it is possible to visualize the area of any target densities, for example the existence of air foams in the samples. Figures 19 and 20 shows the images of spatial distribution of air foams in the SGM. Those images are so called "binary images" under threshold operation, which is one of the most popular technique in the image processing analysis (Reid et al., 2000). Here, a threshold value of CT-value = 0 which can be considered to be the density of water as described before is chosen for the area of low density including air foams and thus, the area of the CT-value less than zero is presented with white color in three-dimensional space of the specimen. Figure 19 shows those results for Sample A and Sample B, which are the cases of surface active agent. As easily realized from these images, the amount of white color area for Sample A is much larger than those for Sample B and thus, it can be considered that some of the air foams in Sample B were contracted. These results show the effect of sampling depth as a result of water pressure and overburden pressure in the ocean. Figure 20 shows the same results as Fig.19 and those are the cases of Sample C and Sample D which are the cases of protein. The amount of the air foams for both cases are decreased as the case of Sample B and besides, the size of the air foam for Sample C and Sample D is much larger than that of Sample B. It is considered that those large foams are produced by gathering some of the air foams. Therefore, the air foams made by protein is

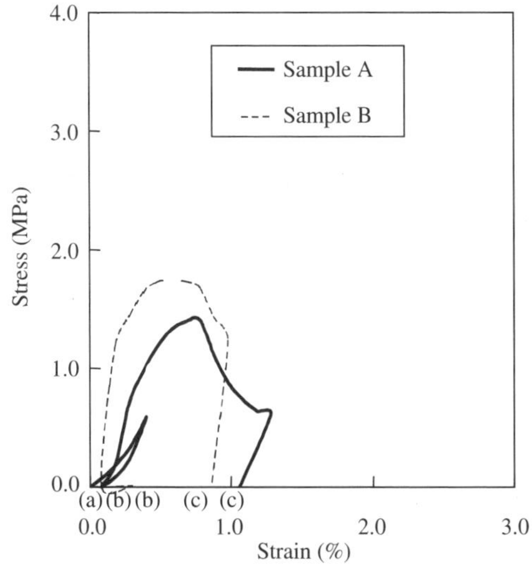

Figure 21. Stress–strain relationship for surface active agent case.

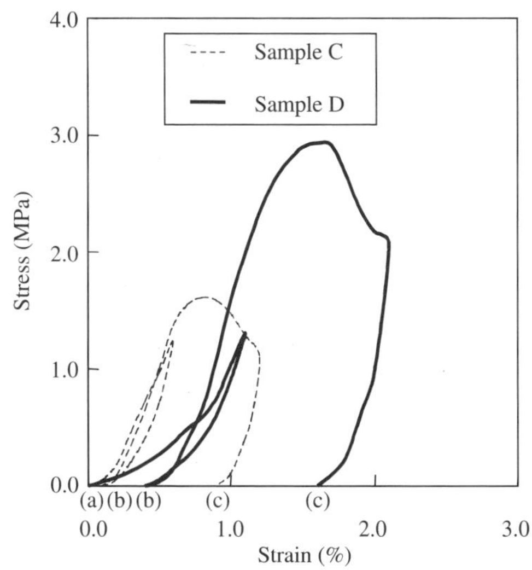

Figure 22. Stress–strain relationship for protein case.

easily broken or contracted compared with those samples of surface active agent.

3.2.3 *Mechanical property*

A series of unconfined compression test were conducted for all the samples (Sample A, Sample B, Sample C and Sample D). The nondestructive tests using X-ray CT scanner were also conducted at the stress conditions of initial, pre-peak and post-peak, respectively. Figure 21 shows the results of stress–strain

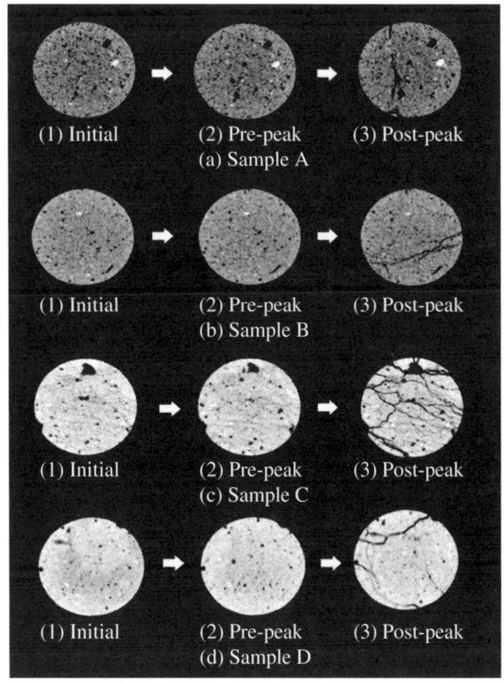

Figure 23. Change of CT image during unconfined compression.

relationship for Sample A and Sample B while Figure 22 shows those for Sample C and Sample D. The points (a), (b) and (c) in the figure show the scanning points of initial, pre-peak and post-peak conditions, respectively. It is noted that those locations are the conditions of zero stress because the specimen was released from the unconfined compression apparatus in order to be scanned. Comparing those results, the peak stresses for all the cases are not much changed with almost the same strain levels except the case of Sample D although the density for the cases of surface active agent are much smaller than those for the cases of protein. For the case of Sample D, the stiffness of the soil is much smaller than the case of Sample C at the beginning of compression. This can be considered that there may be a local weak area due to gathering some of the air foams and this area is contracted after compression. Thus, the peak stress for Sample D may be considered to become a large value with relatively large strain level. However, it is noted here that the number of test results is very limited in this study, so that more test data should be expected in order to convince this discussion.

The CT image in each cross section is obtained based on the distribution of CT-values after scanning the specimen. The scanning of one cross section takes about 5 minutes. Figure 23 shows one of the cross

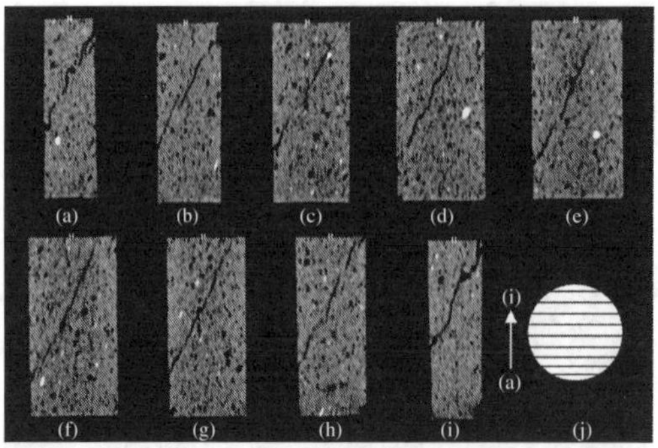

Figure 24. Vertical cross sectional image for Sample A.

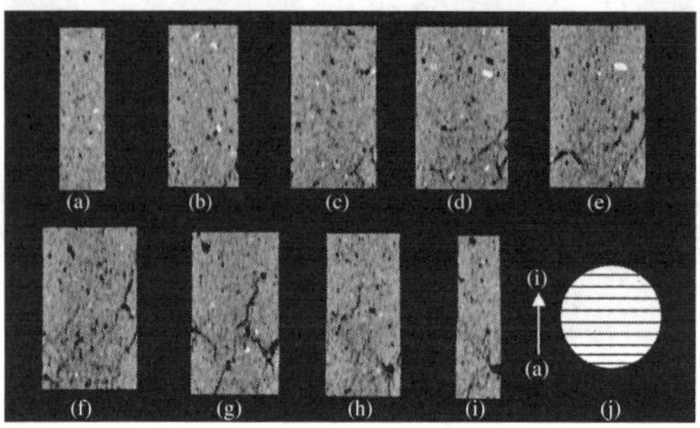

Figure 25. Vertical cross sectional image for Sample B.

sectional images of all the samples for initial, pre-peak and post-peak conditions, respectively. Here, those were chosen at the central height of each sample. As a whole, although there is no change until at the pre-peak condition, the strain localization appears at the post-peak condition for all the samples. But the way of appearance of this localization in this cross section is different among all the samples, in which the samples of surface active agent show relatively single dominant localization and those of protein show complicated localizations. And it is also interesting to note that the progress of those failure surfaces is not monotonic but intermittent for all the samples. Figures 24 and 25 show vertical cross sectional images for Sample A and Sample B at the post-peak condition. Nine images of equally slices are presented for each condition, in which the location of each vertical cross section is indicated in the horizontal cross sectional image shown in Figs 24(j) and 25(j). For the case of Sample A, there is a dominant strain localization while the case of Sample B shows rather complicated localization around the bottom of the specimen. Figures 26 and 27 show the same results as Figs 24 and 25 for the cases of Sample C and Sample D. Those images show much complicated failure patterns compared with the samples of surface active agent. There are many strain localizations and those behavior are the same as rock materials. Furthermore, it can be found that the strain localization for Sample D started from the circumference of the specimen and those have not been reached to the center of the specimen although all other samples such as Sample A, Sample B and Sample C were totally failed.

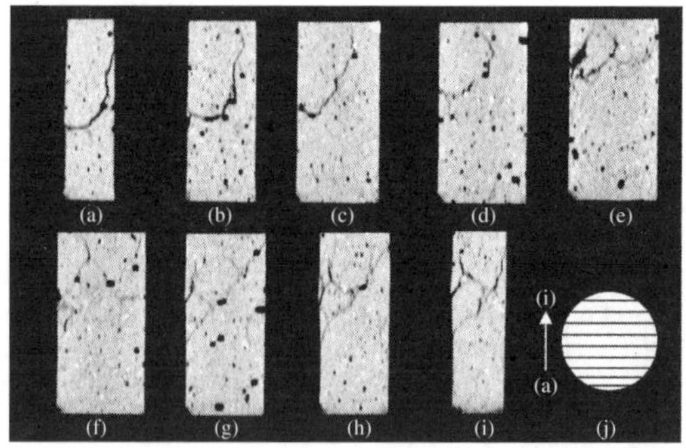

Figure 26. Vertical cross sectional image for Sample C.

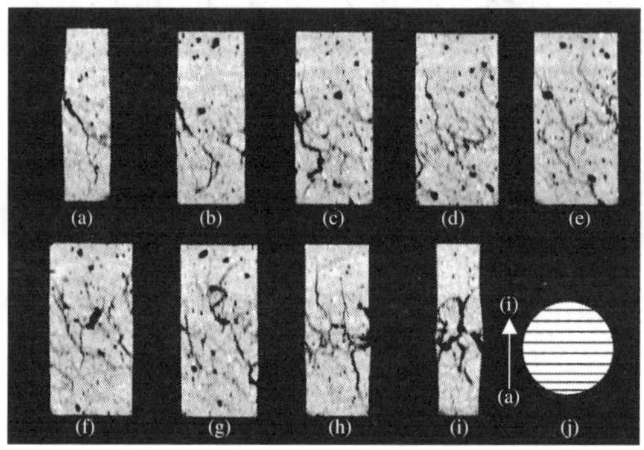

Figure 27. Vertical cross sectional image for Sample D.

3.2.4 *Change of density in the SGM*

In order to evaluate the changes of soil properties in the SGM, more quantitative discussion is expected. Here, the change of the density in the SGM is evaluated quantitatively using the results of CT scanning. As described before, the CT images are constructed using the spatial distribution of CT-values and CT-value can be converted to the density of the material. The following equation of the characteristic curve, which is the relationship between the density and the CT-value of SGM, is used:

$$\textit{CT-value} = 1181\rho_t - 1179 \qquad (5)$$

where *CT-value*: average CT-value in each cross section whose thickness is 1.0 mm and ρ_t: average wet

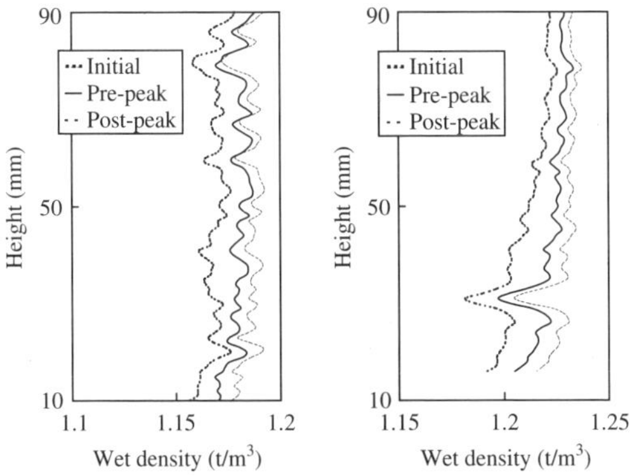

(a) Sample A (b) Sample B

Figure 28. Distribution of density for surface active agent case.

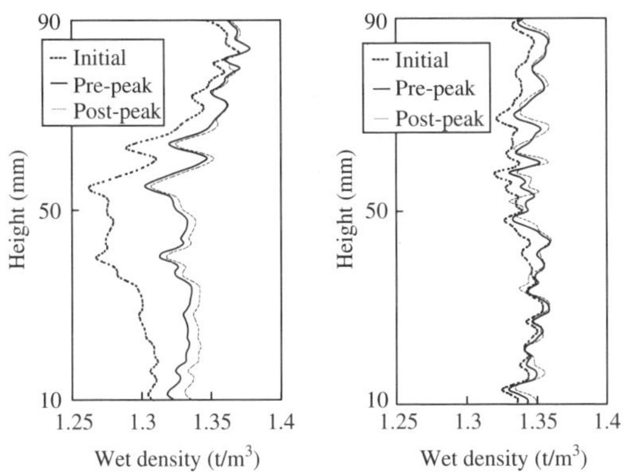

(a) Sample C (a) Sample D

Figure 29. Distribution of density for protein case.

density. Figure 28 shows the change of the density distribution from the initial condition to the post-peak condition for Sample A and Sample B using Eq.(5). Likewise, Fig.29 shows the same results for Sample C and Sample D. The density distribution in the SGM is decreased monotonically with keeping the same shape of the distribution as the strain is increased for Sample A and Sample B. But, the density for Sample C and Sample D is decreased drastically and locally as well at the post-peak condition when these results are compared with those of Sample A and Sample B which are shown in Fig.28. Those results convince that the samples using surface active agent fail like a soft soil while those of using protein show brittle failure such as rock. And it is also concluded that the strain localization is affected by the initial condition of non-homogeneity of the density because the shape of the density distribution in the specimen does not change from the initial condition to the post-peak condition.

It is also noted that the number of test results is very limited in this study, so that more test data should be expected in order to convince these discussion.

3.2.5 *Summary*

The conclusions drawn from this study are shown as follows:

(1) The distributions of both wet density and air foams were investigated visually in three dimension and those were evaluated quantitatively;
(2) It was observed that the air foams made by different types of air orientation methods show different size and volume of air foams in the soil after curing process and this is more notable for the case of protein;
(3) The change of the density due to unconfined compression is caused by the effect of strain localization growth but not the existence of air foams and the progress of shear banding is not monotonic but intermittent;
(4) The SGM by the use of surface active agent fails like a soft soil while that by protein shows brittle failure such as rock; and
(5) The distribution of the density in the SGM was evaluated quantitatively under unconfined compression and it was concluded that the strain localization in the SGM is affected by the initial condition of non-homogeneity of the density.

3.3 *Soil-structure interaction*

Earth reinforcement technique has been widely used around the world and so far many research projects for both experimental and analytical aspects such as model testing and numerical analysis have been conducted. But the modeling of interaction between soil and reinforcement is still on going issues and its real behavior has not been observed precisely.

The objective of this study is to visualize the behavior of soil-reinforcement interaction using industrial X-ray CT scanner. Here, a new pull-out testing apparatus for the use in the system of X-ray CT scanner is developed and a series of pull-out tests is conducted for grid type of reinforcement. Then, the pull-out box in the apparatus is scanned at several steps of pull-out displacement and a number of cross sectional images for the interaction behavior in each step are obtained. Three-dimensional images are also reconstructed by summing up all the images in each step. Here, the sheet type of the reinforcement is also examined in order to evaluate the effect of the reinforcement geometry on the soil behavior around the reinforcement. Based on those results, the change of the density in the soil around the reinforcement materials during pull-out displacement is observed and the effect of the geometry of reinforcing material on that behavior is also discussed.

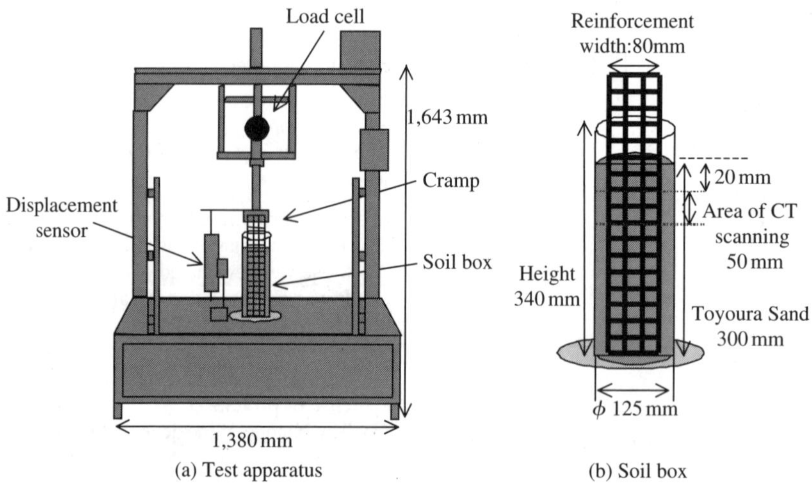

Figure 30. Pull-out test apparatus.

Table 4. Soil property of Toyoura Sand.

Maximum dry density (t/m^3)	1.61
Minimum dry density (t/m^3)	1.35
Relative density (%)	100

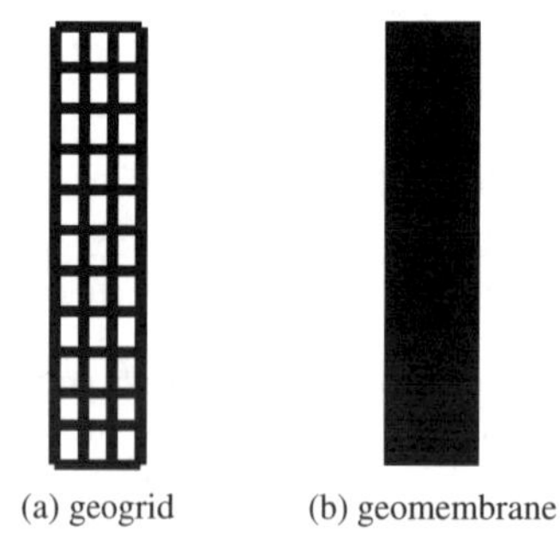

Figure 31. Types of reinforcement.

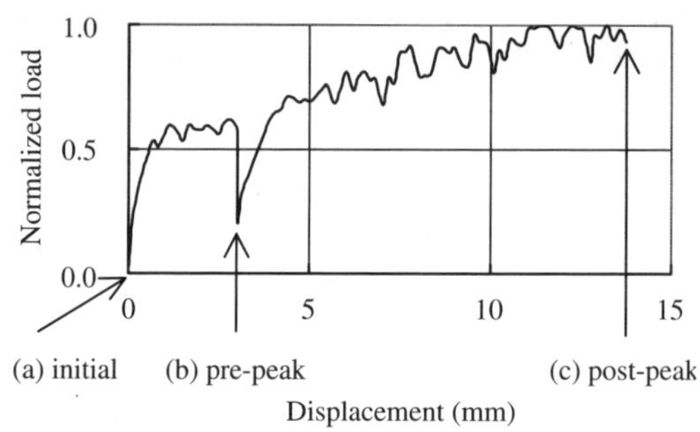

Figure 32. Pull-out force–displacement relationship for the case of geogrid.

3.3.1 *Pull-out test and CT scanning*

Figure 30 shows a pull-out testing apparatus which was newly developed by the author. Figure 30(a) shows the total apparatus while Fig.30(b) shows the soil box part in which the size of the reinforcement and the area of scanning are denoted. Toyoura sand was used and its soil property is shown in Table 4. Two different types of reinforcing materials were used which are grid type and sheet type. Those are shown in Fig.31. In the test, following process was conducted:

(1) After installing the reinforcement in the soil, a series of CT scanning are conducted as a initial condition.
(2) Then the pull-out loading is applied at the head of the reinforcement under displacement control (1 mm/min). This loading is stopped at one pull-out displacement level (pre-peak condition) and start CT scanning with every 1 mm thickness. The total number of scanning was 50.
(3) After scanning the soil box, the loading is reapplied and same scanning is conducted at the next strain level (post-peak condition) which is the condition of relatively large displacement for the reinforcement.

Figure 32 shows the pull-out force–displacement relationship for the case of geogrid, in which the scanning points are indicated in the figure. It is noted here that stress relaxation was occurred as shown in this figure and this was caused by stopping the pull-out test during CT scanning.

3.3.2 *Results and discussion*

Figure 33 shows one of cross sectional image at the depth of 35 mm from the surface of the ground for

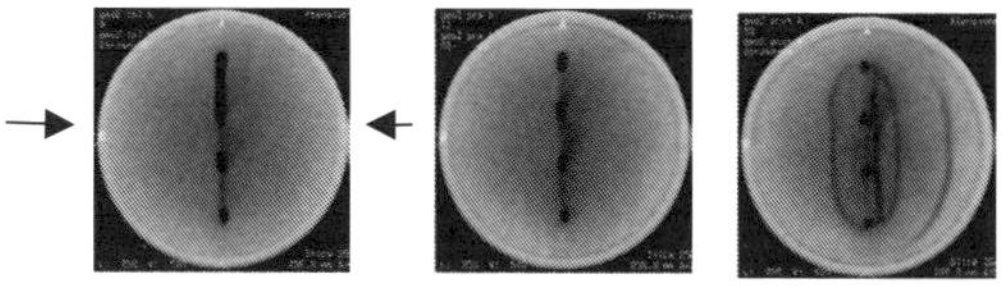

(a) initial (b) pre-peak (c) post-peak

Figure 33. Cross sectional images for the case of geogrid.

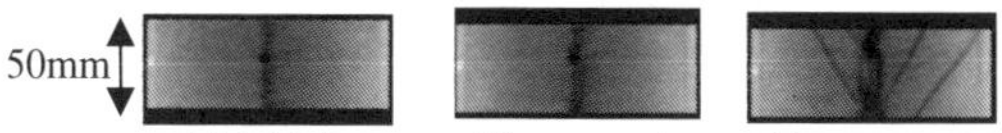

(a) initial (b) pre-peak (c) post-peak

Figure 34. Vertical cross sectional images for the case of geogrid.

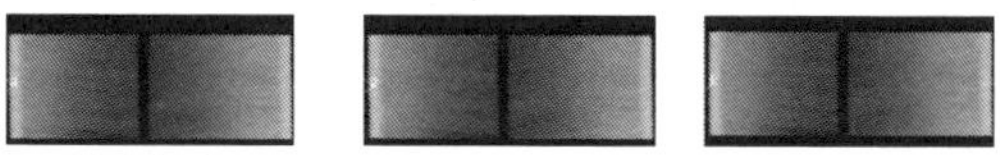

(a) initial (b) pre-peak (c) post-peak

Figure 35. Vertical cross sectional images for the case of geomembrane.

three different strain levels and the change of the density is shown by gray level distribution. As easily realized from those figures, the reinforcement makes the soil density variable even from the initial condition. Figure 34 shows the vertical cross sectional images for those three cases at total depth of 50 mm from 20 mm below the surface. These are reconstructed using all the horizontal cross sectional images and the clear shear zones can be observed at the large strain level as shown in Fig.34(c) in which there is not much change between initial and pre-peak strain levels. Figure 35 shows the same images as Fig.34 for the case of sheet type of reinforcement under the same pull-out test. There is no change of the density around the reinforcement in the ground, so that the geometry of the reinforcement makes the interaction behavior different. Figure 36 shows three-dimensional reconstruction images for those three strain levels in which the subtraction image between two images is also shown in this figure. As realized from these figures, the shear banding due to pull-out loadings is clearly occurred around the reinforcement with not single zone but multiple ones in three-dimension. Figure 37 shows special three dimensional images which are reconstructed in order to emphasize the area of shear banding. This is enable to visualize the inside behavior of the ground. Thus, it is confirmed that the industrial X-ray CT scanner has a possibility of characterizing the effect of the reinforcement in the soil and it may produce the valuable information about modeling of interaction between soil and reinforcement.

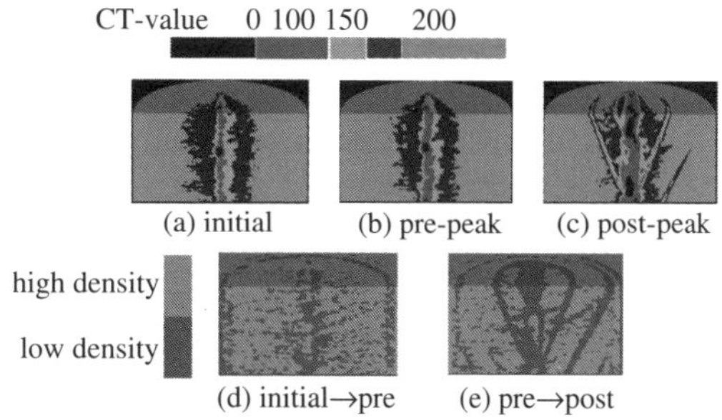

Figure 36. 3-D reconstruction images for the shear zone in the soil.

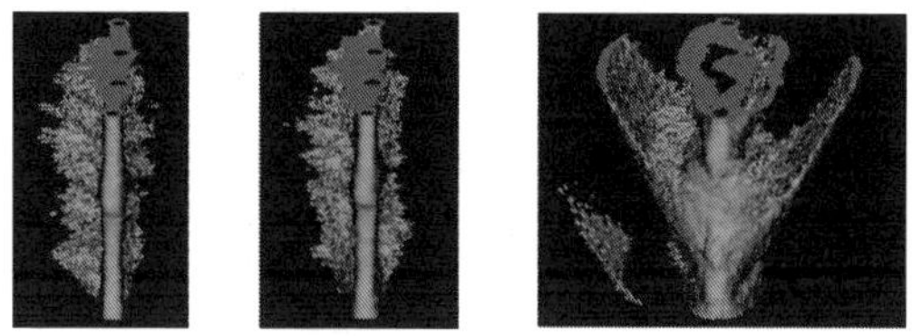

(a) initial (b) pre-peak (c) post-peak

Figure 37. Special 3-D reconstruction images for the shear zone in the soil.

3.3.3 *Summary*

A series of pull-out test was conducted for geogrid type of reinforcement. And a number of cross sectional images for the interaction behavior in each loading step were obtained using industrial X-ray CT scanner during pull-out forces. The same pull-out test for sheet type of the reinforcement was also examined and the effect of the geometry of the reinforcement on the interaction behavior between soil and reinforcement was discussed.

3.4 *Seepage and drying*

Light weight soil is one of composite soils which have originally been developed for the purpose of reducing the self-weight or applied loading due to embankment and reclamation on the soft ground. Methods of stabilized light weight soil which is composed of any soils, cement and light materials such as air foams and expanded polystirol (EPS) beads is one of this technique. Recently, this method has been widely used as a countermeasure method against increase of the solid waste such as dredged slurry from construction activities in Japan. One of the typical applications for this method is the use of backfill materials for quay walls at seaport for the purpose of the reduction of its weight on soft ground. A Supper Geo-Material, which is known by the name of SGM, has been developed by

Table 5. Mixing condition.

	Mass (kg/m^3)	Volumetric fraction (L)
Dry mass	367.0	136.0
Water	624.0	606.0
Cement	100.0	32.8
Air foam	9.3	222.5
Total	1100.3	999.8

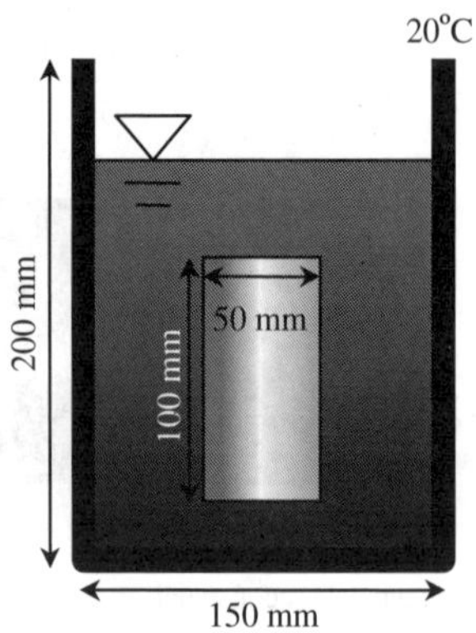

Figure 38. Seepage test.

the research group (Tuchida et al. (1996)). This material is made by mixing dredged slurry from the ocean with cement and air foam and is mixed at the construction site. Thus, it is very difficult to check the quality of the material and its performance. Especially, SGM has been used for water front construction along the coastal area and besides, this material is used in the ocean. Under these circumstances, the hydraulic properties such as seepage and drying of the SGM are very important and this should be controlled for the purpose of the long term performance of this material.

The purpose of this study is to evaluate hydraulic property of mixed soil with air foam using X-ray CT scanner. A series of seepage and drying tests are conducted for in-situ light weight soils which were sampled at the trial construction site of new Kumamoto Seaport, Japan. And the effect of air foams on seepage and drying are investigated qualitatively and quantitatively as well.

The specimen used in this study was in-situ SGM which is a light weight soil by mixing dredged slurry with cement and air foam. This was sampled at the trial construction site at new Kumamoto Seaport. Table 5 shows mixing condition of those in-situ light weight soil and those were mixed using special mixing plant at the construction site. Here, the air foam consists of the orientation by surface active agent was used. The dredged slurry used for this soil was Ariake Clay which

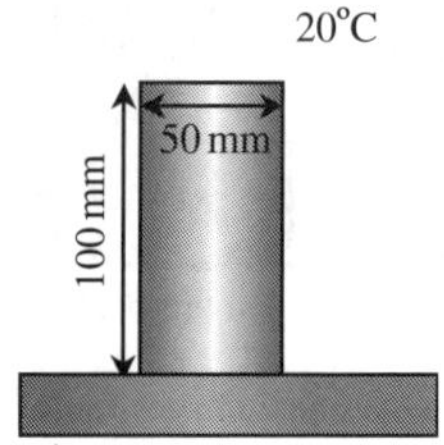

Figure 39. Drying test.

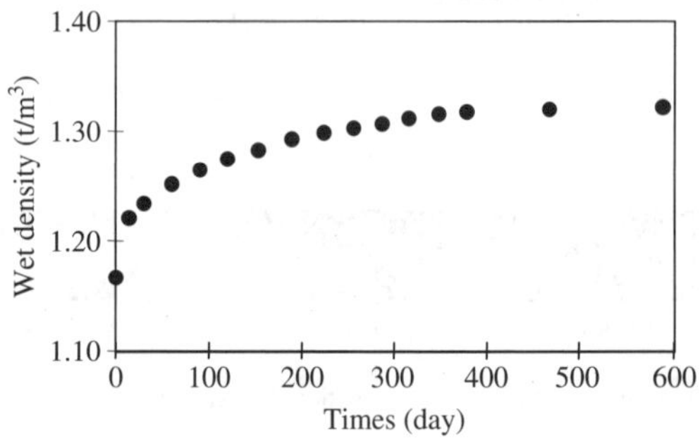

Figure 40. Change of wet density of the specimen.

is know as a soft clayey soil deposited around the Kumamoto Seaport located in Ariake Bay of Kyushu Island in Japan. The target of the density after curing process of 28 days was expected to be the value of 1.1 t/m^3. The precise contents of in-situ light weight soil will be delivered by the reference by Otani et al. (2002).

3.4.1 *Seepage test*

The size of the specimen was fixed to be a diameter of 50 mm with the height of 100 mm in this test. Figure 38 shows the view of seepage test. The specimen was submerged in the container under constant temperature of 20°C. The specimen was scanned at every 1 mm thickness along its height and total of scanning cross section was 100. The total elapsed time of this test was 19 months and the scanning was conducted step by step in each certain time with measuring weight and volume in order to calculate average density of the specimen.

3.4.2 *Drying test*

As shown in Fig.39, the specimen was left in the room of constant temperature of 20°C for drying test and CT scanning was conducted at each elapsed time which is the same way as seepage test.

3.4.3 *Test results*

Figure 40 shows the density change during seepage test. It was found that the density of the specimen was increased with the increase of elapsed time but the

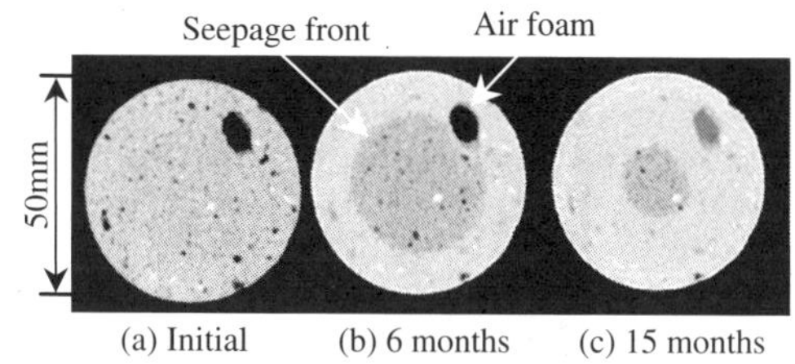

Figure 41. Cross sectional image due to seepage test.

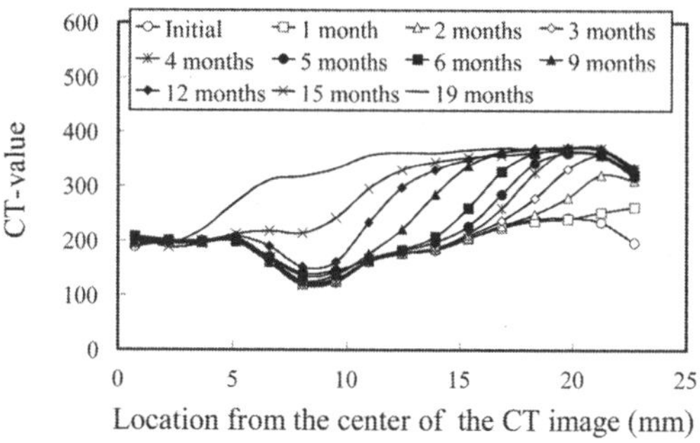

Figure 42. Change of CT-value distributions.

velocity of the seepage was gradually decreased. Figure 41 shows X-ray CT images of the specimen at the middle of height for three different elapsed times, which are initial, 6 months and 15 months. It is noted here that the white color shows relatively high density regions while the black color shows that of low density in the CT image. Thus, it was observed that the seepage front of the water was extended gradually to the center of the specimen axi-symmetrically. Here, there is a large black region in the CT image and it is realized as a relatively large air void. The shape of the air void did not change by the period of 6 months since the seepage test had started. However, it is observed that the specimen was submerged after 15 months later because the change of the color in the air void from black to gray. And also, the size of the air foam became small after 15 months and 19 months as well. Figure 42 shows the distribution of the mean CT-value in the submerged regions. The position, which the mean CT-value started to increase, pointed out the seepage front. Furthermore, it is found that the slope of the curve around seepage front area was constant even 12 months later but the slope of the curve became smaller 15 months later. This means that the seepage speed became slow after seepage in the soil. Thus, the seepage condition in the light weight soil was evaluated visually and quantitatively based on X-ray CT data.

In order to estimate the change of void ratio in the specimen during seepage test, an image analysis what

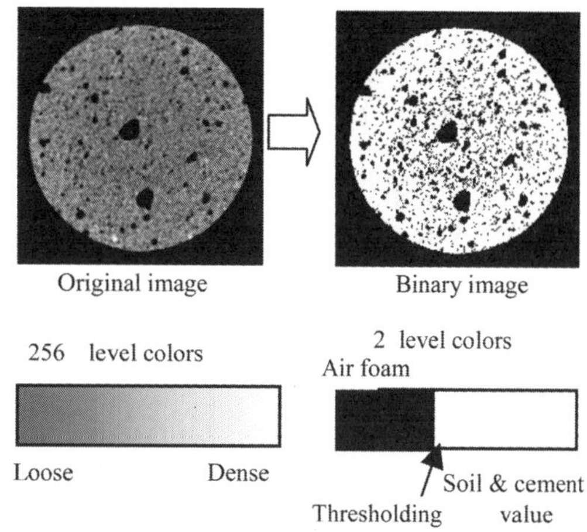

Figure 43. Binary image processing analysis.

is called "binary image processing" was conducted. This technique is to divide the region of material of cement with soil from the regions of air void. Figure 43 presents the basic idea of so called "thresholding technique" in the image processing analysis. The process of obtaining the thresholding value for CT-value is shown as follows:

(a) The air void ratio was calculated based on the mixing condition
(b) The CT-value for the thresholding between air foams and soil with cement was assumed and the volume of air foams is calculated in the arbitrary cross sectional image and
(c) If the average volume of the air foams in the specimen after the calculation at the process of (b) was not equal to the one obtained for the process of (a), the trial thresholding value should be changed. Then, the process is restarted from the process (b) until the calculated average value of air foams is close enough to the value obtained at the process of (a).

Figure 44 shows the distribution change of mean air void ratio along the height of the specimen during seepage testing. Consequently the reduction of air voids in light weight soil was evaluated quantitatively based on X-ray CT data.

Figure 45 shows the same figure as Fig.40, which shows the change of the density during the process of drying. Total elapsed time was about 600 hours and the specimen itself shows many cracks with its shrinkage. Figure 46 shows the cross sectional images at 3 different elapsed times. As easily realized from these images, the black region which shows the area of drying became larger from circumference of the specimen. And it is interesting to note that the velocity of the drying is much higher than that of seepage in the soil.

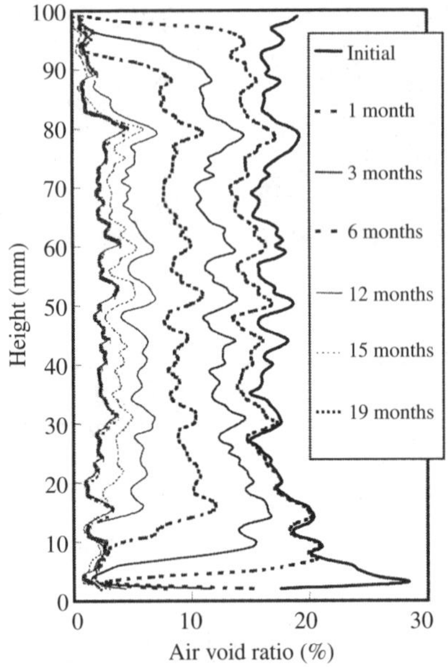

Figure 44. Distributions of the air voids.

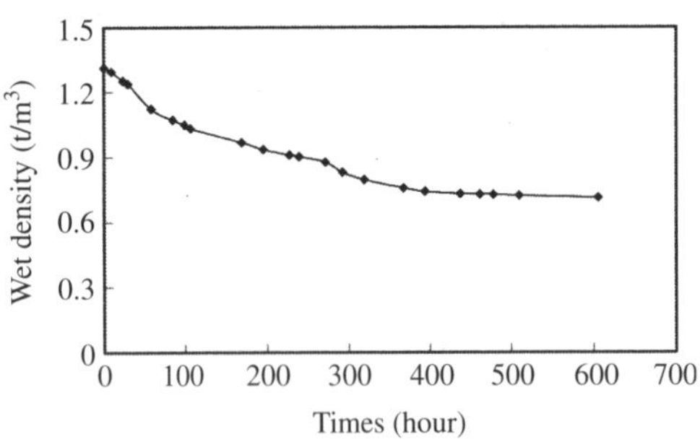

Figure 45. Change of wet density of the specimen.

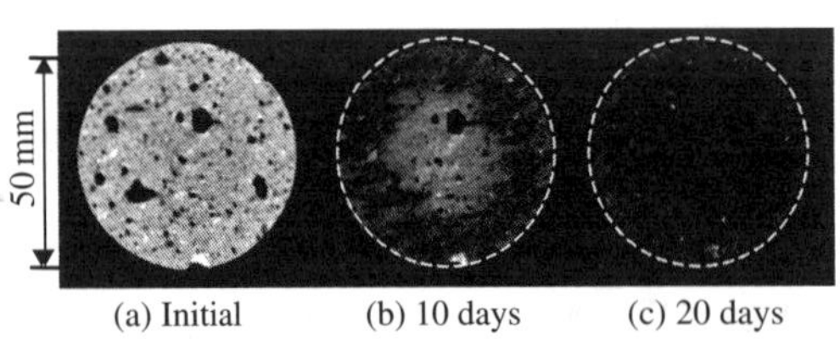

Figure 46. Cross sectional images for drying test.

Figure 47 shows one of cross sectional image after drying. As easily realized, there are many cracks in the soil and the decrease of the soil strength is expected by drying this type of soil. Figure 48 shows the same figure as Fig.42 which shows the change of the average CT-value at the central height of the specimen

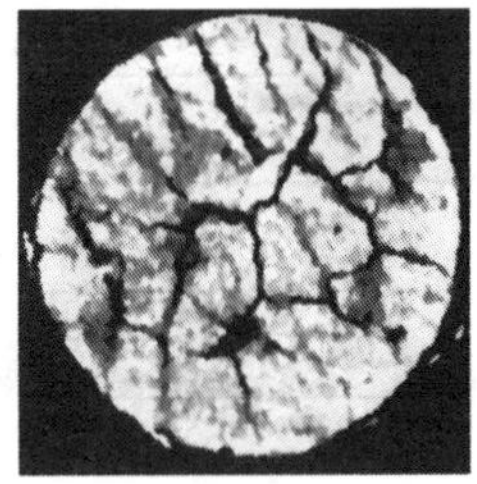

Figure 47. Cross sectional image for drying specimen.

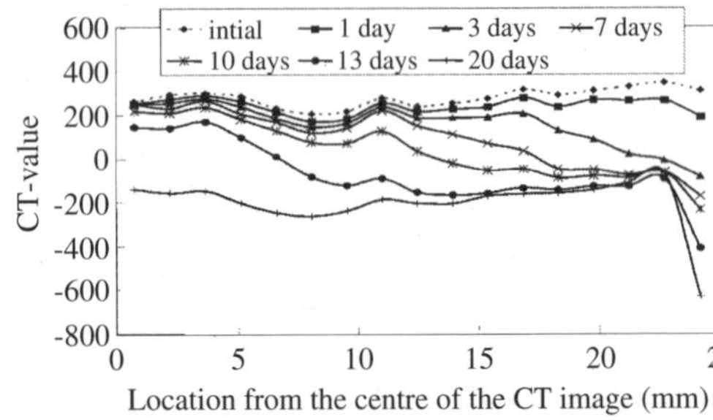

Figure 48. Change of CT-value distributions.

during drying. This figure shows that the density decreases as the drying proceeds in the soil from circumference of the specimen.

3.4.4 *Summary*

The conclusions from this study were drawn as follows:

(1) The behaviors of seepage and drying in the mixed soil can be well observed using industrial X-ray CT scanner.
(2) It was observed that the volume and property of air foams played an important role for seepage behavior.
(3) The velocity for drying in the soil is much quicker than that of seepage and as far as material control is concerned, the drying should be paid attention because of appearance of cracking.

4 DEVELOPMENT OF NEW TRIAXIAL COMPRESSION TEST APPARATUS

In the preliminary efforts, characterization of failure in soil under unconfined compression was investigated; however, the unconfined compression tests and the CT scanning were not conducted simultaneously due to the lack of a special compression apparatus suitable for use with an X-ray CT scanner.

The objective of this research is to develop a new triaxial compression test apparatus suitable for use with

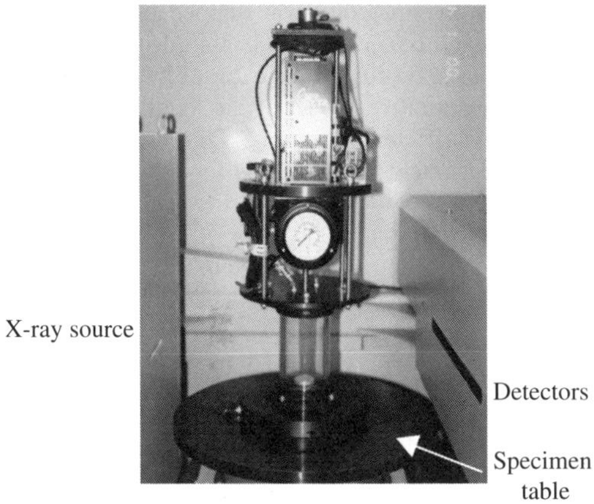

Photo 2. New triaxial compression test apparatus.

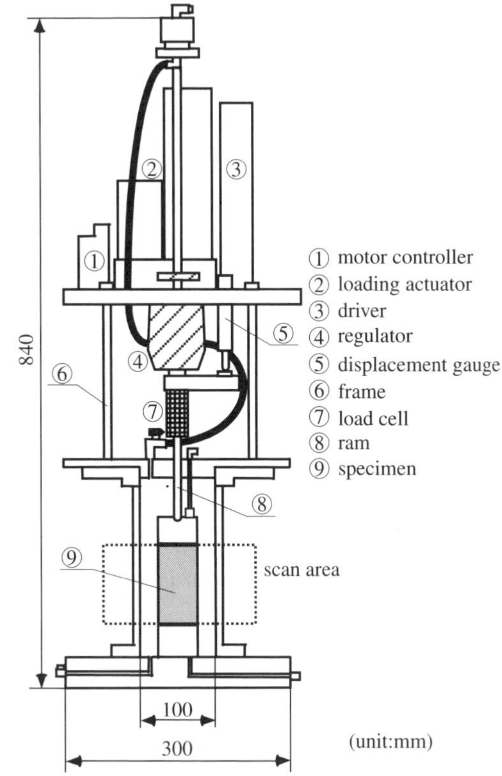

Figure 49. Diagram of the new test apparatus.

an industrial X-ray CT scanner and to characterize failure in sand using this new system. Firstly, the performance of the new triaxial compression apparatus is verified, by which the accuracy of the loading system and the resulting stress–strain relationship are confirmed using a dummy specimen (a spring). Then, results obtained using this system are compared with those of a conventional triaxial compression test apparatus. This new test apparatus is then used in unison with an X-ray CT scanner. A series of nondestructive measurements are conducted during triaxial compression in which the compression apparatus is placed within the X-ray CT scanner device. A large number of horizontal CT scanning images are obtained and the progressive failure of the soil is followed by visualization. It is thus demonstrated that an industrial X-ray CT scanner could be used effectively in conjunction with this new triaxial compression apparatus in geotechnical engineering applications.

4.1 *Features of the new apparatus*

Due to the high voltage rating of 300 kV for the X-ray tubes of industrial X-ray CT scanners, all scanning operations had to be performed in a room with lead shielding. Accordingly, all compression testing, as well, had to be conducted on the specimen table in the shield room as shown in Fig.7 and all operations were controlled remotely from outside this room. A new triaxial compression test apparatus was specifically developed for use with an industrial X-ray CT scanner under the above conditions. The arrangement of this apparatus is shown in Photo 2 and its features are detailed in Fig.49. The specifications of this apparatus are noted in Table 6 and explained in detail as follows:

Table 6. Specification of new triaxial compression test apparatus

Loading system	Stepping motor (strain controlled)
Maximum capacity of loading	100 (kg)
Minimum loading speed	0.005 mm/step (0.3%/min)
Confining pressure	400 (kPa)
Size of soil specimen	f = 50 mm H = 100 mm
Test conditions	UU, CU and CD test (but CD test for clay is exception)

(1) To function on the specimen table, which moves transversely and rotationally during scanning, the apparatus must be compact and lightweight (not more than 100 kg) and is thus mostly constructed of duralumin.
(2) The applied load reacts only on the pressure cell wall, which is made of acrylic and is counteracted in the apparatus; thus the weight of the apparatus itself must only be applied to the specimen table.
(3) In order to scan the specimen horizontally during triaxial compression, there should be no obstacles (e.g., steel bars) around the compression cell because such materials would interfere with X-ray

CT imaging. Figure 50(a) demonstrates the effect of such interference in which three stainless steel bars were used with a conventional triaxial compression cell. Figure 50(b) shows the same image obtained using the new triaxial compression cell, demonstrating improved clarity.

(4) All the operations for this apparatus were conducted remotely using a personal computer from outside of the shield room and the whole loading process was recorded electronically.

(5) Loading was stopped during the scanning operation, which takes about 5.0 min for one cross sectional image.

(6) Figure 49 shows an operational setup in which all the equipment used for measurements with their leads on the top of the apparatus are positioned to avoid interference with the imaging processing.

4.2 *Verification*

Initially, the loading system was verified using a dummy specimen consisting of a spring. This specimen had a diameter of 50.0 mm and height of 100.0 mm and a spring constant of 82.9 N/mm. The test was conducted using strain control so that the input velocity of applied displacement and the value of load transfer were monitored during the test. Figure 51 shows the confirmation of the velocity of the applied displacement. To demonstrate the accuracy of the results, the loading test was repeated five times. For the compression test with the CT scanner, the loading has to be stopped during specimen scanning; thus it is noted that the loading procedure was stopped at strain levels of 3.0 mm and 6.0 mm for 30.0 min during compression. All of the results had an error of less than 1.0%, thus the quantitative aspect of the loading system is considered sufficiently accurate. Figure 52 shows the load–displacement relationships for these five tests. The uniqueness of these results is evident and the stiffness values were within an error of 1.0%; therefore, the reliability of the loading system was verified and the reproducibility of the tests was demonstrated.

4.3 *Test procedure*

The triaxial compression test under CD (Consolidated Drained) conditions was conducted using Toyoura Sand with a minimum dry density of 1.33 t/m^3, maximum dry density of 1.65 t/m^3 and relative density of 65.3%. The test procedure was as follows:

(1) After consolidating the specimen at the same pressure as the confining pressure, the soil specimen was scanned at its initial condition before applying the compression force.

(2) The specimen was compressed under strain control and was unloaded at strain level intervals of 3.0%. To avoid the effect of stress relaxation, the

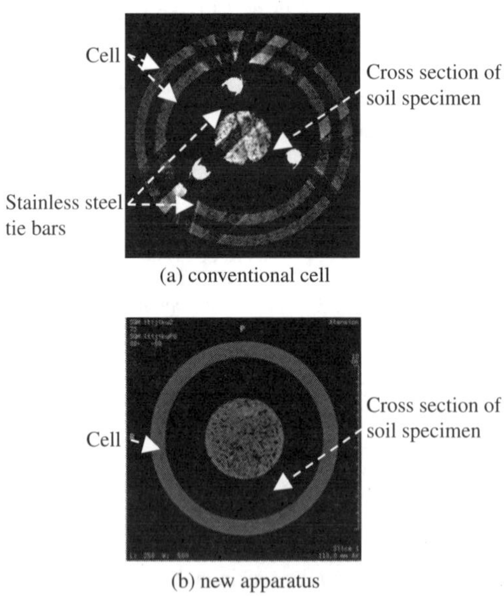

Figure 50. CT image using different types of compression cells.

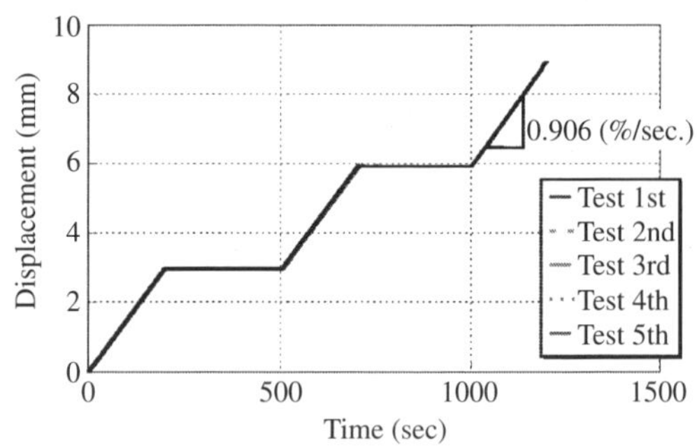

Figure 51. Verification of loading system (velocity of the loading).

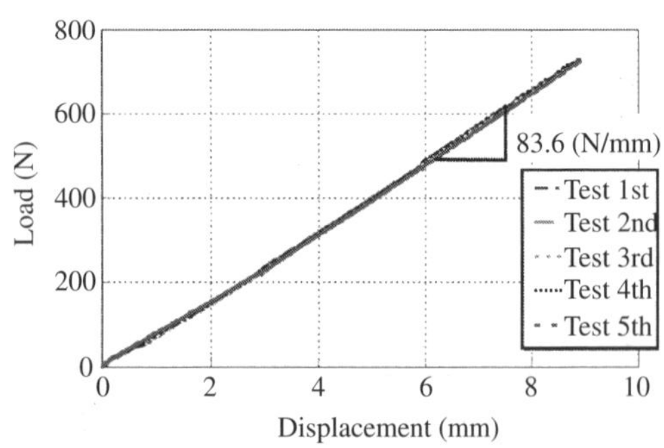

Figure 52. Verification of loading system (load–displacement relationship).

specimen was unloaded until the deviator stress reached zero, then the nondestructive test using the X-ray CT scanner was conducted. After scanning was finished, the specimen was reloaded until the strain level reached 6.0%. A total of six cross sections were scanned, which were located at heights of 10.0, 25.0, 40.0, 55.0 and 70 mm from the bottom of the specimen.

(3) The same process used in step 2, above, was continued step wises at 3% axial strain intervals until a strain level of 15.0% was obtained.

4.4 *Features of the new apparatus*

A series of drained tests were conducted using Toyoura Sand in accordance with the procedures described above. Figure 53 shows the stress–strain relationship with volumetric strain from the results of one test in which the deviator stress is plotted as a function of axial strain where the confining pressure was 49.0 kPa and the density was set to 1.52 t/m^3. Steps A, B, C, D and E in Fig.11 are the locations of strain levels 3.0, 6.0, 9.0, 12.0 and 15.0%, respectively, where the CT scanning was conducted. There was a peak stress at a strain level of about 7.0% and it is evident that the volume of the specimen decreases in the interval from the beginning of the test to the strain level of 3.0% and increases thereafter. It takes 5 min to scan one slice of CT image, so to avoid X-ray attenuation disturbance during loading, the specimen was unloaded until the deviator stress reached zero. This testing method produced stable images; however, further research is needed to improve upon the processional accuracy of the stiffness and strength measurements. The total behavior of the results as shown in Fig.53 is cyclic in nature and does not differ with those of conventional methods. These results confirm the effectiveness of the proposed apparatus.

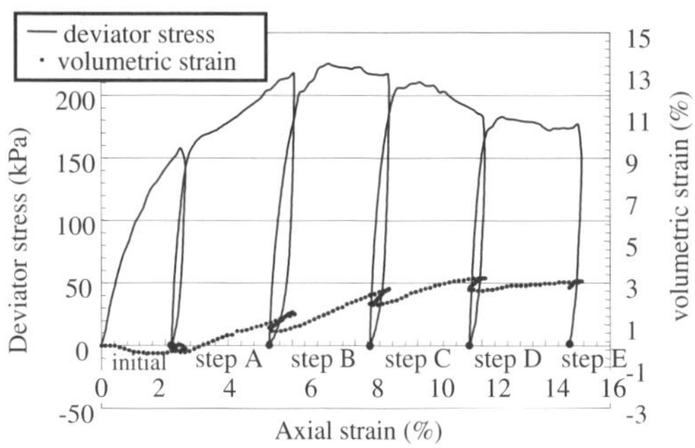

Figure 53. Stress–strain relationship with volume change.

4.5 *Visualization of progressive failure in sand*

Figure 54 shows the images for all strain levels at the six cross sections. The dark areas (indicating relatively low density) around the center of each cross section at the initial condition indicate that the specimen was not homogeneous due to insufficient saturation.

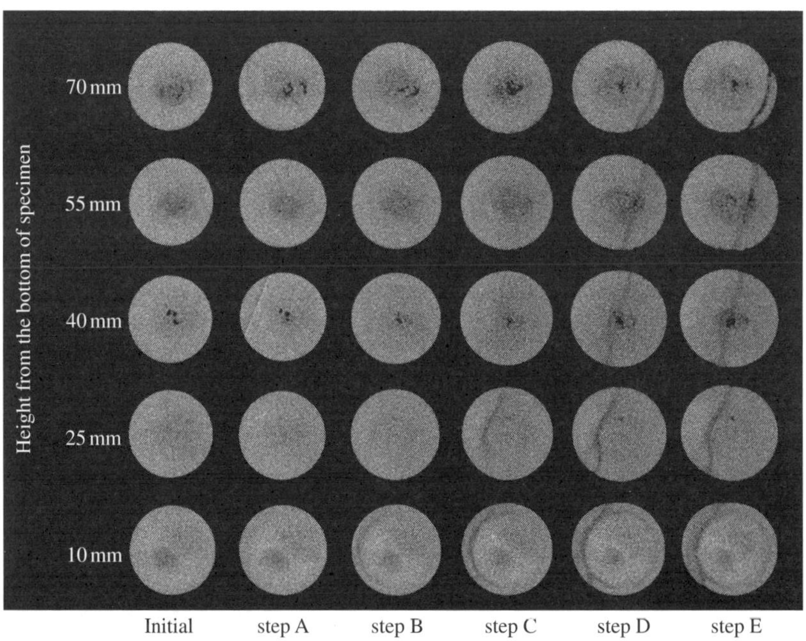

Figure 54. Cross sectional images of specimen.

Meanwhile, a different type of low-density area appears in the images from step B at the height of 10 mm, which is indicative of strain localization. It is easily understood from Fig.54 that local shear banding starts from the bottom of the specimen at the strain level of step B immediately prior to the peak stress shown in Fig.53, although the shear band cannot be observed from outside of the specimen. The shape of this local shear band in the cross section is the same as that on the circumference at the bottom of the specimen and this strain localization propagates upwards as the strain increases. It is also evident that the total failure surface, which results from the progression of local failures, appears after the peak stress condition occurs, which corresponds to the strain level at step D. Thus, the following conclusions are summarized from the results shown in Fig.54 for this specimen as follows:

(1) The local shear band appeared before the peak stress occurred in the soil, and this behavior could not be visually observed on the outside of the specimen.
(2) The local shear band propagated from the bottom of the specimen to the top.
(3) The shape of strain localization was not entirely on a plane surface, but rather curved in each cross section.
(4) The total failure surface appeared after the peak stress in the soil occurred.

The distributions of CT-values for all the strain levels (from the initial condition to step E) for a half cross section in the specimen at a height of 25.0 mm are shown in Fig.55. The density at a location about 15.0 mm from the center decreases locally as the strain level increases and this phenomenon shows the progress of the shear band in the cross section. It is interesting to note that the starting point of the decrease in density at that area is observable even at the strain level of step B, although the CT image shown in Fig.54 (at 25 mm with step B) did not show any localization in that cross section. Thus, a more precise understanding of the progress of the shear band is possible using the CT-value distribution in the specimen. Furthermore, the change in location of the left edge in this figure indicates the volume change of the specimen, and the CT-value at the edge is approaching −1000, which corresponds to the density of air. Figure 56 shows a computer graphic image of the total failure surface in the soil derived from the six cross sectional images at the end of the test, which is the step E strain level. The shape of the failure surface is clearly reconstructed and it is easily realized that this is not on a plane surface, but rather an irregular curved surface. It is interesting to note that the shapes of the total failure surface at the cross sections at both the top and bottom of the specimen are the same as those at the circumference. The possibility that the shape of the specimen influences this development is considered; thus further testing with other specimen shapes would be expedient to further our understanding of failure phenomena in soils.

Even though the number of cross sectional images used in this study was small, the graphical images obtained made it possible to qualitatively assess the characteristics of the failure surface in three-dimensions. However, it should also be noted that evaluations of a more quantitative nature would be possible by increasing the number of scanning slices.

4.6 *Summary*

Triaxial compression testing is a standard methodology for determining soil design parameters. However, it has recently been realized that failure in soils is caused by progressive strain localization and that this behavior is greatly affected by the boundary conditions and the three-dimensional characteristics of a soil specimen. Precise nondestructive methods of

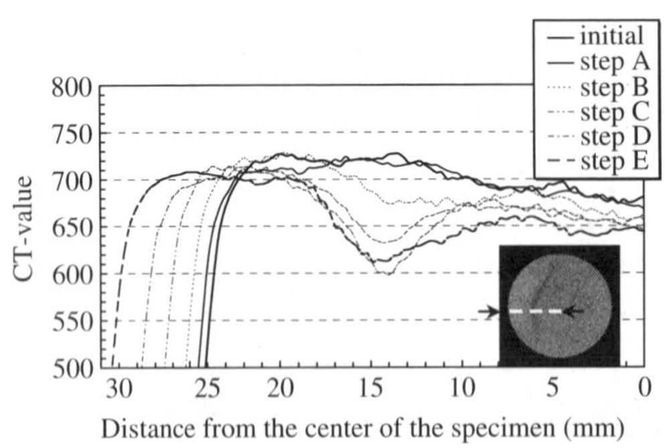

Figure 55. Distribution of CT-values for half cross sections at a height of 25.0 mm.

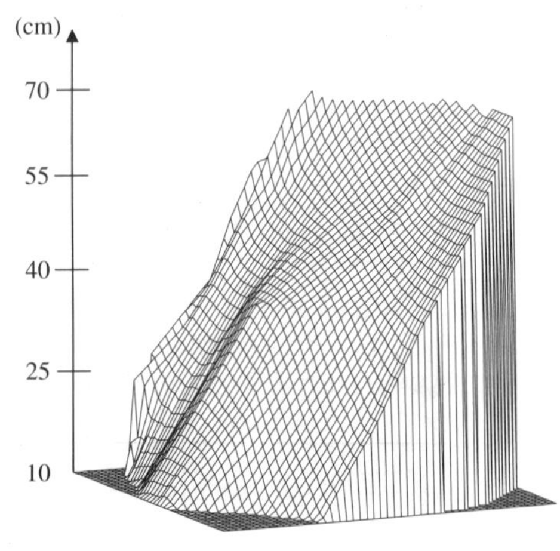

Figure 56. Graphical image of failure surface.

observation are thus necessary to accurately model soil behavior.

In this research a new triaxial compression test apparatus was developed for use with an X-ray CT scanner and utilized to investigate progressive failure with strain localization during triaxial compression by three-dimensional imaging. The features of this new apparatus are summarized as follows:

(1) It is lightweight and compact so as to be used directly on the specimen table of the X-ray CT scanner in the shield room.
(2) To avoid interruption of the propagation of X-ray photons in the soil, there are no obstacles around the triaxial cell such as steel frames and leads of measuring equipment.
(3) All testing is controlled automatically using a computer program because all operations must be conducted in an isolated shield room (for protection from X-rays).

The following conclusions were drawn based on test results:

(1) The newly developed triaxial compression test apparatus provided verifiable results.
(2) Progressive failure with strain localization was visualized using CT images. Because it takes 5 min to scan one CT image slice, the specimen was unloaded until the deviator stress reached zero to avoid disturbance of X-ray attenuation during loading. Stable high quality images were obtainable by this method; however, further work is needed to develop more precise methods for quantitative purposes.
(3) The shape and characteristics of the soil failure surface were qualitatively assessed even with only a small number of scanning slices. It is considered that more quantitative results can be obtained by increasing the number of scanning slices.

The newly developed triaxial compression apparatus made it possible to evaluate progressive failure in soil with an industrial X-ray CT scanner using a nondestructive method.

5 MORE POSITIVE USAGE OF X-RAY CT DATA

5.1 *Application to numerical analysis*

In this study, three-dimensional rigid plastic finite element method (RPFEM) is conducted for the purpose of simulating the failure mechanism of the mixed soil under confined compression. Here in the analysis, the results of CT scanning which is the spatial distribution of the density in the specimen are used in order to perform the non-homogeneity of the soil. In RPFEM analysis, not only the strength of the soil but also the shape of failure zone are obtained, and those numerical results are compared with those of unconfined compression tests. Note that the precise contents of RPFEM are shown in the references of Tamura et al. (1987) and Yamamoto and Otani (2002).

5.1.1 *Test results*

A series of unconfined compression test was conducted for mixed soil which is made by mixing dredged slurry with cement and air foams under certain mixing condition. During unconfined compression test, the soil specimen was scanned at 6 different cross sections in the specimen for initial and nine strain levels. The paper by Otani et al. (2002) should be referred for more details of this soil and the test. Figure 57 shows one of test results for stress–strain relationship. Stress relaxation is realized in this figure and this was caused by CT scanning. Figure 58 shows one of cross sectional image obtained by CT scanning. Generally, CT images are presented with shaded darker or black for lower density region and light gray or white for high density one for all the subsequent black and white images. The total number of gray level is 256 for this

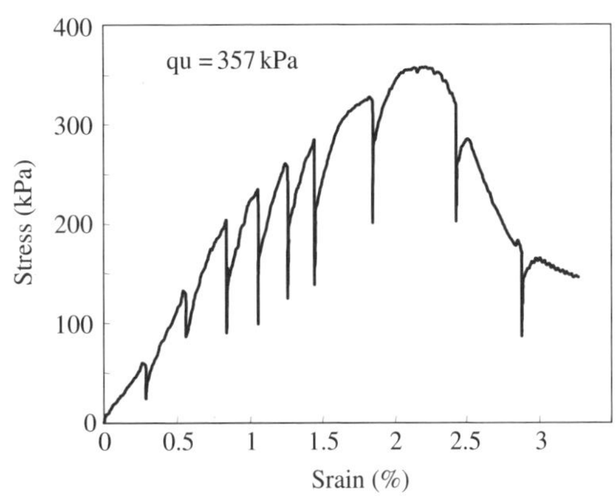

Figure 57. Stress–strain relationship.

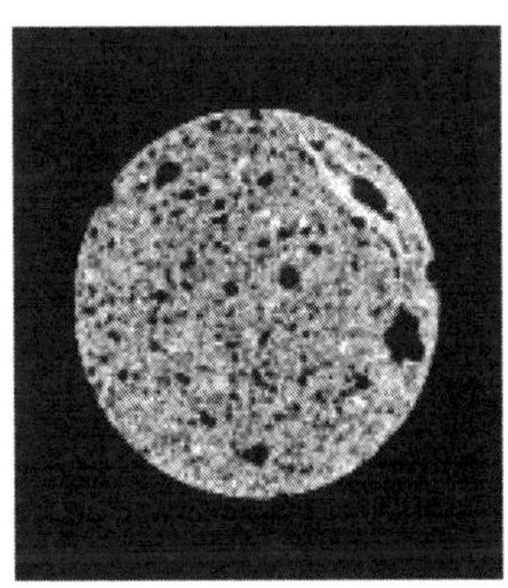

Figure 58. X-ray CT image.

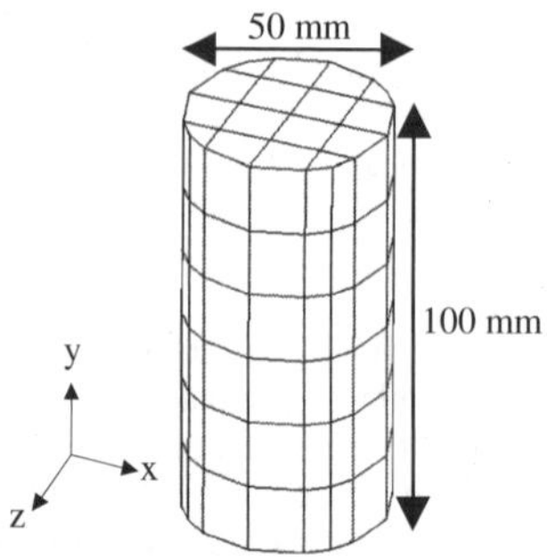

Figure 59. Finite element mesh for unconfined compression test.

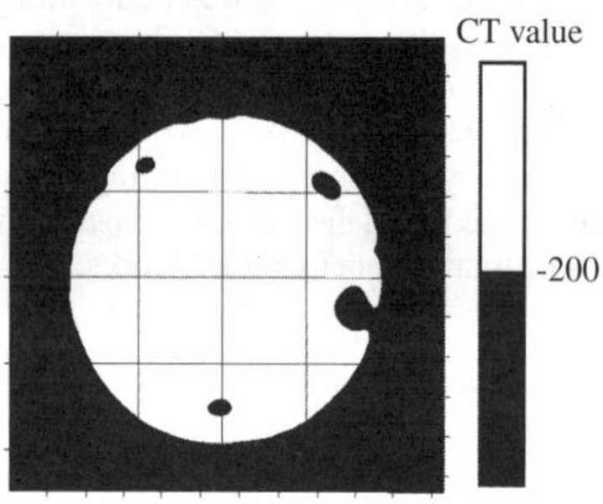

Figure 60. Binary image.

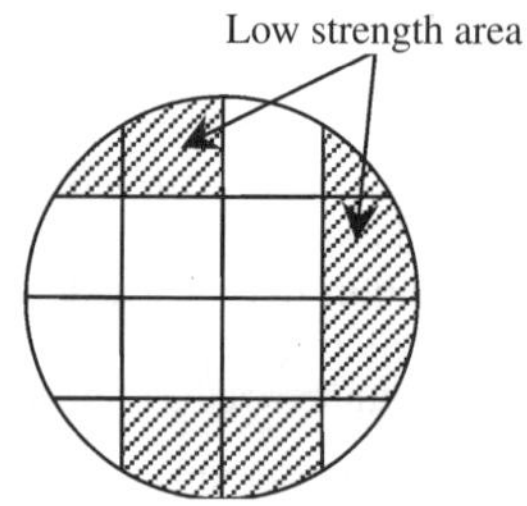

Figure 61. Strength distribution.

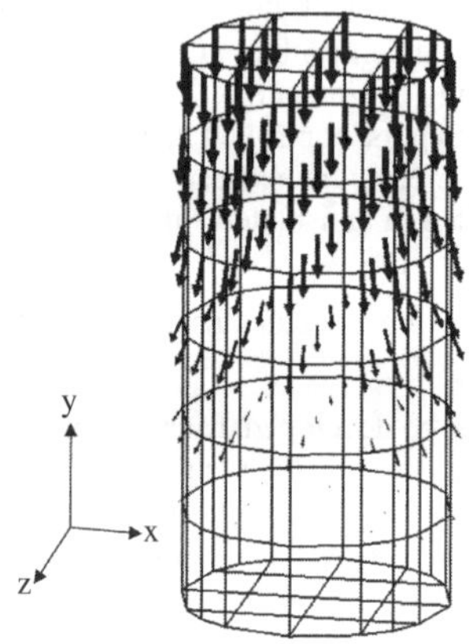

Figure 62. Velocity field for homogeneous condition.

distribution. It is also noted that the images are reconstructed by so called "CT-value", so that the image can also be considered as a spatial distribution of this CT-value.

5.1.2 *Evaluation of initial imperfection by CT image*

The spatial distribution of CT-value is used for evaluating the non-homogeneity in the soil for the analysis. This result is reflected to the spatial distribution of the strength value, c in the analysis because this is the only parameter for RPFEM in this study. Figure 59 shows 3-D finite element mesh used for the analysis of unconfined compression test. The size of the specimen is the same as test condition and total number of element is 96, in which the total number of nodes is 175 with 6 layers. The boundary conditions are set as follows: (1) The bottom of the specimen is fixed; (2) The top of the specimen is applied vertical velocity as a loading condition under displacement control and the lateral direction is fixed; and (3) The side of the specimen is totally free because of unconfined compression test. Figure 60 shows binary image for Fig.58, in which the threshold value is set to be a CT-value of -200 and the area of white color shows relatively high density while that of black area shows low density. The mesh shown in the figure indicates each element size. The cohesion, c of the element where the area of black color exists is obtained by reducing the strength value using some certain factors. This modeling is shown in Fig.61 and is used for all the elements. Thus, the non-homogeneity of the cohesion in the soil is evaluated as an initial imperfection condition.

5.1.3 *Results and discussion*

In order to discuss the effect of proposed model of non-homogeneity, the case of homogeneity is also analyzed, in which the unique cohesion, c is set using the test result of unconfined compression strength as shown in Fig.57. Figure 62 shows the result of velocity field for homogeneous case. The velocity vector is equally distributed around the circumference of the specimen and those are gradually decrease towards the bottom of the specimen. Besides, it is difficult to evaluate the real failure mechanism. Figure 63 shows the same result as Fig.62 for the case of non-homogeneity consideration as described in previous section. The dominant failure mechanism can be seen by the distribution of velocity field. Figure 64 shows the reconstructed CT image for the unconfined compression test and this seems very similar to the computation result as shown in Fig.63.

5.1.4 *Summary*

Based on the results obtained from this study, it is concluded that the failure of the mixed soil can be well evaluated using 3-D rigid plastic finite element analysis with considering the non-homogeneity of the density based on the results of CT scanning. And the possibility of the effectiveness of this analysis method is convinced. The more quantitative determination of density change should be expected for the next step of this study.

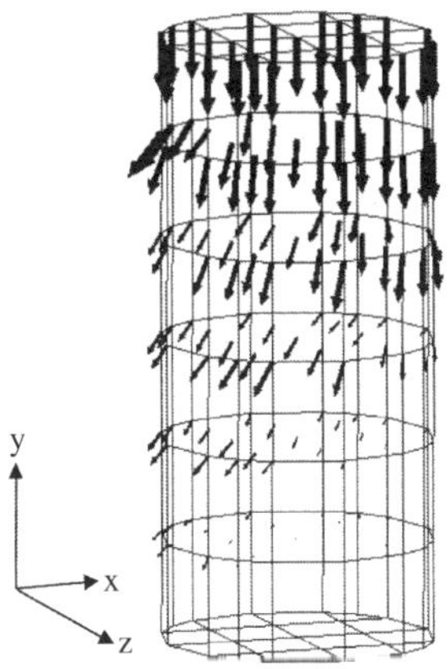

Figure 63. Velocity field for non-homogeneous condition.

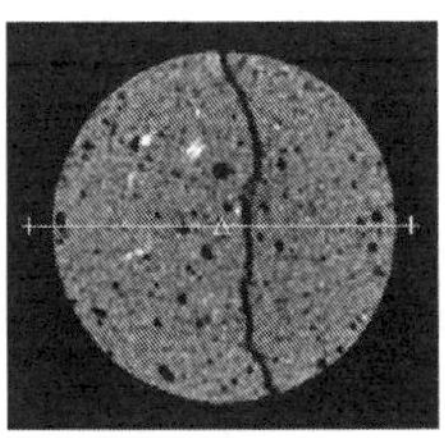

(a) horizontal image

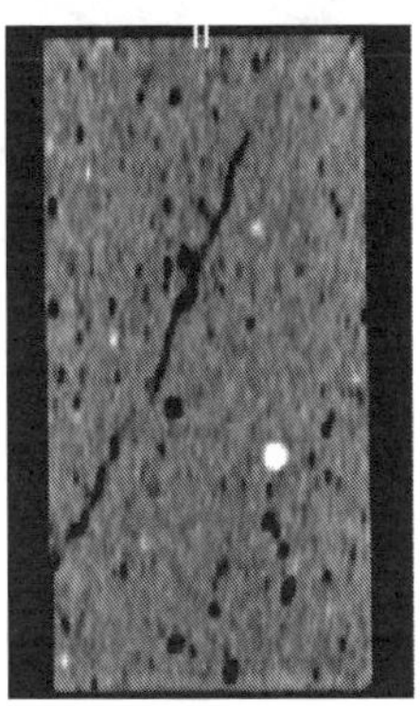

(b) vertical image

Figure 64. CT image of mixed soil after compression.

5.2 *Evaluation of particle crushing in soils*

The ground right beneath the pile tip is generally under the condition of high confining pressure and soil particle can often be crushed due to high pressure. They are also so called "crushable soils" such as calcareous sand, decomposed granite, and Sirasu and those are relatively easy to break due to the shape and mineral formation for the particle. The bearing capacity due to pile loading on this kind of ground is complicated because of the local dilatancy and the pile settlement due to particle crushing. Research activities so far related to particle crushing can be categorized into two groups which are (1) basic characteristic of particle crushing and (2) the effect of particle crushing on the bearing capacity of any kinds of foundations. The studies by Miura and O-hara (1979), Fukumoto (1992), Lade et al. (1996), McDowell et al. (1996), Nakata et al. (1999) and Takei et al. (2001) are the category of former group and those for the latter one are de Beer (1963), Miura (1985), Yasufuku and Hyde (1995), and Leung et al. (1996). But those are mostly based on the experimental studies with sampling technique in order to check the existence of particle crushing in the soil.

The purpose of this study is to evaluate the particle crushing of the soil using the results of X-ray CT scanning without any destruction and sampling. First of all, an idea of evaluating particle crushing is proposed with simple verification using the model ground by a large number of aluminum rods. Then, a series of model pile loading tests are conducted for the materials of non-crushable and crushable soils. Based on the results of CT scanning for those model grounds of the loading test, the proposed method for evaluating particle crushing is examined. Finally, the effectiveness of the proposed method for finding the existence of particle crushing is confirmed based on all the results.

5.2.1 *Idea of evaluating particle crushing*

Figure 65 shows fundamental idea of particle crushing from the CT image, which shows the relationship between the sizes of voxels and those of soil particles. Before particle crushing are induced, there will be a number of soil particles with different diameters that are larger or smaller than the size of one voxel as shown in Figs 65(a) and (b). Hence, it can be considered that the variance of CT-values in one region should be large enough because of the large variation of particle sizes with that of various voids. Then, the range of the particle size reduces after particle crushing. For these reasons, it can be assumed that the variance of CT-values in a certain region becomes smaller when the soil particles are crushed.

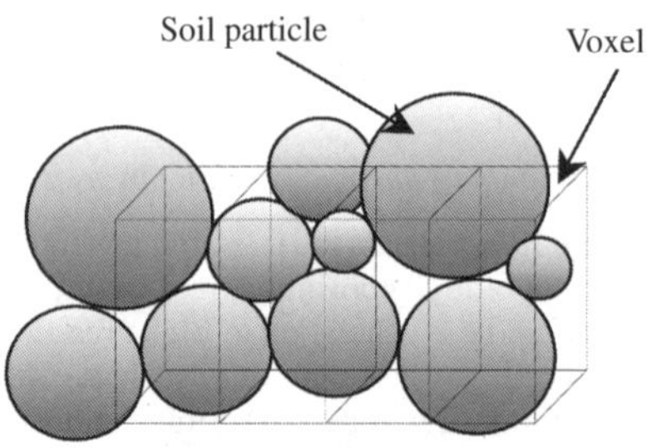

(a) Particles vs. Voxel

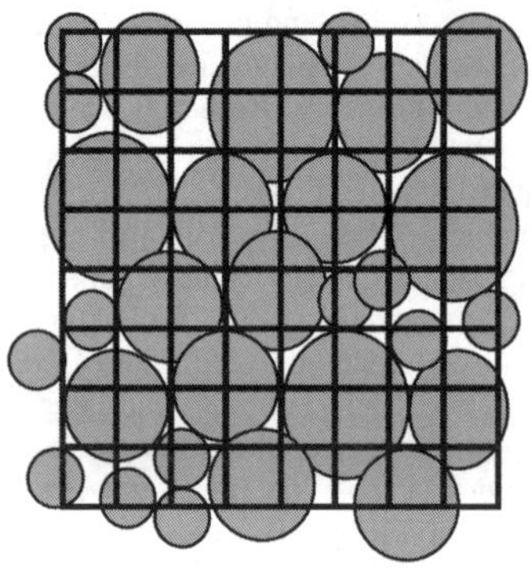

(b) Plane view of particles vs. Voxel

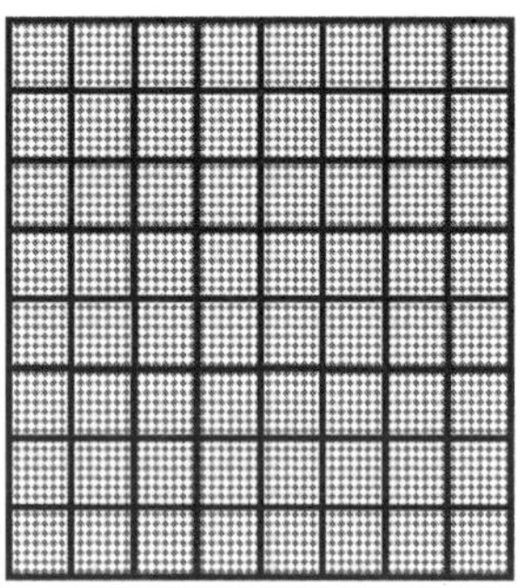

(c) Plane view of particles vs. Voxel
after particle breakages

Figure 65. Concept of particle crushing observed by X-ray CT image.

Coefficient of variation (COV) is often a preferred and convenient non-dimensional measure of dispersion or variability. When the mean CT-value and its standard deviation are calculated in the region of interest (ROI), the coefficient of variation for the CT-values can be expressed as following equation:

$$v = \frac{\sigma_{ROI}}{CT_{mean}} \tag{6}$$

where v is COV of CT-values, σ_{ROI} is standard deviation in the ROI and CT_{mean} is the mean CT-value in the ROI. Therefore, it is considered that the value of COV is decreased when the particles are crushed in the soil.

In order to verify above idea, four samples made of aluminum rods using two sizes of its diameter, which

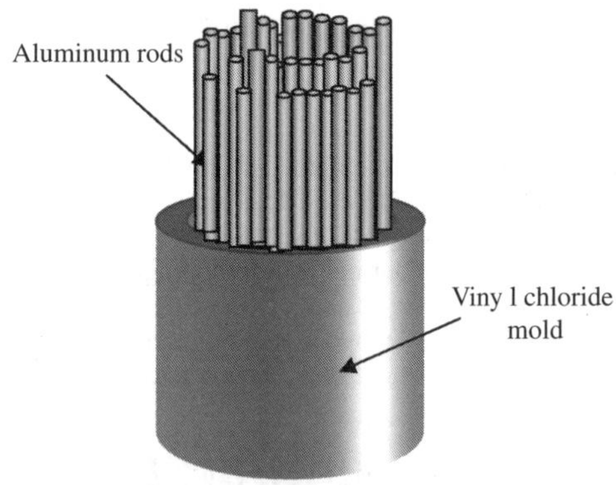

Figure 66. Aluminum rods sample.

Table 7. Density of aluminum rods samples.

	Diamter of Al rod (mm)	Density (t/m^3)	
		(2)	(1)
Case 1	3	1.95	2.31
Case 2	1.6	2.14	2.36

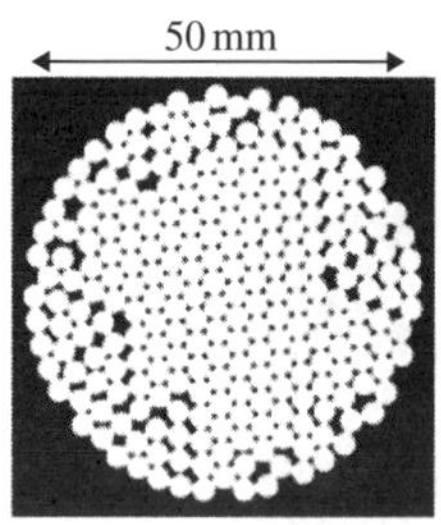

(1) Dense condition

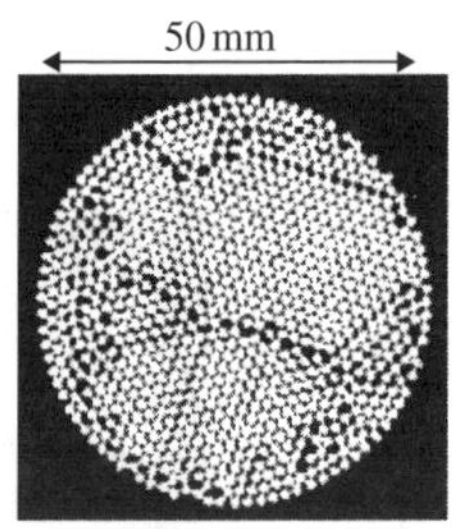

(1) Dense condition

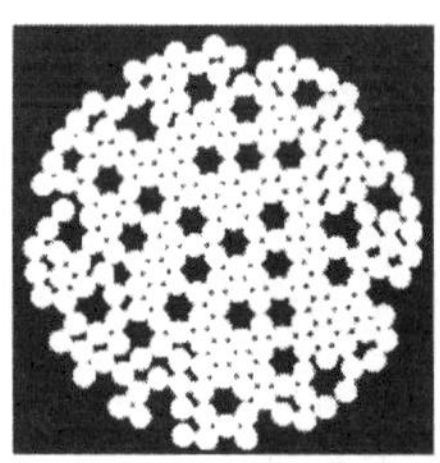

(2) Loose condition
(a) Case 1

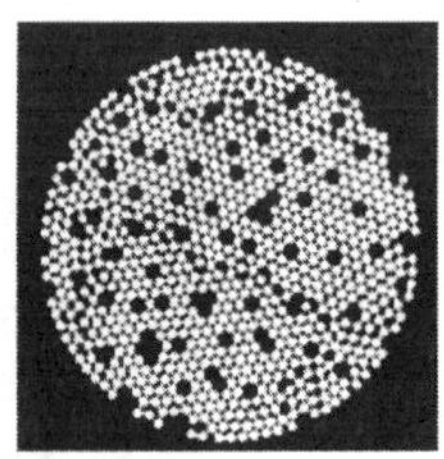

(2) Loose condition
(b) Case 2

Figure 67. X-ray CT images of each aluminum rod sample.

Table 8. Coefficient of variations for four X-ray CT images of aluminum rods samples.

	Case 1 (3 mm)		Case 2 (1.6 mm)	
	(2)	(1)	(2)	(1)
Density (t/m^3)	1.95	2.31	2.14	2.36
COV	1.07	0.43	0.82	0.36

Table 9. Density and fine grained ratio of each sample.

	Case 1	Case 2	Case 3	Case 4	
Tensity density (t/m^3)	1.43	1.42	1.63	1.63	
Each grain contents (%)	70	50	30	0	2 mm~4.75 mm 850 μm~2 mm
	30	50	70	100	425 μm~850 μm 250 μm~425 μm 106 μm~250 μm 75 μm~106 μm
Mean size of particle (mm)	1.47	1.42	1.38	0.43	

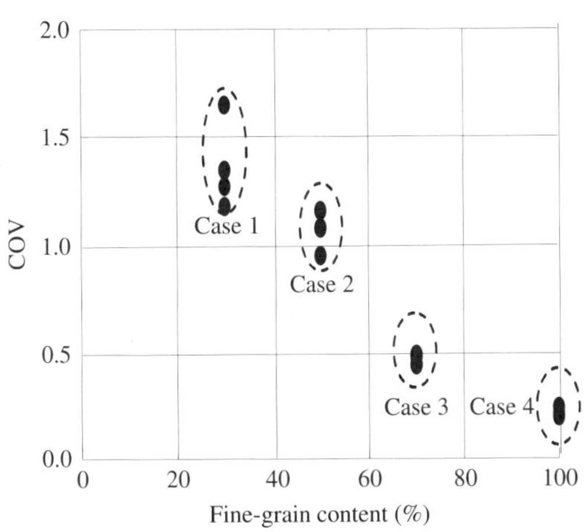

Figure 68. Reduction of variation coefficient due to increase of fine-grain contents.

are 3 mm and 1.6 mm, were used. Figure 66 shows one example of the sample made of aluminum rods. Here, a large number of aluminum rods were packed in a vinyl chloride mold whose size was the diameter of 50 mm and four samples of different densities were prepared. Table 7 shows the densities per unit area of the four samples made of single size of the rod. As easily realized, the cases of loose and dense packing were prepared in each size of the rod. Figure 67 shows cross sectional CT images for those four samples. Figure 67(a) shows the case of 3 mm rods (Case1) while Figure 67(b) shows that of 1.6 mm (Case 2). Both cases consist of the cases of loose and dense packing. Table 8 shows the COV values for all the cases. As easily realized from this table, the value of COV decreases as density increases. Therefore, it is confirmed that the increase of the volume of fine-grained particles affects the decrease of the COV due to particle crushing.

Next, in order to clarify the relationship between the COV and fine-grains content, four kinds of samples with different content of fine grain soil particles were prepared. Decomposed granite was used in this test and each soil with dry condition was set in the vinyl chloride mold. Table 9 shows the specifications of four samples. Each sample was scanned and the COV of CT-values in the ROI was calculated. Figure 68 is the relationship between the COV of CT-values and the ratio of fine-grains content. Although the density of the samples for Case 1 and Case 3 were equal to those of Case 2 and Case 4, respectively, the COV for Case 4 was the smallest of all the cases. It is therefore confirmed that particle crushing can be evaluated by knowing the decrease of COV.

5.2.2 *Test procedure and results*

In order to implement the proposed idea of particle crushing, a series of model loading tests were conducted. Figure 69 shows an apparatus of pile loading test. The size of model ground was 120.0 mm diameter and 305.0 mm depth. Model pile was made of aluminum with a diameter of 30.0 mm. In order to check the effect of particle crushing, decomposed granite as a crushable material and "Garnet" as a non-crushable material were used. Figure 70 shows distribution curves of grain size for these two materials. The maximum

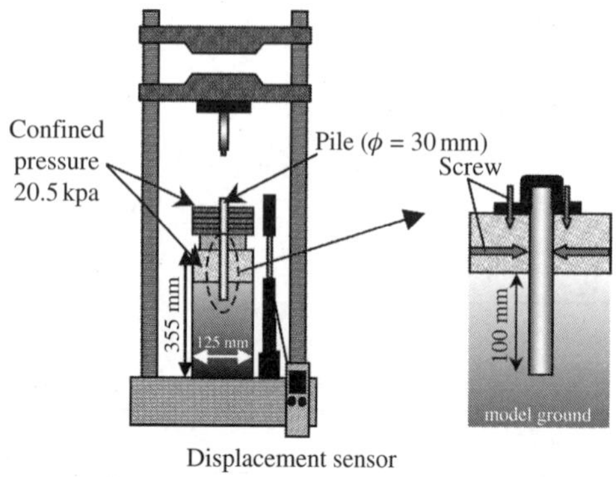

(a) Model ground and loading apparatus (b) Zoom up

Figure 69. Schematic pile loading test apparatus.

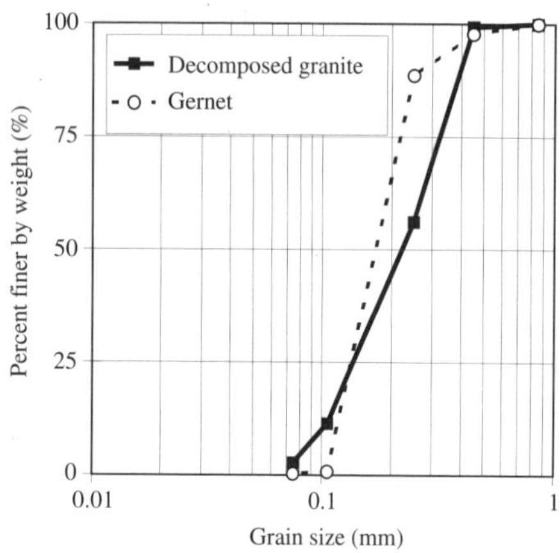

Figure 70. Distribution of particle grain size.

diameter of these grains was controlled to be less than 1.0 mm. In the test, a confined pressure was applied at the ground surface using dead load as shown in Fig. 69(a). Vertical loading was applied to the pile top by a compression apparatus and its loading speed was 1.0 mm/min. Then, an X-ray CT scanning was performed at every 1.0 mm thickness of the ground beneath the pile tip. This procedure was repeated with increased vertical loading.

Figure 71 shows load–settlement relationship at the pile top. The scanning points are shown in the figure and the settlement was normalized by the diameter of

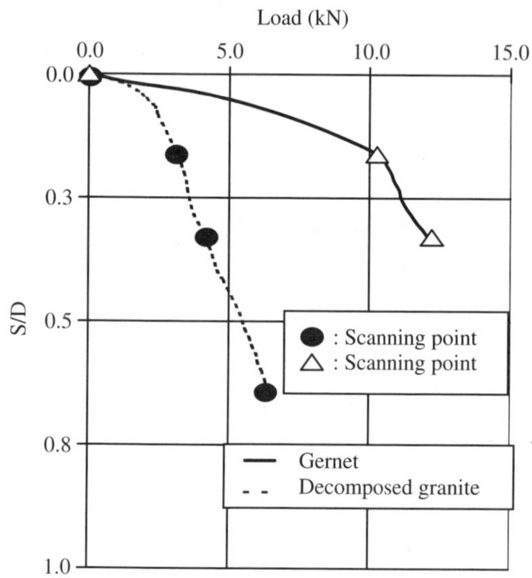

Figure 71. Load–settlement relationship.

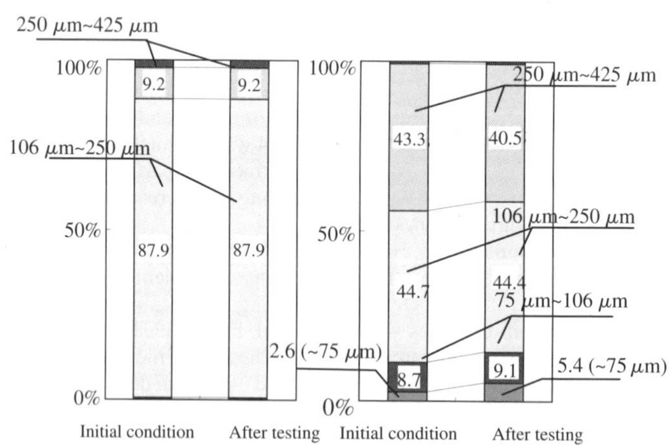

(a) Garnet (b) Decomposed granite

Figure 72. Residual ratio of particle grain size.

the pile. The grain size analysis was conducted for both grounds of decomposed granite and Garnet around the area of right beneath the pile tip at the end of the test. Figure 72 shows the residual ratio of particles for both of grounds at the initial and the end of the test. As easily realized, it was found that the volume of particle size less than 105μm is increased after the test for the case of decomposed granite while that for Garnet does not change, so that it is obvious that the particle crushing was occurred for the case of decomposed granite.

Figure 73 shows the ROI for sampling CT-values in the model ground. Figure 74 shows the distribution of the mean CT-value and the COV in the ROI for the case of Garnet ground at the settlement level of S/D = 0.4. Figure 75 shows the same results for the case of decomposed Granite ground. As shown in Fig.74, the CT-values increased after the pile loading for the case of Garnet and the same result was obtained for the case of the decomposed granite. However, when the distributions of COV for the case of Garnet are compared with those of decomposed granite, the decrease of COV is obvious for the case of decomposed granite while that for the case of Garnet is not found. Therefore, it is again confirmed that particle crushing can be evaluated by checking the decrease of COV.

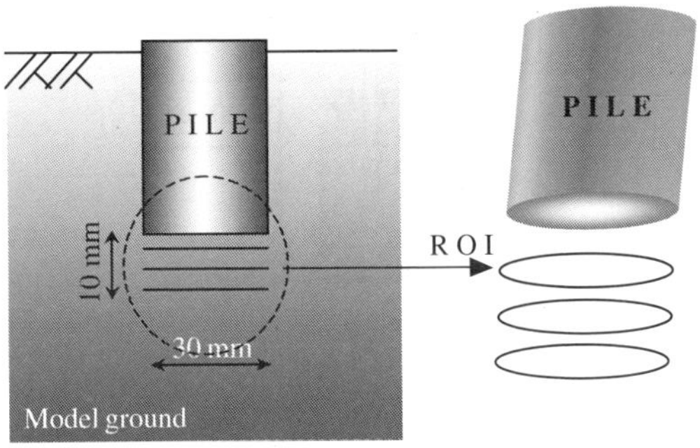

Figure 73. Region of interesting (ROI).

5.2.3 *Discussion*

In general, the reduction of COV means that the density became uniform. From a viewpoint of image processing, it can be explained that the uniformity of the density is equal to make X-ray CT image with an technique of smoothing. Fig. 76 shows the relationship between smoothed image processing and the change of particle size. Here, a large number of particles with two different diameters are imaged. It is assumed that COV in 3 × 3 voxels is A as shown in Fig.76 (a), and the COV in the case of Fig.76(b) is B. The value of A is larger than that of B. The change of Fig.76(a) into Fig.76(b) can be realized as particle crushing in the CT-image. When Fig.76(a) was treated by the smoothed image processing, the value of COV, A, will be close to the value of B. Finally, the COV of Fig.76(a) will become B at the condition of Fig.76(c). Meanwhile, the number of voxels in Fig.76(c) becomes larger than 3 × 3. The number of voxels is

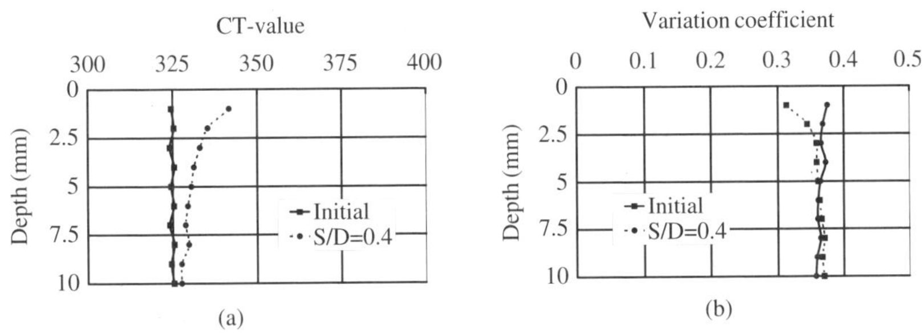

Figure 74. Mean CT-value distribution and variation coefficients for Garnet.

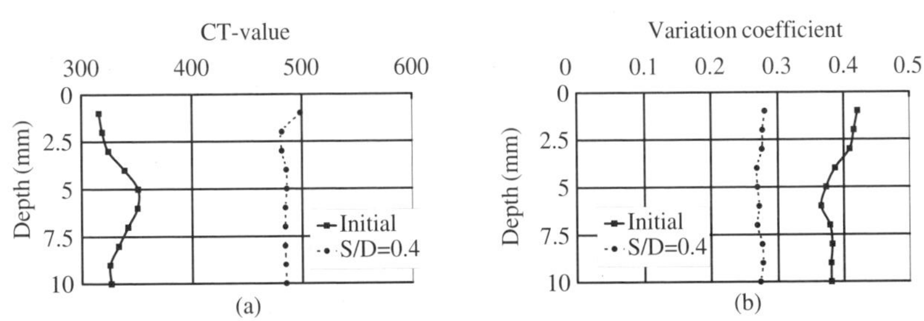

Figure 75. Mean CT-value distribution and variation coefficients for decomposed granite.

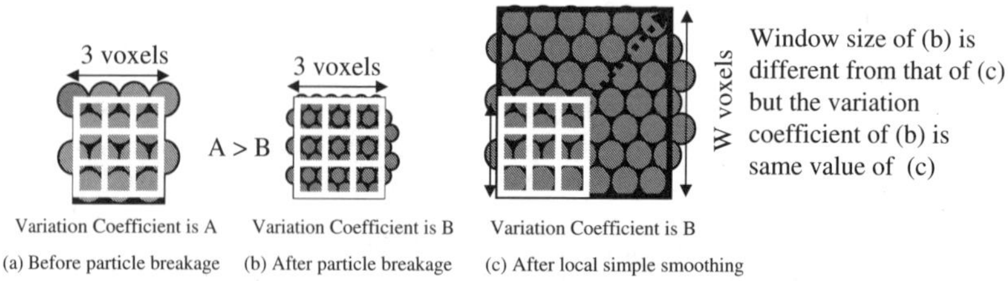

Figure 76. Concept for estimation of particle crushing using change of window size.

called "Window size". As a result, it can be said that the change in the window size is equal to the change of particle size in the CT image.

5.2.4 *Summary*

An idea of evaluating particle crushing in the ground due to vertical pile loading was proposed as one of effective use of X-ray CT results. It can be said that this idea is totally different from previous studies on the topic of particle crushing. The conclusions drawn from this study are summarized as follows:

(1) During the process of particle crushing, the density of soil approaches a state of uniformity.
(2) Particle crushing can be investigated by checking a reduction of COV during an increase of the density using the results of X-ray CT scanning.
(3) As far as CT image is concerned, it can be said that the change in the window size in the image processing analysis is equal to the change of particle size.

6 BEARING CAPACITY MECHANISM UNDER VERTICAL PILE LOADING

There are different types of vertically loaded pile foundations such as steel pipe pile, cast-in-place pile, under-reamed pile and so on. And it is considered that a search for the failure pattern of different tip shape of piles is important for the design of pile foundations especially for the limit state design. So far, there are many failure patterns such as those proposed by Terzaghi, Meyerhof and Vesic (Lambe and Whitman (1969)). But those have been proposed for the purpose of design calculation and are not based on close observation of real behavior. Besides this behavior itself appears at the certain depth in the ground so that it is difficult to check such behavior. The objective of this paper is to visualize and characterize failure patterns under vertical loading on different types of pile foundations using X-ray CT method. First of all, a series of model loading tests for the model piles of three different tip shapes (normal pile, under-reamed pile and pipe pile) is conducted and the model ground in each case is scanned at the area of certain depth around and below pile tip.

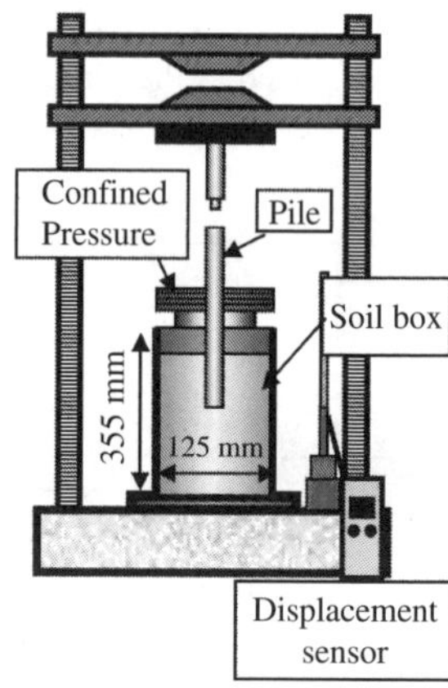

Figure 77. Model test apparatus.

6.1 *Test procedure*

A series of model loading tests for three different model piles was conducted using a conventional loading apparatus as shown in Fig.77. It is noted that the soil box in the apparatus made by PVC including piles (embedded depth of 100 mm), which is the size of 355 mm height with 125 mm diameter, was moved to the specimen table of the CT scanner when CT scanning is conducted. The model piles were made of aluminum under consideration of material absorption for X-ray. Here, normal pile (diameter of 20 mm), under-reamed pile (diameter of 30 mm) and pipe pile (diameter of 20 mm) were selected in order to investigate the effect of different tip shape on the failure patterns and those are shown in Fig.78. Soil used in this test was Toyoura Sand with min. dry density = 1.35 t/m^3, max. dry density = 1.61 t/m^3 and relative density = 100%.

In the test, the dry density was fixed to the value of 1.61 t/m^3 for all the cases using multiple sieves and the overburden pressure of 18.1 kPa was applied by dead load in order to conduct relatively large confining pressure as the condition of deep foundations. The vertical load was applied at pile head under displacement control and the test was stopped at the settlement of 10 mm. For the CT scanning, initial and the stage at after 10 mm settlement were scanned with every 1 mm thickness for maximum depth of 60 mm below the pile tip.

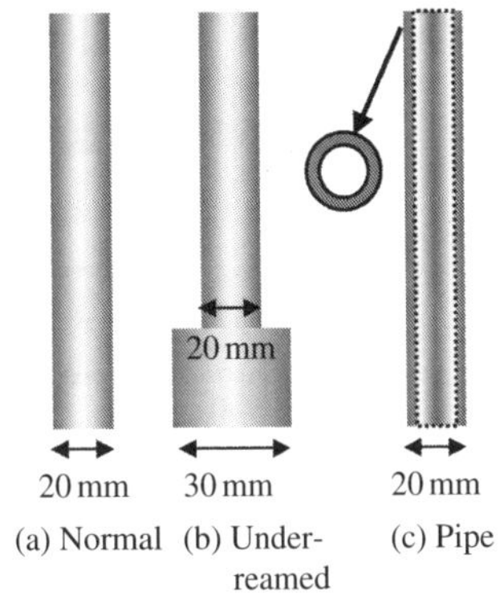

Figure 78. Model piles.

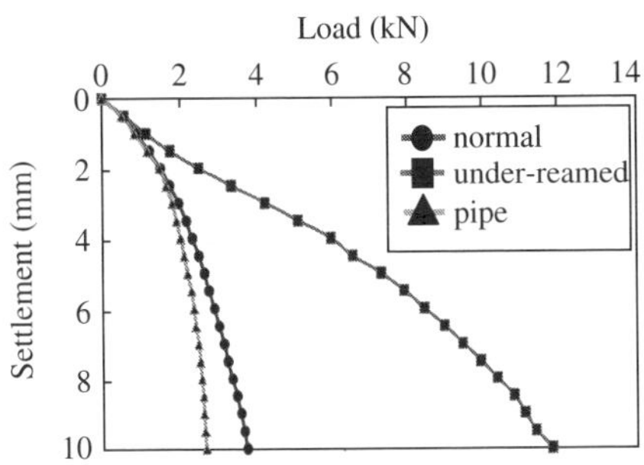

Figure 79. Load–settlement relationship.

6.2 *Results and discussion*

Figure 79 shows load–settlement relationships for all the cases. There are no peak loads for any of the cases, so that failure may be considered to be progressive failure rather than total failure. It is also realized that the case of under-reamed pile shows much higher capacity than the other cases. Fig.80 shows the cross sectional images for after 10 mm settlement at the depth of within 2 mm below the pile tip and the cross sectional image at the same lication as before loading (initial condition) is also shown in this figure for three cases. Figure 81 shows the distribution of CT-value at the cross section along two white arrows shown in Fig.80, in which the distribution of CT-value between initial and after 10 mm settlement is compared. As easily realized, the density around the circumference of the pile at the tip is decreased as the pile is penetrated, which is the appearance of the area of ring shape with black color in the image. This difference is easily realized from Fig.80. And, it is interesting to note on Fig.81 that the both cases of normal and under-reamed piles show the decrease of the density only around the pile but the case of pipe pile shows

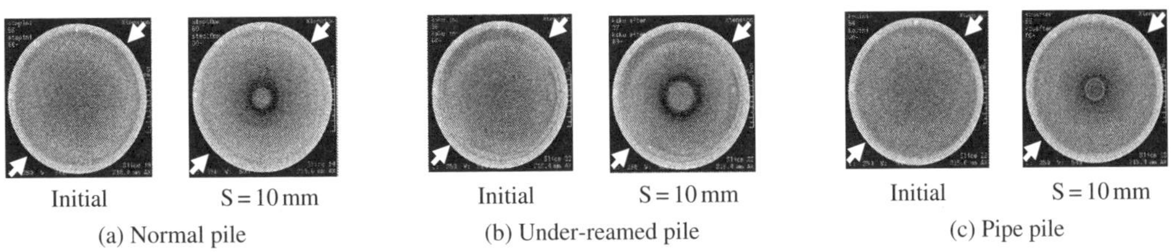

Figure 80. Horizontal cross sectional images.

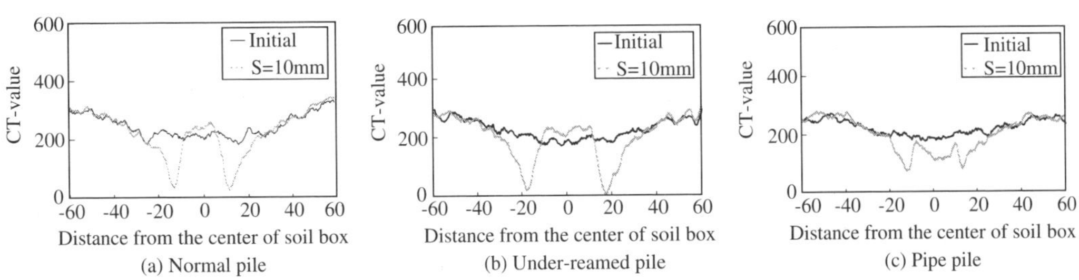

Figure 81. Distributions of CT-value.

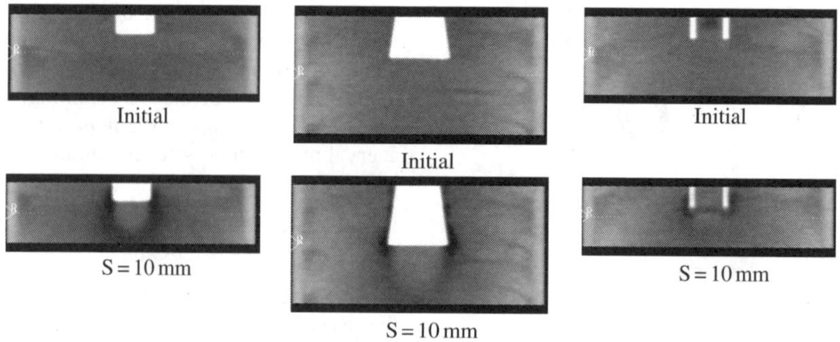

(a) Normal pile (b) Under-reamed pile (c) Pipe pile

Figure 82. Vertical cross sectional image.

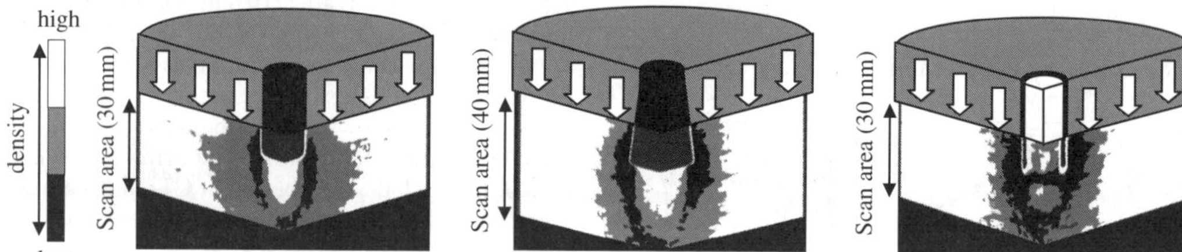

(a) Normal pile (b) Under-reamed pile (c) Pipe pile

Figure 83. 3-D reconstruction images.

another low density area at right under the pile tip because of the hollow shape of pile. Since the large number of cross sectional images are obtained for each case, a vertical cross sectional image or three dimensional image can be also reconstructed. Figure 82 shows vertical cross sectional images for three cases, in which the area of white color indicates the material of piles. It can be realized that there is a finite high density area right below the pile tip for the cases of normal and under-reamed pile, which is shown as the area of light gray color, and those are surrounded by the banded low density area which is the area of black color. The area of low density is also essential around the circumference of the pile. The case of pipe pile is somehow different from other cases. The area of high density below the tip does not appear and there is a banded area of low density in the hollow part of the pile. The tendency of the density change around the circumference of pile is the same as those of normal and under-reamed piles. Figure 83 shows reconstruction images in three-dimension for all the cases. These images are reconstructed by the change of the density using the colors of black and white gradation in the image. It is more clearly shown that the area of high density right below the pile tip is surrounded by the banded area of low density for both cases of normal and under-reamed piles. For the case of pipe pile, more complicated low density area is observed, especially at right under the pile tip. It may be considered that those banded areas of low density are the areas of strain localization. And it is also confirmed based on the results of 3-D images for all the cases that the shape of the failure pattern seems to be axi-symmetric.

Finally, it is concluded that the failure patterns for vertically loaded pile foundation could be well investigated using X-ray CT method.

6.3 *Summary*

Failure patterns for different types of pile foundations were visualized using industrial X-ray CT scanner. The following conclusions are drawn from this study:

(1) The normal and under-reamed piles show similar failure patterns except its size;
(2) Although the area of high density around right under the tip was observed for the cases of normal and under-reamed piles, there was no such area for the case of pipe pile;
(3) The density around the circumference of the pile decreases due to the settlement of pile;
(4) The progress of failure pattern during pile loading could be investigated visually; and
(5) The shape of failure pattern seems to be axi-symmetric.

The future prospects for this study are described as follows:

(1) The quality of the model loading test should be improved such as the confinement for deep foundation and installation method of model pile;
(2) The obtained failure patterns by X-ray CT scanner should be used quantitatively for conducting the bearing capacity calculation by limit equilibrium theory; and
(3) Other types of piles such as the pile with tip shape of cone will be examined.

It is confirmed that those results make the quantitative discussion of the failure patterns possible and as far as the limit equilibrium method has been used for the design of pile foundation in practice, those observations could be appreciated.

7 CONCLUSIONS

Industrial X-ray CT scanner was installed at Kumamoto University, Japan in 1996 and since then, a large number of application studies have been done from relatively fundamental aspects to boundary value problems. The previous purpose of these researches were to find our what kind of application is appropriate for X-ray CT scanner.

The application studies which have introduced in this paper were listed as follows:

(1) Characterization of soil behavior;
 1.1 Failure of undisturbed overconsolidated clay
 1.2 Failure of mixed soil with dredged slurry, cement and air foam
 1.3 Soil-structure interaction
 1.4 Seepage and drying
(2) Development of new triaxial compression test apparatus;
(3) More positive use of X-ray CT data; and
 3.1 Application of numerical analysis
 3.2 Evaluation of particle breakage in soils
(4) Bearing capacity mechanism under vertical pile loading.

Based on these results, following conclusions including the future aspects are drawn:

(1) So called CT-value is only one output and this value is well correlated with material density. But as far as geomaterials are concerned, the behaviors of shearing and compression are dominant. Therefore, the proper way of converting from CT-value to these behaviors is necessary in order to discuss more precise behavior of geomaterials using X-ray CT scanner. This is one reason which we need proper image processing analysis, especially for geomaterials;
(2) The development of special apparatus especially for the system of X-ray CT scanner is important in order to conduct more precise and valuable discussion on the behavior of geomaterials;
(3) The deformation property is very important for soils even the failure of soils is discussed. As far as X-ray CT scanning is concerned, it is well understood that the location of CT scanning should be fixed under the process of deformation. Under these circumstances, the application of seepage or drying takes advantage because the location of CT scanning never changes even after certain time; and
(4) Under the reason above (3), the application of geoenvironmental study such as seepage or diffusion of contaminant water in the soils may be proper application in geotechnical engineering. Therefore, the application to environmental research should be appreciated as one of future prospects.

Finally, it is evident from all the discussion here that the X-ray CT scanner promises to be a powerful tool even for geomaterials and geotechnical engineering field.

ACKNOWLEDGEMENT

The contents of this paper were mostly done under the Ph.D. study by Dr. Toshifumi Mukunoki who is my former Ph.D. student at Kumamoto University and now at Queen's University, Canada. The author would like to give my sincere thank you to him for his hard working during his doctoral study. And the system of X-ray CT scanner used in our studies is a property of the group of Rock Engineering at the Department of Civil and Environmental Engineering, Kumamoto University, Japan. The author would like to express his gratitude to the head of this group, Prof. Katsuhiko Sugawara, who gave me the opportunity to use this valuable apparatus. The author also would like to give his gratitude to Prof. Yuzo Obara of Kumamoto University and Prof. Katsuhiko Kaneko of Hokkaido University, Japan for their kind encouragement on all the research topics related to the application of X-ray CT scanner in geotechnical engineering. Finally, the author would like to give his gratitude to his Master's student, Mr. Takahiro Sato who gave the author his enormous help for the preparation of this manuscript.

REFERENCES

Anderson, S.H. and Hopmans, J.W. 1994. Tomography of Soil-Water-Root Processes. *SSSA Special Publication* Number 36, Soil Science Society of America.

de Beer, E.E. 1963. The scale effect in the transposition of the results of deep-sounding tests on the ultimate bearing capacity of piles and caisson foundations, *Geotechnique*, 13(1): 39–75.

Desrues, J., Chambon, R., Mokni, M., and Mazerolle, F. 1996. Void ratio evolution inside shear bands in triaxial sand specimens studied by computed tomography. *Geotechnique*: 46(3): 529–546.
Fukumoto, T. 1992. Particle breakage characteristics of granular soils, *Soils and Foundations*, 32(1): 26–40.
Hagiwara, T. and Nanba, T. 1990. Generation of Proximity Function for Naturally Fractured Reservoir Simulator Using X-ray CT Scanner System, *Proc. Eleventh Workshop for the IEA*, Collaborative Project on EOR, Paris.
Hounsfield, G.N. 1972. A method of and appratus for examination of a body by radiation such as x-ray or gamma radiation, *Patent Specification* 1283915, The Patent Office.
Kak, A.C. and Slaney, M. 1987. *Principles of Computed Tomographic Imaging*. IEEE PRESS, pp.49–110.
Kasahara, J. and Tomoda, Y. 1993. *An Introduction to Computerized Geoscience*, University of Tokyo Press: 180–185 (in Japanese).
Kruse, G.A.M. and Bezuijen, A. 1998. The use of CT scans to evaluate soil models. *Proc. of centrifuge* '98, Balkema: 79–84.
Lade, P.V., Yamamuro, J.A., and Bopp, P.A. 1996. Significance of particle crushing in granular material, *ASCE*, 122(4): 309–316.
Lambe, T.W. and Whitman, R.V. 1969. *Soil Mechanics*, John Wiley & Sons: 502.
Leung, C.F., Lee, F.H., and Yet, N.S. 1996. The role of particle breakage in pile creep in sand, *Can. Geotech. Journal.*, 33(6): 888–898.
McDowell, G.R., Bolton, M.D. and Robertson, D. 1996. The fractal crushing of granular materials, *J. of the Mechanics and Physics of Solids*, 12(44): 2079–2102.
Miura , N. and O-hara, S. 1977. Particle-crushing of a decomposed granite soil under shear stresses, *Soils and Foundations*, 19(3): 1–14.
Miura, N. 1985. Point resistance of piles in sand, *Proc. 11th ICSMFE*, San Francisco, 3: 1445–1448.
Nagao, M. and Matuyama,T. 1978. Edge Preserving Smoothing. *CGIP*, 9: 394–407.
Nakata, Y., Hyde, A.F.L., Hyodo, M. and Murata, H. 1999. A probabilistic approach to sand particle crushing in the triaxial test, *Geotechniuqe*, 49(5): 567–583.
Otani, J., Obara, Y. and Mukunoki, T. 1997. Characterization of failure in soils using X-ray CT scanner. *Proc. of Int. Symp. on Deformation and Progressive failure in Geomechanics, Nagoya* '97: 311–314.
Otani, J., Mukunoki, T. and Obara, Y. 2000. Application of X-ray CT method for characterization of failure in soils, *Soils and Foundations*, 40(2): 111–118.
Otani, J., Mukunoki, T. and Kikuchi, Y. 2002. Visualization for engineering property of in-situ light weight soils with air foams. *Soils and Foundations* 42(3): 93–105.
Reid, T.R. and Harrison, J.P 2000. A semi-automated methodology for discontinuity trace detection in digital images of rock mass exposures, *International Journal of Rock Mechanics & Mining Sciences*, 37: 1073–1089.
Sugawara, K, Obara, Y., Kaneko, K., Koike, K., Ohmi, M. and Aoi, T.1997. Visualization of Three-Dimensional Structure of Rocks Using X-Ray CT Method, *Proc. of Asian Conf. on Rock Mechanics*, Seoul: 769–774.
Sugawara, K., Kojima, R., Obara, Y., Sato, A. and Shimada, H. 1998. Crack Opening Analysis by Means of The X-Rays CT, *Journal of the mining and materials processing Institute of Japan,* 114(12): 881–887(in Japanese).
Takei, M., Kusakabe, O., and Hayashi, T. 2001. Time-dependent behavior pf crushable materials in one-dimensional compression tests, *Soils and Foundations*, 41(1): 97–121.
Tamura, T., Kobayashi, S. and Sumi, T. 1987. Rigid-plastic finite element method for frictional materials. *Soils and Foundations* 27(3): 1–12.
Tani, K. 1997. X-ray computed tomography technique to observe shear banding in dense sands, Deformation and Progressive Failure in Geomechanics, *IS Nagoya* '97, Pergamon: 315–320.
Tuchida, T., Takeuchi, D., Okumura, T. and Kishida, T. 1996. Development of light weight fill from dredging, *Proc. of Environmental Geotechnics*: 415–420.
Verhelst, F., Vervoort, A., Bosscher, D., and Marchal, G. 1995. X-ray computed tomography: Determination of heterogeneties in rock samples. *Proceeding of International Congress on Rock Mechanics*, Japan 1: 105–108.
Yasufuku, N. and Hyde, A.F.L. 1995. Pile end-bearing capacity in crushable sands, *Geotechnique*, 45(4): 663–676.
Yamamoto, K. and Otani, J. 2002. Bearing capacity and failure mechanism of reinforced foundations based on rigid-plastic finite element formulation, *Geotextiles and Geomembranes*, 20: 367–393.

Following references are the list of papers written in English by the group of geotechnical engineering at Kumamoto University on the topic of application of X-ray CT scanner in geotechnical engineering.

1997

Otani, J., Obara, Y. and Mukunoki, T. 1997. Characterization of failure and density distribution in soils using X-ray CT scanner, *Proc. of China-Japan Joint Symposium on Recent Development of Theory & Practice in Geotechnology*: 45–50.
Otani, J., Obara, Y. and Mukunoki, T. 1997. Characterization of failure in soils using X-ray CT Scanner, *Proceedings of International Symposium on Deformation and progressive failure in Geomehanics, IS Nagoya* '97: 311–314.

1999

Otani, J., Mukunoki, T. and Kikuchi, Y. 1999. Evaluation of engineering property of in-situ light weight soil using X-ray CT scanner, *Proc. of the Eleventh Asian Regional Conference on Soil Mechanics and Geotechnical Engineering*, ISSMGE, Korea: 57–60.
Otani, J., Mukunoki, T., Obara, Y. and Minoura, K. 1999. Mechanism of bearing capacity in crushable ground due to pile loading using X-ray CT scanner, *Proc. of APCOM '99 Fourth Asia-Pacific Conference in Computational Mechanics*: 891–896.
Mukunoki, T., Otani, J. and Kikuchi, Y. 1999. Evaluation of engineering property of in-situ light-weight soil using X-ray CT scanner, *Proc. of Second Japan-China Joint Symposium on Recent development of theory and practice in geotechnology*: 292–299.

2000

Otani, J., Mukunoki, T. and Obara, Y. 2000. Application of X-ray CT method for characterization of failure in soils, *Soils and Foundations*, 40(2): 111–118.

Mukunoki, T., Otani, J., Nagatome, T. and Kikuchi, Y. 2000. Evaluation of engineering property of in-situ light weight soil with air foam using X-ray CT Technique, *Proc. of Coastal Geotechnical Engineering in Practice*, IS Yokohama 2000: 681–686.

Otani, J., Mukunoki, T., Obara, Y. and Sugawara, K. 2000. Application of X-rays CT to Soil and Rock Engineering, *Proc. of An International Conference on Geotechnical & Geological Engineering*, GeoEng2000, Melbourne, CD-ROM: paper\pf\0297. pdf.

2001

Otani, J., Mukunoki, T. and Obara, Y. 2001. Evaluation of progressive failure in soils using industrial X-ray CT scanner, *Proc. of the 10th International Conference on Computer Methods and Advances in Geomechanics*, 7–12 January: 245–250.

Otani, J., Mukunoki, T. and Obara, Y. 2001. Development of new triaxial compression test apparatus for geomaterials on industrial X-ray CT Scanner, *Proc. of XVth International Conference on Soil Mechanics and Geotechnical Engineering*: 231–234.

Otani, J., Miyamoto, K., Mukunoki, T. and Hirai, T. 2001. Visualization of interaction behavior between soil and reinforcement using X-ray CT, *Proc. of Landmarks in Earth Reinforcment, IS Kyushu* 2001: 117–120.

Otani, J., Hoashi, H., Mukunoki, T., Obara, Y. and Kaneko, K. 2001. Evaluation of failure in soils under unconfined compression using 3-D rigid plastic finite element analysis, *Proc. of 1st Asian-Pacific Congress on Computational Mechanics*, Sydney, Australia, November:1: 445–450.

2002

Otani, J., Mukunoki, T. and Obara, Y. 2002. Characterization of failure in sand under triaxial compression using industrial X-ray CT scanner, *International Journal of Physical Modeling in Geotechnics*. 2: 15–22, 2002.

Otani, J., Mukunoki, T. and Kikuchi, Y. 2002. Visualization for engineering property of in-situ light weight soils with air foams, *Soils and Foundations,* 42(3): 93–105.

Mukunoki, T., Otani, J., Obara, Y., Sugawara, K. and Hirata, A. 2002. New methodology using X-ray CT data to characterize the engineering property of geomaterials, *Proc. of the 5th North American Rock Mechanics Symposium [NARMS] and 17th Tunneling Association of Canada [TAC] conference*: 397–402.

Mukunoki, T. and Otani, J. 2002. Evaluation of particle breakage using X-ray CT data, *Proc. of 1st International Workshop on New Frontiers in Computational Geotechnics*, Banff, Canada, November: 111–118.

2003

Otani, J. and Kikuchi, Y. 2003. Evaluation of hydraulic property of mixed soil with air foam using X-ray CT method, *Proc. of the Second Asian Conf. on Unsaturated Soils*, April: 71–74.

Otani, J., Hironaka, J. and Mukunoki, T. 2003. Visualization of failure pertterns under vertically loaded foundation using X-ray CT method, *Proc. of Asian Regional Conference*, Singapore, August: 973–976.

Otani, J., Kikuchi Y. and Kukunoki, T. 2003. Investigation of progressive failure in composite soils using X-ray CT scanner, *Proc. of First Japan-U.S.A. Workshop on Testing, Modeling and Simulation in Geomechanics,* Boston, June (to appear).

Mukunoki, T., Otani, J and Sugawara, K. 2003. Estimation of particle crushing using X-ray CT, *Soils and Foundations* (to be submitted).

X-ray CT for Geomaterials; Soils, Concrete, Rocks – Otani & Obara (eds.)
© 2004 Swets & Zeitlinger. Lisse, ISBN 90 5809 666 1

Recent advances of X-ray CT and its applications for rock material

A. Vervoort, M. Wevers, R. Swennen & S. Roels
K.U. Leuven, Leuven, Belgium

M. Van Geet
SCK-CEN, Waste & disposal, Mol, Belgium

E. Sellers
CSIR Division of Mining Technology, Johannesburg, South Africa

ABSTRACT: During the last 10 to 20 years, the X-ray computerized tomography has shown to be useful, as a research tool for rock investigations or as a research tool to better understand and quantify physical phenomena in rock material. As rock material is by definition a heterogeneous medium and as it contains different constituents, artefacts do occur. For quantitative measurements these artefacts have to be minimised as much as possible. Several applications are presented in the area of rock mechanics, mining, petroleum and environmental engineering, but also results on porous building materials are presented.

1 INTRODUCTION: OVERVIEW OF APPLICATIONS FOR ROCK MATERIAL

The X-ray computerized tomography (CT) is a non-destructive technique that allows visualisation of the internal structure of objects, determined mainly by variations in density and atomic composition. Initially, it was a technique applied in the medical field. Today it has many applications for the study of all types of materials (e.g. Coenen & Maas (1994); Duliu (1999); Baruchel et al. (2000); Wevers et al. (2001)), including soils and rocks. This paper focuses on applications for rock material.

As a large contrast exists between solid phases and gaseous or liquid phases, the technique is in first instance useful to visualise open fractures and pores. When these features are filled with air or another gas, the contrast is the largest. Hence, numerous applications are situated in the area of fracture mechanics, reservoir engineering, environmental engineering and gas or liquid transport in general. Some recent publications in this field, excluding the work presented further in detail (see paragraph 3), are for example:

a) Determination of open fractures:
Verhelst et al. (1995b) determined fracture openings of natural or induced fractures using a medical scanner and taken into account the artefacts present. Their work was mainly based on a calibration technique using glass samples. The investigated rock was sand- and siltstone. Vandersteen et al. (2003) carried on with similar work, but using a micro-CT-scanner. They applied their technique on crinoidal limestone.

b) Determination of porosity and open pores:
Coles et al. (1996) scanned the same sandstone samples in a medical and a micro-CT-scanner. The latter clearly gave more accurate results with respect to porosity and pore distribution. They used this data to calculate permeability values, which compared well with plug permeability values. Dehghani & Kamath (2001) used a CT-scanner to determine the porosity distribution in carbonate cores. The dry core (solvent-cleaned and air-dried) was first scanned, followed by a saturation with 0.5 mol% KCl and scanned again. Bazin (2001) used a CT-scanner to visualise wormhole-dissolution in three-dimension, as part of a larger study of acid fracturing and matrix acidizing of limestone. Hidajat et al. (2002) used micro-CT images to develop a 3D image of the porosity in sandstone. This technique was compared to the labour-intensive technique of thin sections. Jones et al. (2003) investigated sandstone using a micro-CT-scanner, mainly to visualise the microstructures and the pores. They also quantified stress induced grain crushing and pore collapse. Karacan et al. (2003) studied also the porosity under an applied load. They investigated limestone

and placed samples inside a X-ray-transparent triaxial cell.

c) Determination of fluid flow and liquid content: Cook et al. (1993) studied wellbore processes such as mud invasion and mud/shale interaction around the wellbore, by conducting experiments inside a scanner. Shale and sandstone samples were studied for various mud compositions. Dehghani & Kamath (2001) CT-scanned carbonate cores to map the initial oil saturation distribution and scanned the samples again after a high-temperature blowdown experiment. Géraud et al. (2003) studied a very low porosity granite and investigated the fluid flow and capillary wetting in this rock type, using a medical scanner. Hirono et al. (2003) studied the fluid flow in fault-related rocks. They placed a permeameter cell inside a medical scanner and they used KI-solutions as a contrast medium, as it has a high X-ray attenuation. Rousset-Tournier et al. (2003) studied the drying process of water in sandstone samples, using a medical scanner. They showed that the location of water in the pore network depends on the method of initial saturation. Ruiz de Argandona et al. (2003) studied free water absorption in limestone with time, using a medical scanner. The effect of layering in the rock material was quantified.

To visualise individual pores and/or fractures, the minimum resolution is a crucial parameter. The resolution is linked to the voxel size and is influenced by the source and detectors characteristics, the geometry and the object size. While the medical CT-scanners have generally a resolution between 1 mm × 1 mm × 1 mm and 60 μm × 60 μm × 1 mm depending on the zoom-factor used, the resolution of a micro-focus CT can be of the order of 10 μm × 10 μm ×10 μm. However, the characteristics of the source (e.g. energy and width of beam) affects directly and indirectly the resolution.

A X-ray CT-scanner can also be used to visualise the difference between various solid materials. Of course, the contrast between them is smaller than for a liquid or gas phase. Again some recent examples, excluding the work presented further in detail (see paragraph 3), are for example:

Coles et al. (1996) used a micro-CT to differentiate between quartz, siderite and feldspar. They used SEM data to verify the results obtained. Verhelst et al. (1995a & 1996) have used a medical CT-scanner in combination with 2D-colour image analysis of polished surfaces to establish a three-dimensional model of the maceral (vitrinite, inertinite and liptinite) distribution and mineral content (mainly pyrite) of coal. By this technique, it was also possible to estimate the density of the individual maceral components. Caers et al. (1997) have used a medical X-ray CT-scanner to distinguish between two types of filled fractures within coal strata samples. One type consisted mainly of carbonate cements, while the other consisted mainly of kaolenite. A relation with the rock mechanical strength parameters of the fractures was established. Tivey (1998) and Spiess et al. (2001) studied iron-bearing minerals and distinguished various solid phases. Taylor et al. (2000) studied diamonds using X-ray CT. Carlson et al. (2003) used high resolution (100 μm) and ultra-high resolution (10 μm) scanners to determine the distribution of different minerals in rock samples and to visualise them in 3D. For example a 3D reconstruction was made of plagioclase, pyroxene, glass and voids in basalt. Flisch & Becker (2003) visualised sand dykes, dropstones and plant remains in sedimentary material.

The above list of examples, which is far from being complete, shows that the number of possible applications of CT-scans for rock material is very large. On the one hand, a significant part of these applications helps in better visualising and, hence, understanding physical phenomena like fluid flow, saturation, wetting, drying, etc. in rock material, but also processes like fracturing, pore collapse, grain crushing, etc. These applications are still mainly situated in the field of fundamental and practical research. On the other hand, other applications are less research oriented, but more practical in nature. The most common of such applications is the scanning of core material (either in tube/packed or not), prior to cutting or re-coring. The CT-scans assist the operator in determining in a qualitative way the sections of a core that are suited for further testing, namely sections without damage, inclusions, fractures, cavities, etc. Some of the applications, mentioned above, that are these days rather situated in a research environment can become in the short to middle term industrial applications. The determination of pore and mineralogical distributions is probably the first application that will evolve from a research to a practical tool, partly because the current classical techniques are time consuming and sometimes subjective (e.g. point counting).

2 X-RAY COMPUTERIZED TOMOGRAPHY, PRINCIPLES

The X-ray technique allows visualising in a non-destructive way the interior of non-transparent objects. These objects are illuminated with X-rays and the change in transmitted X-ray intensity is measured. For monochromatic X-rays, the relationship between the intensity of the incident and attenuated X-rays (I_0 and I respectively) is expressed by Beer's law:

$$\frac{I}{I_0} = \exp(-\mu \cdot t) \tag{1}$$

where t represents the thickness of the object and μ the attenuation coefficient. The latter depends mainly on the density and atomic number of the object and the used X-ray energy:

$$\mu = \rho \cdot \left(a + b \frac{Z^{3.8}}{E^{3.2}} \right) \tag{2}$$

where ρ represents the bulk density, Z the bulk atomic number of the material, E the X-ray energy and where a and b are energy-dependent coefficients. As the X-ray source is not monochromatic, the relation between the attenuation coefficient μ and the other parameters is more complex (Curry et al. (1990)). This relationship is illustrated in Figure 1. The normal operating range of a CT-scanner is situated between 30 and 200 keV.

A conventional X-ray radiograph shows an object from one angle only and shadows from X-ray absorbing material along the ray paths are superimposed onto each other. Crucial information is lost in this way. In a CT-scanner, either the object is positioned inside the circle of a revolving X-ray tube, or the object is rotated for a fixed position of the X-ray source and detectors at the diametrically opposite side. For both set-ups, the CT-scanner sends X-rays at numerous different angles through the object and the attenuation of the rays are recorded at the opposite side. The slice of the object intersected by the X-rays is divided into a grid of volume elements (voxels). In each voxel the attenuation coefficient is assumed to be constant. The scanners' computer calculates the linear attenuation coefficient in all the voxels, based on the measured attenuations of the different X-ray paths. These linear attenuation coefficients are assumed to relate to the bulk densities.

Some of the applications presented further (see paragraph 3) were studied using a multi-slice medical CT scanner (model: Siemens Volume Zoom). The scan spiral parameters were selected to have a radiation dose determined by 140 KeV and 180 mAs, a slice width of 0.5 mm, a collimation of 0.5 mm and a rotation time of 1 s. A standard medical reconstruction algorithm designed for the human inner ear was used. The reconstructed slice width was also 0.5 mm with an increment of 0.2 mm. Two Siemens reconstruction kernel settings were used – the ultra sharp u90u and the medium smooth u30u.

The other applications made use of one or two microfocus computer tomography systems available at the Department of Metallurgy and Materials Engineering (K.U. Leuven), being the desktop SkyScan 1072 computerized microtomograph (for small objects of a diameter of up to 1 or 2 cm) and the AEA Tomohawk CT system on the Philips HOMX 161 microfocus system (for larger objects up to a diameter of 5 to 8 cm). In microfocus computer tomography the resolution of a system can be in the order of 10 μm × 10 μm × 10 μm, but it depends on the object size; e.g. for a 20 mm diameter core, it is situated between 58 and 78 μm (Wevers et al. (2001)).

Various types of artefacts can occur during the reconstruction. Beam hardening is one of them. It is a consequence of the polychromatic X-rays used in a CT. The differential attenuation of photons (see Figure 1) within the investigated object leads to the rapid attenuation of the lowest energy photons and hence to the gradual increase of the mean energy. Beam hardening or cupping effect is the anomalous decreasing attenuation toward the centre of a homogeneous object (see Figure 2). It can be reduced by a mathematical correction at some stage in the reconstruction process, by going to higher source energies or filtering the low energy content of the incident radiation with metal filters placed between the X-ray source and the object (Baruchel et al. (2000); Van Geet et al. (2000)). Other artefacts are ring artefacts and star or streak artefacts. Ring artefacts are caused by inhomogeneities of the detector and are minimised by randomly moving the object and with it the field of

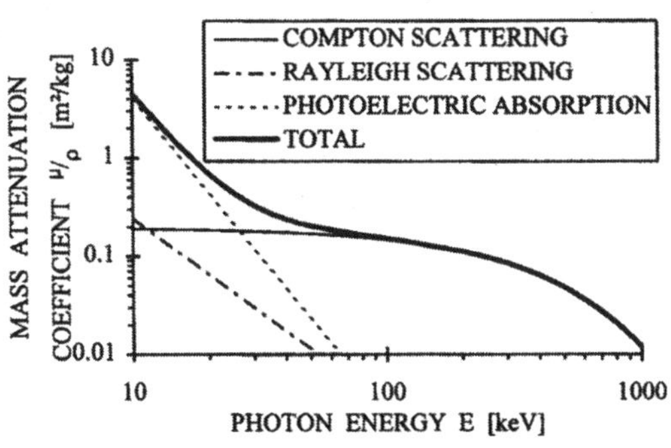

Figure 1. The contribution of the different attenuation processes in the mass attenuation coefficient in function of the photon energy.

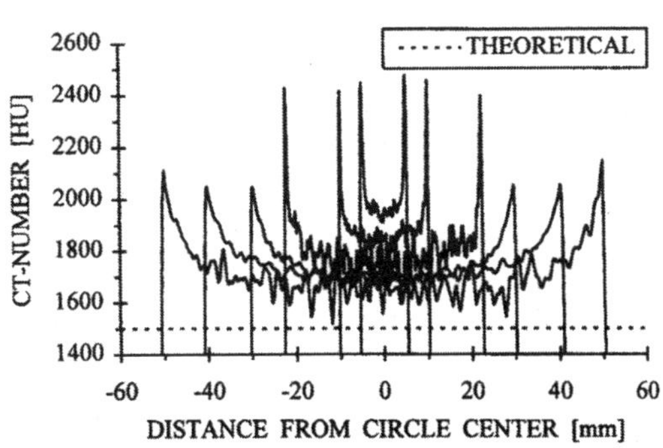

Figure 2. CT-numbers along the diameter of a set of circular homogeneous glass samples.

detector used (Skyscan (1997); Burch et al. (1998)). Star or streak artefacts are caused by secondary radiation that augments the noise and creates the artefacts. Metal filters such as aluminium or copper placed in front of the detector can suppress to a major extent the star artefacts because they help to reduce the secondary radiation. However, some of the primary radiation will also be attenuated and as a consequence the contrast will be lowered (Baruchel et al. (2000)). All these artefacts have to be avoided or at least minimised, if some internal feature of a material needs to be determined accurately in size or if the material needs to be characterised based on density measurements for instance.

3 RECENT APPLICATIONS FOR ROCK MATERIAL

In paragraph 1, an overview is given of applications of the X-ray CT, discussed in the literature, but without going into detail. The list of references is certainly not exhaustive. It shows, however, that even for rock material only, the number of different applications is large, that CT-scans have advantages above other techniques, that they give valuable results for a wide range of rock material, that successful applications are realised using medical scanners, as well as micro-CT-scanners, and that it is a technique that is being used worldwide in different industrial and research environments. In this paragraph, the authors present a few own examples in more detail. All examples were realised by one or more of the CT-scanners available at the K.U. Leuven (various medical scanners at the university hospital Gasthuisberg and two micro-CT-scanners of the Department of Metallurgy and Materials Engineering).

3.1 *Visualisation of induced fractures in rock mechanical studies*

The main task of a rock mechanical engineer is to estimate beforehand the behaviour of the rock mass around an excavation. For this task, the rock behaviour characteristics have first to be quantified (e.g. stress-strain curves and failure envelopes). Second, based on this information, but also on experience, the reaction of the rock mass is estimated. More and more, sophisticated numerical simulation codes are being developed to assist the rock mechanical engineer with this estimation. In the early days of numerical simulations, most calculations were limited to the linear elastic domain. For the calculation of the stress levels, only the elastic modulus and Poisson coefficient were needed. Now codes have become available, allowing the calculation of plastic and time dependent deformation (e.g. Barla & Barla (2001); Bonini et al. (2001); Eberhardt (2001)), but also of individual newly induced fractures (e.g. Dyskin & Germanovich (1993); Malan & Napier (1995); Potyondy et al. (1996); Van de Steen et al. (2003)). For these codes, numerous input parameters are needed and most of them cannot be determined (easily) by laboratory experiments. Hence, the values of these parameters are often determined by back-analysis. For the codes simulating the growth of individual fractures, it is crucial to be able to visualise induced fractures in laboratory experiments. Hence, the CT-scanner becomes a useful tool in this process of back-analysis.

3.1.1 *Failure of limestone sample in poly-axial cell*

In Figure 3, a first simple example is given of a cubic limestone block that was tested in a poly-axial cell till failure, and simulated afterwards using the boundary element code DIGS (see also Vervoort (2003) and Vervoort et al. (2003) for more details on these experiments and Napier & Pierce (1995) for information on the numerical simulation code DIGS). The size of the cubes is about 30 mm and a medical scanner was used. On both images (CT-scan and simulation), V-type fractures are clearly visible, whereby the fractures make an angle of 60° to 70° between the normal on the fracture plane and the direction of the major principal stress orientation. However, some parallel fractures are present, but also some macro-fractures with an entirely different orientation are observed (e.g. perpendicular to the major principal stress). On the image of the laboratory sample, one would conclude, based on the orientation of the main fractures (V-type), that they are a shear type of failure. The simulations show that more than a third of the failure is tensile driven.

Although CT-scans give a good image of the major fractures, thin sections or SEM images give other and more detailed information. In Figure 4, an example is given of a microphotograph of the same sample, after some thin sections were prepared. It is now obvious that the fractures visible on the CT-scans are rather fractured zones, with a width that varies between 0.05 and 0.2 mm. From Figure 4, it is clear that some shear displacement has occurred along the fracture dipping to the left, after the two fractures dipping to the right were formed. Apart from the wide macro-fractures, some thin fractures are also present and some cleavage planes inside crystals have been activated. In Figure 5, a SEM image of a tensile fracture induced in a Brazilian test of a limestone core is presented. It is clear that the macro-fracture has followed the cleavage planes in a step wise way (Van de Steen et al. (2002)).

3.1.2 *Failure of scale model of mining excavations*

A second, more elaborated, example is presented in Figures 6 to 8 (see also Sellers et al. (2003a, b)).

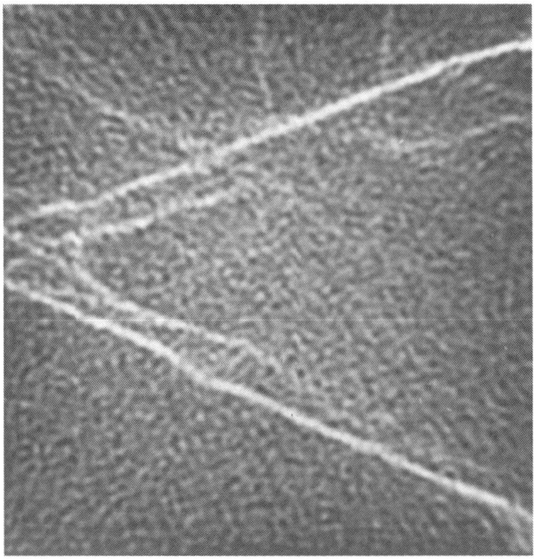

(a)

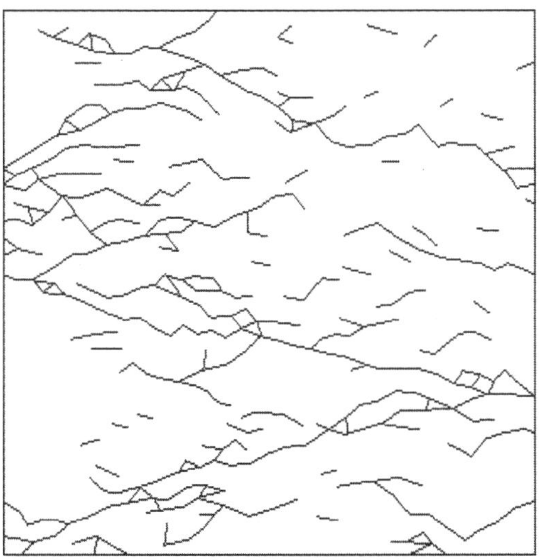

(b)

Figure 3. Fracture pattern (a) visualized by CT-scanning and (b) calculated by DIGS in a limestone sample loaded till failure in a poly-axial cell [parallel to plane of largest deviatoric stress; horizontal direction: parallel to major principal stress; side length: 30 mm].

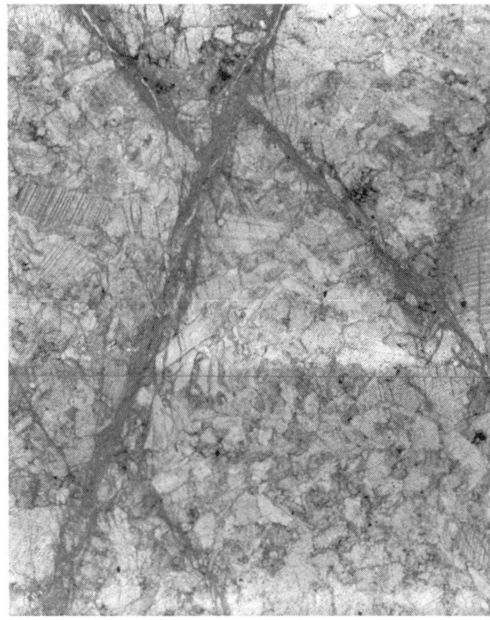

Figure 4. Microphotograph of a crystalline limestone sample loaded till failure in a poly-axial cell [parallel to plane of largest deviatoric stress; vertical direction: parallel to major principal stress; width of picture corresponds to 1.9 mm].

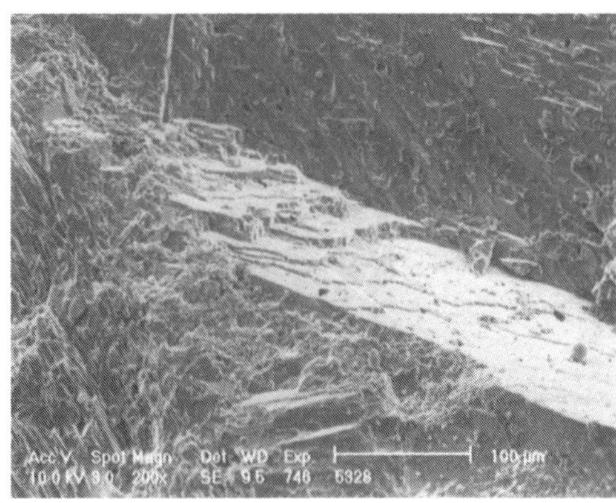

Figure 5. SEM image of macro-fracture induced in a Brazilian test (tensile failure).

A series of experiments were conducted in the laboratory on cubic samples of quartzite in order to be able to study the development of foundation, roof and pillar failure for different mining geometries in the deep level gold mines in South Africa. Mining and tunnelling at great depths (e.g. more than 1000 m) leads to considerable fracturing of the rock surrounding the excavation (Hagan (1990); Handley et al. (1997); Durrheim et al. (1998)). The presence of large blocks caused by mining induced fracturing, or the intersection of these fractures with pre-existing geological discontinuities increases the potential for rockfalls that are hazardous to workers and can interrupt production (Jaeger & Ryder (1999)). Rockbursts may occur when the stresses induced around the mining excavation exceed the strength of the solid rock or

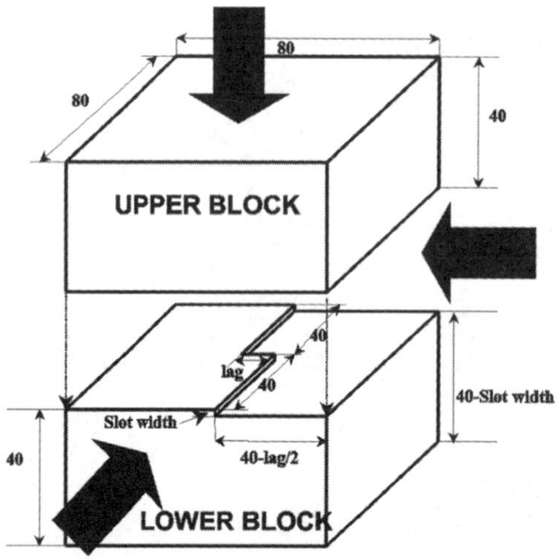

Figure 6. Cubic sample with mine layout tested in a poly-axial cell (dimensions in mm), after Sellers et al. (2003a).

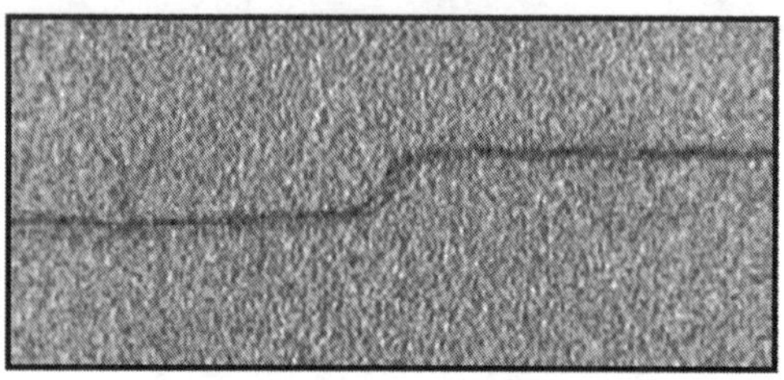

(a)

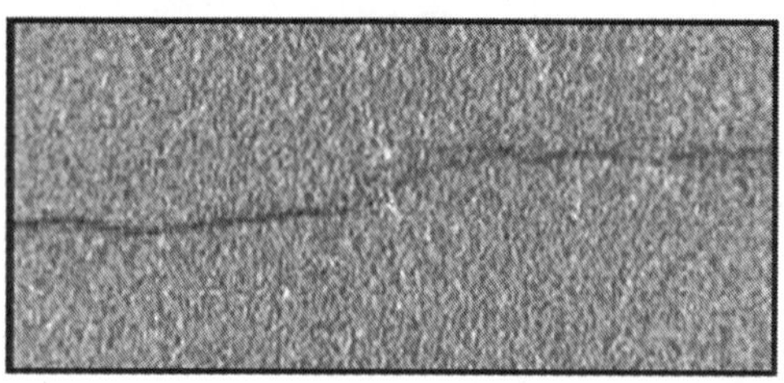

(b)

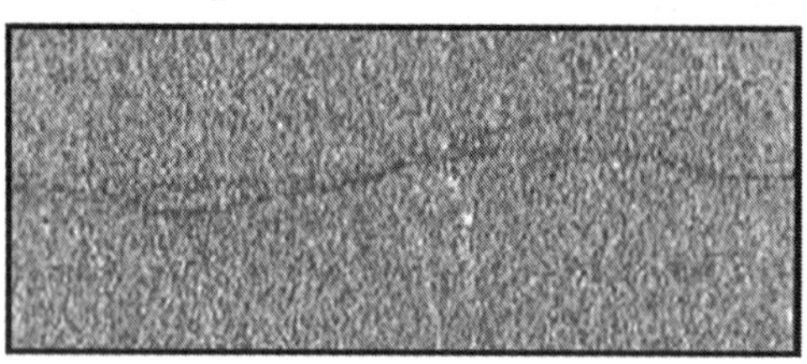

(c)

Figure 7. CT-scans of a rock sample showing how the fracture traces (dark lines) follow the general shape of the layout at vertical distances of (a) 0.5 mm, (b) 10 mm and (c) 30 mm above the slot with a lag of 10 mm.

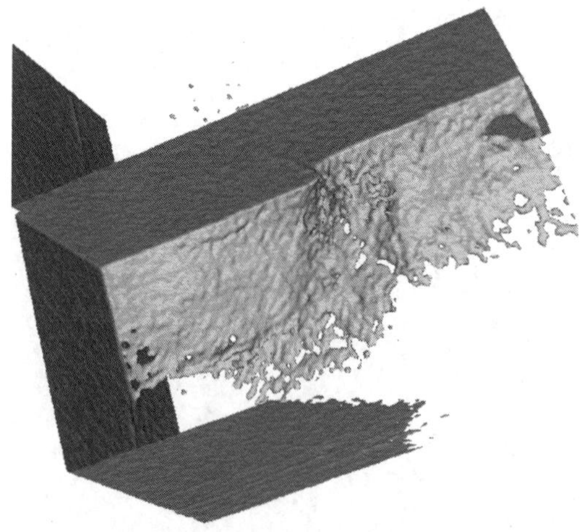

Figure 8. Three-dimensional reconstruction of the fracture pattern in a block with a lag of 10 mm.

when they are sufficiently high to trigger slip on pre-existing discontinuities such as faults or dykes. Understanding three-dimensional fracture processes around deep level gold mines is important to be able to predict the rock mass response to planned excavation shapes.

The aim of the experiments was to provide basic situations that could be used to prove newly developed three-dimensional numerical models. Good comparisons between the observed and modelled failure planes should lead to confidence in the application of the models to underground situations. The models were monitored using acoustic emission to determine the failure processes during loading. However, it was important to be able to visualise the failure planes within the samples. The experimental configuration consisted of cubic samples that were tested under poly-axial stress states. Slots cut into the samples simulated tabular mine openings and acted as stress raisers for the initiation of fractures (see Figure 6 for an example). To overcome the practical problems related to cutting the samples in sections, but to still accurately describe the fracture paths in three dimensions, the tested and fractured samples were scanned using medical X-ray computerized tomography.

Visualization software was written based on standard visualization techniques (Schroeder et al. (1997)). Three orthogonal sections of the scanned grid can be viewed simultaneously to enable the researcher to follow fracture paths within the sample. The CT scans clearly show the fractures within the sample, as illustrated in Figure 7. The plan views of the fractures for a lag length of 10 mm are shown for three distances above the slot, visualising the way that the fracture surface transforms inside the sample. At a distance of 0.5 mm above the slot, the fracture follows the face well, including the lag. However, further above the slot, the fracture evolve to a more linear feature and it is difficult to recognise the lag of the face. Parallel fractures are also observed.

Three-dimensional views of the fracture planes can be reconstructed using image processing and visualization techniques. The VTK visualization package (Schroeder et al. (1997)) is an open source software library that can be accessed using scripting languages to provide interactive visualization modules. The data file containing the image representing the voxel grid of a scanned sample was exported from the CT scanner and imported into the visualization software. This process requires large amount of memory and disk storage space, as there are 1.25×10^8 voxels in the scan of a single 80 mm cubic sample. Approximately 250 Mb of storage and 1.1 Gb of memory are required. The resolution of the scan is therefore selected based on the amount of data that can be manipulated with the available computer resources. A "marching cubes" algorithm was used to obtain an isosurface contour of densities below a selected threshold value of CT number from the voxel grid. The three-dimensional fracture picture of Figure 8 demonstrates the insight that can be obtained when viewing a digital reconstruction of the entire fracture pattern (sample with a 10 mm lag). Figure 8 illustrates how the fracture curves below the leading panel, especially in the region adjacent to the other panel. In the underground situation, this would represent a great hazard. Due to the relatively low dip of the fracture at this point, the process of fracture formation and any subsequent slip displacement in this region would transmit seismic waves directly upwards at the edge of the panel and the gully. As the gully is a main access way and a region with a high probability that workers are present, there is considerable risk of injury or loss of life.

3.2 *Quantitative analysis of reservoir rocks*

3.2.1 *Visualisation of natural open fractures (cleats) in coal*

Probably the most important factor controlling the possibilities of coalbed methane extraction and/or CO_2 injection in coal layers relates to the natural fracture (cleat) system within the coal seam (Gayer & Harris (1996)). A complete 3D-characterisation of the fracture network is needed to understand and predict the flow through rocks, as well as some of its rock mechanical characteristics. Hence, the possibilities of a micro-CT scanner were evaluated for such a characterisation by scanning a small coal sample. A sample of 8 mm in diameter was drilled from the core of the Peer borehole (KB 206), at a depth of 1155.66 m (Dusar & Verkaeren (1992); Caers et al. (1996); Van Geet et al. (2002b)). This sample was not impregnated.

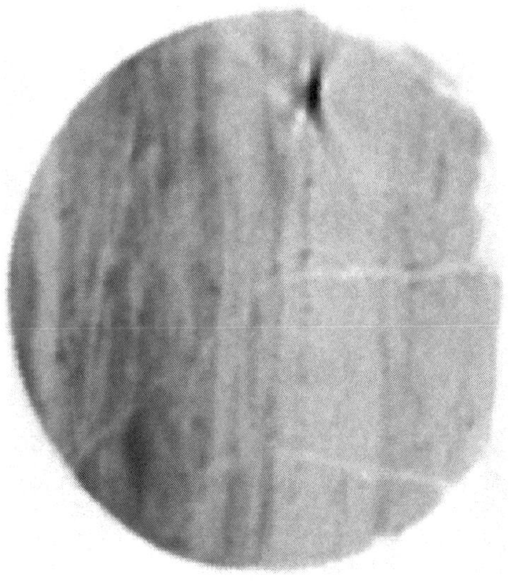

Figure 9. Micro-CT slice through a natural coal sample of 8 mm in diameter. [High attenuation materials are represented in dark (e.g. pyrite); Air-filled cleats can be seen as thin white lines].

This should result in a maximum contrast between air-filled cleats and coal components. Whenever an air-filled fracture occurs in a material, the density and atomic number lower at the fracture location. Consequently, lowering in the attenuation coefficient can be observed. Apart from visualising these fractures within a 3D-volume, it is necessary for quantitative purposes to measure the aperture along the fracture. When an attenuation profile through a fractured material is observed, one can notice that the profile does not reflect the true values, i.e. air. This deviation from the real attenuation values is caused by the limited resolution of the instrument and the reconstruction procedure.

Figure 9 visualises one slice of the studied sample. In this sample the cleats (white lines) are visible. However, classical image processing techniques could not be used to extract the entire location of the cleats. Consequently, a Matlab-algorithm was written (see Van Geet (2001) and Van Geet & Swennen (2001) for more details). This algorithm needs a starting point and direction as input. From this starting point all neighbouring pixels in the given direction are analysed and the one with the smallest difference in attenuation value is chosen. This procedure for 1 slice was repeated for 100 sequential slices. Consequently, the cleat distribution within the 3D-volume can be visualised (Figure 10). In this particular sample, only two separate cleat planes can be defined, i.e. one very small cleat and one larger and conjugated cleat (see also Van Geet & Swennen (2001) and Van Geet et al. (2002b) for more details). The distribution of the cleat

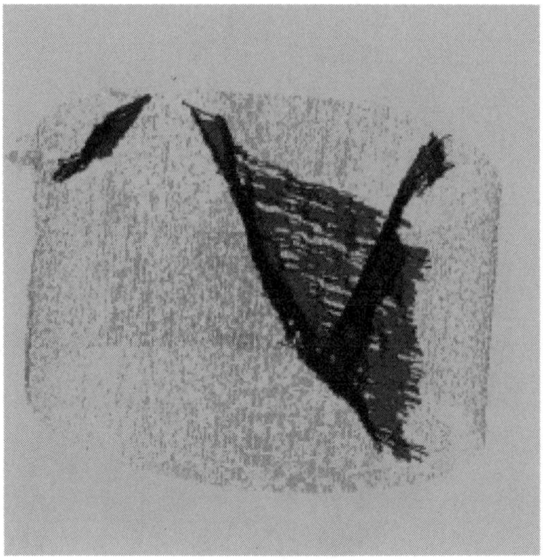

Figure 10. Visualisation of the 3D-distribution of the cleats (dark planes) within the analysed coal sample [diameter: 8 mm]. Two cleats can be distinguished, namely one small cleat (I, at left) and one larger and conjugated cleat (II, at right).

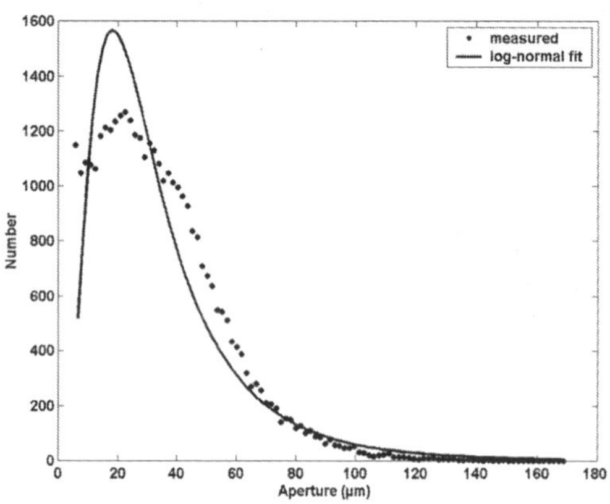

Figure 11. Histogram of the cleat apertures as measured in the whole volume for cleat II.

apertures of cleat II is given as an example in Figure 11. The data display a lognormal distribution (see also Van Geet & Swennen (2001)). After log-transformation the measured cleat apertures show some skewness towards small cleat apertures. This is in agreement with former studies, where a lognormal distribution of a natural cleat aperture seems most appropriate (Johns et al. (1993); Pyrak-Nolte et al. (1997) and Keller (1998)).

3.2.2 *Porosity measurements of sedimentary rock*

Porosity of reservoir rocks is an important petrophysical characteristic. It is one of the basic parameters in simulation studies for predicting reservoir quality. Various techniques are available for porosity measurements and visualization. Petrophysical measurements are performed on volumetric samples, whereas classical geological petrography using a petrographical microscope is restricted to 2D analysis. This leads to a discrepancy between petrographical and petrophysical studies. The microfocus X-ray computerized tomography should be able to link petrography and petrophysics. Results for porosity measurements of a limestone are compared with results obtained by other techniques (see also Van Geet (2001); Van Geet et al. (2000 and 2003)).

Many carbonate reservoirs consist predominantly of pure limestone, i.e. calcite, enabling the use of a linearisation procedure to exclude beam hardening artefacts. A homogeneous monocrystalline calcite crystal was used as a calibration sample. The deviation from a linear correlation between measured intensity and thickness of the calcite was fitted with a fifth order polynomial, which was then used for correcting beam hardening. Visual inspection showed a complete elimination of the effect of beam hardening in calcite crystals and calcareous mudstones. Once beam hardening was corrected, the measured linear attenuation coefficient can be correlated with density or porosity of the object. Because the linear attenuation coefficient reflects the mean attenuation of the whole voxel, the measured data include total porosity, including microporosity related to voids that are not visible as individual pores. A calcite crystal was used for calibration (0% porosity). To determine the possibilities of quantifying porosity, a sample containing porous and nonporous zones was used. The limestone sample is 8 mm in diameter, derived from a turbiditic oil reservoir formation of the Ionian Zone, Albania (Van Geet et al. 2002a). It contains a porous zone at the top, with a dark colour due to oil impregnation. The bottom part is non-porous, due to early diagenetic calcite cementation, and lacks any oil impregnation. About 300 micro-CT-slices were scanned for this sample, perpendicular to the longitudinal axis of the cylindrical object. The mean attenuation coefficient was measured in every slice to calculate the mean density, which was subsequently converted to porosity.

To verify the micro-CT results, image analysis was carried out with reflected light microscopy on a polished surface to measure porosity along a trace parallel to the longitudinal axis of the object (a magnification of 2.5 and of 10 was used). Note that with this approach it was not possible to differentiate isolated pores from connected pores that make up the network porosity that can be accessed by fluids. However, this differentiation is also not possible for micro-CT-derived

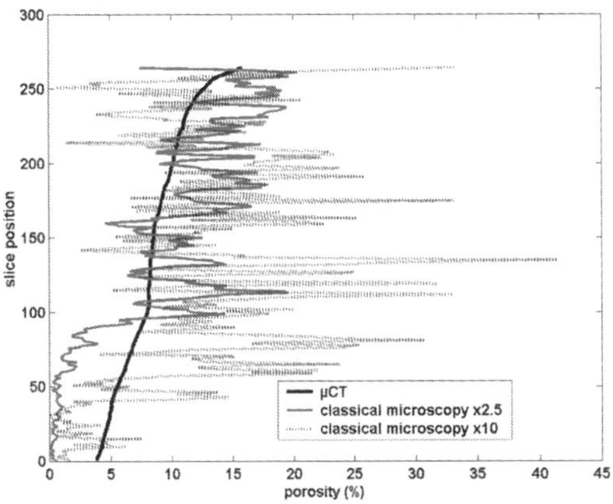

Figure 12. Evaluation of porosity measurements by micro-CT and classical reflected light microscopy carried out on a polished surface (Cretaceous turbidite, Ionian Zone, Albania). [This sample comprises an originally oil-impregnated zone (slice numbers above 120) and a non-impregnated section (slice numbers below 120)]

porosity measurements. Discrimination between porosity and limestone was done by thresholding. The measured porosity profiles obtained by both techniques are plotted in Figure 12. Although different types of information are compared (two dimensional versus three dimensional), a similar trend is found in all measurements, with a particularly good correlation between the micro-CT results and optical microscopy measurements at the highest of the two magnifications that were used. At this magnification, micro-porosity is incorporated as well, which is also included in the micro-CT data. This shows that micro-CT can clearly be used for total porosity measurements in limestone samples after calibration.

Micro-CT scanning has the additional advantage of allowing visualization of the largest pores in three dimensions, providing information about their interconnectivity. To evaluate this, a turbidite limestone reservoir sample composed of several bands of porous (oil-impregnated) and non-porous zones was scanned. Figure 13 illustrates the micro-CT results for this sample as a kind of radiograph in which limestone is made transparent (here light grey) and porosity is shown as dark grey features. It is clear that a banded structure and bedding can be seen, illustrating that micro-CT data provide information about macro-porosity distributions, in addition to total porosity measurements.

3.3 *Visualisation of moisture flow*

Previous examples have either practical implications for the mining or for the oil-gas industry. In this section, X-ray is used to study the deterioration processes in porous building materials. Most of these

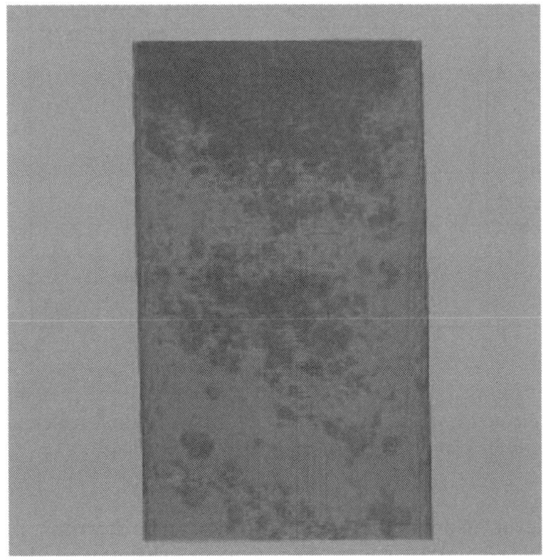

Figure 13. 3D visualisation of the distribution of macroporosity for a turbiditic carbonate sample of the Ionian Zone, Albania, based on micro-CT-analysis. [The carbonate is made "transparent" (i.e. light grey) and the macroporosity is visualised as darker grey sections by means of thresholding, within a fuzzy outline of a cylindrical sample (diameter: 8 mm). Inclined laminae with higher porosities alternate with non-porous laminae]

deterioration processes are strongly related to the presence of moisture. Examples are calcium leaching, frost damage, crystallisation and hydration of salts. Therefore, a better insight in the moisture transport phenomena is a first step towards the understanding of the associated deterioration mechanisms. As an example, the water imbibition in homogeneous, heterogeneous and cracked materials is studied using the X-ray projection method. Although the examples shown are for artificial materials, the technique can also be applied on natural building materials. The specimens are studied at different time steps. By subtracting a reference image (e.g. sample at dry state) from these images, information of the evolution of the moisture content in space and time is gained. Therefore, the X-ray projection method is not only applicable to determine the moisture diffusivity of porous building materials, but also to analyse moisture transport in cracked and heterogeneous porous media. A micro-CT-scanner has been used, but for a fixed position source-sample-receiver.

Before studying the moisture content and flow, the optimal sample thickness was determined. The optimal sample thickness of a sample can be defined as the thickness resulting in the highest possible resolution (Van Besien et al. (2003)). This has been determined for various materials and for water, as illustrated in Figure 14 for a calcium silicate plate. For each energy

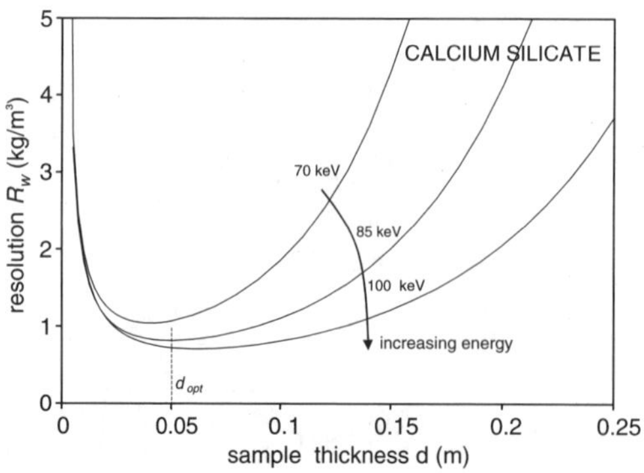

Figure 14. Resolution R_W as a function of sample (calcium silicate plate) thickness and incident X-ray energy.

level, an optimal sample thickness can be determined. Increasing the source energy results in a better resolution and meanwhile the optimal sample thickness shifts towards higher values. So it seems that a high X-ray energy is advantageous. However, the X-ray source proved to be unstable at high voltages. Also the object in the apparatus warms up during radiation with high energies, encouraging evaporation. 85 keV proved to be a good compromise between stability of the source and resolution. The optimal sample thickness corresponding to a X-ray energy of 85 keV was determined as 50 mm for calcium silicate with a corresponding resolution R_W of 0.8 kg/m^3.

In Figure 15, water uptake in a calcium silicate plate with time is presented for a free uptake experiment. Calcium silicate is mainly composed of the synthetic mineral xonotlite and is a very homogeneous material. Hence, the moisture diffusivity using a Boltzmann-transformation of subsequent measured moisture profiles can be determined (Hall & Hoff (2002)). To reduce possible scatter and increase the accuracy at each step in time, a one-dimensional moisture profile is determined as the averaged moisture profile of a bandwidth of 20 pixels in the middle of the image (see Figure 15).

However, the X-ray projection is mainly useful for heterogeneous or cracked material, as for such material the moisture front is much more irregular, as illustrated in Figures 16 and 17. In Figure 16, a snapshot about 2 minutes after the start of the free water uptake is presented for a material with micro-cracks present (cellular concrete). These micro-cracks act as preferential wetting paths, as they suck up the water much faster than the bulk material. As no continuous path of micro-cracks probably exist, the preferential wetting stops after a while and at that moment redistribution from the water-filled micro-cracks to the surrounding matrix seems the major process. This results in an equalisation of the moisture front (after 1 to 1½ hours). Figure 17 shows an example of a brick sample with a fracture

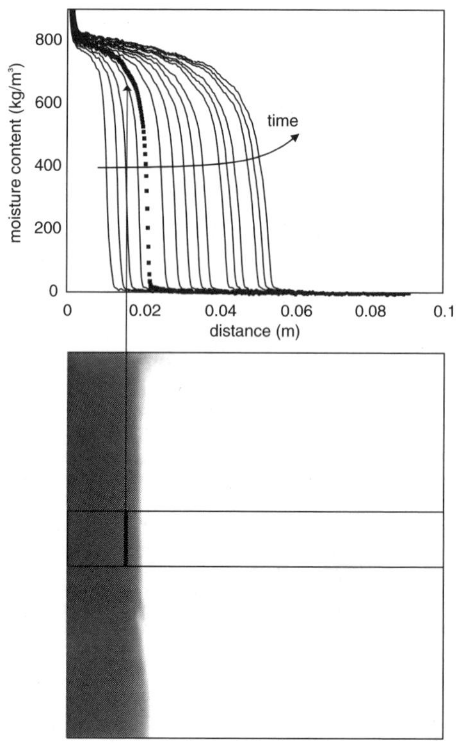

Figure 15. Subsequent moisture profiles (top) for a calcium silicate plate determined from quantitative moisture profile images (bottom), as obtained by the X-ray projection method in a free uptake experiment [water uptake from the left].

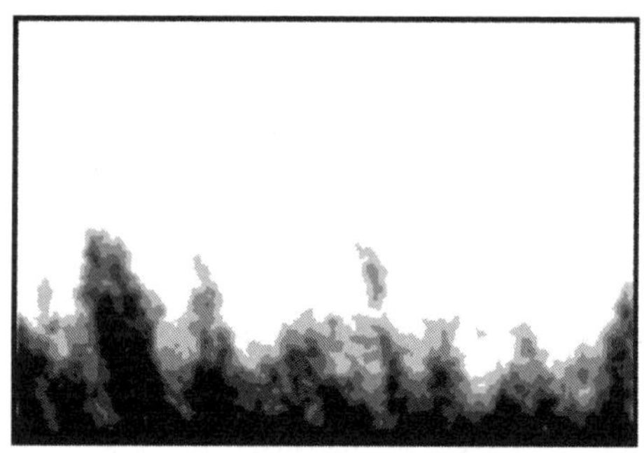

Figure 16. X-ray image after about 2 minutes of the two-dimensional moisture distribution for cellular concrete showing micro-cracks [The baseline of image measures 52 mm; water uptake from the bottom].

(opening of approximately 0.1 mm) across the entire sample. Besides the moisture distribution inside the bulk material, the X-ray projection method is also able to visualise the filled part of the fracture (at about

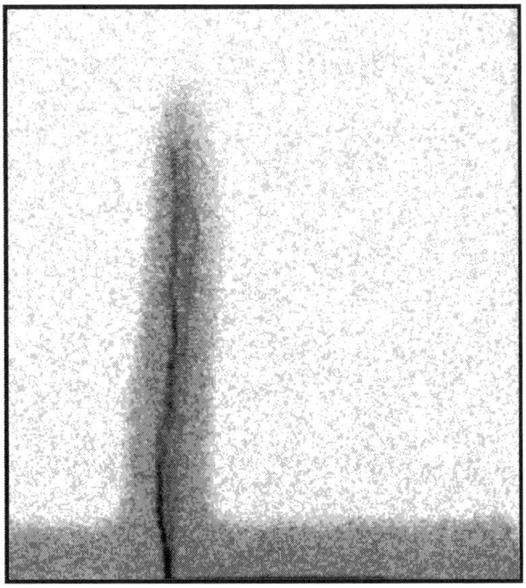

Figure 17. X-ray image of water uptake in a fractured brick sample taken after 33 seconds [The estimated fracture aperture is 0.1 mm; the baseline of image measures 80 mm; water uptake from the bottom].

30 seconds). The waterfront in the fracture quickly reaches the opposite side of the specimen (after 2½ minutes). Afterwards, the fracture acts as an extra water source for the surrounding matrix over the total height of the specimen. Further details can be found in Roels et al. (2003).

4 CONCLUSIONS

The references given in paragraph 1, as well as the own examples by the authors in paragraph 3 show that the X-ray CT technique is useful for the study of rock material, which is most often heterogeneous (e.g. different minerals, presence of pores, fractures, cavities, etc.). The heterogeneous nature of the rock is present at various scales. During recent years, researchers are becoming more and more aware that the behaviour at a micro-scale (e.g. millimetre scale) may have an effect on the large scale behaviour of a rock mass. Two examples to illustrate this: fracture initiation around an excavation is certainly influenced by the presence of various small weak elements and the overall flow of a liquid or a gas can certainly be restricted by the presence of some thin impermeable layers. Also, a two-dimensional model is often insufficient to properly understand physical phenomena. Hence, it is important to create three-dimensional models at small scale and to visualise the microstructure of the rock material in detail at that scale.

X-ray computerized tomography is a technique that can provide such information in a relatively short time span. To produce valuable results with this technique, it is however important to properly understand the physical background of the technique and to limit the effects of artefacts and other inaccuracies. In this way, X-ray CT helps in understanding physical phenomena at small scale, like for example fracture initiation and growth, pore collapse, grain crushing, wetting and flow transport. This better understanding is beneficial for a wide range of industries, e.g. mining, petroleum and gas extraction, environmental engineering, building materials, etc.

REFERENCES

Barla, G. & Barla, M. 2001. Numerical simulations of squeezing behaviour in tunnels. In: *Proceedings of the 2nd International FLAC Symposium on Numerical Modeling in Geomechanics*, Lyon (France), October 2001, Balkema, 323–328.

Baruchel, J., Buffière, J.-Y., Maire, E., Merle, P. & Peix, G. 2000. *X-ray tomography in Material Science, General Principles*. Hermes Science Publications, Paris 2000, ISBN 2-7462-0115-1, 15–21.

Bazin, B. 2001. From matrix acidizing to acid fracturing: a laboratory evaluation of acid/rock interactions. *SPE Production & Facilities*, February 2001, 16(1), 22–29.

Bonini, M., Barla, M. & Barla, G. 2001. FLAC applications to the analysis of swelling behaviour in tunnels. In: *Proceedings of the 2nd International FLAC Symposium on Numerical Modeling in Geomechanics*, Lyon (France), October 2001, Balkema, 323–328.

Burch, S.F., Ramsay, A.T. & Whittaker, J. 1998. *Tomohawk user manual for Leuven University: a user manual produced for Leuven University*, Belgium, AEA Technology, OXON, 89 pp.

Caers, J., Swennen, R. & Dusar, M. 1996. Diagenetic history of Westphalian A and B fluvio-deltaic deposits: an example from the KB206 Peer borehole (Campine Basin, NE-Belgium). *Zentralblatt fur Geologie une Palaontologie*, 1996, 11/12, 1211–1236.

Caers, J., Swennen, R. & Vervoort, A. 1997. Petrography and X-ray computerized tomography applied as an integral part of a rock mechanical investigation of discontinuities. *Transactions of the Institute of Mining and Metallurgy, Section B, Applied Earth Sciences*, January–April 1997, Vol. 106(1), B38–B45.

Carlson, W.D., Rowe, T., Ketcham, R.A. & Colbert, M.W. 2003. Applications of high-resolution X-ray computed tomography in petrology, meteoritics and palaeontology. In Mees, F., Swennen, R., Van Geet, M. & Jacobs, P. (eds) *Applications of X-ray computed tomography in the geosciences*. Geological Society, London, Special publications, 215, 7–22.

Coenen, J.C.G. & Maas, J.G. 1994. Material classification by dual energy computerized X-ray tomography. In: *Proceedings of the International symposium on computerized tomography for industrial applications*, 120–127.

Coles, M.E., Hazlett, R.D., Spanne, P., Muegge, E.L. & Furr, M.J. 1996. Characterization of reservoir core using computed microtomography. *SPE Journal*, September 1996, Vol. 1(3), 295–301.

Cook, J.M., Goldsmith, G. & Auzerais, F. 1993. X-ray tomography studies of wellbore processes under in situ stress conditions. *International Journal of Rock Mechanics and Mining Sciences*, Vol. 30(7), 1091–1094.

Curry, T.S., Dowdey, J.E. & Murry, R.C. 1990. *Christensen's physics of diagnostics radiology*, 4th ed., Philadelphia, Lea and Febiger.

Dehghani, K. & Kamath, J. 2001. High-temperature blowdown experiments in a vuggy carbonate core. *SPE Journal*, September 2001, Vol. 6(3), 283–287.

Duliu O.G. 1999. Computer axial tomography in geo-sciences: an overview. *Earth-Science Reviews*, 48, 265–281.

Durrheim, R., Haile, A., Roberts, M.C.K., Schweitzer, J.K., Spottiswoode, S.M. & Klokow, J.W. 1998. Violent failure of a remnant in a deep South African gold mine. *Tectonophysics*, 289, 105–116.

Dusar, M. & Verkaeren, P. 1992. Methane description in closed collieries: examples from Belgium. *UNECE workshop on the recovery and end use of coalbed methane*, Katowice (Poland), 1992, Report C-4, 1–13.

Dyskin, A.V. & Germanovich, L.N. 1993. A model of crack growth in microcracked rock. *International Journal of Rock Mechanics and Mining Sciences*, 1993, 30(7), 813–820.

Eberhardt, E. 2001. Numerical modelling of three-dimension stress rotation ahead of an advancing tunnel face. *International Journal of Rock Mechanics and Mining Sciences*, 2001, 38(4), 499–518.

Flisch, A. & Becker, A. 2003. Industrial X-ray computed tomography studies of lake sediment drill cores. In Mees, F., Swennen, R., Van Geet, M. & Jacobs, P. (eds) *Applications of X-ray computed tomography in the geosciences*. Geological Society, London, Special publications, 215, 205–212.

Gayer, R. & Harris, I. 1996. *Coalbed methane and coal geology*. Geological Society of London, Special Publication, 109, London (UK), 344 p.

Géraud, Y., Surma, F. & Mazerolle, F. 2003. Porosity and fluid flow characterization of granite by capillary wetting using X-ray computed tomography. In Mees, F., Swennen, R., Van Geet, M. & Jacobs, P. (eds) *Applications of X-ray computed tomography in the geosciences*. Geological Society, London, Special publications, 215, 95–105.

Hagan, T. 1990. Pillar foundations studies on a deep level South African gold mine. *Rockbursts and seismicity in mines*. Fairhurst (ed.) Balkema. 65–70.

Hall, C. & Hoff, W.D. 2002. *Water transport in brick, stone and concrete.* Spon Press, London.

Handley, M., Selfe, D., Viera, F. Maccelari, M. & Dede, T. 1997. Current position of strike stabilizing pillars and bracket pillars – guidelines for deep tabular orebodies. *J. South Afr. Inst. Min. Metal.* 103–116.

Hidajat, I., Rastogi, A., Singh, M. & Mohanty, K.K. 2002. Transport properties of porous media reconstructed from thin-sections. *SPE Journal*, March 2002, Vol. 7(1), 40–48.

Hirono, T., Takahashi, M. & Nakashima, S. 2003. Direct imaging of fluid flow in fault-related rocks by X-ray CT. In Mees, F., Swennen, R., Van Geet, M. & Jacobs, P. (eds) *Applications of X-ray computed tomography in the geosciences*. Geological Society, London, Special publications, 215, 107–115.

Jaeger, A.J & Ryder, J. 1999. *A handbook on rock engineering practice for tabular hard rock mines*. The Safety in Mines Research Advisory Committee (SIMRAC) Johannesburg.

Johns, R.A., Steude, J.S., Castanier, L.M. & Roberts, P.V. 1993. Non-destructive measurements of fracture aperture in crystalline rock cores using X-ray computed tomography. *Journal of Geophysical Research*, 98, B2, 1889–1900.

Jones, K.W., Feng, H., Lindquist, W.B., Adler, P.M., Thovert, J.F., Vekemans, B., Vincze, L., Szaloki, I., Van Grieken, R., Adams, F. & Riekel, C. 2003. Study of the microgeometry of porous materials using synchroton computed microtomography. In Mees, F., Swennen, R., Van Geet, M. & Jacobs, P. (eds) *Applications of X-ray computed tomography in the geosciences*. Geological Society, London, Special publications, 215, 39–49.

Karacan, C.O., Grader, A.S. & Halleck, P.M. 2003. Evaluation of local porosity changes in limestone samples under triaxial stress field by using X-ray computed tomography. In Mees, F., Swennen, R., Van Geet, M. & Jacobs, P. (eds) *Applications of X-ray computed tomography in the geosciences*. Geological Society, London, Special publications, 215, 177–189.

Keller, A. 1998. High resolution, non-destructive measurement and characterization of fracture apertures. *International Journal of Rock Mechanics and Mining Sciences*, 35, 1037–1050.

Malan D.F. & Napier J.A.L. 1995. Computer modelling of granular material microfracturing. *Tectonophysics*, Vol. 248, 21–37.

Napier, J.A.L. & Peirce, A.P. 1995. Simulation of extensive fracture formation and interaction in brittle materials. In: *Proceedings of the 2nd International Conference on mechanics of jointed and faulted rock*, Vienna (Austria), 63–74.

Potyondy, D.O., Cundall, P.A. & Lee, C. 1996. Modeling of rock using bonded assemblies of circular particles. In: Aubertin M. (ed.), *Proc. Second North American Rock Mechanics Symposium*, Montreal. Balkema, Rotterdam, 1996, 1934–1944.

Pyrak-Nolte, L.J., Montemagno, C.D. & Nolte, D. 1997. Volumetric imaging of aperture distributions in connected fracture networks. *Geophysical Research Letters*, 24, 2343–2346.

Roels, S., Vandersteen, K. & Carmeliet, J. 2003. Measuring and simulating moisture uptake in a fractured porous medium. *Advances in water resources*, Vol. 26, 237–246.

Rousset-Tournier, B., Mazerolle, F., Géraud, Y. & Jeannette, D. 2003. Rock drying tests monitored by X-ray computed tomography – the effect of saturation methods on drying behaviour. In Mees, F., Swennen, R., Van Geet, M. & Jacobs, P. (eds) *Applications of X-ray computed tomography in the geosciences*. Geological Society, London, Special publications, 215, 117–125.

Ruiz de Argandona, V.G., Rodriguez-Rey, A., Celorio, C., Calleja, L. & Suarez del Rio, L.M. 2003. Characterization by X-ray computed tomography of water absorption in a limestone used as building stone in the Oviedo Cathedral (Spain). In Mees, F., Swennen, R., Van Geet, M. & Jacobs, P. (eds) *Applications of X-ray computed tomography in the geosciences*. Geological Society, London, Special publications, 215, 127–134.

Schroeder, W., Martin, K. & Lorensen, B. 1997. *The Visualization Toolkit. An object-oriented approach to 3D graphics*. Prentice Hall.

Sellers, E., Vervoort, A. & Van Cleynenbreugel, J. 2003a. Three-dimensional visualization of fractures in rock test samples, simulating deep level mining excavations, using X-ray computed tomography. In Mees, F., Swennen, R., Van Geet, M. & Jacobs, P. (eds) *Applications of X-ray computed tomography in the geosciences*. Geological Society, London, Special publications, 215, 69–80.

Sellers, E., Vervoort, A. & Drummond, M. 2003b. Insight into pillar failure in experimental samples using CT visualization. In: *International Workshop on X-ray CT for Geomaterials GeoX2003*, Kumamoto (Japan), November 6–7 2003, A.A. Balkema, Rotterdam (in press).

Skyscan, 1997, Skyscan 1072 *Desktop Microscope-microtomograph: instruction manual*. Skyscan, Aartselaar, 43 pp.

Spiess, R., Peruzzo, L., Prior, D.J. & Wheeler, J. 2001. Development of garnet porphyroblasts by multiple nucleation, coalescence and boundary misorientation-driven rotations. *Journal of Metamorphic Geology*, 19, 269–290.

Taylor, L.A., Keller, R.A., Snyder, G.A., Wang, W.Y., Carlson, W.D., Hauri, E.H., McCandless, T., Kim, K.R., Sobolev, N.V. & Bezborodov, S.M. 2000. Diamonds and their mineral inclusions, and what they tell us: A detailed "pull-apart" of a diamondiferous eclogite. *International Geology Review*, 42, 959–983.

Tivey, M.K. 1998. Documenting textures and mineral abundances in minicores from the TAG active hydrothermal mound using X-ray computed tomography. In Herzig, P.M., Humphris, S.E., Miller, D.J. & Zierenberg, R.A. (eds) *Proceedings of the Ocean Drilling Pogram, Scientific Results*, Vol. 158, 201–210.

Van Besien, T., Roels, S. & Carmeliet, J. 2003. Analysis of moisture flow in porous materials using microfocus X-ray radiography. *Physics D: Applied Physics* (in review).

Van de Steen B., Vervoort A. & Sahin K. 2002. Influence of internal structure of crinoidal limestone on fracture paths. *Engineering Geology*, Vol. 67, 109–125.

Van de Steen, B., Vervoort, A., Napier, J.A.L. & Durrheim, R.J. 2003. Implementation of a flaw model to the fracturing around a vertical shaft. *Rock Mechanics and Rock Engineering,* Vol. 36(2), April 2003, 143–161.

Vandersteen, K., Busselen, B., Van den Abeele, K. & Carmeliet, J. 2003. Quantitative characterizations of fracture apertures using microfocus computed tomography. In Mees, F., Swennen, R., Van Geet, M. & Jacobs, P. (eds) *Applications of X-ray computed tomography in the geosciences*. Geological Society, London, Special publications, 215, 61–68.

Van Geet, M., Swennen, R. & Wevers, M. 2000. Quantitative analysis of reservoir rocks by means of microfocus X-ray computer tomography. *Sedimentary Geology*, 132, 25–36.

Van Geet, M. 2001. *Optimisation of microfocus X-ray computer tomography for geological research with special emphasis on coal components and fractures characterisation.* PhD-thesis, KULeuven, Leuven, Belgium.

Van Geet, M. & Swennen, R. 2001. Quantitative 3D-fracture analysis by means of microfocus X-ray computer tomography (μCT): an example from coal. *Geoph. Research Letters*, 28, 17, 3333–3336.

Van Geet, M., Swennen, R. Durmishi, C., Roure, F. & Muchez, Ph. 2002a. Paragenesis of Cretaceous to Eocene carbonate reservoirs in the Ionian fold and thrust belt (Albania): relation between tectonism and fluid flow. *Sedimentology*, 49, 697–718.

Van Geet, M., David, P. & Swennen, R. 2002b. Three dimensional coal characterisation (maceral, mineral and cleats) by means of X-ray microfocus computer tomography (μCT). *Polish Geol. Institute Spec. Papers* (Proceedings of the IV European Coal Conference), 7, 263–270.

Van Geet, M., Lagrou, D. & Swennen, R. 2003. Porosity measurements of sedimentary rocks by means of microfocus X-ray computed tomography (μCT). In Mees, F., Swennen, R., Van Geet, M. & Jacobs, P. (eds) *Applications of X-ray computed tomography in the geosciences.* Geological Society, London, Special publications, 215, 51–60.

Verhelst, F., Swennen, R., Vervoort, A., Marchal, G. & Dusar, M. 1995a. X-ray computerized tomography of heterogeneities in Westphalian A & B coal strata (Peer Coalbed methane project; Campine basin, NE Belgium). *Zbl. Geol. Paläont.* Teil I, 1995, H.11/12, 1119–1124.

Verhelst, F., Vervoort, A., De Bosscher, Ph. & Marchal, G. 1995b. X-ray computerised tomography, determination of heterogeneities in rock samples. In: *Proceedings of the "8th International congress on rock mechanics (ISRM)"* (Tokyo (Japan); September 25–30 1995), 105–108.

Verhelst, F., David, P., Fermont, W., Jegers, L. & Vervoort, A. 1996. Correlation of 3D-computerized tomographic scans and 2D-colour image analysis of Westphalian coal by means of multivariate statistics. *International Journal of Coal Geology*, Vol. 29, January 1996, 1–21.

Vervoort, A., Halleux L. & Grégoire, C. 2003. Crinoidal Limestone: Observation of Discontinuities from Micro- to Macro-scale. In: P. Degryse and J. Elsen (eds) *Industrial Minerals – Resources, Characteristics and Applications. Aardundige Mededelingen* 13, Universitaire Pers Leuven, 49–58.

Vervoort, A. 2003. Effect of tri-axial loading and unloading on fracturing of rock. In: *Proceedings of 3rd International Symposium on Rock Stress*, Kumamoto (Japan), November 4–6 2003, A.A. Balkema, Rotterdam (in press).

Wevers, M., de Meester, P. & Swennen, R. 2001. Microfocus X-ray computer tomography in materials research. *The Journal of the British Institute of Non-Destructive Testing*, Vol. 43(10), 2001, 658–663.

Soils

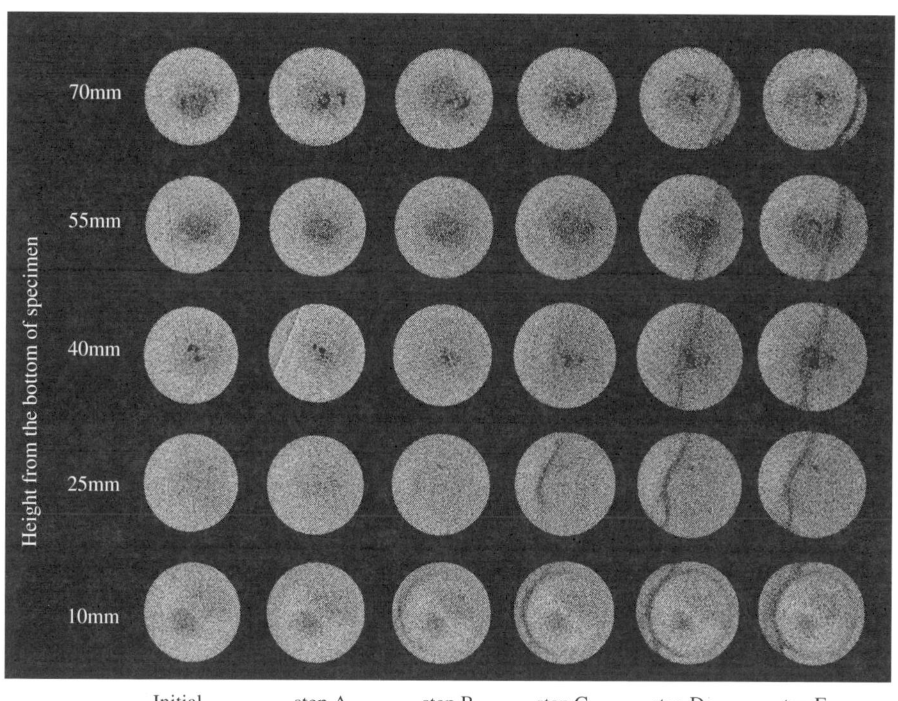
Height from the bottom of specimen
70mm
55mm
40mm
25mm
10mm
Initial
step A
step B
step C
step D
step E

X-ray CT for Geomaterials; Soils, Concrete, Rocks – Otani & Obara (eds.)
 ISBN 90 5809 666 1

Artifacts of X-ray CT data in the analysis of geomaterial properties

T. Mukunoki
GeoEngineering Centre at Queen's-RMC, Queen's University, Kingston, Ontario, Canada

J. Otani & Y. Obara
Department of Civil and Environmental Engineering, Kumamoto University, Kumamoto, Japan

K. Kaneko
Graduate School of Engineering, Hokkaido University, Hokkaido, Japan

ABSTRACT: Two key issues, the *beam hardening effect* and the *partial volume effect*, which qualitatively analyze X-ray CT images, have been investigated in previous studies. Both factors always affect the assessment of the X-ray CT image. The objective of this study is to clarify the basic properties of X-ray CT data in the analysis of geomaterial properties. This paper deals with artifacts due to changing the power voltage of the X-ray tube and the partial volume effects caused by variation in the occupation ratio of soil particles in a voxel.

1 INTRODUCTION

The X-ray Computed Tomography (CT) method is an inverse analysis in which one numerically obtains two-dimensional density information based on X-ray beam attenuation in the object (Avinash and Malcolm 1987). This numerical density spread is called the "CT-value", and an X-ray CT image is composed of these CT-values. The X-ray CT method has been practically applied for medical diagnostics. Recently, it has become applicable as nondestructive test methods in the several industrial fields such as petroleum technology, geology/geotechnical engineering, paleontology and petrology/rock engineering.

In the geotechnical field, the X-ray CT scanner has been used to analyze physical properties, flow patterns/hydraulic properties of air, water/solutions and changes of physical properties due to external forces. For instance, in Peyton *et al.* 1992 and Zeng *et al.* 1996, undisturbed soil cores were scanned and macro pore diameters, and bulk density was evaluated based on image processing analysis and statistical analysis of CT data. Anderson and Hopmans 1994, and Otani *et al.* 2002a assessed the distribution of air voids in X-ray CT images. They distinguished air voids from sands, sand packs and core samples of improved clay soil using the thresholding technique. Several other important studies should be mentioned: visualization of water seepage in rocks and soils (Anderson *et al.* 1992, Hejis *et al.* 1995, Sugawara *et al.* 1998, and Otani *et al.* 2001b), air permeation (Wong and Wibowo 2000) and oil permeation (Wang *et al.* 1985) in sand and diffusivity of heavy ions in clay gels (Nakashima 2003).

As assessments of mechanical properties, Desrues *et al.* 1996, Alshibli *et al.* 2000, Wong 2000, Otani *et al.* 2000, Otani *et al.* 2002a and Alshibli *et al.* 2003 studied the change of pore structure and density evolution in soil and cracks for rocks at residual condition. Otani *et al.* 2002b developed the triaxial compression test apparatus for the industrial X-ray CT scanner and assessed the progressive failure of sand specimens. The X-ray CT scanner has been successfully applied in several studies. However, two key issues, the *beam hardening effect*, and the *partial volume effect*, must be understood in the analysis of X-ray CT imaging.

Beam hardening effect causes the edges of an object to appear brighter than the center, even if the material is the same throughout. The level of beam hardening effect depends on the relationship between performance of the X-ray CT scanner and an object's size/material density. Partial volume effect indicates inherent resolution limitations. This will be discussed in the context of smaller scale elements such as micro pores and cracks in soil and rock materials, elements which are smaller than voxel dimensions. A voxel is a minimum element of an X-ray CT image. To analyze the X-ray CT images of geomaterials, the CT operator should consider artifacts because of the beam hardening effect, and the partial volume effect.

The objective of this study is to clarify the beam hardening effect and the partial volume effects on X-ray CT data in the analysis of geomaterial properties. The X-ray CT system and related concepts are explained in the following section. Then, the beam hardening effect assessed at different power voltages, and the partial volume effects are investigated based on CT-values of soil particle with several grain sizes.

2 X-RAY CT SCANNER

2.1 *System of industrial X-ray CT scanner*

In general, there are four types of X-ray CT scanner (Avinash and Malcolm 1987, Otani *et al.* 2000b, Ketcham and Carlson 2001). The X-ray CT scanner installed in Kumamoto University uses a translating-rotational fan beam geometry. The specification of this system is shown in Table 1. In this apparatus, the collimated X-ray beam is moved around the circumference of the specimen by rotating and translating the specimen table. The data is processed and the cross sectional images are reconstructed using an engineering workstation.

Table 1. The specification of X-ray CT scanner.

Scan type	Traverse/Rotation
Supplied Voltage for X-ray beam	300 kV/200 kV
Number of detectors	176 channels
Maximum size of the specimen	D: 400 mm × H: 600 mm
Thickness of X-ray beam	0.5 mm, 1 mm, 2 mm
Spatial resolution	0.2 mm (diameter of the hole) for 20 mm thickness of steel

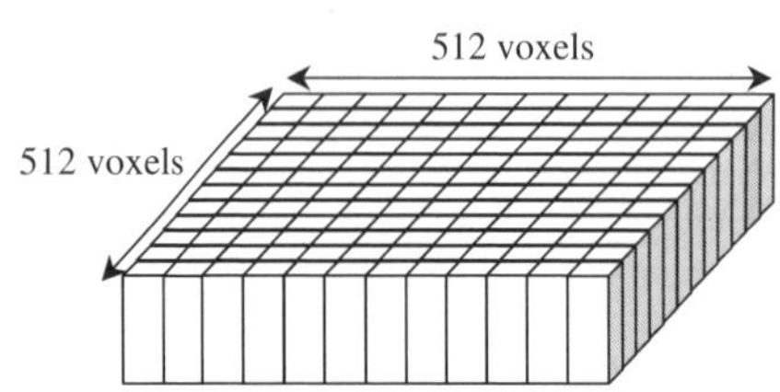

(a) X-ray CT image (voxels)

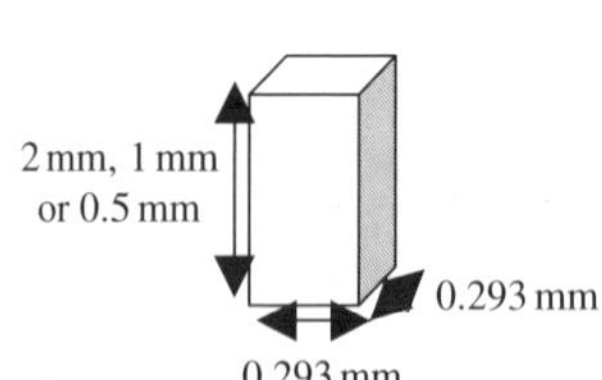

(b) Voxel

Figure 1. Concept of X-ray CT image.

2.2 *CT-value*

In the image processing analysis, a CT-value is defined as:

$$\text{CT-value} = (\mu_t - \mu_w)\,\kappa/\mu_w \tag{1}$$

where μ_t is the coefficient of absorption at scanning point; μ_W is the coefficient of absorption for water; and κ is the material constant. It is noted that this material constant is fixed to a value of 1000. Thus, the CT-value of air should be −1000 because the coefficient of absorption for air is zero. Likewise, the value for water is 0 from the definition of equation (1). Since the coefficient of X-ray absorption is proportional to the material density, the CT-value should be proportional to the material density. Otani *et al.* (2000b) reported that there were linear relationships between bulk densities for several geomaterial and CT-values. The CT-values are processed as voxels and these values are reconstructed as two-dimensional (2-D) images.

2.3 *X-ray CT images*

Figure 1 illustrates an X-ray CT image. The scanning space is divided by 512 × 512 voxels. The total number of color levels on the X-ray CT image is 256. Three-dimensional (3-D) images can be reconstructed by superposing 2-D images. Volume rendering with respect to only interesting elements of the subject can be created. Otani *et al.* (2000b) extracted the CT-values of shear zones developed locally in clay specimen at the residual state in 3 dimensions.

2.4 *Thresholding value*

Figure 2 illustrates the color resolution in an X-ray CT image. Although it seems that image (a) is different from image (b), they have exactly same CT-values as shown in Figure 2 (I). This sample has the range of CT-values from 0 to 500. The CT-value of image (a) thresholds from to 0 to 500, on the other hand those of image (b) threshold from −1000 to 500. It is noted that image (b) is smoothed due to having wide range of CT-values to display; therefore image (b) loses the visual accuracy. It hence is important to know the distribution of CT-values as shown in Figure 2 (II) and then, to define and adjust the thresholding value as the need arises.

3 ARTIFACTS

3.1 *Scanning condition*

The X-ray CT scanner used in this study has several functions such as changing the power voltage of the

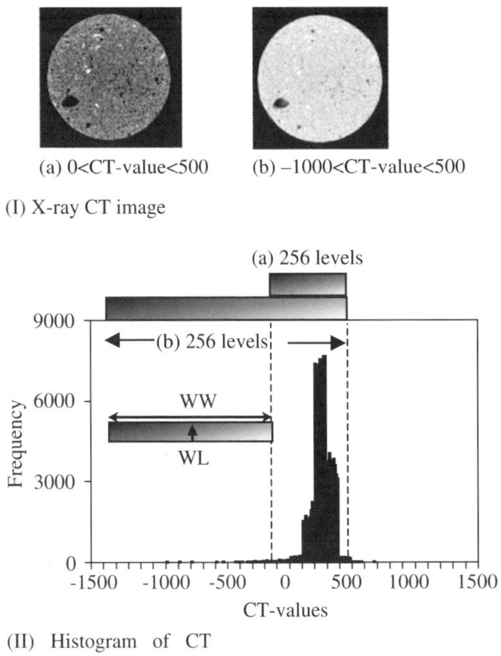

Figure 2. Histogram of CT-value (Adopted Otani *et al.* 2002).

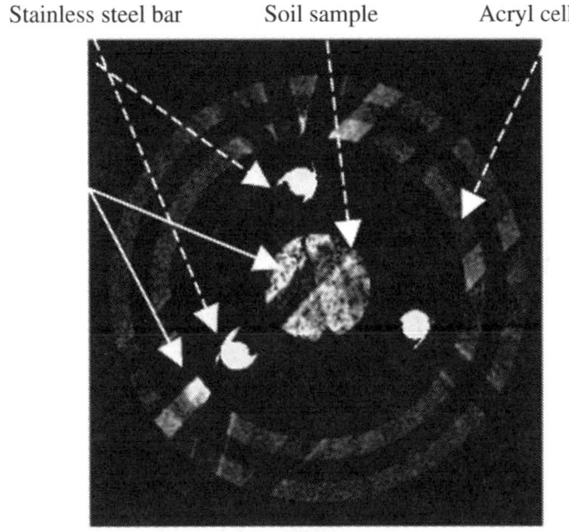

Figure 3. X-ray CT image of the conventional triaxial compression test apparatus with artifacts (Otani *et al.* 2001).

X-ray tube (200 kV or 300 kV), and changing the scanning area ($\phi = 150$ mm or 400 mm), scanning pitch, fan angle of X-ray beam and scanning width (2 mm, 1 mm or 0.5 mm) (see Table 1). The scanning width indicates the thickness of a collimated X-ray beam and it corresponds to the thickness of a voxel (see Fig. 1). A scanning area of $\phi = 150$ mm and a scanning width of 1.0 mm was selected in this study. The dimension of a voxel is therefore $0.293 \times 0.293 \times 1.0\,\text{mm}^3$.

3.2 *Beam hardening effect*

The most frequently encountered artifact in the X-ray CT scanning is the beam hardening effect, which causes the edges of an object to appear brighter than the center, even if the material is the same throughout. The artifact derives its name from its underlying cause – the increase in mean X-ray energy, or "hardening" of the X-ray beam as it passes through the scanned object. Since a lower energy X-ray beam is attenuated more readily than a higher energy X-ray beam, a polychromatic beam passing through an object loses the lower energy parts of its spectrum. In the X-ray CT images of a sufficiently attenuating material, this process generally manifests itself as an artificial darkening at the center of long beam path, and a corresponding brightening near the edges of objects. In objects with roughly circular cross sections this process can cause the edge to appear brighter than the interior, but in irregular objects it is commonly difficult to differentiate between beam hardening artifacts and actual material variations. For instance, Figure 3 presents an X-ray CT image of conventional triaxial test apparatus at the power voltage of 300 kV. An acryl cell, clay sample and three tie bars made of stainless steel exist in the scan area. The tie bars absorb the energy of the X-ray beam so much that artifacts are present. The X-rays which pass through the object are attenuated by Compton scattering and photoelectric absorption. Ketcham and Carlson (2001) reported that Compton scattering is dominant at high X-ray energies up to 5–10 MeV and photoelectric absorption is dominant at low energies up to approximately 50–100 keV. It was reported that attenuation of the X-ray beam by Compton scattering should be negligible. Figures 4 and 5 give X-ray CT images of cement mortar with three different diameters, which were scanned by a power voltage of 200 and 300 kV, and their CT-value distributions were measured along a diameter. These images in Figure 4 are displayed using the same threshold value (450–950). In the X-ray CT images of samples with the diameter of 100 and 140 mm scanned by power voltage of 200 kV, artifacts can be observed in the outline of the sample due to an increase in specimen diameter. An X-ray CT image at 300 kV with a diameter of 140 mm also has artifacts. The CT-values for a specimen with a 50 mm diameter distribute almost uniformly (see Figure 5 (a)). However, it is clear that beam hardening effects were caused in the Figure 5 (b) and (c). As shown in Figures 5 (b) and (c), beam hardening effect is lessened at 300 kV compared to 200 kV. Because X-rays generated at 200 kV have lower energy than those at 300 kV, the beam hardening is more prominent. In Ketcham and Carlson (2001), the

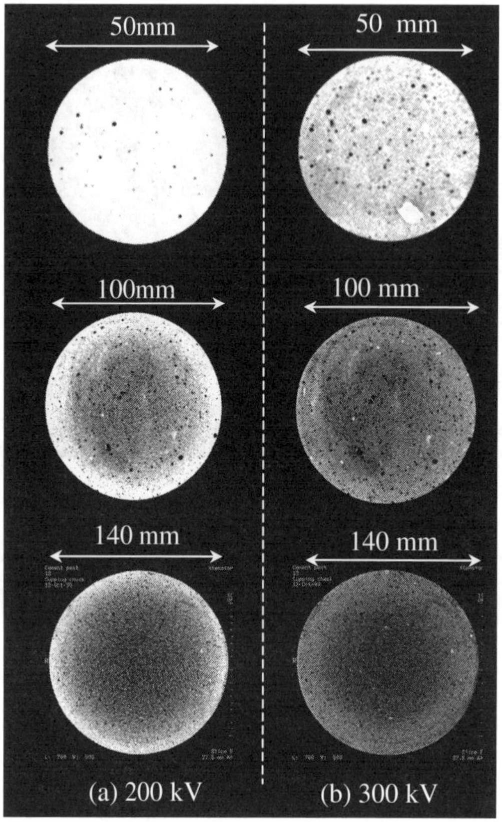

Figure 4. X-ray CT images scanned at two different power voltages.

relationship between the magnitude of power voltage and the beam hardening effect was studied. An X-ray beam with higher energy propagates more effectively than that with lower energy; however it is less sensitive to changes in material density and composition. The intensity of the X-ray beam directly affects the signal to noise (S/N) ratio and thus image quality. Although higher intensities reduce the beam hardening effect, they often require a larger object. As seen in Figure 5, the distribution of the CT-values at both power voltages has no significant difference except for the edge of the object. The use of a 300 kV power voltage in the X-ray tube is suitable for analyzing geomaterials in this study.

3.3 *Optimization to beam hardening effect*

Beam hardening changes the CT-value of objects depending on its location in an image. Thus, the attempt to utilize a single CT-value range to identify and quantify the extent of a particular material can become problematic. One measure that is sometimes taken is

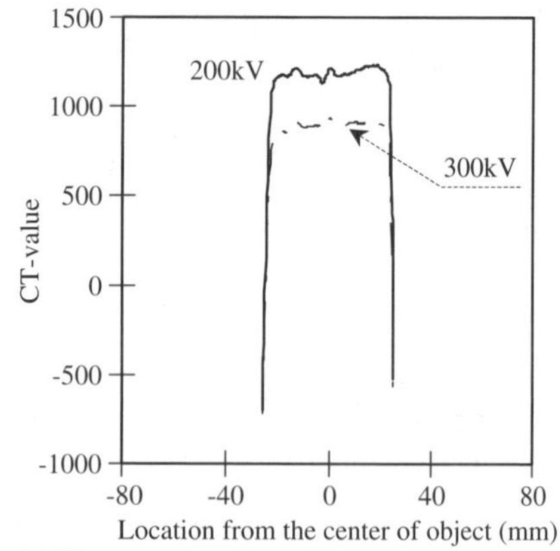

(a) 50 mm

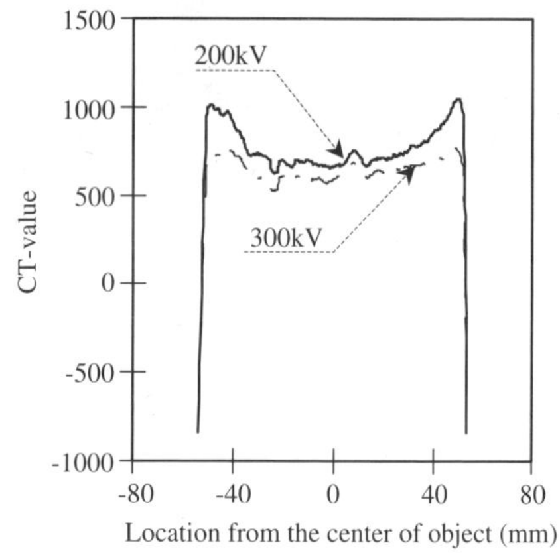

(b) 100 mm

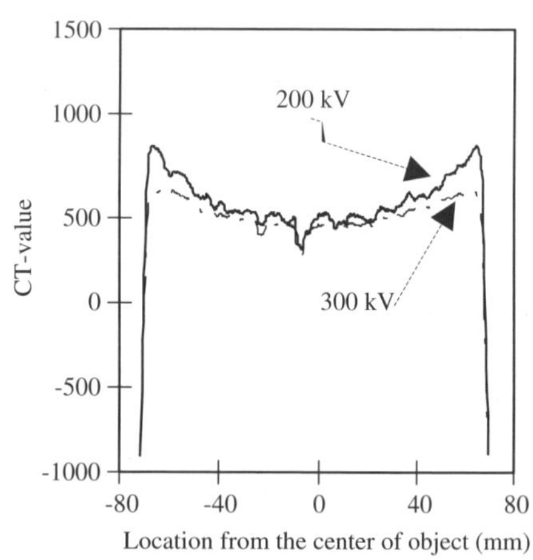

(c) 140 mm

Figure 5. Evaluation of beam hardening effect.

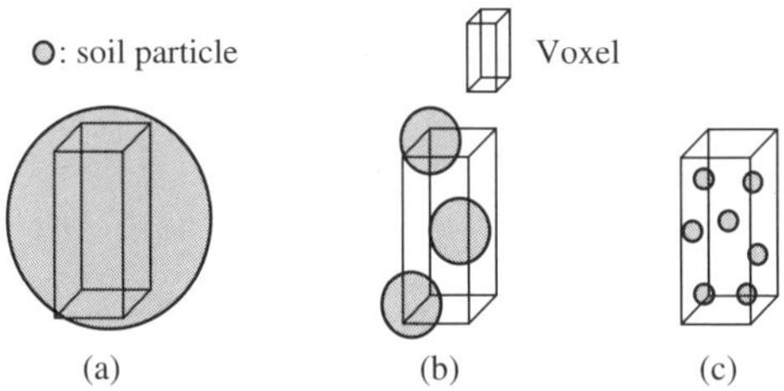

Figure 6. Factor of partial volume effect (Adopted Otani *et al.* 2002a).

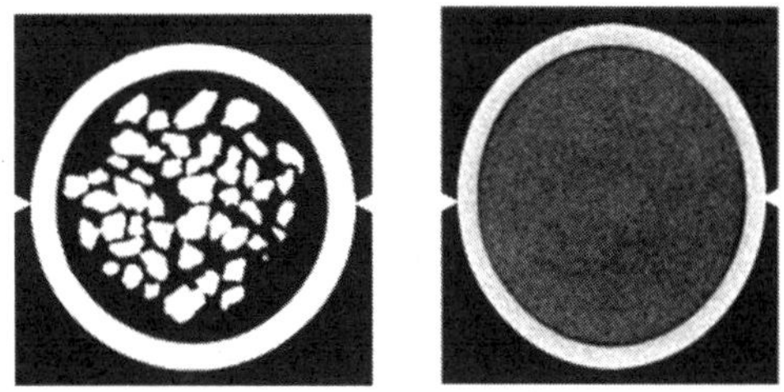

(a) 2.00–4.75 mm
(0<CT-value<500)

(b) 75–106 μm
(0<CT-value<250)

Figure 7. X-ray CT images of soil particle with each grain size.

the removal of the outer edge of the image so that the center can be analyzed (see Figure 4). Although this technique removes the worst part of the problem, the artifact is continuous and thus even subsets of the image are affected. If the cross-sectional area of the object changes from slice to slice, the extent of the beam hardening effect also changes, making such a strategy prone to error.

There are a number of possible remedies for beam hardening, ranging from sample and scanning preparation to data processing. For small samples, the effects of beam hardening are lessened and can therefore be ignored. Most geomaterials of interest cause enough attenuation so that beam hardening is noticeable. However, higher beams which are generated by more than 300 kV are less sensitive to attenuation contrasts in materials, and thus may not provide sufficient differentiation between elements of interest.

3.4 *Partial volume effects*

Since each voxel in a CT image represents the attenuation properties of an object, the resulting CT-value represents an average of their properties. If the specific voxel contains both air and soil particles, the CT-value will not represent the true structure of soil particles. All material boundaries are blurred to some extent, and thus any one voxel can affect the CT-values of surrounding voxels because the X-ray CT method has inherent resolution limitations. This concept is termed the partial volume effect. Although the factors described above can make CT-values more problematic to interpret quantitatively, they also represent an opportunity to extract unexpectedly fine-scale data from CT images.

Figure 6 illustrates the relation between soil particles and voxel dimension (Adopted Otani *et al.* 2002a). This diagram indicates; (a) a soil particle is larger than size of a voxel, (b) a soil particle is larger than base area of a voxel and (c) a soil particle is much smaller than size of a voxel. Otani *et al.* 2002a investigated the relationship between voxel dimensions and pore space in the soil material and evaluated the pore size

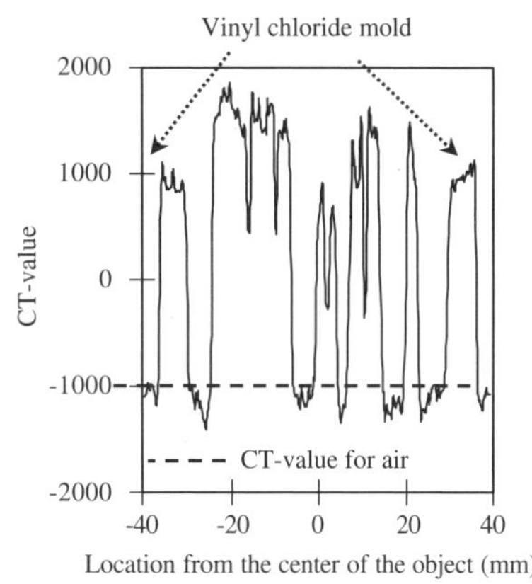

(a) 2.00–4.75 mm

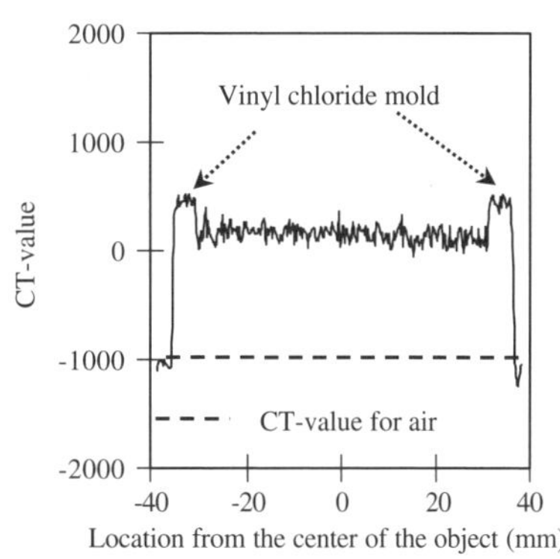

(b) 75–106 μm

Figure 8. CT-value distribution.

based on an X-ray CT binary image. Since the CT-value is proportional to the material density, the CT-value should be different in each situation in Figure 6. Figure 7 (a) and (b) are X-ray CT images with the average soil particle size larger than 4.75 mm and 106 μm respectively. Figure 8 shows CT-value distributions between arrows as shown in Figure 7 (a) and (b).

Table 2. Mean CT-value and standard deviation of soil sample with each grain size.

Size of soil particles (mm)	Average CT-value	Standard deviation
−0.075	25.2	5.4
0.075–0.106	158.9	10.0
0.106–0.250	210.6	26.9
0.250–0.425	769.9	60.7
0.425–0.850	1130.3	191.7
0.85–2.00	1463.4	156.6
2.00–4.75	1448.5	140.5

The average diameter of grain size scanned is larger than the size of a voxel.

However, the CT-value distribution in Figure 8(b) represents a smaller variation than that of Figure 8(a). The average grain size is smaller than the voxel dimension and it is therefore difficult to distinguish soil particles from pore spaces. Table 2 presents mean CT-values and standard deviations of soil samples with varying of grain sizes. Grain sizes with a mean CT-value of more than 1000 and a standard deviation greater than 100 are larger than dimension as a voxel. However, a sample with fine grains would have smaller CT-values and standard deviations than that of a sample with a large grain size. Since the resolution of X-ray CT images depends on the size of a voxel, the grain size of soil samples should be selected to comply with the voxel dimensions of the scanner used.

4 CONCLUSIONS

In this paper, the basic properties of the X-ray CT scanner were outlined. The beam hardening effect and the partial volume effect in the analysis of geomaterials was also discussed.

Since the beam hardening effect is present during X-ray propagation through an object, the CT-value affected by the beam hardening effect must be scrutinized. For small samples the effects of beam hardening are small and can therefore be ignored as long as the CT-value at the center of long ray path has no significant variation. Although it is possible to apply an X-ray beam with the sufficient energy to reduce the beam hardening effect, the X-ray CT image obtained will lose its sensitivity to changes in material density and composition.

The visual resolution of the X-ray CT image depends on the voxel dimension. Partial volume effects must be considered when analyzing CT-values and X-ray CT images. In the case of aggregate materials such as soils, the small disparity between grain size and voxel dimension means that the partial volume effect is significant. Examining the calibration between partial CT-values and grain size can solve this issue.

REFERENCES

Alshibli, K.A., Sture, S., Costes, C., Frank, M.L., Lankton, M.R., Batiste, S.N. and Swanson, R.A. 2000. Assessment of Localized Deformations in Sand Using X-Ray Computed Tomography, *Geotechnical Testing Journal, GJODJ*, Vol. 23, No. 3: 274–299.

Alshibli, K.A., Batiste, S. and Sture, S. 2003. Strain Localization in Sand: Plane Strain versus Triaxial Compression, *Journal of Geotechnical and Geoenvironmental Engineering*, 129 (6): 483–494.

Anderson, S.H., Peyton, R.L., Wigger, J.W. and Ganzer, C.J. 1992. Influence of aggregate size of solute transport as measured using computed tomography, *Geoderma*, 53: 387–398.

Anderson, S.H. and Hopmans, J.W. 1994. Tomography of soil-water-root processes, SSSA special Publication number 36, Soil Science Society of America.

Avinash, C.K. and Malcolm, S. 1987. Principles of Computerized Tomographic Imaging, Published under the sponsorship of the IEEE Engineering in Medicine and Biology Society.

Desrues, J., Chambon, R., Mokni, M. and Mazerolle, F. 1996. Void ratio evolution inside shear bands in triaxial sand specimens studies by computed tomography, *Geotechnique*, 46 (3): 529–546.

Heijs, W.J., Anton Lange, J., de Schoute, J.F.Th. and Bouma, J. 1995. Computed tomography as a tool for non-destructive analysis of flow patterns in macroporous clay soils, *Geoderma*, 64: 183–196.

Ketcham, A.R. and Carlson, D.W. 2001. Acquisition, optimization and interpretation of X-ray computed tomographic imagery: application to the geosciences, *Computer & Geosciences*, 27: 381–400.

Nakashima, Y. 2003. Diffusivity measurement of heavy ions in Wyoming montmorillonite gels by X-ray computed tomography, *Journal of Contaminant Hydrology*, 61: 147–156.

Otani, J., Mukunoki, T., Obara, Y. and Sugawara, K. 2000a. Application of X-ray CT to Soil and Rock Engineering, Proceedings of an international conference on Geotechnical & Geological Engineering, CD-ROM: \paper\pf\0297.pdf.

Otani, J., Mukunoki, T. and Obara, Y. 2000b. Application of X-ray CT Method for Characterization of Failure in Soils, *Soils & Foundations the Japanese Geotechnical Society*, 40 (2): 113–120.

Otani, J., Kikuchi, Y., Mukunoki, T. and Yamagata, N. 2001b. Evaluation of hydraulic property of light weight soil with air foams, Proc. of the International Workshop on lightweight Geo-Materials, pp. 159–164.

Otani, J., Mukunoki, T. and Kikuchi, Y. 2002a. Visualization for engineering property of in-situ light weight soils with air foams, *Soils & Foundations the Japanese Geotechnical Society*, 42 (3): 93–105.

Otani, J., Mukunoki, T. and Obara, Y. 2002b. Characterization of failure in sand under triaxial compression using a industrial X-ray CT scanner, *IJPMG-International Journal of Physical Modeling in Geotechnics*, 1: 15–22.

Peyton, R.L., Haeffner, B.A., Anderson, S.H. and Ganzer, C.J. 1992. Applying X-ray CT to measure micropore diameters in undisturbed soil cores, *Geoderma*, 53: 329–340.

Pralle, N., Bahner, M.L. and Benkler, J. 2001. Computer tomographic analysis of undisturbed samples of loose sands, *Canadian Geotechnical Journal*, 38: 770–781.

Sugawara, K., Obara, Y., Kaneko, K., Koike, K., Ohmi, M. and Aoi, T. 1997. Visualization of Three-Dimensional Structure of Rocks Using X-Ray CT Method, Proc. of the 1st ARMS, Vol. 2, Seoul, Korea, pp. 769–774.

Sugawara, K., Kojima, R., Obara, Y., Sato, A. and Shimada, H. 1998. Crack opening analysis by means of the X-rays CT, *Journal of the Mining and Material Processing Institute of Japan*, 114 (12): 881–887 (in Japanese).

Wang, S.Y., Huag, Y.B., Pereria, V. and Gryte, C.C. 1985. Applicaton of computed tomography to oil recovery from porous media, *Applied Optics*, 24 (23): 4021–4027.

Wellington, S.L. and Vinegar, H.J. 1987. X-ray Computerized Tomography, *Journal of Petroleum Technology*, 39 (8): 885–898.

Wong, R.C.K. 2000. Shear Deformation of Locked Sand in Triaxial Compression, *Geotechnical Testing Journal, GTJODJ*, Vol. 23, No. 2: 158–170.

Wong, R.C.K. and Wibowo, R. 2000. Tomographic Evaluation of Air and Water Flow Patterns in Soil Column, *Geotechnical Testing Journal, GTJODJ*, Vol. 23, No. 4: 413–422.

Zeng, Y., Ganzer, C.J., Peyton, R.L. and Anderson, S.H. 1996. Fractal Dimension and Lacunarity of Bulk Density Determined with X-ray Computed Tomography, *Soil Science America Journal*, 60: 1718–1724.

X-ray CT for Geomaterials; Soils, Concrete, Rocks – Otani & Obara (eds.)
© 2004 Swets & Zeitlinger. Lisse, ISBN 90 5809 666 1

Original free Mathematica® programs for the calculation of transport properties of porous media

Y. Nakashima
National Institute of Advanced Industrial Science and Technology, Tsukuba, Japan

T. Yamaguchi
KGT Inc., Tokyo, Japan

ABSTRACT: We developed some original Mathematica® programs to calculate the transport properties (porosity, surface-to-volume ratio of the pore space, tortuosity of the pore structure, and permeability) of isotropic porous media using X-ray CT images. The programs were reviewed in this paper, and the application to the microfocus CT images of randomly packed sand grains was demonstrated. The programs are available for free download on the author's web site (URL = http://staff.aist.go.jp/nakashima.yoshito/progeng.htm).

1 INTRODUCTION

Groundwater and contaminants migrate in water-saturated porous geo-materials (e.g. soils and rocks). The estimate of the transport properties (e.g. diffusion coefficient and porosity) of these geo-materials is thus important in terms of groundwater hydrology. X-ray computed tomography (CT) enables us to acquire data on the three-dimensional (3-D) pore structure of the geo-materials. Computer programs to calculate the transport properties using the acquired digital CT images are needed. However, to our knowledge, there were few free programs publicly available on the Internet. Thus we have developed such programs for Mathematica® version 4 or later, available for free download at http://staff.aist.go.jp/nakashima.yoshito/progeng.htm.

To facilitate the study on the porous media using X-ray CT and personal computers, the following package-type Mathematica® programs were reviewed in this paper: Kai3D.m, RW2D.m, RW3D.m, and DMAP.m. Processing methods of the program outputs to estimate the porosity, surface-to-volume ratio of the pore space, tortuosity, and permeability are also described. The application of the programs to the 3-D images of a sand grain pack obtained by microfocus X-ray CT was demonstrated.

2 DESCRIPTION OF PROGRAMS

All programs are listed in Table 1. They are package-type programs and for Mathematica® version 4 or later. Users are required to prepare the CT image data on the porous media as text files (not binary files) without headers. Thus, for example, the conversion of TIFF images into text files is needed using the Graphic Converter software (http://www.lemkesoft.de/en/graphcon.htm).

Table 1. List of the original Mathematica® programs.

Program name	Function
Kai3D.m	Cluster labeling
RW2D.m	2-D random walk
RW3D.m	3-D random walk
DMAP.m	3-D mapping of tortuosity and porosity

Kai3D.m is a cluster labeling program to examine the connectivity of pore voxels (Watanabe et al. 1999, Nakashima & Watanabe 2002). Some pores in porous media are connected to form a single large percolation cluster responsible for the macroscopic transport of materials; other pores are isolated and contribute to neither macroscopic diffusion nor Darcy flow. The cluster labeling allows us to characterize such pore clusters. The algorithm of the cluster labeling obeys Hoshen & Kopelman (1976), and the cluster neighborhood rule is based on Ikeda et al. (2000). Kai3D.m reads the 3-D images as a set of contiguous slices (2-D images), and calculates the volume and surface area for each pore cluster. The surface-to-volume ratio of pore is an important transport property because it is related to the pore diameter (Guéguen & Palciauskas 1994). Users can calculate the surface-to-volume ratio of each pore cluster using the program output.

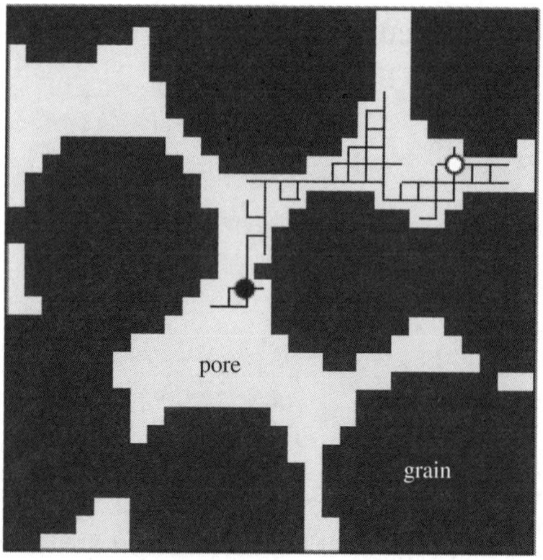

Figure 1. Example of the 2-D lattice-walk trajectory in a porous medium over 200 time steps obtained using RW2D.m. The image system is 30 × 30 voxels. The initial and final positions of the walker are marked by solid and open circles, respectively.

RW2D.m, RW3D.m, and DMAP.m are random walk programs to simulate the diffusion of non-sorbing species in the pore (Watanabe & Nakashima 2001, 2002, Nakashima & Yamaguchi 2003). The random walkers should be non-sorbing because the purpose is to calculate the geometrical tortuosity and the undesirable effects of the sorption of walkers on the solid surface should be eliminated. An example of the random walk trajectory is shown in Figure 1. The random walk algorithm used is the lattice walk in a simple cubic lattice (e.g. Stauffer 1985), and walkers migrate on the discrete voxels whose gray-levels correspond to pore space. A voxel is chosen randomly as a start position of the lattice walk trial at $\tau = 0$ where τ is the dimensionless integer time. The walker executes a random jump to one of the nearest unoccupied sites; τ is incremented by unit time after the jump so that the time becomes $\tau + 1$. If the randomly selected site or voxel is occupied by an obstacle or solid, the jump is not performed, but the time becomes $\tau + 1$.

The main output of RW2D.m and RW3D.m is a mean-square displacement of the walkers (text file):

$$\langle r(\tau)^2 \rangle = \frac{1}{n}\sum_{i=1}^{n} r_i(\tau)^2 \qquad (1)$$

where $<r^2>$ is the mean-square displacement, n is the number of runs of the random walk, and $r_i(\tau)$ is the distance between the walker's position at time τ and that at $\tau = 0$ for the ith run. The diffusion coefficient, D, is related to the time-derivative of $<r^2>$:

$$<r(t)^2> = 2dDt \qquad (2)$$

where t is time and the constant d is 2 for the 2-D space and 3 for the 3-D space. Therefore it is possible to calculate the tortuosity (the ratio of D in the free space to D in porous media) using the mean-square displacement data.

RW2D.m is a 2-D random walk program, and requires a single 2-D image of the pore structure as a text file. RW3D.m simulates a 3-D random walk, and 3-D image data as a set of contiguous 2-D slices are needed. In both programs, a specified number of pore voxels near the center of the image system are chosen randomly as start points of the random walk. If the chosen voxel is pore, the random walk simulation is carried out until τ (i.e. random walk time step) reaches a specified limit. The programs output the trajectory for some random walk trials on the computer display (e.g. Fig. 1).

DMAP.m simulates the "out-diffusion" laboratory experiments. Cubic 3-D CT image data on the porous media should be provided as a set of text files of 2-D square matrices (both the 3-D system size and voxel dimension should be cubic). DMAP.m reads the text files, and executes random walk (lattice walk) in the pore space of the porous media. A specified number of voxels are chosen randomly as start points of the random walk. If the chosen voxel is pore, the random walk simulation is carried out until the walker goes out of the 3-D image system. If the chosen voxel is not pore but solid, the random walk will not be performed. The time required for each walker to escape from the 3-D image system is recorded to calculate the cumulated flux (i.e. integrated number of walkers escaped from the 3-D system by the time τ). The cumulated flux data are used to calculate the tortuosity of the porous media. Although DMAP.m is for the tortuosity calculation, the porosity can also be obtained as a byproduct by counting the hit number of the pore voxels in the random choice of the start positions for the lattice walk (Monte Carlo integral). By dividing the image system into sub-cubes (Fig. 2), DMAP.m allows us to map the 3-D distribution of the tortuosity and porosity for each sub-cube. This is useful to characterize the pore structure of heterogeneous porous media.

3 ESTIMATE OF TRANSPORT PROPERTIES

The methods of estimating transport properties (porosity, surface-to-volume ratio, tortuosity, and permeability) of the isotropic porous media using the

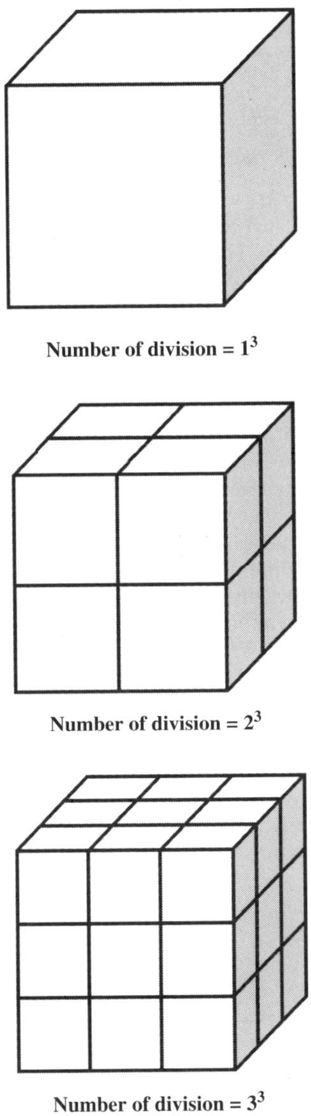

Figure 2. Division of the 3-D cubic image system into sub-cubes in DMAP.m. Tortuosity and porosity are calculated for each sub-cube. Examples for the 1-division, 8-division, and 27-division are shown.

programs are described. The porosity, ϕ, refers to the volume fraction of the pore voxels in the discrete 3-D image of the porous media. The porosity can be obtained as an outcome of the cluster labeling of all pore voxels by Kai3D.m. DMAP.m also allows us to obtain ϕ by counting the hit number of the pore voxels in the random choice of the start positions for the lattice walk trials. The former gives the exact value of ϕ, whereas the latter contains the stochastic fluctuation derived from the Monte Carlo integral method. However, a larger number trial of the random choice of the start positions would reduce this stochastic error.

The surface-to-volume ratio of the pore cluster can be obtained using the cluster labeling results by Kai3D.m. The ratio is calculated by dividing the surface area of the pore cluster by the pore cluster volume. This is an exact value because Kai3D.m examines all voxels in the 3-D image system.

It is also possible to calculate the surface-to-volume ratio by analyzing $\langle r^2 \rangle$ which is the output of RW3D.m. This theory comes from the nuclear magnetic resonance (NMR) laboratory diffusion experiments. It should be noted that D for the random walkers migrating in porous media is no longer a constant, but depends on the diffusion time. The diffusion coefficient is defined as follows:

$$D(t) = \frac{1}{6}\frac{d\langle r(t)^2\rangle}{dt} \tag{3}$$

In the short-time limit, the normalized D in a porous medium with negligible NMR surface relaxivity is expressed theoretically by

$$\frac{D}{D_0} = 1 - \frac{4}{9\sqrt{\pi}}\left(\frac{S}{V}\right)_{\text{pore}}\sqrt{D_0 t} + c_1 t \qquad \text{as } t \to 0 \tag{4}$$

where D_0 is D in the free space (i.e. $\phi = 1$), $(S/V)_{\text{pore}}$ is the surface-to-volume ratio of the pore space, and c_1 is a constant (e.g. Dunn et al. 2002). D_0 is a time-independent quantity. Integrating Equation 3 with respect to t, we have

$$\frac{\langle r(t)^2\rangle}{\langle r(t)^2\rangle\big|_{\phi=1}} = \frac{\int_0^t 6D\,dt}{\int_0^t 6D_0\,dt} = \frac{1}{t}\int_0^t\left(\frac{D}{D_0}\right)dt \tag{5}$$

The substitution of Equation 4 into Equation 5 yields

$$\frac{\langle r(t)^2\rangle}{\langle r(t)^2\rangle\big|_{\phi=1}} = 1 - \frac{8}{27\sqrt{\pi}}\left(\frac{S}{V}\right)_{\text{pore}}\sqrt{D_0 t} + c_2 t \tag{6}$$

where c_2 is a constant. The exact solution (Equation 7) for $\langle r^2 \rangle$ in the free space can be used to translate t into τ (Nakashima & Watanabe 2002):

$$\langle r^2\rangle = 6D_0 t = a^2\tau \tag{7}$$

where a is a lattice constant of the simple cubic lattice (i.e. voxel dimension of the CT image). In conclusion we obtain Equation 8 (as $\tau \rightarrow 0$):

$$\frac{\langle r(t)^2 \rangle}{\langle r(t)^2 \rangle \big|_{\phi=1}} = 1 - \frac{8a}{27\sqrt{6\pi}} \left(\frac{S}{V} \right)_{\text{pore}} \sqrt{\tau} + c_3 \tau \qquad (8)$$

where c_3 is a constant. This is the final expression for the calculation of $(S/V)_{\text{pore}}$ using RW3D.m.

It should be noted that estimating $(S/V)_{\text{pore}}$ using Equation 8 contains inevitable stochastic error derived from the stochastic nature of the random walk. However, a larger number of the random walk trials would reduce this stochastic error. Another problem related Equation 8 is that RW3D.m probes only the pore structure near the center of the 3-D image system because the random walk in RW3D.m always starts from near the center of the image system. Thus $(S/V)_{\text{pore}}$ obtained by Equation 8 is the value for the pore structure located near the center of the system, and the pore structure information near the eight corners of the 3-D image system is omitted. Thus, if the porous medium is heterogeneous, the $(S/V)_{\text{pore}}$ value by Equation 8 is different from the exact value by Kai3D.m.

The tortuosity of the porous media refers to the ratio of D for non-sorbing tracers in the bulk water (i.e. porous media of $\phi = 1$) to D in water-saturated porous media. It is possible to calculate the tortuosity using RW3D.m and DMAP.m.

The tortuosity can be calculated by taking the time-derivative of $\langle r^2 \rangle$ obtained by RW3D.m (Nakashima & Watanabe 2002):

$$\frac{D_0}{D_\infty} = \frac{a^2}{\dfrac{d\langle r(\tau)^2 \rangle}{d\tau}} \qquad \text{as } \tau \rightarrow \infty \qquad (9)$$

where D_∞ is D for the porous medium in the limit of $\tau \rightarrow \infty$.

The tortuosity can also be estimated using the cumulated flux, M, (integrated number of walkers escaped from the 3-D image system) obtained by DMAP.m (Nakashima & Yamaguchi 2003):

$$M(\tau) = M_\infty \left(1 - \sum_{i=1}^{4} E_i(\tau) \right) \qquad (10)$$

where

$$E_1(\tau) = \frac{512}{\pi^6} \exp\left[-K\tau \right]$$

$$E_2(\tau) = \frac{512}{3\pi^6} \exp\left[-\frac{11K\tau}{3} \right]$$

$$E_3(\tau) = \frac{1132544}{18225\pi^6} \exp\left[-9K\tau \right]$$

$$E_4(\tau) = \frac{512}{27\pi^6} \exp\left[-\frac{19K\tau}{3} \right]$$

The quantity M_∞ is the M-value in the limit of $\tau \rightarrow \infty$, and K is related to the apparent diffusivity of non-sorbing species. The tortuosity, D_0/D_∞, is thus:

$$\frac{D_0}{D_\infty} = \frac{K_0}{K} \qquad (11)$$

where K_0 is K for the free space (i.e. porous medium of $\phi = 1$). It should be noted that RW3D.m probes only the pore structure near the center of the 3-D image system whereas DMAP.m averages the tortuosity of the whole system. Thus, if the porous medium is heterogeneous, the tortuosity estimated by RW3D.m is different from that by DMAP.m.

The permeability can be estimated via empirical Carman-Kozeny equation using the simulation results of Kai3D.m, RW3D.m, and DMAP.m. Consider a pipe model for the calculation of the permeability (Fig. 3). The porosity of the system is:

$$\phi = \frac{n\pi r^2 l}{l_0^3} \qquad (12)$$

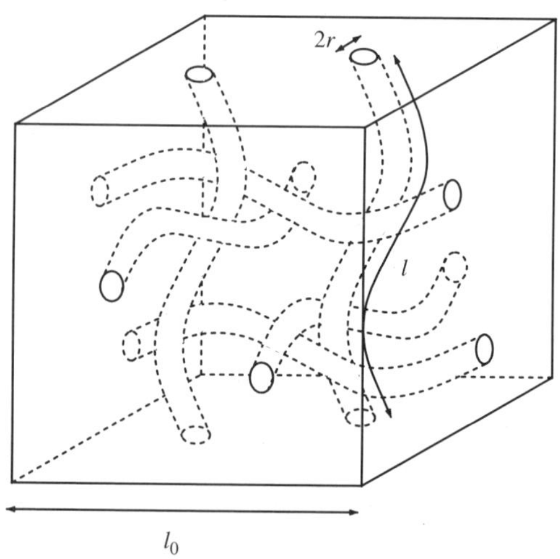

Figure 3. Model of the pore structure in a cubic porous medium for the estimate of the permeability. Cylindrical pipes of diameter $2r$ run orthogonally. The pipe length is l in the cube of l_0^3, and thus the tortuosity of the pipes is $(l/l_0)^2$.

where l is the pipe length, r is the radius of the cylindrical pipe, and n is the number of cylindrical pipes in the l_0^3 cube. The surface-to-volume ratio of the pore, $(S/V)_{pore}$, is defined as the ratio of the cylinder surface area to the cylinder volume:

$$\left(\frac{S}{V}\right)_{pore} = \frac{2\pi rl}{\pi r^2 l} = \frac{2}{r} \tag{13}$$

Assuming the Poiseuille flow in the pipes, the volumetric flux, Q, along a single pipe is given by:

$$Q = \frac{\pi r^4}{8\mu}\frac{\Delta P}{l} \tag{14}$$

where μ is the fluid viscosity, ΔP is the fluid pressure drop along the pipe length, l. The permeability, k, for the orthogonal pipe system is defined as:

$$k = \frac{\frac{n}{3}Q\frac{\mu}{l_0^2}}{\frac{\Delta P}{l_0}} \tag{15}$$

It is assumed that one-third of the pipes are parallel (i.e. run in the same direction), and the factor 3 in Equation 15 is derived from this assumption. The substitution of Equations 12, 13, and 14 into Equation 15 yields:

$$k = \frac{n\pi r^4}{24 l l_0} = \frac{\phi}{6\left(\frac{l}{l_0}\right)^2\left(\frac{S}{V}\right)^2_{pore}} \tag{16}$$

where $(l/l_0)^2 = D_0/D_\infty$ is the tortuosity. This is the final expression of the permeability estimate based on the NMR diffusometry. It should be noted that all quantities in the right-hand side of Equation 16 can be obtained by Kai3D.m, RW3D.m, and DMAP.m.

4 APPLICATION TO A SAND PACK

Kai3D.m, RW3D.m, and DMAP.m were applied to 3-D CT images of a monosized sand grain pack to demonstrate the program performance. The sand pack sample was chosen because well-sorted sandy formations are one of typical aquifers in the earth's crust. The porosity, surface-to-volume ratio, tortuosity, and permeability were estimated for the sand grain pack.

The CT system used was the microfocus cone-beam X-ray CT (ELESCAN®, Nittetsu Co. Ltd., Tokyo, Japan). The acceleration voltage of the X-ray tube was 70 kV, and the tube current was 0.02 mA. The ratio of the detector-source distance to the sample-source distance was 5.0. The field-of-view (FOV) of the 3-D image was $14.5 \times 14.5 \times 7.26\,mm^3$. The number of the projection was 1800, and about 39 minutes was required for the acquisition of the projections. No metal filter for the reduction of the beam-hardening artifact was used. Contiguous 256 2-D slices (512×512 voxels) with an 8-bit gray level were reconstructed using the Shepp-Logan filter. Eighty three minutes were needed for this image reconstruction. The dimension of the cubic voxel was $0.02834^3\,mm^3$ (i.e. $a = 0.02834$ mm).

The sample imaged was granodioritic sand grains collected at the coast of Uchinoura, Kagoshima, Japan. The sand grains are derived from the Osumi granodiorite batholith. The dominant mineral species of the sand were quartz, feldspar, biotite, and cummingtonite. The sand sample was sieved, so that the grain size is 0.85–1.18 mm in diameter, and was packed in a plastic cylinder (Fig. 4). The high-density iron-bearing magnetic minerals are strong X-ray absorbers, and yield undesirable artifacts in the CT images. Thus the magnetic minerals were removed from the sample by a magnet before the CT experiments.

An example of the reconstructed 2-D CT image is shown in Figure 5. The profile of the image intensity is shown in Figure 6. One of the important procedures

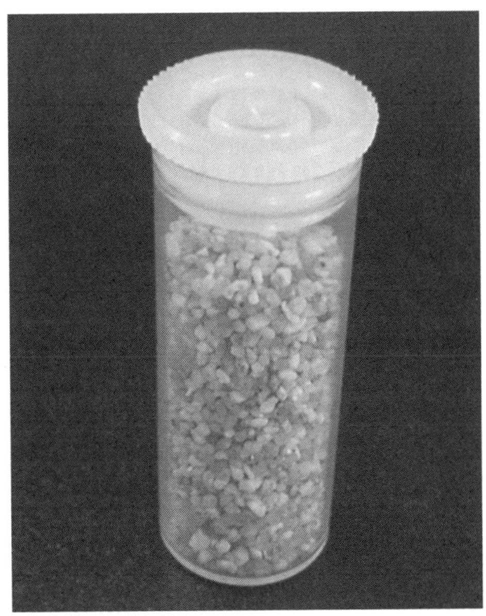

Figure 4. Photograph of the sample for the microfocus X-ray CT. Granodioritic sand grains (grain diameter 0.85–1.18 mm) are packed in a plastic cylinder (outside diameter 16 mm, length 44 mm). The zone about 11 to 18 mm above from the cylinder bottom was imaged to obtain contiguous 256 CT slices.

is to determine the threshold value of the image intensity for the discrimination of the pores from solid grains. On the basis of the histogram (Fig. 7), we determined the threshold to be 58.5, giving a binary square slice (Fig. 8). 256 square slices were used to construct a cubic 256^3 system (Fig. 9), and we ran all programs on this cubic system.

The results by Kai3D.m (Fig. 10) show that there is a single large pore cluster responsible for the macroscopic material transport. Although 323 small pore clusters (obeying a power law distribution with an exponent of 0.79) exist, their total volume in the 256^3 system is 1573 voxels. The small ratio, $1573/256^3 \approx 0.009\%$, indicates that they are negligible in volume.

The simulation results by RW3D.m and DMAP.m are shown in Figures 11–13 and Figures 14–15, respectively. The $(S/V)_{\text{pore}}$ value by Kai3D.m (Fig. 10) is nearly equal to that by RW3D.m (Fig. 13). The tortuosity estimated by RW3D.m (Fig. 12) agrees well with that by DMAP.m. (Fig. 14). The porosity was determined as a byproduct of the DMAP.m run of Figure 14 to be 0.33, which again agrees well with the

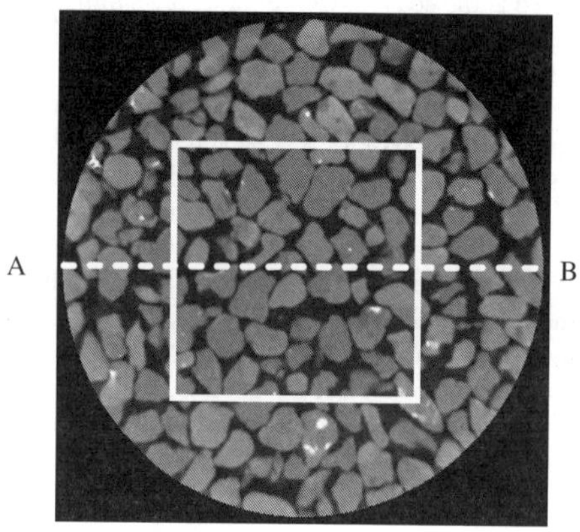

Figure 5. Example of the CT slice (2-D 8-bit image) of the sand grain pack of Figure 4. The image dimension is 512×512 voxels $= 14.5 \times 14.5\,\text{mm}^2$. The line profile along the line AB is shown in Figure 6. The histogram of the voxel intensity of the 256×256 square region (open frame) is shown in Figure 7. The binary image of the square region is shown in Figure 8.

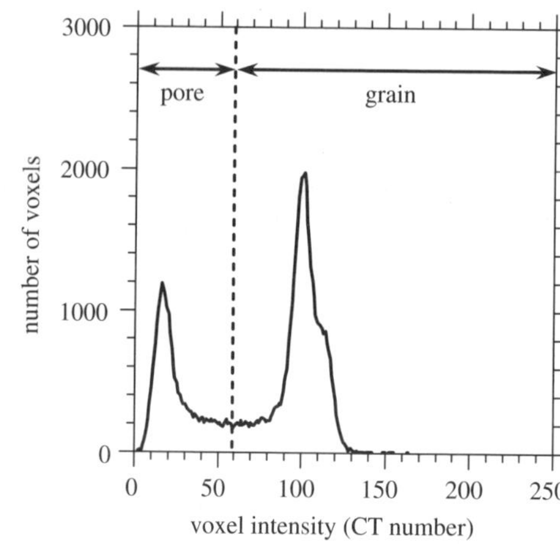

Figure 7. Histogram of the voxel intensity of the square region (256×256 voxels) of Fig. 5. The 8-bit voxel intensities of the peaks of the grain and pore are 101 and 16, respectively. The midpoint, 58.5, of the peaks was chosen as a threshold for the discrimination of the pore from grain (dotted line).

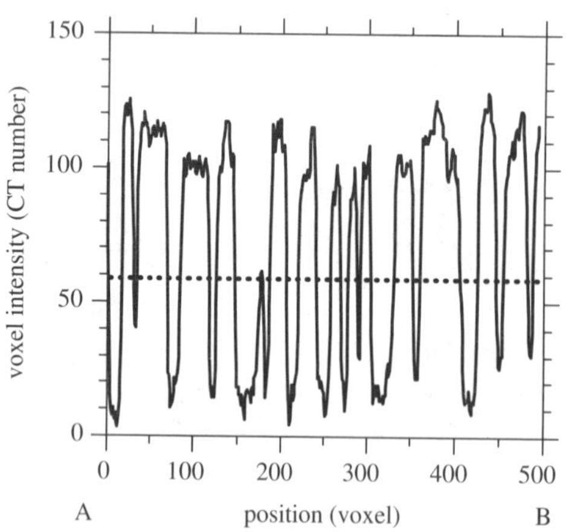

Figure 6. Line profile of the voxel intensity along the line AB of Figure 5. The threshold (58.5) for the discrimination of pore voxels from grain voxels is indicated by a dotted line.

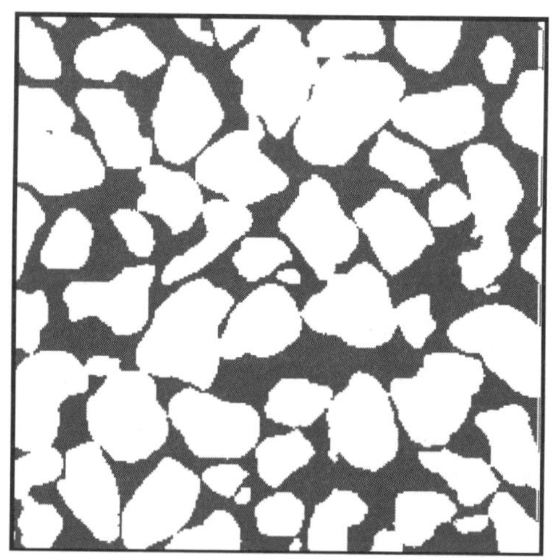

Figure 8. Binary (1-bit) image of the square region (256×256 voxels) of Figure 5 for the threshold of 58.5. Pore voxels are in black and grain voxels are in white.

result by Kai3D.m (Fig. 10). These demonstrate that the simulations were performed in a reliable manner.

The mapping of the porosity and tortuosity (Fig. 15) suggests that there is the small pore-structure heterogeneity derived from the random packing of the sand grains. Using Equation 16, k was estimated to be $2.5 \times 10^{-10}\,m^2$. An inevitable systematic error is incurred in the calculation of $(S/V)_{pore}$ using blocky discrete images (Nakashima & Watanabe 2002). Thus, in Equation 16, the $(S/V)_{pore}$ value was corrected by dividing a factor 1.5 to obtain $1.1 \times 10^4\,m^{-1}$. The estimated permeability is nearly equal to that for randomly packed monodisperse spherical grains of $\phi = 0.33$ and diameter of 1.0 mm ($k = 4.2 \times 10^{-10}\,m^2$; Fand et al. 1987), demonstrating the validity of Equation 16.

We have developed Mathematica® programs to estimate the transport properties of isotropic porous

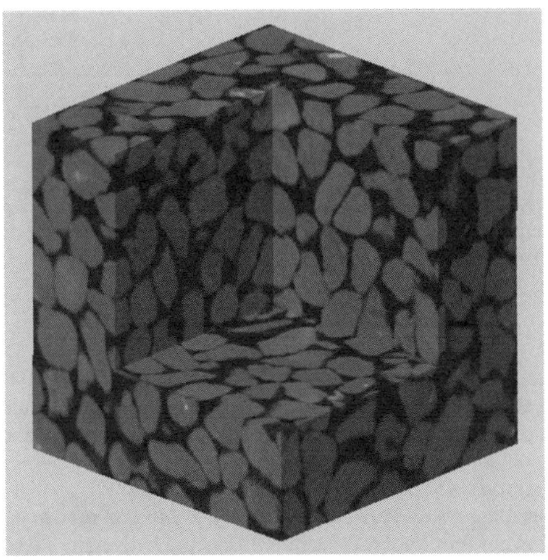

Figure 9. 3-D 8-bit CT image of the sand grain pack. The heavy-element-bearing minerals (e.g. biotite) are bright, quartz and feldspar are gray, and the air-filled pore is black. The system size is $256 \times 256 \times 256$ voxels $\approx 7.3 \times 7.3 \times 7.3\,mm^3$.

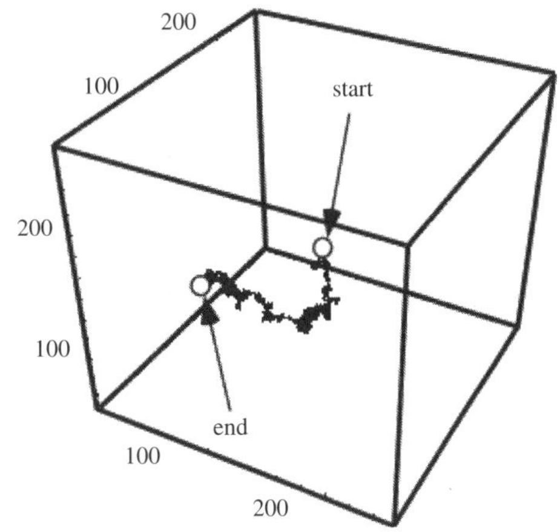

Figure 11. Example of the 3-D trajectory of the lattice-walk through the pore space of Figure 9. The total time step is 5000. The initial ($\tau = 0$) and final ($\tau = 5000$) positions of the walker are marked by open circles.

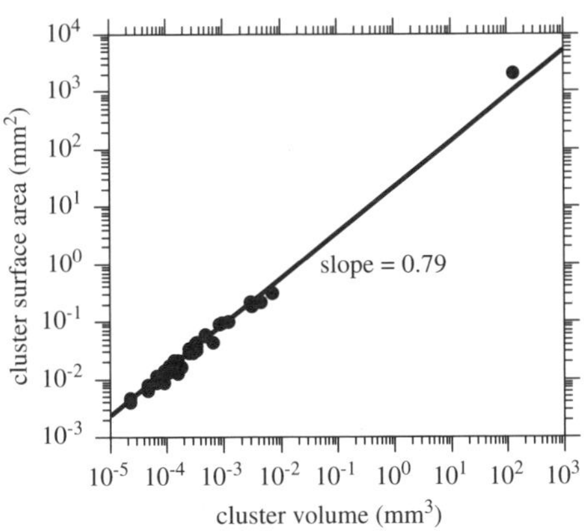

Figure 10. Results of the cluster labeling analysis using Kai3D.m applied to the 3-D image of Figure 9. 324 pore clusters were identified. The porosity, volume, and surface area of the largest pore cluster are 0.33, 128 mm³, and 2068 mm², respectively. Thus, $(S/V)_{pore}$ is $2068/128\,mm^{-1} = 1.6 \times 10^4\,m^{-1}$.

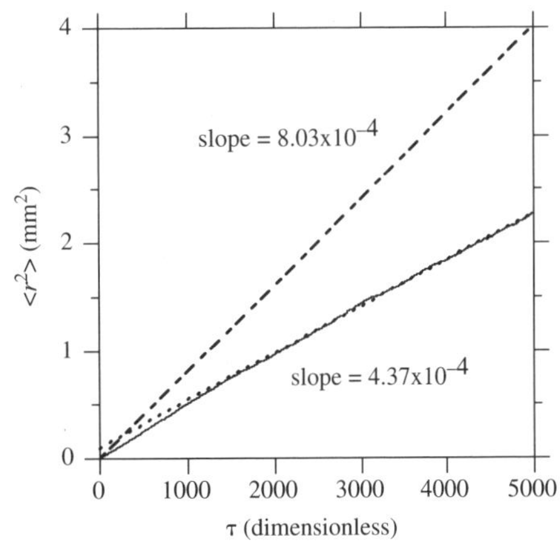

Figure 12. Mean-square displacement of the random walk averaged over 2000 walkers (solid line) calculated by Equation 1. The linear regression analysis (dotted line) was applied to the data points for $\tau > 1000$ to obtain the slope of 4.37×10^{-4}. The exact solution, Equation 7, for the random walk in the free space is also shown by a dash-dotted line (slope $= 8.03 \times 10^{-4}$). Thus the tortuosity is $8.03 \times 10^{-4}/4.37 \times 10^{-4} = 1.8$.

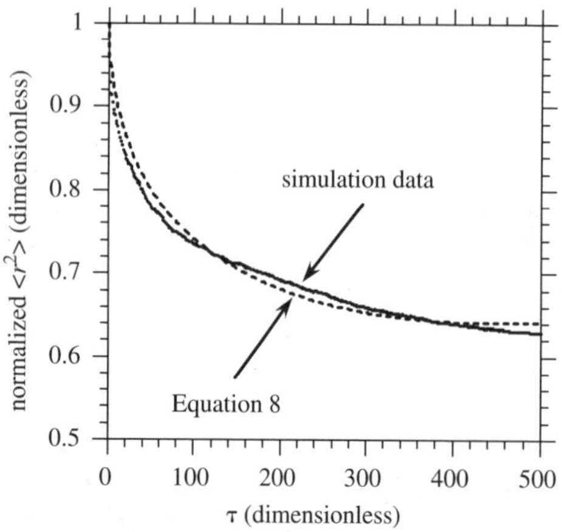

Figure 13. Normalized mean-square displacement of the random walk averaged over 20,000 walkers. The theoretical curve (dotted line), Equation 8, was applied to the data points to obtain $(S/V)_{pore} = 1.7 \times 10^4 m^{-1}$.

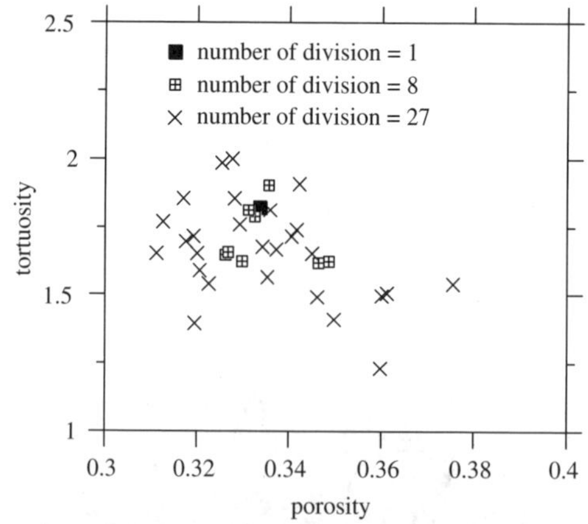

Figure 15. Results of the mapping of the heterogeneity of the pore structure obtained by DMAP.m. The number of the sub-cubes (Fig. 2) is indicated.

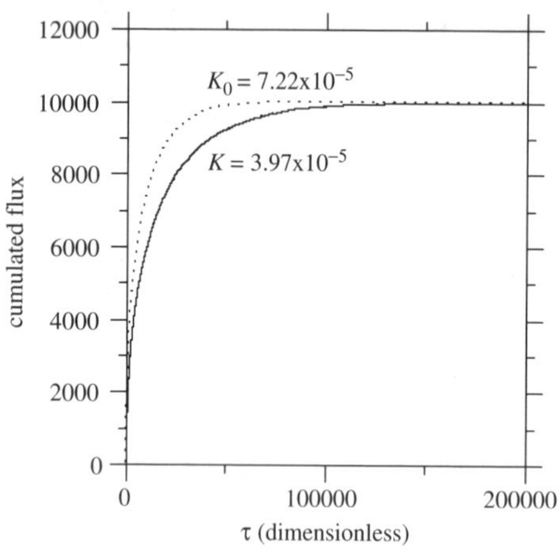

Figure 14. Results of the out-diffusion simulation for the pore space of Figure 9 obtained by DMAP.m (solid curve). The number of division is unity, and the number of walkers is 10,009. Simulation results for the 10,009 walkers in the free space (i.e. porosity 100%) are also shown by a dotted curve. A theoretical model, Equation 10, was applied to the data to obtain the tortuosity value of $K_0/K = 7.22 \times 10^{-5}/3.97 \times 10^{-5} = 1.8$ via Equation 11.

media. The programs are open on the Internet to facilitate study on the porous media using X-ray CT.

REFERENCES

Dunn, K.-J., Bergman, D.J. & Latorraca, G.A. 2002. *Nuclear Magnetic Resonance Petrophysical and Logging Applications*. Amsterdam: Pergamon.

Fand, R.M., Kim, B.Y.K., Lam, A.C.C. & Phan, R.T. 1987. Resistance to the flow of fluids through simple and complex porous media whose matrices are composed of randomly packed spheres. *Journal of Fluids Engineering* (*Trans. ASME*) 109: 268–274.

Guéguen, Y. & Palciauskas, V. 1994. *Introduction to the Physics of Rocks*. Princeton: Princeton University Press.

Hoshen, J. & Kopelman, R. 1976. Percolation and cluster distribution. I. Cluster multiple labeling technique and critical concentration algorithm. *Physical Review* B 14: 3438–3445.

Ikeda, S., Nakano, T. & Nakashima, Y. 2000. Three-dimensional study on the interconnection and shape of crystals in a graphic granite by X-ray CT and image analysis. *Mineralogical Magazine* 64: 945–959.

Nakashima, Y. & Watanabe, Y. 2002. Estimate of transport properties of porous media by micro-focus X-ray computed tomography and random walk simulation. *Water Resources Research* 38: paper number 1272, DOI number 10.1029/2001WR000937.

Nakashima, Y. & Yamaguchi, T. 2003. DMAP.m: A Mathematica® program for the three-dimensional mapping of the diffusivity and porosity of heterogeneous porous media. *Computers & Geosciences* (in review).

Stauffer, D. 1985. *Introduction to Percolation Theory*. London: Taylor & Francis.

Watanabe, Y. & Nakashima, Y. 2001. Two-dimensional random walk program for the calculation of the tortuosity of porous media. *Journal of Groundwater Hydrology* 43: 13–22.

Watanabe, Y. & Nakashima, Y. 2002. RW3D.m: Three-dimensional random walk program for the calculation of the diffusivities in porous media. *Computers & Geosciences* 28: 583–586.

Watanabe, Y., Nakashima, Y. & Ohtani, T. 1999. 3D-image processing program for the calculation of the volume histogram of cavities in rock samples. *Journal of Geothermal Research Society of Japan* 21: 181–188.

X-ray CT for Geomaterials; Soils, Concrete, Rocks – Otani & Obara (eds.)
© 2004 Swets & Zeitlinger. Lisse, ISBN 90 5809 666 1

Development of a time-resolving X-ray tomography system and its application to multi-phase flows

M. Misawa & N. Ichikawa
National Institute of Advanced Industrial Science & Technology (AIST), Tsukuba, Japan

I. Tiseanu
Institute of Atomic Physics, INFLPR Laboratory, Bucharest, Romania

Y. Tomita & Y. Shiroyanagi
Hamamatsu Photonics K.K., Hamamatsu, Japan

ABSTRACT: The proposed time resolving X-ray tomography system is aimed to reduce the scanning time by two orders of magnitude compared with conventional ones for measurement of interface geometry in various forms of multiphase flow. To reduce the scanning time, all mechanically moving parts were eliminated from the system. Instead, multiple X-ray sources and detector elements were installed around the region of interest to complete the scanning operation in 3.6 msec. Scanning time of this order is necessary to resolve transient shape of bubble interface in flowing liquids, which is one of our primary application of interest. Maximum sampling frequency is 263 Hz for scanning over the 50 mm diameter region. In this paper, we will explain the design concept and development of key components of the system and present some of the recent results of interface measurements in multiphase flow.

1 BACKGROUND AND OBJECTIVES

1.1 *Interface measurement in multiphase flow*

Interface geometry is an important quantity for both modeling and numerical simulation of gas–liquid two-phase flow because the interfacial area concentration should be given as a constitutive equation in momentum and energy equations. Since mass, momentum, and energy between the phases are exchanged through the interface, it affects directly to the accuracy of prediction. A mixture of flowing gas and liquid is widely seen not only in industries such as chemical and power plants but also in diffusive fluid flow through underground porous media (Jasti et al., 1990) or of inertially driven ground water flow containing various forms of gas phase (Bear, 1972). In the field of multiphase flow study, an extensive effort was made to measure the amount of interface area in two-phase flow in wide range of parameters. Measurement of transient interface geometry in flow is not easy because the use of visible light technique is often hampered by the strong reflection of light at the irregular shape of interfaces. Also, due to large deformation, the interface area varies for the same value of the void fraction (defined as the ratio of the gas phase area to the liquid phase area in a cross section). In early period, irreversible chemical reaction of CO_2 in air and NaOH in water was employed to measure the time and volume averaged interface area (Sharma et al., 1970). The capacitance probe technique provided measurements of accurate multidimensional interface area in a local point in flow (Revankar et al., 1997). However, the chemical technique cannot provide detailed interface geometry that also changes in time, and the probe technique provides information only at a local point, which makes inappropriate to transient inhomogeneous flow patterns. As an attempt to develop a multi-dimensional, time-resolving technique, a rapid scanning X-ray tomography system was proposed and its prototype was tested (Akai, 1986). In this paper, its design process including reconstruction simulation and key component development will be presented, together with some recent examples of interface visualization of air–water two-phase flow in vertical tubes and of a simplified catalytic fluidized bed facility.

1.2 *Review of tomography measurements in multiphase flow*

Gamma-ray tomography systems were the first to be applied to void fraction measurement in late 1970s as an extension of the gamma densitometer. Kulacki et al. (1980), Schlosser et al. (1980), and De Vuono et al. (1980) designed a tomography system based on a fan beam gamma rays from a ^{137}Cs source and NaI scintillation detectors. They applied the system to the two-phase flow in a 0.15 m diameter vertical tube, the void fraction ranging from 0.1 to 0.46. Kumar et al. (1995) also used a similar system and measured bubbly flow void fraction in 0.1–0.3 m diameter tubes and discussed the effects of tube diameter, gas velocity, nozzle shape, and water quality on the void fraction distribution in a systematic way. Although time consuming, use of monoenergetic gamma ray source with energy selective photon counting detectors helped avoid the scattering and beam hardening problems, which causes errors in X-ray tomography systems. In Japan, however, X-ray tomography systems have been used in void fraction measurement to avoid safety complication of handling high intensity radio isotopes and to make use of tomography techniques then advanced in the medical field. Iizuka et al. (1982) used a X-ray tomography system (TOSHIBA TCT-30) to investigate the capability of flow pattern recognition and reported that the bubbly and annular flow patterns can be distinguished. Ikeda et al. (1983) analyzed the accuracy of tomography void fraction measurement based on comparison with that by the hot film probe and quick-valve methods. An accuracy of 10% is reported, considering the standard deviation of projection data. Encouraged by the success of void fraction measurement in straight vertical tubes, Iizuka et al. (1984), Morooka et al. (1989), and Ishizuka et al. (1995) then applied the X-ray tomography system to fuel rod bundle geometry in adiabatic and diabatic two-phase flow, simulating the flow conditions in nuclear reactors. A part of metallic structure was made of Beryllium to allow transmission of X-rays. The obtained void fraction correlation for rod bundle was able to correlate the existing void fraction data base within an accuracy of 1.3% in average. Recently, Tiseanu et al. (1999) developed a 3D X-ray tomography system and successfully visualized a void fraction distribution in bubbly flow in a 0.08 m tube. The results showed a sharper wall peak profile than previously reported.

Nevertheless, the tomography systems previously mentioned have poor time resolution for measurement of dynamic events. Single scan normally takes on the order of minutes, allowing to acquire only time averaged projections. The proposed rapid scanning X-ray tomography system completes the single scan in 3.6 msec (Misawa et al. 2003), and even in 0.5 msec in the advanced type developed by Hori et al. (1997). Design concept and key components will be described in the next chapter.

2 DEVELOPMENT OF THE TIME-RESOLVING X-RAY TOMOGRAPHY SYSTEM

2.1 *System design*

A tomography system can be evaluated by spatial, density, and temporal resolutions. A single scan should be completed in a few msec to capture the interface moving about 1.0 m/s. This scanning time is not achievable if mechanical motion of the source-detector assembly is involved. The main idea of our rapid scanning tomography system is to replace the mechanical rotation with electrical switching of multiple X-ray sources placed around the measuring object. As shown in Figure 1, pulse X-ray sources and detector pixels are placed around the 50 mm diameter region of interest to perform equivalent scanning motion of existing X-ray tomography systems. Approximately 60 pixels are irradiated by a 24 degree fan beam.

Irradiation of pulsed X-ray sources is controlled by the bias grid voltage that repels the emitted photons when the grid is armed (Figure 2). When the grid disarmed, the electrons pass through the bias grid and accelerated by the high voltage electric field, shooting at the tungsten target to emit X-rays towards the center of the region of interest through a 0.5 mm aluminum window. X-ray beams going through the object are detected by a line sensor placed on a plane slightly above the X-ray focus. This offset is necessary to avoid interaction of beams with fixed detectors, but minimized since it is undesirable in terms of reconstruction theory.

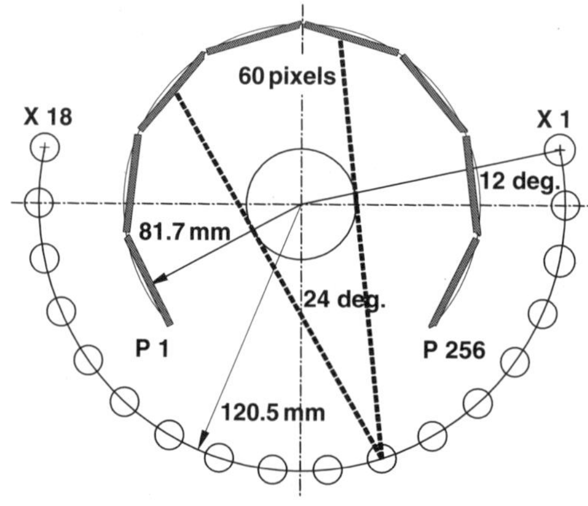

Figure 1. Arrangement of pulse X-ray sources and detector modules for the rapid scanning X-ray CT.

Transient time of pulsed X-ray irradiation is on the order of 5–7 micro sec, which is less significant compared to the total pulse duration of 100–150 micro sec. In this design, 18 pulse X-ray sources are switched on sequentially in order before a single scan is completed in 3.8 msec. The data acquisition system is synchronized with the trigger for each X-ray pulse. Specifications of the rapid scanning tomography system are listed in Table 1. The pulse X-ray source has a capacity of 1.6 kW with its maximum current of 10 mA. As a detector device, CdTe (cadmium telluride) semi-conductor was chosen for its high detection efficiency. From the source ring and detector ring diameters, the magnification factor becomes 1.48. With the present numbers of X-ray sources and detector pixels, spatial resolution is expected to be 2.6 mm. This resolution is compromised by relatively unbalanced numbers of projection angles (equivalent to X-ray sources in this design) and detector pixels per fan beam. A filtered back projection with rebinning process was used in image reconstruction on an off-line computer. The resulting tomography image is presented in a 101 × 101 pixel format of 8 bit gray scale. Computation time is about 3.5 sec per image by a 500 MHz Pentium II PC.

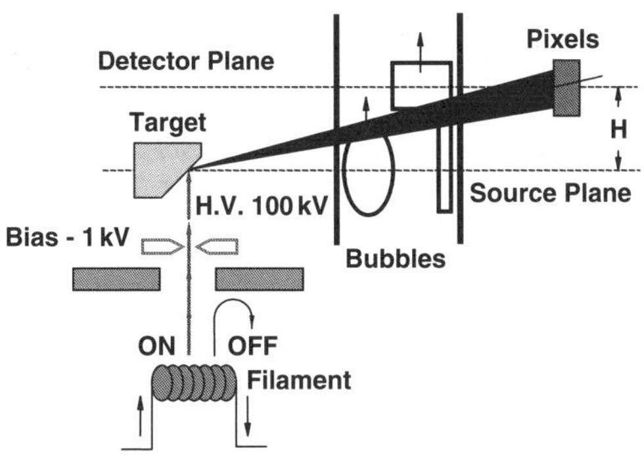

Figure 2. Switching mechanism of multiple pulsed X-ray sources.

Table 1. Design parameters of the rapid scanning X-ray CT.

Number of X-ray sources	18
Acceleration voltage	160 kV max.
Beam current	10 mA max.
Scan time per slice	3.8 msec
Scan rate	263 slices
Beam thickness	5 mm
Number of detectors	256
Detector device	CdTe
No. of detectors /fan beam	60
Maximum object diameter	50 mm
Designed spatial resolution	2.6 mm
Fan beam angle	24 degrees
X-ray source ring diameter	241 mm
Detector ring diameter	163.4 mm
A/D resolution	12 bit
Integration time	0.2 msec. min.
Image reconstruction	FBP
Filter type	Shepp-Logan

2.2 *Simulation*

Prior to hardware development, simulation of image reconstruction was conducted to verify selected design parameters and also to understand causes of artifact in various forms. Given the required spatial and density resolutions (2.0 mm and 200 kg/m^3, respectively) together with the scanning time constraint (<4.0 msec), the number of projections, the number of detector pixels, dimensions of pixels, X-ray voltage and current, and magnification factor are primal parameters to determine. Figure 3 indicates reconstruction results of a 0.05 m diameter area with varying number of detector pixels and projections. It is clear that increasing the number of pixels per fan beam and projections improves the spatial resolution in tomography since the Fourier space is filled densely by fine sampling of projection data. However, as is described later, the number of projection is the same as the number of pulsed X-ray generator in the rapid scanning system. A limitation imposed on the source number comes from the minimum distance of each electron gun to avoid discharge at 100 kV and from the scanning time to irradiate all X-ray sources.

In actual system, electrical and mechanical noise will be superimposed on the projection data. In tomography, noise tends to be enhanced in reconstruction because convolution is a high-pass filtering process. The allowable noise level can be judged by imposing a pre-determined random noise on the projection data.

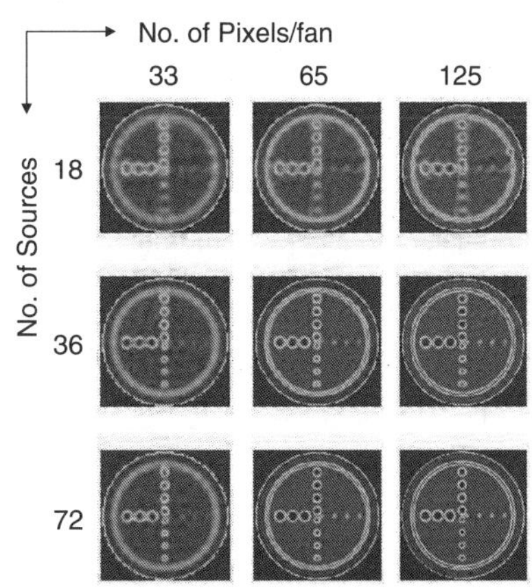

Figure 3. Simulation of image reconstruction with varying numbers of detector pixels and projections (=X-ray sources).

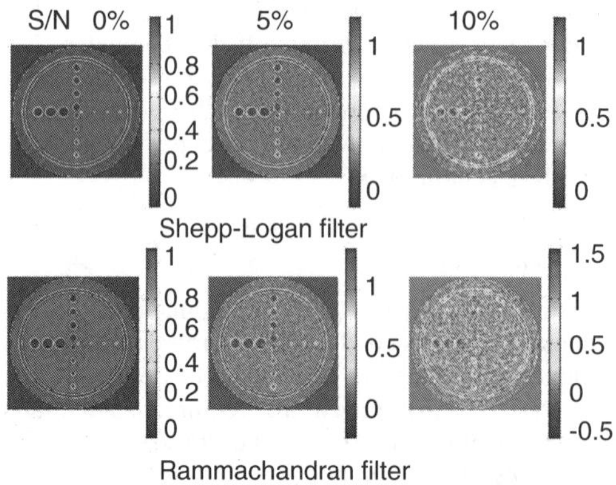

Figure 4. Random noise effect on the reconstructed images in simulation.

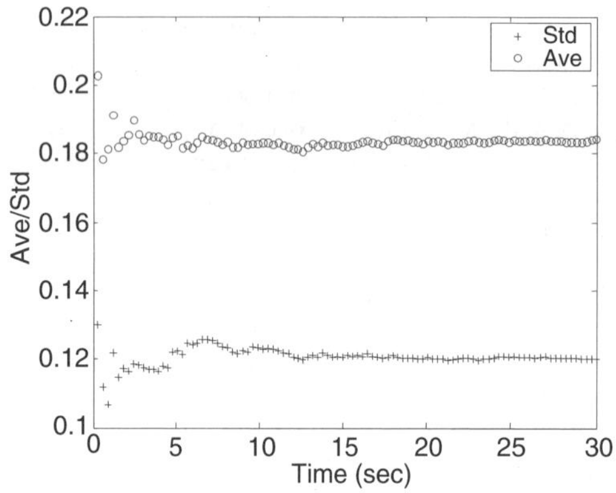

Figure 5. Time variations of standard deviation and average for slug flow void fraction in a 0.1 m tube measured by the wire-mesh sensor. $j_g = 0.42$ m/s, $j_l = 0.21$ m/s.

The tomography images tarnished by random noise of different intensity is shown in Figure 4. Both density and spatial resolutions are deteriorated as the noise intensity increases. In our design, we tried to suppress the noise level less than 5% to satisfy the given requirements. It should be noted that fluctuation in projection data also comes from bubble motion, too, which is inherent physical phenomena in two-phase flow. According to tomographic measurement of slug flow void fraction separately conducted by the wiremesh sensor (Prasser et al., 2001), the average and standard deviation smoothed out after 10 sec (Figure 5), indicating that fluctuating projection is still valid in tomography if the acquisition is long enough to average fluctuation. This result justifies the use of X-ray tomography to two-phase flow measurements as long as the average void fraction is concerned.

One of the major artifacts expected in two-phase flow is motion artifact. Even with the rapid scanning system, the distance traveled by a moving or deforming object within a scanning period is not negligible. Figure 6 shows the simulated motion artifact of ellipsoidal spheres rising at 0.5 m/s in a 50 mm vertical tube. In this simulation, we assumed a scanning period of 3.8 msec for 18 projections and 33 pixels per fan beam. Radiative traces are typical when a part of the sphere was projected at limited angles. To prevent this artifact, the scanning time should be reduced so that the object stays in the thickness of the fan beam during the scanning, or the object velocity should be lower to meet the above condition. In practice, however, the artifact with lower intensity will be dismissed when quantities such as area ratio of bubbles are computed from binarized images. This is possible only for binary mixture of air and water where the density resolution is not an important issue.

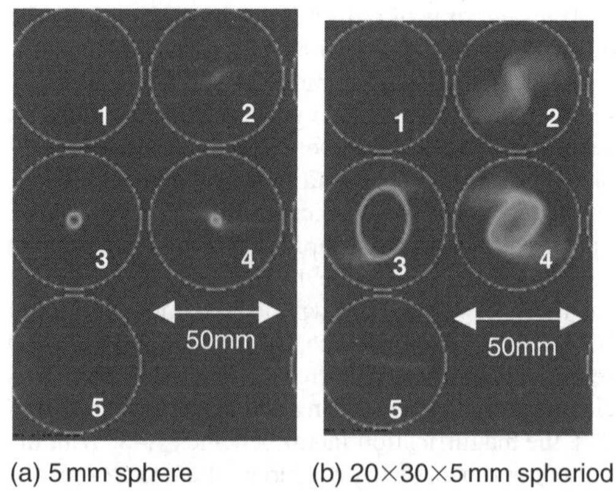

Figure 6. Artifact from simulated rising sphere and spheroid in a 50 mm tube at 0.5 m/s for 18 projections and 33 pixels per fan beam.

2.3 *Semiconductor detector*

Highly efficient photon detection is a key element in the rapid scanning tomography system. Most existing X-ray detectors consist of scintillator and photo diodes, in which the incident X-ray is converted to visible light by the scintillator and then converted to electrical signal by the photo diodes. However, the semiconductor detector converts the X-ray photon directly into hole–electron pairs which can be integrated in signal processing circuits (Figure 7). Among available devices, CdTe semi-conductor was chosen because of its high detection efficiency and operability at room temperature. In one detector module, 32 of 0.3 × 0.8 mm pixels were printed on a 5 × 20 × 1 mm CdTe substrate by photo lithography technique at an interval of 1.425 mm pitch. The 256 detector system consists of 8 sets of such modules. Each pixel is coupled to a charge integration CMOS-IC (Hamamatsu Photonics

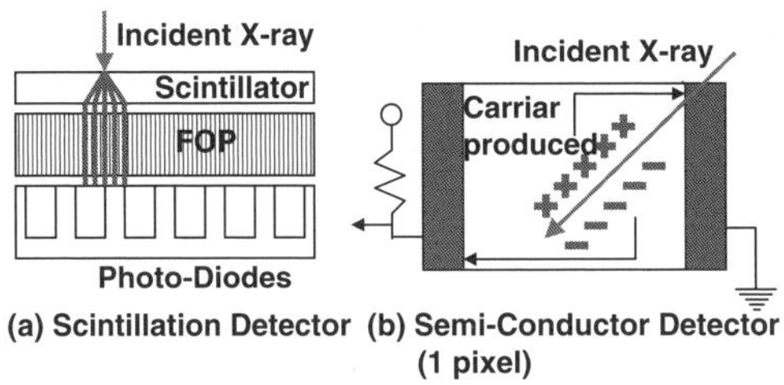

Figure 7. Operation of scintillation detector and semi-conductor detector.

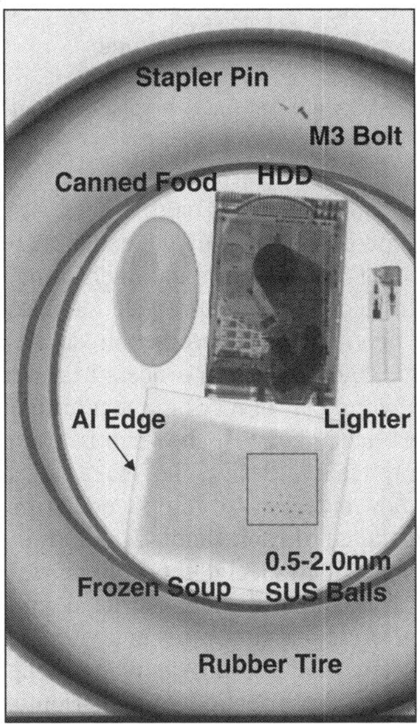

Figure 8. X-ray transmission image of objects moving at 0.33 m/s taken by the developed CdTe detector.

K.K., Japan) mounted on the same module. The projection signal is transferred to a host computer memory through a 12 bit A/D converter for each X-ray pulse irradiation. To test the performance of this detector, modules were aligned as a line sensor format and used to scan some objects on a belt conveyer moving at 0.33 m/s. Figure 8 shows transmission images of various objects such as a rubber tire, hard disk, and canned food. From the clearly defined edges of each moving object, we assured that the developed detector works in rapid X-ray scanning mode.

2.4 *Multi-pulse X-ray generator*

Rapid scanning tomography system requires not only sensitive detectors but also high intensity multi-pulse X-ray sources. The pitch of the X-ray sources should be minimized from spatial resolution requirement while discharge between adjacent X-ray guns must be prevented. In the present design, a common ring anode was designed to include each target for 18 X-ray guns situated beneath the anodes on a semi-circle. Thus, high voltage over 100 kV is uniformly applied to all anodes. The entire structure is built in a vacuum chamber maintained constantly at 10^{-6} Torr by a large diffusion pump. X-ray intensity for each unit can be adjusted by the filament current control individually. The homogeneity of X-ray units is especially important for the rapid scanning system with relatively small number of projections. Sequence of pulse operation is given by an external pulse generator through optical fibers which electrically disconnects from controllers.

3 MEASUREMENT OF INTERFACE

3.1 *Phantom test*

Prior to the fluid measurement test, a plastic phantom with known dimensions was scanned to evaluate the accuracy of the measurement. From the reconstructed images, the interface area and solid volume were calculated and compared with the actual values of the tested phantom. The phantom contained a semi-spherical dome at the top, followed by a 2 mm thick cylindrical tube, and 3–6 mm spherical cavities scattered across the cross section at the bottom. While the phantom was passing through the measuring plane, its cross section was continuously scanned at 263 Hz. In a case of moving velocity at 0.3 m/s, the phantom travels an axial distance of 1.14 mm which is smaller than the thickness of the X-ray fan beam. A total of 105 slices were made for the 120 mm long phantom. An example of resulting reconstructed images are shown in Figure 9. The intensity fluctuation in solid part is due to smaller number of projections (18 projections in this case). At the semi-spherical dome and scattered spherical cavity where the variation of cross section geometry is abrupt, reconstruction consistency is lost and the resulting interface blurs. This blurring can be suppressed if the scanning time is further reduced or the axial geometry mildly varies. The accuracy of interface area and solid volume obtained from binary images are estimated to be 15 and 20%, respectively (Misawa et al., 2001), for velocities less than 1.0 m.

3.2 *Gas–liquid two-phase flow*

Phase distribution of air in still water in a 42 mm diameter tube was then visualized at 263 Hz scanning frequency. Air was introduced through a 4 mm diameter nozzle at regulated flow rates from 0.013–0.091 m/s.

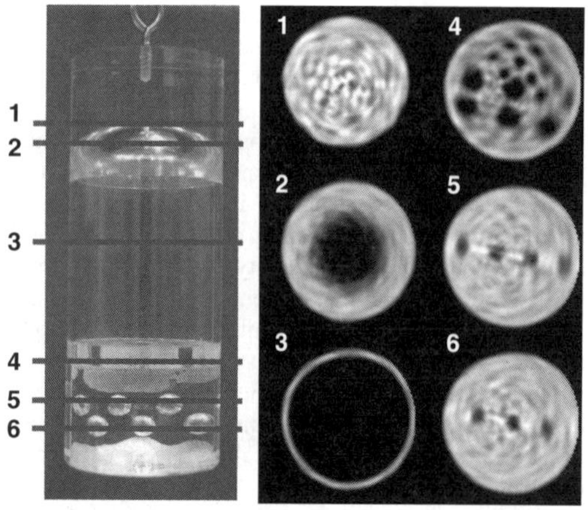

Figure 9. A 40 mm diameter acrylic slug phantom with cavities of different sizes moving at 0.3 m/s.

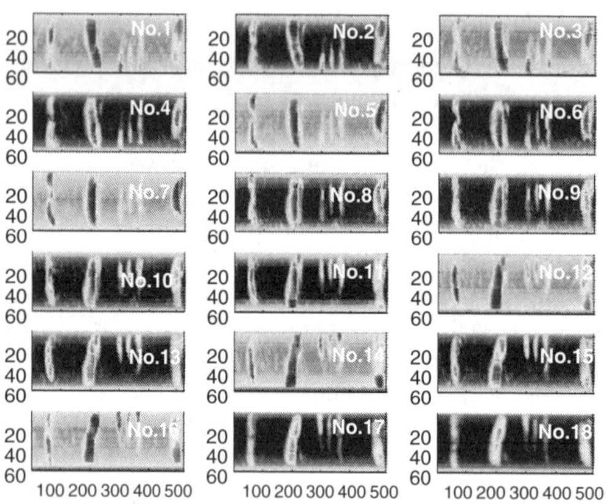

Figure 10. Radiography images for 18 pulsed X-ray sources. Image reconstruction uses this data set.

Mostly slug bubbles were observed for this flow range. A set of projection images per fan beam for individual 18 X-ray sources are shown in Figure 10. Bubble shapes in the images are deformed since the diverging fan beam transmission was projected on to linear detector arrays. It should be noted that the projection images can be used for densitometer if the beam hardening is insignificant, which is the case for water in a 42 mm tube. Time variation of the average void fraction is calculated in relative unit between the intensity values of air and water alone as shown in Figure 11. The water alone signal fluctuates around the level 0, which is considered as a noise level. When air is introduced, the signal fluctuation apparently increases corresponding to density fluctuation due to traversing bubbles. When measurement of the void fraction is suffice in some practical applications, then

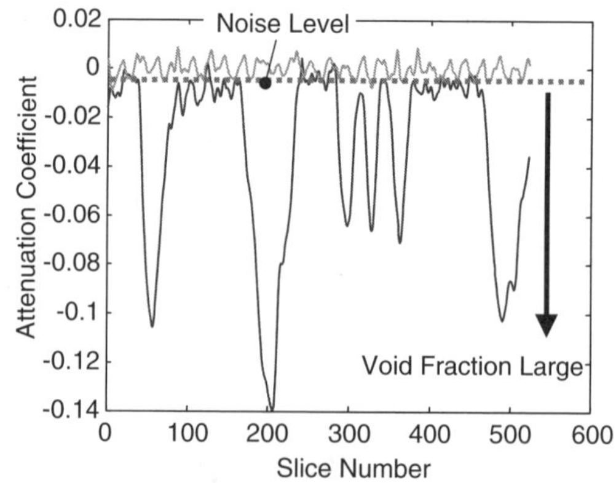

Figure 11. Average void fraction obtained from the radiography images.

only the radiography data can be used without performing time-consuming image reconstruction.

In need of interface measurement, image reconstruction is necessary to reproduce the instantaneous interface geometry. The projection data is used in convolution-backprojection process to generate 1000 tomography images for measurement in about 1.0 sec. The reconstructed image is shown in 101×101 pixels of 8 bit gray scale intensity. The images are stacked in order to show side view of interface distribution. The interval distance of each slice was determined by the average void fraction and the volumetric gas flow rate. Figure 12 shows the reconstructed void distribution for different gas flow rates in continuous 1.0 sec. The side view of the tomography stack represents a time history of cross section void distribution, unlike the instantaneous views by camera. If the relative motion of each bubble is insignificant, the time history image looks like camera view, which is partly true in this experiment.

Next, the concurrent air–water two-phase flow in a 42 mm, 1.5 m long vertical tube was scanned. The X-ray voltage and current were 70 kV and 0.46 mA, respectively. The pulse X-ray was turned on for 100 micro sec and the integration time of the detector was set to 200 micro sec. The average air velocities varied from 0.0 to 0.6 m/s for a constant water velocity of 0.15 m/s. The reconstructed images are shown in Figure 13 for (a) slug flow and (b) bubbly flow. An array of 4 mm nozzles were used for slug flow, while a 100 micron meter pore sintered metal was used for bubbly flow for the same air flow rates. Bubble distribution is successfully reproduced not only in slug flow but also in bubbly flow. Considering the measurement accuracy estimated from the phantom test, the present data may contain approximately 20% error in interface area measurement. The threshold value for extracting air phase was determined by referring to

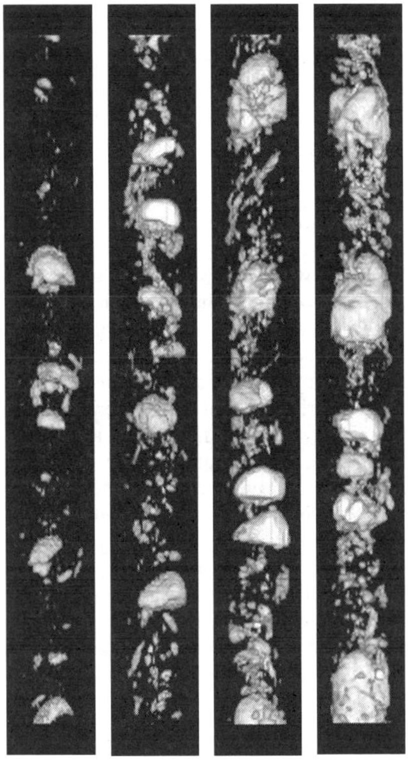

Figure 12. Side view of reconstructed void distribution in still water for different gas flow rates.

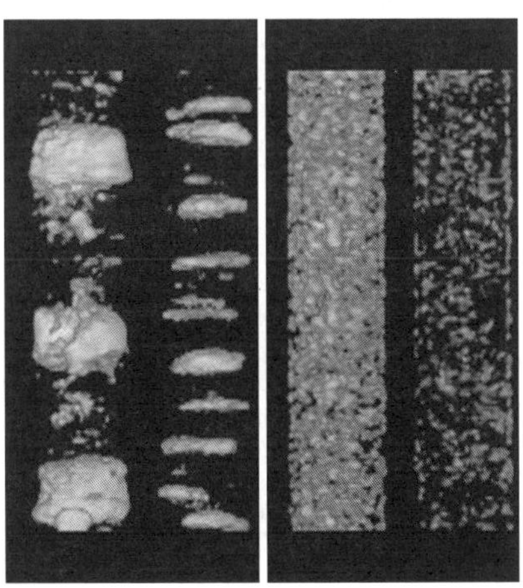

Figure 13. Reconstructed images for concurrent air-water two-phase flow in a 42 mm, 1.5 m long vertical tube. Gas flow rate remained constant ($j_g = 0.15$ m/s).

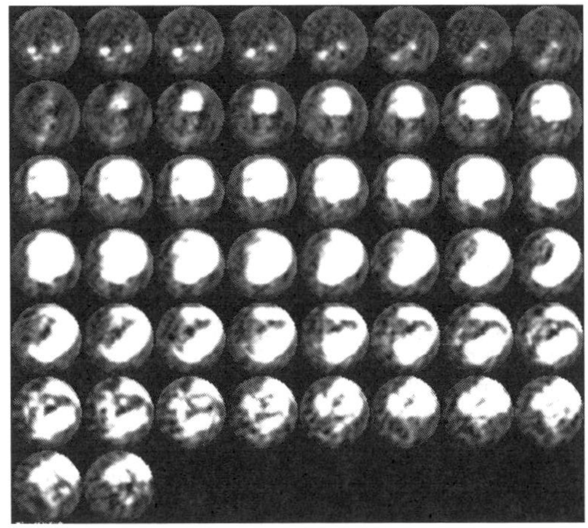

Figure 14. Tomography images of void in a silica-alumina catalyst powder in a 46 mm vertical tube for $j_g = 0.07$ m/s. Image interval is 3.8 msec.

the histogram of image intensity, in which the level was set at the bottom of the noise peak.

3.3 *Voids in fluidized bed*

As long as X-ray penetrates through, the X-ray tomography system is applicable to any composition of materials. One example of fluidized beds widely used in chemical industry is fuel catalytic cracking (FCC) process using alumina-silica powder as a catalyst. In the fluidized bed system, depending on the gas flow rate and characteristics of the catalytic powder, various sizes of bubbles are formed, which are invisible from outside. Since the bubble interface area affects the reaction rate of the system, estimation of the interface area is important. A mixture of SiO_2 and Al_2O_3 (weight ratio: 13% vs. 87%, particle diameter: 36 micro meter in average) was loosely packed in a vertical tube. Regulated air was introduced at the bottom of the tube through a sparger with an array of 1 mm holes facing downward (Kai et al. 2000). The average density of the catalytic powder is about 560 kg/m^3, which allows X-rays penetrate easier than water. Static height of the powder was 0.86 m and the measuring plane of the tomography was set at 0.6 m from the air sparger. Average air flow was controlled from 0.005 to 0.07 m/s. An example of continuous tomography images at $j_g = 0.07$ m/s is shown in Figure 14. The experimental conditions are listed in Table 2. It is interesting to note that similar slug shape bubbles with distinctive interface are formed inside the catalytic powder, but the breakup of bubbles at rear end is more irregular than air–water systems. However, the essential difference is that the fluidized bed system has an emulsion phase where its average

Table 2. Conditions of fluidized bed experiment.

Fluidized bed composition	
Material	$SiO_2 + Al_2O_3$ (13%:87%)
Particle diameter	36 micron meter
Solid density	2600 kg/m^3
Porous density	980 kg/m^3
Packed density	560 kg/m^3
Fluid conditions	
Direction	vertical
Bed height	0.86 m
Tube outer diameter	0.05 m
Tube inner diameter	0.046 m
Measurement level	0.6 m (L/D = 13.0)
Average air velocity	0.005–0.07 m/s
Tomography conditions	
X-ray voltage and current	100 kV, 5 mA max.
Vacuum level	1.2×10^{-6} Torr
Duration	2.0 sec.

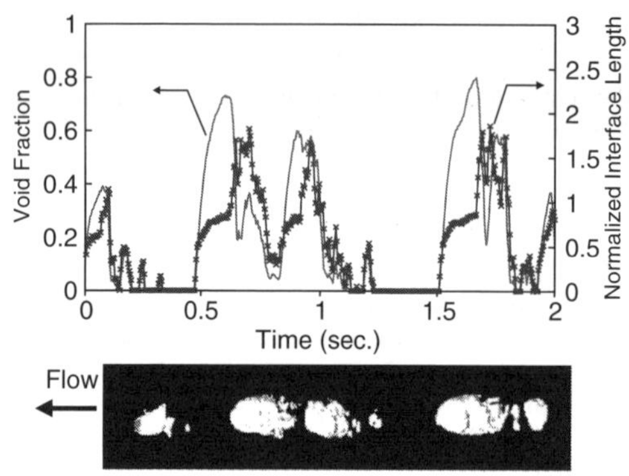

Figure 15. Variations of the void fraction and the normalized interface length for $j_g = 0.07$ m/s.

density falls in between pure powder and air. Since the expected density resolution is rather low in the present system, quantitative assessment of emulsion density may be difficult. Instead, the interface of large slug bubbles can be reproduced since their interface has distinctive density change. After binarization of cross section images, the edge of bubbles in the cross section are traced to compute the interface length. This length divided by the inner perimeter of the tube is referred to as the normalized interface length, which represents planar local concentration of interface area. The void fraction is simply defined as the ratio of the bubble cross section to the flow area. Figure 15 indicates variations of the void fraction and the normalized interface length in a case of $j_g = 0.07$ m/s. It is shown that the interface length becomes larger when the bubble breaks up at the end of bubbles, the region where the chemical reaction is possibly enhanced.

4 CONCLUDING REMARKS

For visualization of interface geometry in unsteady, inhomogeneous two-phase flow, a rapid scanning X-ray tomography system was built based on development of highly efficient semi-conductor detectors and multi-pulse X-ray sources. Preliminary test with plastic phantoms provided measurement accuracy of the volume and interface area. Then it was shown that the system is able to reconstruct dynamic interface geometry in air–water two-phase flow and in the silica-alumina fluidized bed. The results proves that the time resolving tomography works with the present design concept. In addition to visualization, the quantitative database of multi-dimensional, transient interface is useful for verification of 3D numerical codes under development. Although not shown in this paper, the system can be applied to multiphase flow in complicated or irregular channels. Such advantage will be recognized when the system is used for flow in rod bundles or in artificial/natural narrow channels. In geology, time resolving tomography will be suitable for analysis of fluid flow of binary or tertiary phases in irregular channels such as fissures and cracks. We plan to pursue geological applications in which use of the time-resolving tomography merits.

ACKNOWLEDGEMENT

A part of this study was financially supported by the Budget for Nuclear Research of the Ministry of Education, Culture, Sports, Science and Technology, based on the screening and counseling by the Atomic Energy Commission. Also, a part of this study has been performed as a public subscription project of practical and innovative nuclear power development by Institute of Advanced Energy (IAE) and Japan's Ministry of Economics, Trade and Industry (METI).

REFERENCES

Akai, M., 1986. Development of a fast X-ray tomography scanner: *18th meeting of multiphase flow and energy research MFE-No. 18*: (in Japanese)

Bear, J. 1972. *Dynamics of Fluids in Porous Media*: 1–13. New York: Dover Publications.

De Vuono, A.C., Schlosser, P.A., & Kulacki, F.A., 1980. Design of an isotopic CT scanner for two-phase flow measurements: *IEEE Trans. On Nucl. Sci., Vol. NS-27, No. 1*: 814–820.

Hori, K., Fujimoto, T., Kawanishi, K. & Nishikawa, H. 1997. Advanced high-speed X-ray CT scanner for measurement and visualization of multiphase flow: *OECD/CSNI Specialist Meeting on Advanced Instrumentation and Measurement Techniques, 17–20 March 1997, Santa Barbara, USA*.

Iizuka, M., Kimura, H., Morooka, S., Ishizuka, T., Kagawa, T., Osanai, S. & Shiroyama, S., 1982. *Japan J. Nucl. Engineering 24(6)*: 460–465. (in Japanese)

Iizuka, M., Morooka, S., Kimura, H. & Kagawa, T. 1984. Local void fraction measurement of two-phase flow by a X-ray CT scanner: *Japan J. Nucl. Engineering 26(5)*: 421–429. (in Japanese)

Ikeda, T., Kotani, K. Maeda, Y. & Kohno, H. 1983. Preliminary study on application of X-ray CT scanner to measurement of void fractions in steady two-phase flows: *Journal of Nuclear Science and Technology 20(1)*: 1–12.

Ishizuka, T., Inoue, A., Kurosu, T., Aoki, T., Ninokuchi, M., Yagi, M., Morooka, S., Hoshide, A. & Yoshimura, K. 1995. Void fraction correlation for rod bundle systems: A fuel assembly void fraction correlation based on X-ray CT measurements: *Japan J. Nucl. Engineering 37(2)*: 133–143. (in Japanese)

Jasti, J., Jesion, G., & Feldkamp, L. 1990. Microscopic imaging of porous media using X-ray computer tomography. *SPE Paper 20495; Proc. 65th Annual Technical Conf. and Exhibition of the Soc. Petroleum Engineers, New Orleans 1990.*

Kai, T., Misawa, M., Takahashi, T., Tiseanu, I., Ichikawa, N. & Takada, N. 2000. Application of fast X-ray CT scanner to visualization of bubbles in fluidized bed: *J. Chemical Engineering of Japan 33(6)*: 906–909.

Kukacki, F.A., Schlosser, P.A., De & Vuono, A.C. 1980. A preliminary study of the application of reconstruction tomography to void fraction measurements in two-phase flow: *ANS/AASME/NRC Int. Topical Metg. On Nuclear Reactor Hydraulics NUREG/CP-0014, Vol. 2*: 904–922.

Kumar B.S., et al. 1995. A gamma ray tomographic scanner for imaging void fraction distribution in bubble columns: *Flow Meas. Instru. 6(1)*: 61–73.

Misawa, M., Takada N., Ichikawa, N. & Akai, M., 2001. Interface measurement of moving objects by using a fast X-ray CT scanner: *J. Visualization, 21(2)*: 38–44. (in Japanese)

Misawa, M., Tiseanu, I., Ichikawa, N. & Akai, M. 2003. Ultra-fast X-ray tomography for multi-phase flow interface dynamic studies: *KERNTECHNIK, 61(3)*: 85–90.

Morooka, S., Ishizuka, T., Iizuka, M. & Yoshimura, K., 1989. Experimental study on void fraction in a simulated BWR fuel assembly (Evaluation of cross-sectional averaged void fraction): *Nucl. Eng. And Design, Vol. 114*: 91–98.

Prasser, H.-M. Scholz, D. & Zippe, C. 2001. Bubble size measurement using wire-mesh sensors: *Flow Measurement and Instrumentation, 12(4)*: 299–312.

Revankar, S.T., et al. 1997. *Int. J. Heat and Mass Transfer* 36(12): 2997–3007.

Schlosser, P.A., De Vuono, A.C., Kulacki, F.A. & Munshi, P. 1980. Analysis of high-speed CT scanners for non-medical applications: *IEEE Trans. On Nucl. Sci. Vol. NS-27, No.1*: 788–794.

Sharma, M.M., et al. 1970. *British Chem. Eng., 15(4)*: 522.

Tiseanu, I. & Simon, M. 1999. High-resolution cone-beam tomography for two-phase flow diagnostics: *Proc. of 2nd International Symposium on Two-Phase Flow Modeling and Experimentation, 23–26 May 1999, Pisa, Italy.*

X-ray CT for Geomaterials; Soils, Concrete, Rocks – Otani & Obara (eds.)
© 2004 Swets & Zeitlinger. Lisse, ISBN 90 5809 666 1

Detection of 3-D irregular grain shape of Toyoura sand at SPring-8

T. Matsushima & H. Saomoto
Institute of Engineering Mechanics and Systems, University of Tsukuba, Ibaraki, Japan

K. Uesugi
JASRI/SPring-8, Hyogo, Japan

A. Tsuchiyama
Department of Earth and Space Science, Graduate School of Science, Osaka University, Osaka, Japan

T. Nakano
Geological Survey of Japan, Ibaraki, Japan

ABSTRACT: 3-D granular fabric of Toyoura sand were detected by a micro X-ray CT at BL20B2 in SPring-8 and the obtained data were analyzed in this paper. The high-resolution X-ray CT system enables us to observe the fabric of the grains, whose diameter is ranging from 0.1 mm to 0.2 mm, with spatial resolution of 13 μm. After determining a threshold CT value to distinguish the grains from voids, a grain identification method to separate each grain from the others is examined. Additionally some results on contact area between the grains are demonstrated.

1 INTRODUCTION

It is well known that the mechanical properties of sand are strongly affected by its irregular grain shape. For instance, an assembly of angular grains exhibits much higher shear strength and lower fluidity than that of round grains. However, it is still unclear how to evaluate this grain-shape effect. This lack of the knowledge causes the wide spread of empirical laws in geotechnical engineering and powder engineering fields. Therefore, more intensive research for this subject is required for efficient structural and material design.

Experimental researches on this matter so far always have encountered the difficulty how to measure the 3-D grain shapes. X-ray CT is a powerful method to do that, but standard sands frequently used in geotechnical laboratory tests have their mean diameter of about 0.1 mm to 0.5 mm, which is less than the resolution of usual medical or industrial X-ray CT devices. Micro X-ray CT using a synchrotron radiation facility is one of the very few exceptions (Bonse and Busch 1996). In particular, the high flux density X-ray beam available in SPring-8, the world's largest third-generation synchrotron radiation facility, is naturally well collimated and monochromatic, and these features make very high spatial resolution of X-ray CT possible (about 1.5 μm and 13 μm at beamlines BL47XU and BL20B2, respectively (Uesugi et al. 1999, 2000)).

A basic procedure to detect and digitalize 3-D grain shapes from an assembly at BL20B2 is described in the first half of this paper. Considering the limitation of specimen size (0.5 mm and 5 mm in BL47XU and BL20B2, respectively), the system at BL20B2 is suitable for analyzing a sufficient number of grains at once. The key issue is how to identify each grain from the CT image of granular assembly, because the grains in the CT image are usually connected to each other at their contact points. In this paper we adopt an "erosion" process to separate each grain from the others, and the eroded pixels are then attributed to one of the identified grains inversely. The performance of this method is examined in the second half of this paper.

2 X-RAY CT SYSTEM AT BL20B2 IN SPRING-8

The X-ray CT system (SP-μCT) at BL20B2 consists of an X-ray light source, double crystal monochromator, high precision stages and high resolution X-ray image detector (Figure 1) (Uesugi et al. 1999, Tsuchiyama et al. 2000). The X-ray is monochromatized with a

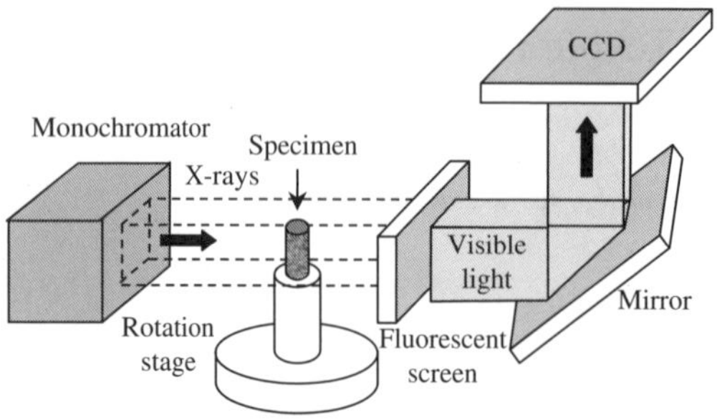

Figure 1. X-ray CT system in SPring-8.

Si (311) double crystal monochromator. The available X-ray energy at the sample stage is 9–72 keV. The transmitted images are detected by X-ray image detector, which consists of thin scintillator, optic system and CCD camera. The format of the CCD camera is 1000 by 1018 and the effective pixel size of the detector is 5.8 μm by 5.8 μm.

The X-ray energy used in the following experiment was 25 keV, and the explosion time was 12 seconds. The image was taken every 0.5 degree for 180 degrees rotation, that means 360 images for one specimen. Additionally an image of direct beam without a specimen was taken for every 10 images with a specimen by the aid of high-precision horizontal displacement stages.

3 SAMPLE PREPARATION

We conducted a series of experiment with different standard sands including Toyoura sand Ottawa sand and Hostun sand together with glass beads (nearly spherical grains), but this paper concerns the results on Toyoura sand.

Toyoura sand, a Japanese standard sand, is composed of the grains whose diameter ranges 0.1 to 0.2 mm (the mean diameter D50 is 0.167). Its grain shape is categorized as "sub-angular" (Figure 2(a)), and over 90% of its mineral content is quartz.

Three types of specimen with different porosity (dense, medium dense and loose) were prepared in cylindrical vessels whose inner and outer diameters are 3.5 mm and 4.5 mm, respectively (Figure 2(b)). The dense specimen was made by tamping with a rod layer by layer to make the specimen as dense as possible. The loose specimen was prepared with a special funnel that can be inserted in the vessel. Firstly we put the funnel in the vessel and placed the sand in the funnel. Then the funnel was slowly pulled out so that the loosest condition corresponding to the maximum void ratio test (JSF T161-1990, JSSMFE 1990) is attained. The medium dense specimen was prepared by soft tamping.

After the CT imaging, the weight of the specimen was measured and the void ratio (volume of void/volume of grain) was calculated.

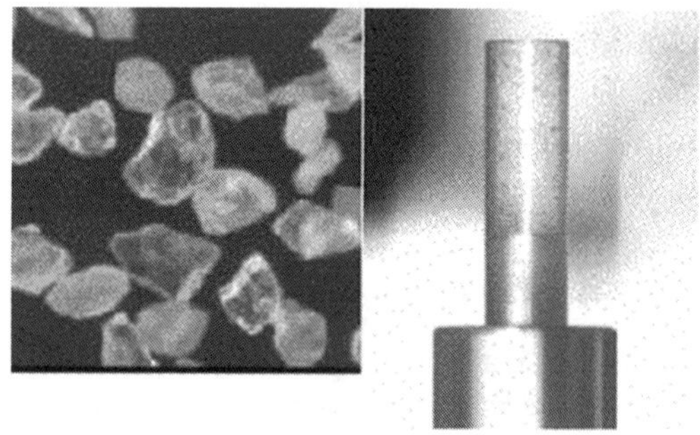

(a) Grain image by a microscope (b) A specimen

Figure 2. Toyoura sand and a sample used in X-ray scanning.

4 CT RECONSTRUCTION AND BINARIZATION

The reconstruction of CT image (Figure 3) was conducted with a program based on the convolution back projection (CBP) method (Nakano et al. 2000). The inclination of rotation axis was considered to obtain clear images. Figure 3 shows examples of the CT images converted to 8-bit images. The pixel intensity 0 and 100 in the images correspond to the CT values (the value of linear attenuation coefficient (LAC) of X-ray obtained by CT reconstruction) of 0 and 3.663 cm^{-1}, respectively. The latter value is the LAC of quartz (SiO_2) at 25 keV. Since Most of Toyoura sand grains consist of quartz, the grains in Figure 3 are mainly colored in monotonic gray. Slightly brighter grains than quartz are feldspars. Very few grains have rather white, which indicates that they consist of more heavy minerals.

Figure 4 shows the frequency of LAC within a central part of the specimens. All curves have the same peak value around 3.22 cm^{-1} in CT value. This is consistent with the CT value–LAC relation for the X-ray CT system (SP-μCT) at BL20B2 (CT value $\propto$ $9.8870 \pm 0.0039 \times$ LAC for LAC $< 20\,cm^{-1}$) (Tsuchiyama 2003).

In order to distinguish sand grains from void, the threshold LAC value (or pixel intensity) should be determined in rational manner. Figure 5 shows the computed void ratio with different threshold value. Compared to the void ratio from the measurement of specimen weight, it turns out that the good threshold value is about 2.23 cm^{-1}, which corresponds to about 60 in pixel intensity. This result is in good agreement with the eye judgment from the cross sectional CT images, as shown in Figure 6. The figure includes bright lines, that is a result of edge detection by this threshold value, which fits well with the real edge of the grains. However, it should be noticed that many grains are connected with each other via their contact

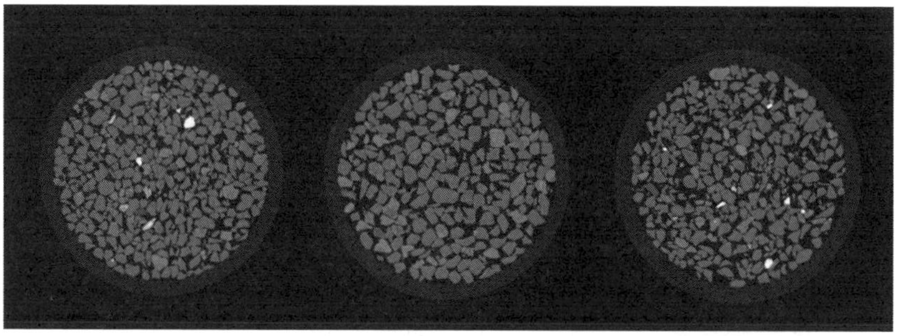

(a) Dense specimen (b) Medium dense specimen (c) Loose specimen

Figure 3. Reconstructed cross sectional CT images.

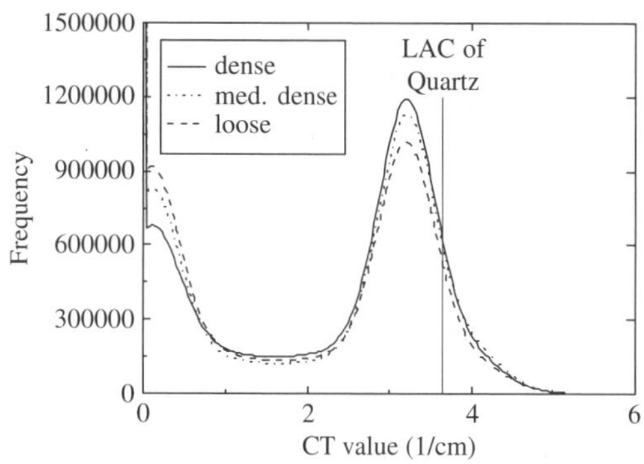

Figure 4. Frequency of CT value.

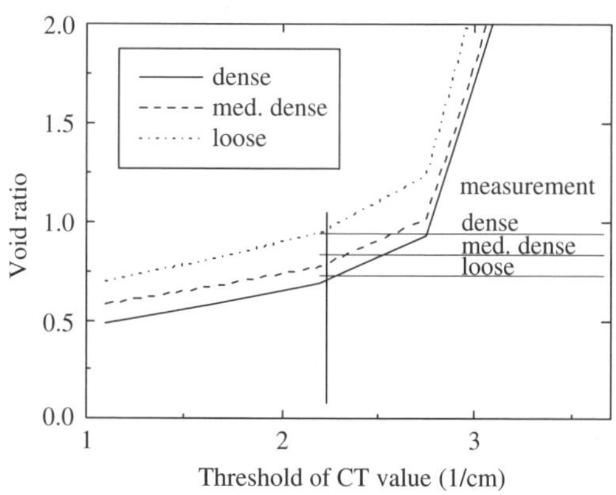

Figure 5. Computed void ratio from CT image.

points with such adequate threshold value. Applying "cluster labeling" analysis (Stauffer 1985, Nakano and Fujii 1989) into our 3-D CT data results in that almost all grains are connected together. Therefore, it is necessary to separate them into individual grains, which is termed "grain identification".

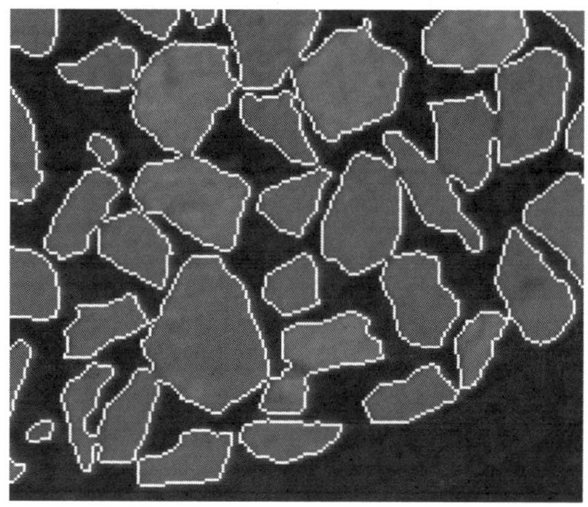

Figure 6. Result of edge detection scheme (threshold pixel intensity is 60).

5 GRAIN IDENTIFICATION

At first, we adopt so called "erosion" process to separate each grain from the others. Figure 7 shows a 2-D schematic illustration of this process. Actual process is done in 3-D. White pixels represent the solid grains and black pixels signify the voids. In the adopted erosion process any white pixel having at least one neighboring pixel in black (adding "*" in the figure) is changed into black. Therefore the pixels composing the grain edge will be eliminated and the grain becomes smaller (eroded).

Figure 8 shows its application into a part of cross section of CT image of dense Toyoura specimen for several times. One can recognize that the single erosion process cannot make all the grains separated. Applying the process for three times, a completely separated condition seems to be attained. However, this process may eliminate some real small grains. Since Toyoura sand grains are very poorly-graded, this may not occur so frequently. Even though it occurs, it can be checked in the following process.

After a sufficient number of erosion processes, the remaining "core" pixel clusters are considered as individual grains. Then the next step is to attribute the eroded pixels to the identified grains. In order to do that, we prepare in advance a list of eroded pixels for each erosion process. Then the lists are inversely used in the attribution process to find the neighboring core pixel cluster. If some pixels are next to plural core clusters, they are attributed to all of these clusters. It is clear from Figure 7 that some eroded pixels are not directly next to the remaining core clusters. Therefore, this attribution process is repeatedly conducted even for the single erosion process. Several pixels were never attributed by the repetition. Most of them may come from the image noise, but some could be considered as a result of "lost" grains due to the erosion processes. In fact such pixels were not so many in the process of our data, and they were neglected in this study.

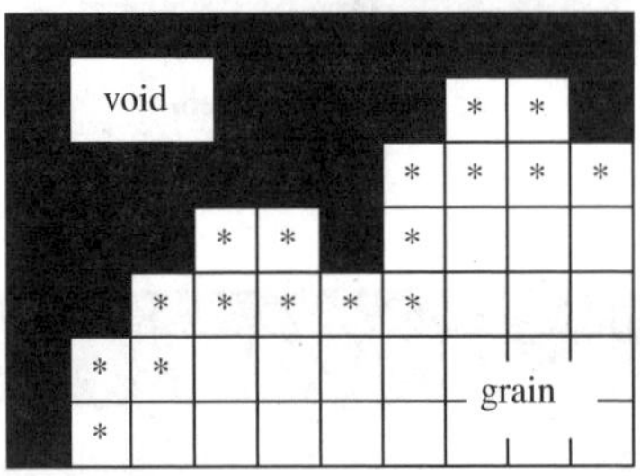

Figure 7. Erosion process.

In this way, the original binary image is translated into the information of 3-D granular assembly. Figure 9 shows the result of grain identification. A pixel with different gray scale indicates different grain. It is shown that the grain identification is successfully made in case that three successive erosion processes are applied before the attribution process. However, some pixels seem to be wrongly attributed as indicated by a circle in Figure 9(a), and it is necessary to develop a method for checking such errors automatically.

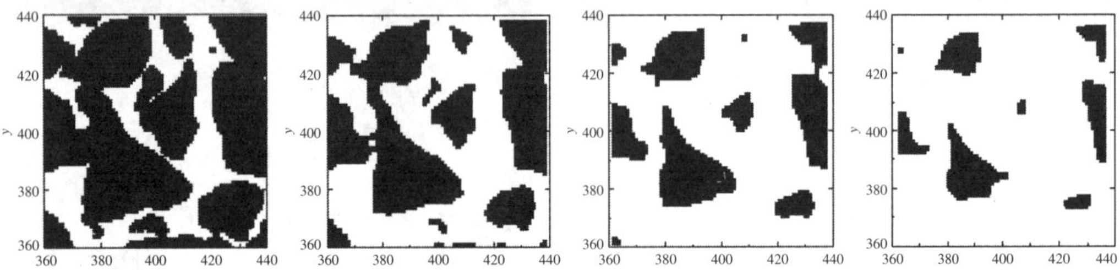

(a) Initial binary image (b) Image after one erosion process (c) After second process (d) After third process

Figure 8. Cross sectional image after erosion process (z = 140).

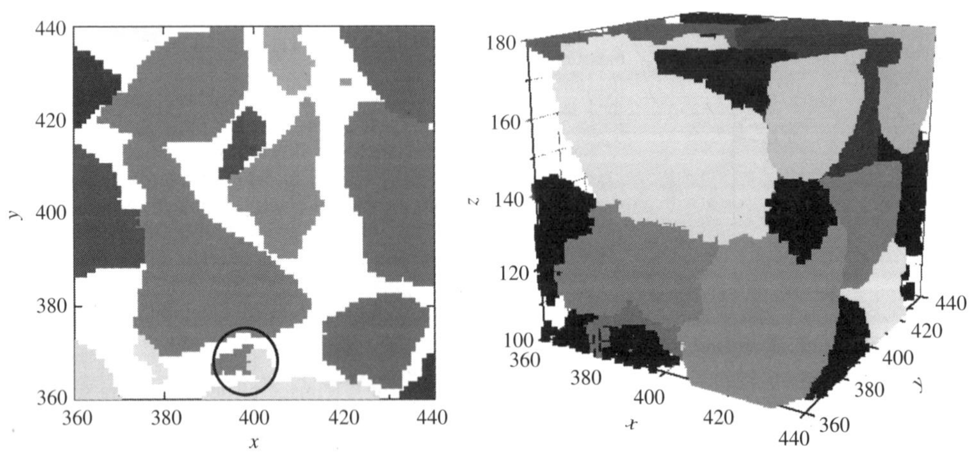

(a) Cross sectional image (z = 140) (b) 3-D image

Figure 9. Result of grain identification by three times of erosion process plus attribution process (different color indicates different grain).

6 SOME PROPERTIES OF GRAINS AND THEIR PACKING STRUCTURE

After the grain identification it becomes possible to analyze the volume and shape of each grain as well as the number and the orientation of contact points between grains. Evaluation of such properties helps us to prove the accuracy of grain identification method to some extent.

Figure 10 shows the grain size distribution computed from the grain information; the volume of each grain is computed from the number of total pixels attributed to the grain and its representative diameter is defined from that of the sphere of the same volume. The vertical axis is not a percent passing by weight but that by number of grains. The figure also contains the range of grain diameter of Toyoura sand based on sieving data. One can recognize that three-times erosion processes gives the most reasonable result of all, while the result by applying single erosion process is similar to that without the process; most of grains are still connected to each other. It is noted that some grains intersect the boundary of analyzing domain and their diameter is under-estimated. This may cause the 20% of grains having the diameter smaller than 0.1 mm in the result by three-times erosion processes. Also, a few grains are still not separated even after the three-times erosions, which leads to the existence of the grains having the diameter bigger than 0.2 mm.

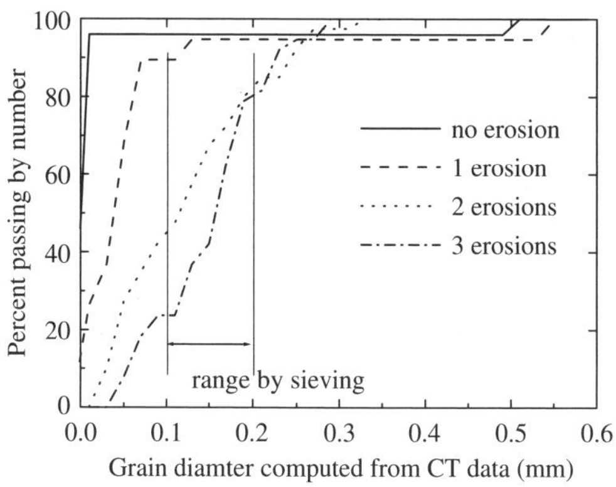

Figure 10. Grain size distribution.

Figure 11 is some examples of the spatial configuration of contact areas between grains. They are defined by a set of pixels which are attributed to different grains but are next to each other. It turns out that they have very irregular shapes; some are elongated and some are located dispersedly. This is due to the irregular shape of the grains. If they were spheres, the contact points should be circular-shaped. Further study is necessary to remove the processing errors, but this kind of contact area observation, which has never done before, helps us

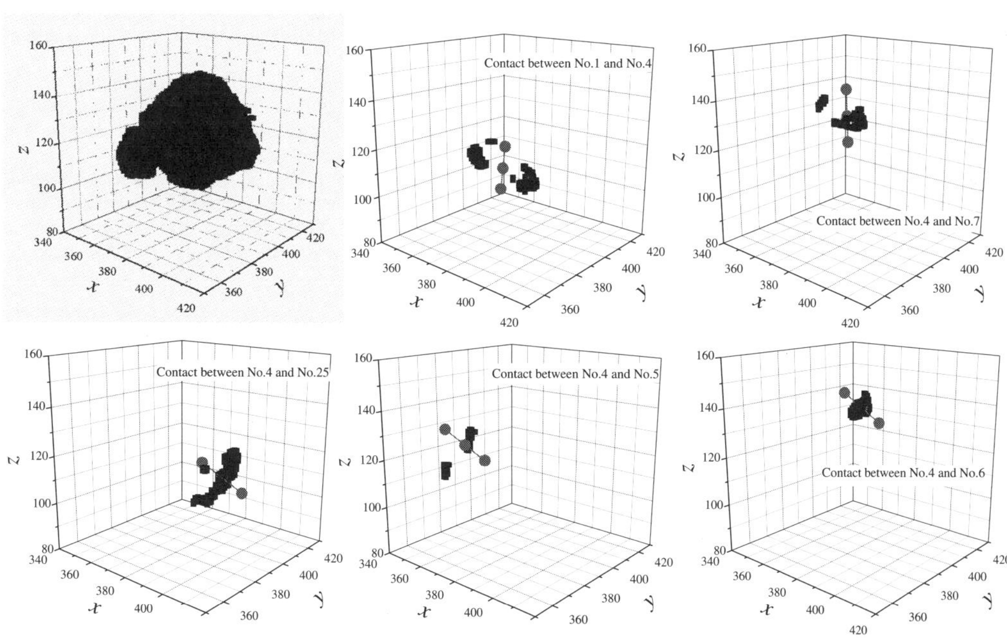

Figure 11. Example of spatial configuration of contact area between grains. (Top-left figure shows a grain image, and others show the contact areas together with the computed contact normals of the grain.)

to make clear the moment transmission mechanism between the irregularly-shaped grains and the grain-shape effect on shear strength of granular assembly.

7 CONCLUSION

X-ray CT is a powerful tool to investigate the microstructure of granular materials. In particular, The system in SPring-8 is suitable for the analyses of commonly-used standard sands.

This paper concerns the method of grain identification from the CT image of an assembly of irregularly-shaped grains. The results proved the performance of the proposed method to some extent. More detailed examination on the method will be necessary for quantitative discussion.

Our experiment in SPring-8 in 2003A period dealt with several standard sands such as Ottawa sand and Hostun sand together with glass beads, whose results will be presented elsewhere. The quantitative comparison among them will help a better understanding of the grain shape effect on mechanical behavior of granular assembly.

ACKNOWLEDGEMENT

The authors gratefully acknowledge Prof. J. Desrues of Laboratoire 3S, Universite Joseph Fourier for advising TM to use a synchrotron radiation facility for X-ray CT of standard sands. The authors would like to thank Mr. M. Iidaka, technician of Institute of Engineering Mechanics and Systems, University of Tsukuba for making a special vessel and funnel for the experiment. Mr. K. Toda and Mr. Y. Kawamura are also acknowledged for their help in conducting the experiment in SPring-8.

The experiment was carried out at the SPring-8 with the approval of the Japan Synchrotron Radiation Research Institute (Proposal Number 2003A0127-NDL2-np). This work is supported by a grant-in-aid of Japan Society for the Promotion of Science (No. 14750409).

REFERENCES

Bonse, U. and Busch, F. 1996. X-ray computed microtomography (μCT) using synchrotron radiation (SR), *Prog. Biophys. molec.*, 65, 133–169.

JSSMFE (Japanese Society of soil Mechanics and Foundation engineering) 1990. *Method of Soil Testing*, (in Japanese).

Nakano, T. and Fujii, N. 1989. The multiphase grain control percolation: its implication for a partially molten rock, *J. Geophysics. Res.*, 94, 15653–61.

Nakano, T., Nakashima, Y., Nakamura, K. and Ikeda, S. 2000. Observation and analysis of internal structure of rock using X-ray CT, *Jour. Geol. Soc. Japan*, 106, 5, 363–378.

Stauffer, D. 1985. Introduction to percolation theory, Taylor & Francis, Philadelphia, PA, USA.

Tsuchiyama, A., Uesugi, K. and Nakano, T. 2000. A study of three-dimensional structures of rocks and minerals using a high-resolution x-ray CT method – Primitive materials in the solar system and chondrules, *Journal of Geography*, 109, 6, 854–858 (in Japanese).

Tsuchiyama, A., Uesugi, K., Nakano, T. and Ikeda S. 2003. Quantitative evaluation of attenuation contrast of X-ray computed tomography images using monochromatized beams, *American Mineral.*, submitted.

Uesugi, K., Tsuchiyama, A., Nakano, T., Suzuki, Y., Yagi, N., Umetani, K. and Kohmura, Y. 1999. Development of microtomography imaging system for rocks and mineral samples, Proc. SPIE, Developments in X-ray Tomography II, 3772, 214–221.

Uesugi, K., Suzuki, Y., Yagi, N., Tsuchiyama, A. and Nakano, T. 2000. Development of high spatial resolution X-ray CT system for rocks and mineral samples. Proc. Nuclear Instruments and Methods, Sec. A.

Uesugi, K., Suzuki, Y., Yagi, N., Tsuchiyama, A. and Nakano, T. 2001. Development of high spatial resolution X-ray CT system at BL47XU in SPring-8. *Nuclear Instruments and Methods in Physics Research A*, 467–468, 853–856.

X-ray CT for Geomaterials; Soils, Concrete, Rocks – Otani & Obara (eds.)
© 2004 Swets & Zeitlinger. Lisse, ISBN 90 5809 666 1

Microscopic investigation from crack propagation to shear band of a gravel soil at uniaxial compression by CT image

S. Kiyama & S. Aoyama
Graduate School of Agriculture, Kyoto University, Japan

ABSTRACT: The image given from the X-ray CT of a gravel soil is analyzed in order to acknowledge the mechanism of the growth of crack–shear band relation and macro pore structure occurs during uniaxial compression. Especially, the geometry major axis on the cracks generated by shear is examined. The cracks having more than a certain major axis exist with the consistent manner on their direction against the compression line. The boundary scale for crack growth is confirmed. It is concluded that the cracks allocated within the final slide angle are involved to the serious damage of soil structure.

1 INTRODUCTION

One of the great characteristic of the gravel contained soils may be the generation of crack or macro pore space due to either the interlocking like structure sustained by gravels collapses or not. The sliding between gravels develops the crack growth and sometimes the corresponding interlocking between gravels makes macro pore, which may locally permit big storing of water and air in the pore. In other words, this links the more excessive difference of permeability and other mechanical properties so that the stability is jeopardized, than the case of fine soils. Therefore, the quantification of the inner structure geometry is requested with a certain precision.

In this research, X-ray CT method is adopted to analyze the fundamental solid structure geometry of a sheared soil sample. Especially, the macro pore and crack, which are capable of detecting from image, is quantified and the crack propagation mechanism is investigated. Some researches are also reported to acknowledge characteristics on the localized deformation of geomaterials. Khalid et al investigated the above problem to have the successive localized deformation images. Although the medical CT is elaborate for medical diagnosis because target is limited to the internal organs, the industry CT is developed, in general, for the wider utilization so that it is difficult to estimate local material density finely. The problem actually surfaces for the composite or non-uniform materials. The authors previously examined the scale dependency of uniformity of compacted gravel soil by the local fractal analysis, the spatial correlation factor and FFT. The relation micro crack – uniform scale of gravel soil given from the previous study is also considered.

2 TEST SCHEME

2.1 *Material*

A prepared material has the following characteristics; $D_{max} = 9.5$ mm, $D_{50} = 2.01$ mm, the weight fraction of gravel = 40%, fine = 27%, U_c (coefficient of uniformity) = 2159. A cylinder shaped sample with 10 cm diameter and 20 cm height is made by 5 layers compaction with the standard compaction energy. The averaged dry density is 21.08 N/m^3, the degree of saturation is 87.5%. This corresponds to the dry side of 95% maximum dry density. The sample is lapped with the Saran Wrap to prevent of drying.

2.2 *Uniaxial test and CT*

Uniaxial compression test is performed at the axial strain rate of 0.25%/min. Here adopted an industrial CT apparatus is, SMX-225CT(Shimadzu Co. Ltd., Japan), whose specification is shown in Table 1. CT scanning is independently conducted from the uniaxial compression in the present laboratory environment. This shows that all the crack that generates during compression test cannot be observed clearly. However, it can be thought that the subsequent crack development that governs the mechanical stability, as the chief purpose of this study, is recognized with the residual crack visualized in image.

Table 1. Specification of CT apparatus.

X-ray incident radiation	30–225 (kV), 0.01–1 (mA), 225 W
Min. focus scale	4 (μm)
Max. sample size	φ 140, h 250 mm (CT)
Max. image matrix	1024^2

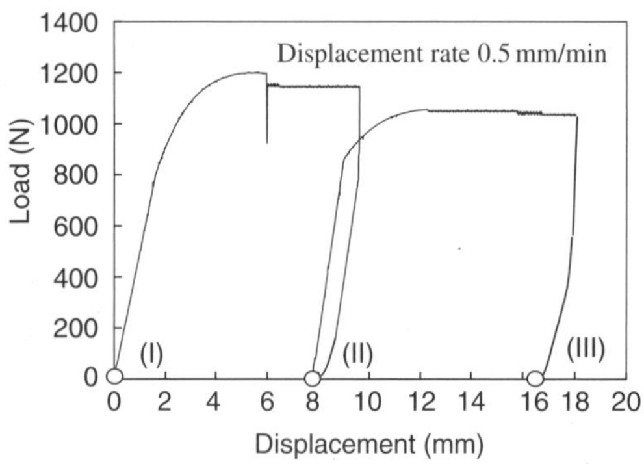

Figure 1. Uniaxial compression test.

Table 2. Scanning information for the test.

X-ray incident radiation	150 (kV), 160 (μA)
Projection area	119.500^2 (mm^2)
Image matrix	512^2
Slice width, total number	1 (mm), 201 (times)
Scanning rate	2 (min/slice)

Figure 1 shows the performed axial load – displacement relation and three scanning points, i.e., the before test; stage (I), post peak; stage (II) and the after test; stage (III). The CT images are given from the sample subjected to stress relaxation. The scanning condition is surmised in Table 2. The basic image pixel represents 0.2334 mm, the analyzed image constitutes of 8 bits, gray color of 256 gradations. In this paper, the geometrical measurement of crack and pore is limited in the two dimensions. It takes a lot of time more than 6 hours to have CT image at a stage.

3 CT IMAGES

3.1 *Compacted sample*

A set of three dimensional appearance and a vertical section of compacted gravel soil is shown in Figure 2. Higher density component like as gravel is visualized with light color. The sufficiently recognizable image is given in gravel shape. On the other hand, dark color or black expresses the pore space. For the finer soil part, it may not be enough to quantify their particle's linkage because of the wider projection area. However, it is found that the compacted layer is discernible

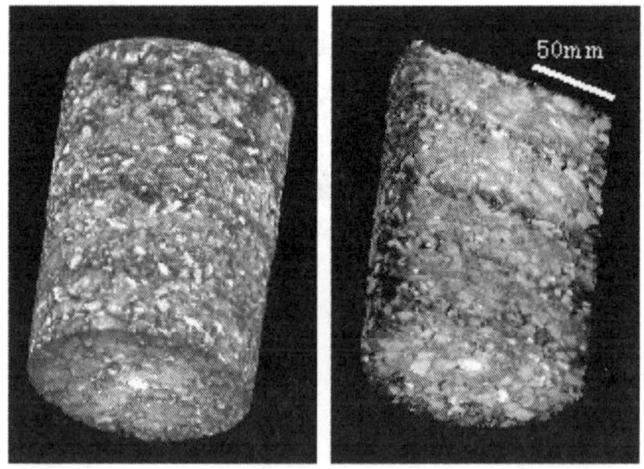

Figure 2. 3-D image of compacted gravel soil.

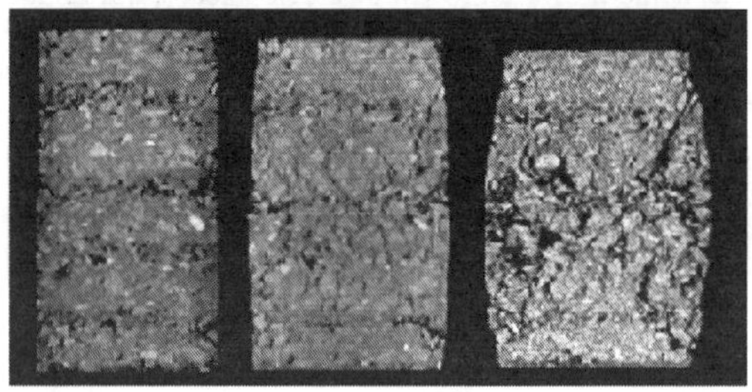

Figure 3. Original image of vertical cross section; starting from the left, (I) initial, (II) post peak, (III) final state. Chart is 256-tones.

clearly, which suggests that the serious crack or macro pore generated during shear can be visualized.

3.2 *Local development of crack and interlocking*

Original images of a vertical section of sample given from the compression test are shown in Figure 3. As loading goes on, four horizontal joints between the gravel soil layers diminish (see stages (II), (III)), alternatively a lot of cracks interconnect to produce the shear lines with X character or wedge shape. At the post peak stage (II), the thin shear line is confirmed. It seems that the horizontal joint pore space, which is seated on the orthogonal plane to compression axis, is not influenced on the direction of shear plane.

Next, the original image is corrected to the two tones image in order to quantify the spatial void distribution (Figure 4). The operation to extract void is manually done with proper noise cleaning by the trial-and-error method. Successful correction is conducted for all the images, so that the thickness of shear plane and the generation of macro pore changes at each compression stages (II), (III).

Figure 5 is prepared to investigate the void behavior by compression in detail. The marked circle A represents the case of growing up to the macro pore having

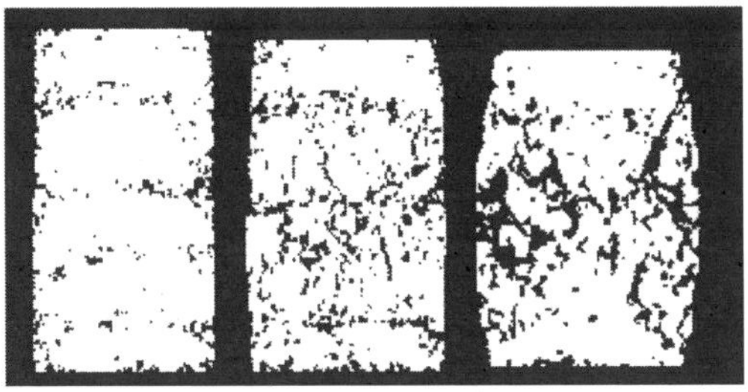

Figure 4. Corrected image with 2-tones. Black area is visually identified crack.

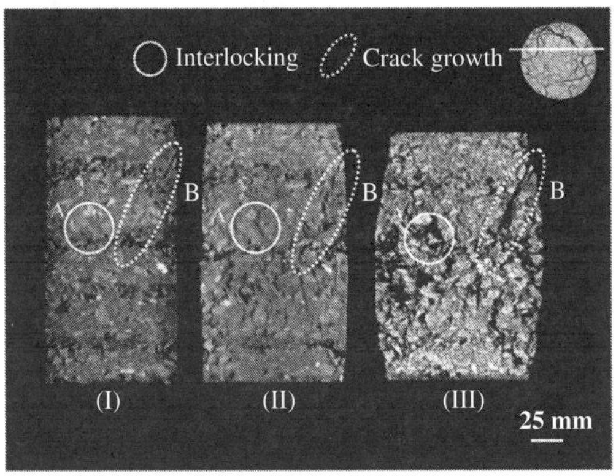

Figure 5. Interlocking and crack growth during shear.

the maximum length of 24 mm at the final stage (III). It should be noted that the final macro pore comes along once after the shear plane generates. This phenomenon to produce interlocking structure conditionally occurs by the combination of the gravel sliding and the gravel distribution in the neighborhood. When the grain content becomes larger, the tendency may be distinguished.

As shown with the ellipse B in Figure 5, the crucial for the strength is the existence of cracks that link each other and contribute to develop the bigger shear plane. The tip of fatal shear plane locates at the rapid change point of geometrical shape.

It is found that for the gravel soil mass the compression process can create the shear plane formed by crack propagation and the macro pore supported by the interlocking between gravels. The crack behavior of gravel soil briefly summarised in Figure 6.

3.3 *Directional character of crack*

Horizontal images at all the compression stages are shown in Figures 7, 8. From the images of Figure 7 at the upper side of wedge, the most clear crack circle is confirmed along the wedge boundary. The secondary

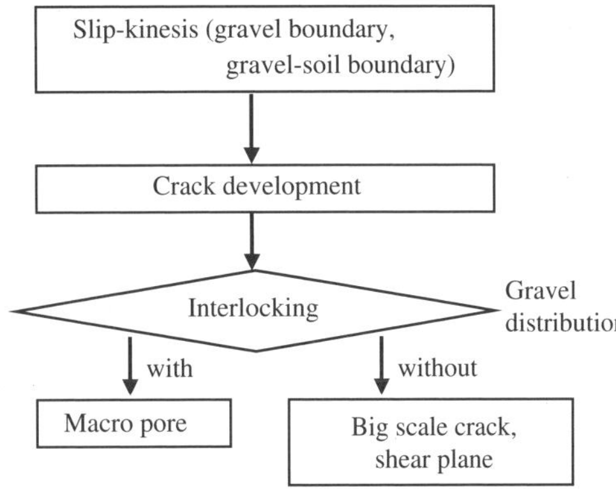

Figure 6. Schematic flow to micro crack behavior.

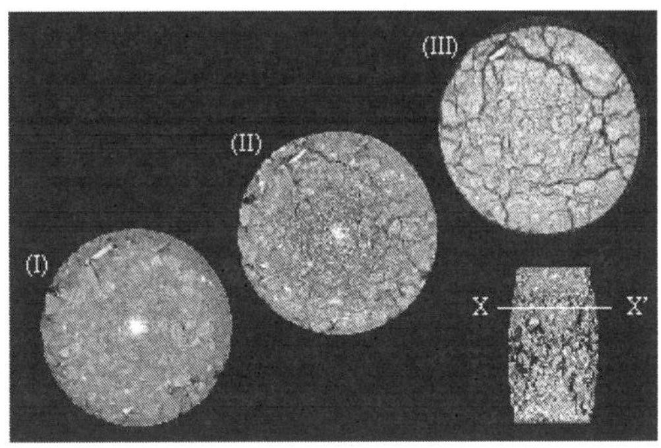

Figure 7. Slice images at a upper side of vertical section.

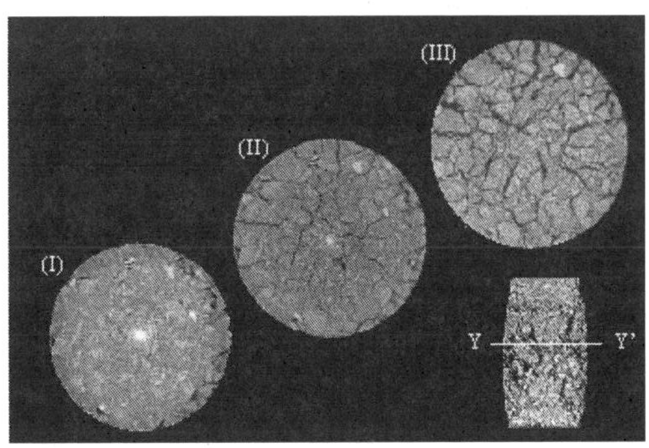

Figure 8. Slice images at the middle height.

crack along the grain boundary is also seen on the horizontal plane.

In the top of wedge, i.e., the middle height, cracks develop to radiate in all directions (Figure 8). Assuming that the stress concentration and lateral deformation is the biggest at the top of wedge, the maximum scale of horizontal crack development may occur.

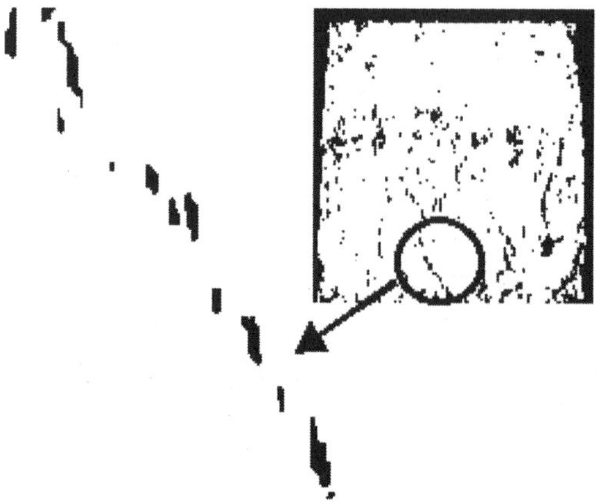

Figure 9. Typical micro crack to form shear line.

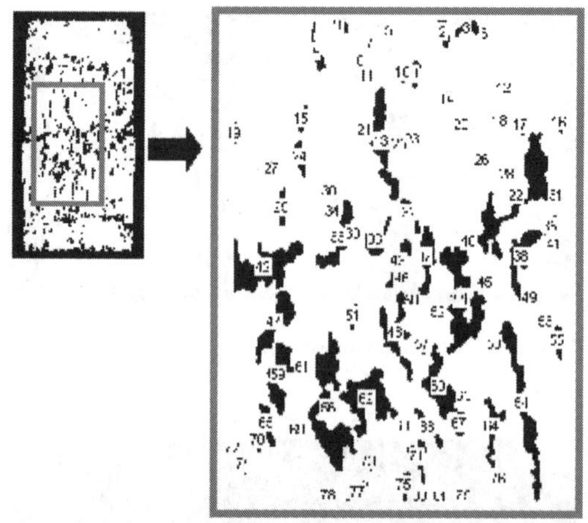

Figure 10. Labeling of cracks at the post peak stage (II).

Table 3. Geometry of micro crack to form shear band.

Geometry unit	Maximum length L (mm)	Pore area A (mm^2)	Orientation form vertical (°)	Degree of circularity ($4\pi L^2/A$)	Distance of gravity points between pores (mm)
Average	3.70	4.03	97.02	0.54	2.99
S.D.	2.78	4.38	21.41	0.18	1.03
Min.	1.24	0.59	42.43	0.24	1.04
Max.	10.36	14.17	106.89	0.85	5.16

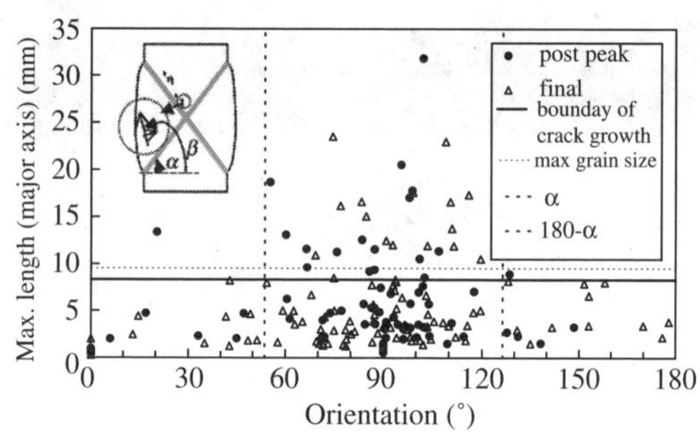

Figure 11. Typical micro crack to form shear line.

4 IMAGE ANALYSIS OF DOMINANT MICRO CRACK GROUP FOR FAILURE

4.1 *Definition of dominant micro crack*

Although there is a infinite number of micro crack in each images, it is thought that the typical micro crack group which links to grow up a certain big crack, exists on the thin shear line. In order to acquire the proper information on the micro cracks–shear line relation, the following methodology is introduced. The micro crack group that allocates more or less digestedly but also the farthest vertical section from the vertical image having the most clear shear line, is chosen as the contributor to crack growth. This may be convenient technique to analysis with a few of image data. The example of micro crack image that comes up for the study is shown in Figure 9.

The geometrical properties of the corresponding micro cracks are collected in Table 3.

All the micro cracks keeps the major axis almost vertical which is suitable for the compression direction. The average major crack length corresponds to about 40% length of the maximum grain size. The distance of each micro crack is relatively equal with the 0.31 times of the maximum grain size. The orientation of the discontinuous micro crack is 53.67 degree, which nicely correlate with the angle of the final shear plane. It is found that the slip by shear firstly occurs in the discontinuous micro cracks and then to links them to generate the fetal shear line.

4.2 *Development of dominant micro crack*

The behavior of any micro cracks between compression stages (II), (III) is analyzed in order to classify objectively either the dominant micro crack or not. The selected vertical cross section is the same coordinate, which may be slightly error because of the crack moves in three-dimensional space.

Figure 10 represents a example of labeling of any cracks at the post peak stage (II). It is thought that the relation of the length of major axis – its orientation is important to understand the mechanism of crack development. Figure 11 easily shows the following facts. The cracks that grow up to the more major length than 8.3 (mm) is oriented within a certain angle

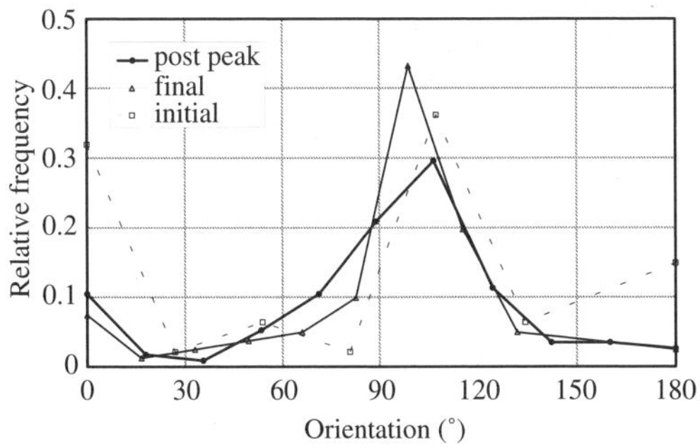

Figure 12. Relative frequency – orientation of cracks among the three stages.

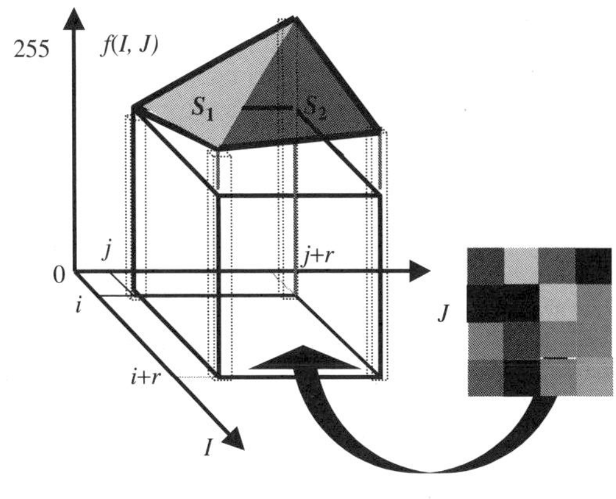

Figure 13. Estimation of the image surface area.

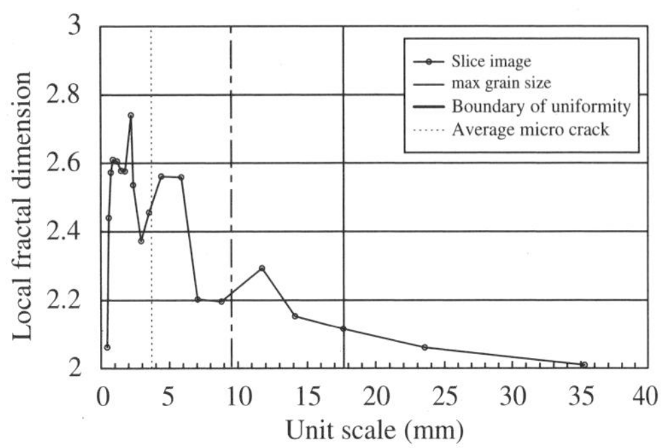

Figure 14. Local fractal dimension of a slice image of compacted sample.

range. In Figure 11, the boundary length shown with the horizontal dot line is equivalent to the 0.84 times as the maximum grain size. It seems that this length expresses the boundary between the micro crack and developed crack. The angle range of developed crack finely corresponds to the one of the final shear plane. From the fact, the criterion of either micro crack develops or not is defined as,

Cracks develop, when $\alpha < \beta < \pi/2 - \tilde{\alpha}$.

Cracks don't develop, or disappear, when β is other than those above.

where β is angle of major axis of the crack, α is the angle of shear plane from horizontal. The relative frequency on the orientation of crack's major axis at the each stage is shown in Figure 12.

5 MICRO CRACK SCALE AND UNIFORMITY SCALE OF COMPACTED MASS

5.1 *Texture analysis for variation of density*

It may be difficult to evaluate the spatial density distribution precisely because there is no absolute way of the direct calibration of the local density. However, it is easy to evaluate the image pattern from color variation in image. There is a method of local fractal analysis to quantify the texture of image.

In the fractal analysis of image, Fractal dimension is defined the following formula, and is in the range from 2 to the less real number of 3.

$$H = -\log\{N(r)/r\} \quad (1)$$

where H is the fractal dimension, N is the division number of surface $S(r)$ that expresses the image shading of the square area with a certain scale,

$$N(r) = S(r)/r^2 \quad (2)$$

The procedure to calculate the fractal dimension is as follows. First, calculate the image surface $S(r)$ for different scale r as shown in Figure 13. $f(I, J)$ expresses the brightness at image coordinate (I, J). The $S(r)$ assumes to be sum of $S_1(r)$ and $S_2(r)$ here as shown in Figure 13. Each $S_i(r)$, (i = 1, 2) is calculated from the brightness number (0–255 here) at the apex of triangle. Second, evaluate the gradient of $\log\{S(r)\} - \log(r)$, A (<0). Finally, the fractal dimension H is given as $(2 - A)$. When H is equal to 2, it means the flat image, i.e., monotone. The complicated texture has a higher H value.

5.2 *Scales of uniform density and micro crack*

The inflection point of fractal dimension – scale curve is defined as the uniform scale boundary. From the previous examination on sand, gravel soils with different gravel weight fraction (20, 40, 60%), it is found that materials having higher coefficient of uniformity U_c become smaller scale for the uniformity. For example, the scale of 17.64 mm is thought as the boundary scale either the uniform scale or not for the compacted gravel soil that contains 40% gravel in the weight (Figure 14).

As presented before, the average scale of micro cracks of 3.7 mm that set the stage for the fetal shear band, is very small of 0.2 times comparing with the uniform scale of this material. It may be concluded that the micro crack is sufficiently small scale not to recognize in homogenous scale of initial healthy soil sample. The geometry of the sample shape is rather an important factor to explain the mechanism to develop from micro crack to shear band. Anyway, the observation of microscopic structure by innovative CT method conducts to the serious solution how the localized deformation goes on.

6 CONCLUSIONS

Remarks in this study are summarized as follows.

A soil sample contains of 40% gravel weight has a local macro pore and shear band given by the development of micro crack during the uniaxial compression. Especially, it is found that the macro pore caused by interlocking structure of gravels may locate at the mid-height where permits the maximum deformation.

The orthogonal pore of joint space between soil layers to the compression axis disappears during the shear and doesn't influences mechanical stability.

The condition of micro crack to grow up is that its orientation of major axis is wedged between conjugated shear lines for the compression direction.

The micro crack having the potential to form shear plane allocates not only discontinuously but digestedly in some measure. The maximum grain size becomes a rough standard to confirm the development of crack.

The investigation presented here will be extended to extend in the three-dimensional field.

REFERENCES

Khalid, A.A. et al. 2000. Assessment of Localized Deformation in Sand Using X-ray Computed Tomography, *Geotechnical Testing Journal* 23(3): 274–299.

Kiyama, S., Kimura H. & Aoyama S. 2001. Mesoscopic Structure Analysis of Gravel Soils and Measurements of Their Complexity Based on the X-ray CT Image, *Proceeding of National Symposium on Mechanical Properties of Gravel Soils* 124: 199–208 (in Japanese), Committee on Mechanical Properties of Gravel Soils (ed.), *Japanese Geotechnical Society*.

X-ray CT for Geomaterials; Soils, Concrete, Rocks – Otani & Obara (eds.)
© 2004 Swets & Zeitlinger. Lisse, ISBN 90 5809 666 1

Characterization of permeability on light weight soil with air foam using X-ray CT scanner

Y. Kikuchi
Port and Airport Research Institute, Yokosuka, Japan

J. Otani & K. Tokunaga
Kumamoto University, Kumamoto, Japan

T. Mukunoki
Queen's University, Ontario, Canada

ABSTRACT: New geo-material made by mixing dredged slurry with air foam and cement is proposed to use for construction of water front structures. The characteristics of such materials can be influenced by the sea water when it is used in water front structure. Because the material can be weathered if the water is absorbed to it, pollution of ground and sea water can be occurred by the water through the material. These effects are mainly affected by the permeability of the material and it is the most important part to check the permeability of the material for utilizing it. In this paper, discussion of the permeability of light-weight soil (LWS) made-up of dredged slurry mixed with air foam and cement is made.

1 INTRODUCTION

Light-weight soils (light-weight super geo-materials, LWS) are geotechnical materials made of high water content clays mixed with air foam and cementing materials. They are characterized that the unit weights are light and their shearing strengths are strong. Such characteristics are favorable to backfilling materials for reducing the earth pressure to structures.

As LWS is intended to be used under water table in port area, a part of air included in the material can be exchanged for water during the long period. This kind of problem will be caused not only by water pressure but by its permeability. The problems as the strength reduction of the material by contact with sea water or the ground water pollution through the material alkaline may occur if we use LWS. These kinds of phenomena are mainly related to the permeability of LWS.

As LWS is a new material composed from saturated clay, cement, and air foam, less information has been given. The air included in LWS is in bubble state. Each bubble stays its position after the LWS solidified. Though LWS is in unsaturated state, permeability mechanism of it is different from ordinal unsaturated soil. Photo 1 shows the X-ray scanned image of the cross section of LWS. The black part shows large bubbles and the white part shows cement concentrated zone and the gray part shows the mixture of small bubbles and clay material.

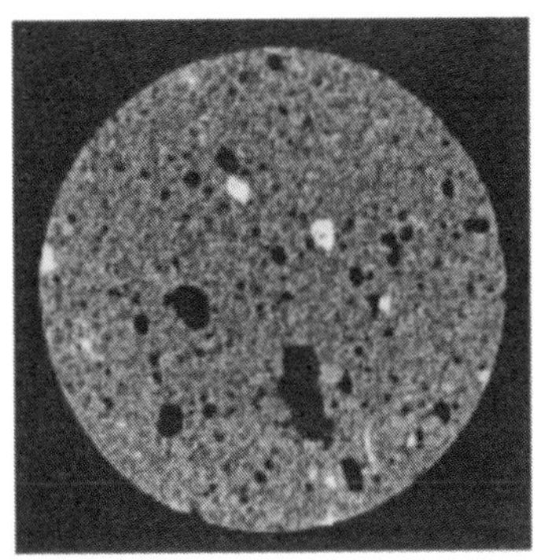

Photo 1. CT image of LWS.

Purpose of this study is to clarify the permeability characteristics of LWS. At first, permeability experiment results are shown, and a hypothesis of the mechanism of the permeance. Then seepage experiment is done and check the change of water content with X-ray scanner and find out the absorption mechanism. Finally, another permeability experiment is done and check the mechanism of the permeance with X-ray scanner.

Table 1. Physical properties of Kawasaki clay.

Density	ρ_s	2.678 g/cm^3
Liquid limit	w_L	52.1%
Plastic limit	w_P	23.0%

Table 2. Mixing condition for LWS.

	Mass (kg/m^3)	Volumetric fraction (l/m^3)
Dry mass	442	164
Water	574	574
Cement	75	24
Air foam	9	238
Total	1100	1000

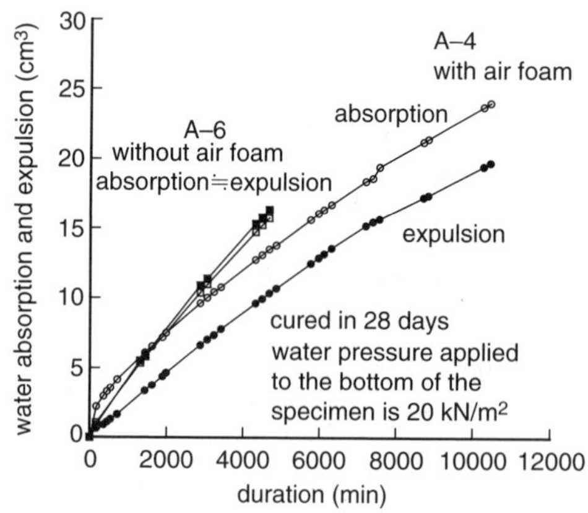

Figure 1. Difference of water absorption and expulsion by existing of air foam.

2 PERMEABILITY EXPERIMENT

2.1 *Specimen preparation*

Marine clay dredged in Kawasaki Port is used for main material in this experiment. The physical properties are shown in Table 1. The mixing condition for making LWS is shown in Table 2. The target unconfined strength at 28 days cured q_{u28} is 200 kN/m^2.

The mixture is filled up to the mold. It is put into the pressure cell filled with water before solidified for cured in the pressure simulating the under water condition. The pressure in the cell is 0, 50, 100 kN/m^2. Curing duration is between 14 days and 28 days.

2.2 *Permeability experiment with triaxial apparatus*

The experiment procedure is as follows. At first, the specimen cured in 100 mm high and 50 mm diameter mold with 0 kN/m^2 curing pressure is set into the triaxial cell without trimmed. Then the cell pressure is applied to the certain level and start consolidation. The consolidation duration is 3 days.

After consolidation ended, the pressure is applied to the volume change burette connected to the bottom of the specimen. Then the water is let into the specimen. Absorption and expulsion volume of the water is measured by using volume change burettes connected to both the bottom and top of the specimen during the water flow. Water flow continues for a week.

The specimen made of the same amount of cement and water content without air foam is conducted permeability test for checking the effect of air foam. Figure 1 shows the relation between duration and water absorption and expulsion. The difference of the two specimen conditions in air foam is included or not. The water content of the both specimen is almost the same. The specimen includes air foam in the case A-4 and does not include air foam in case A-6. Water pressure gradients of both tests are about 20. Figure 1 shows that when the specimen does not include air foam, the amount of absorption and expulsion of the water is almost the same and absorption and expulsion velocities are almost constant. The other hand, when the specimen includes air foam, the velocity of water absorption is very fast and the water content increases in the beginning, but the water content goes to constant later. The expulsion rate with air foam is smaller than that without air foam. These two test results show that the permeability decided from the water absorption and expulsion – "apparent" permeability – in the case without air foam is larger than that in the case with air foam even the smaller void ratio in the case without air foam. This result shows that the air foam is impermeable media.

In this test results shows that the volume of air is changed in the test. And the flow of the water in the specimen is affected by the compressibility of the pore. The consolidation of soil including compressive fluid is expressed as follows:

$$\frac{\partial(\rho v)}{\partial z}+\frac{\partial(\rho n)}{\partial t}=0 \tag{1}$$

$$v=-\frac{k}{\rho g}\frac{\partial u}{\partial z} \tag{2}$$

in which ρ: density of the pore fluid, z: distance, t: time, v: apparent velocity of the fluid, n: porosity $(=e/(1+e))$, k: coefficient of permeability, u: absolute pressure of the pore fluid, g: gravity acceleration.

Considering the condition $\sigma=\sigma'+(u-1)=$ *const.* and $(\partial^2u/\partial z^2) >> (\partial u/\partial z)^2$, following equation is derived.

$$\alpha\frac{\partial u}{\partial t}=\frac{k}{m_v\rho g}\frac{\partial^2 u}{\partial z^2} \tag{3}$$

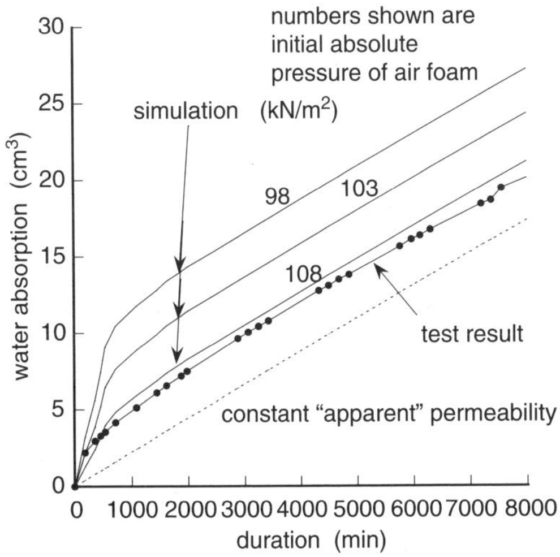

Figure 2. Comparison of test result and simulation.

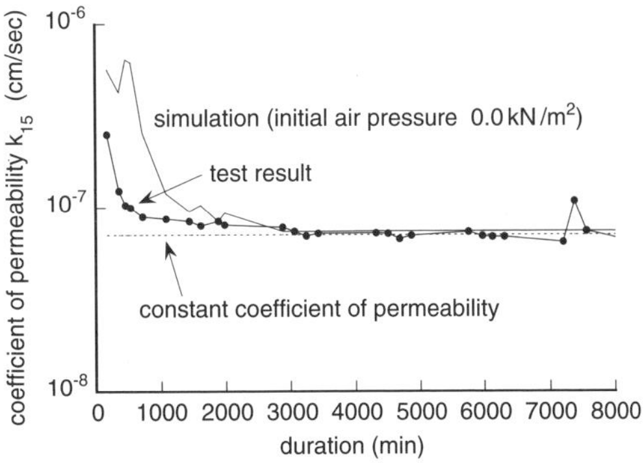

Figure 3. Comparison of test result and simulation in "apparent" coefficient of permeability.

in which $\alpha = 1 + n(C'_w/m_v)$, C'_w: compressibility of pore fluid, m_v: coefficient of volume change for saturated soil.

Verruijt(1969) showed C'_w is expressed as follows if the compressible fluid can be modeled as the mixture of water and air.

$$C'_w = \frac{1 - S_r}{u} + S_r C_w \tag{4}$$

in which C_w: compressibility of water, S_r: rate of saturation.

It is reasonable that LWS can be treated as the material with compressible fluid to consider the permeability of LWS.

Figure 2 shows the several simulation results of the flow test in the condition with different initial pore pressure. Figure 2 shows the change of amount of water absorption to the specimen against time. The result of this simulation shows that the coefficient α in the equation (3) should be suitably selected. The coefficient α is a parameter of m_v and pore pressure u. The simulation results of several initial pore pressures are shown in figure 2, because the selection of initial pore pressure has the large effect for simulation results comparing to m_v and the bubble included in LWS might be pressured (Kikuchi et al. 1995). By the comparison between simulation results and test data, the model used here can simulate the flow test phenomena except the precise estimation of the absolute volume of the water absorption.

Figure 3 shows the simulation and test result of the "apparent" permeability. The simulation results shown in Figure 3 are made in the case that initial pore pressure is assumed 0 kN/m^2. The time when "apparent" permeability becomes almost constant is almost the same. This result also shows this model can explain the phenomena.

2.3 *Permeability test in constant rate consolidation test (CRC)*

Constant ratio consolidation tests (CRC) is also done. This test is a kind of consolidation test. By this test, a coefficient of permeability of the geotechnical material is estimated.

The permeability and void ratio are known to have a strong relation in saturated soil. Air foam in LWS is highly impermeable as mentioned in 2.2. Figure 4 shows the corrected relation between the permeability and void ratio. In the correction, void of the air foam is excluded for calculating the void ratio. The permeability of LWS shown in figure 4 is calculated with equation (3) and with considering that the cross sectional area of air foam is excluded for calculating the effective cross sectional area for water flow. Here, we define this permeability is "true" permeability. Figure 4 shows that the relations between coefficient of permeability and void ratio of LWS with air foam and of LWS without air foam estimated by triaxial apparatus agree well. This result shows that this kind of correction can represent the permeability of LWS with air foam in a macro point of view.

Figure 4 also shows that the relation between permeability and void ratio of the Kawasaki clay used for main material in LWS and the corrected relation estimated by CRC. As Kobayashi et al. (1990) show that there is a linear relation between the permeability in logarithm and void ratio, the permeability of Kawasaki clay is extrapolated in the figure. The estimated relation by CRC is almost parallel to the relation in Kawasaki clay. And from the relation in LWS shown in figure 4, the permeability of LWS is rather small because of mixing cement. Terashi et al. (1983) show that the reduction

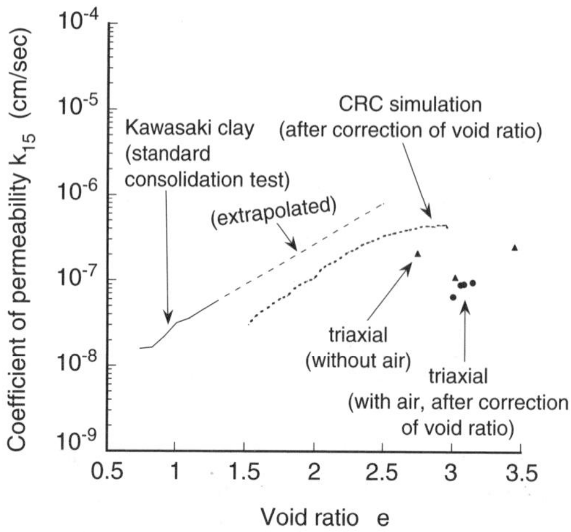

Figure 4. Coefficient of permeability of LWS.

of permeability is affected not only by grain distribution but also by void ratio. Addition of 75 kg/m^3 cement to clay make one or two order reduction of permeability (Terashi et al. 1983). The result shown in this study shows that the reduction of permeability ranges from 1/30 to 1/4.

3 SEEPAGE TEST

3.1 *Specimen preparation*

The specimen used in this test is in-situ LWS which was sampled at the trial construction site on Kumamoto Port. Table 3 shows the mixing condition of those in-situ light weight soil and those were mixed using special mixing plant at the construction site. Here, the air foam consists of the surface active agent was used. The dredged slurry used for this soil was Ariake clay which is known as a soft clayey soil deposited in Ariake Bay. The target of the density after curing process of 28 days was expected to be the value of 1.1 t/m^3. The sampling depth was 0.9 to 1.0 m. It is noted that the density after cured 28 days was 1.17 t/m^3 and this value was a little higher than expected.

This material is trimmed to a diameter of 50 mm with the height of 100 mm in this test. The soaked light weight soil was kept in the water of constant temperature which was 20°*C*. Therefore, water could seep into the soil specimen from not only its side but also from both bottom and top ends. In this test, the weight of the specimen and its volume were measured for a long period. And besides, the specimen was scanned at every 1 mm of the thickness from bottom to the top in each time of those measurement. This test was continued in 19 months.

Table 3. Mixing condition for LWS in 3.

	Mass (kg/m^3)	Volumetric fraction (l/m^3)
Dry mass	367	136
Water	624	606
Cement	100	33
Air foam	9	225
Total	1100	1000

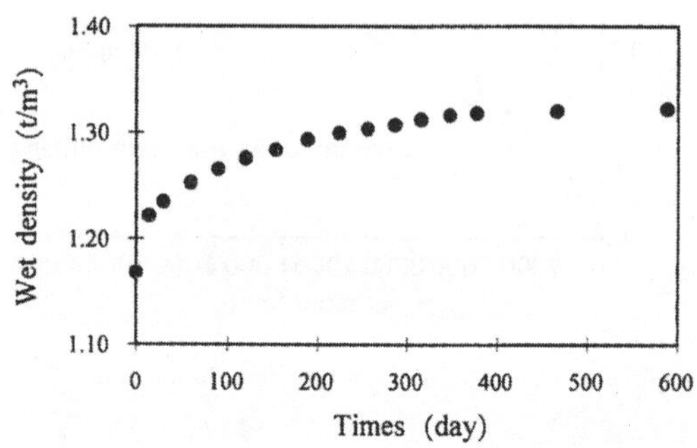

Figure 5. Change of wet density.

3.2 *Test results*

Figure 5 shows the change of wet density during seepage test. It was found that the density of the specimen was increased with the increase of elapsed time but the velocity of the change of the density was gradually decreased.

Figure 6 shows X-ray CT images of the specimen at the middle of height at several different elapse times which are from initial to 19 months. It is noted here that the light part shows relatively high density regions while the dark part shows that of low density in the CT image. Thus it is observed that the seepage front of the water was extended gradually to the center of the specimen axi-symmetrically. Here, there is a large black region in the X-ray CT image and it is realized as an relatively large air void. The shape of the air void did not change by the period of 6 month since the seepage test had started. However, it is observed that the water seep into the air foam after 6 months later because the color of that changed from black to gray.

Figure 7 shows the change of CT-values around the large air void shown by the arrows in figure 6. Up to 6 month, the CT-values of the central part of air void is less than −1000. After 9 month, CT-values are suddenly changed to around 0. In this case, the CT-value of water is 0 from the definition. This change means the void is filled with air up to 6 month, but is filled with water after 9 month. From figure 6, color of the surrounding area of the air void is already changed at 6 month. Then the void was filled with water. It means at first the water seeped in around the air void.

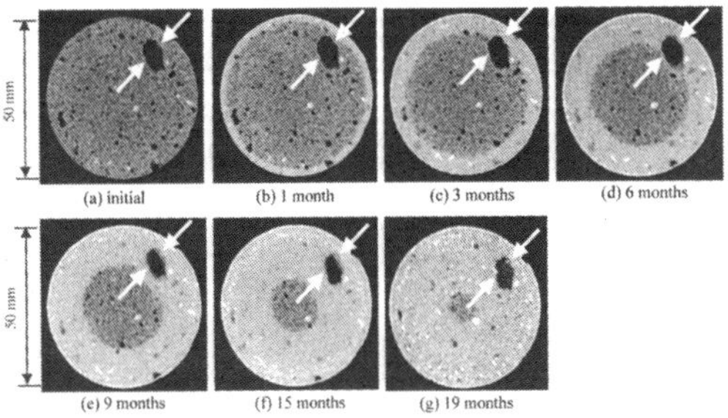

Figure 6. Change of X-ray image according to seepage duration.

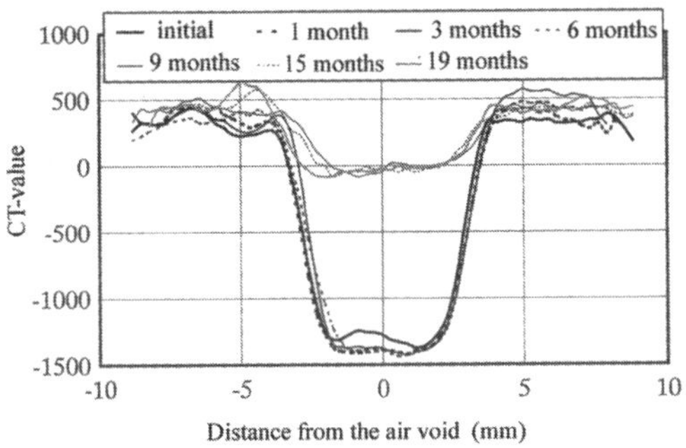

Figure 7. Change of CT values around the air void shown in figure 6.

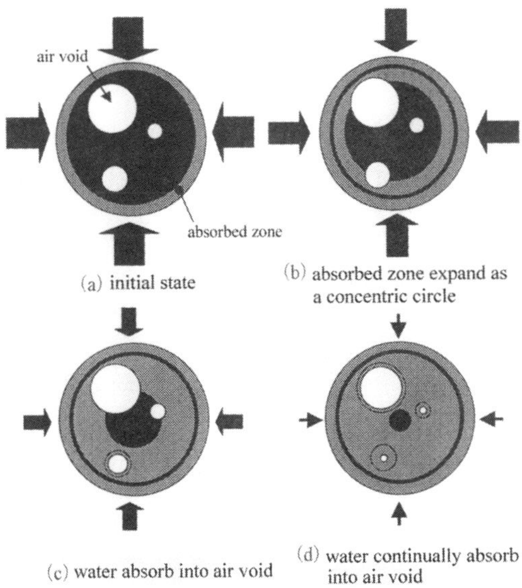

Figure 8. Image of mechanism of absorption to LWS.

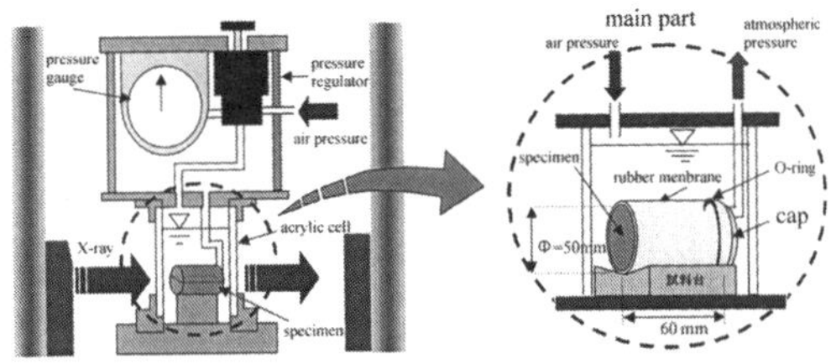

Figure 9. Outline of the permeability test apparatus used in this study.

Here we summarize the mechanism of the seepage (Otani et al. 2001). Figure 8 shows the image of the mechanism of the seepage. (a) Seepage goes a concentric circle. Water seeps to the area without of air at first. (b) The air void will be filled with water after the air void is surrounded by the absorbed area.

4 PERMEABILITY EXPERIMENT IN X-RAY CT SCANNER

4.1 *Testing method*

Two types of LWS with air foam are used in this study. One was sampled from the actual construction site. Main material of it is Kawasaki Clay. The other was prepared in the laboratory. Main material of it is Ariake Clay.

Figure 9 shows the apparatus used in this study. The dimension of the specimen is 50 mm in diameter and 60 mm in height. The specimen is laid in the pressure cell and sealed in side by rubber membrane. To confirm the sealing and minimize the void between the specimen and the membrane, the silicon type glue is used. The one end where the water expel is covered with porous stone and a cap which has a pipe to make the water expel to the outside of the cell. The other end is open for free absorption of the water to the specimen.

1 atm and 3 atm is used for cell pressure. By this apparatus, the water is expected to flow one dimensionally from the open end to the capped end. To visualize the flow of water, X-ray scanner is used.

4.2 *Test results*

Figure 10 shows the X-ray scanned image of the cross section of the center of the cylinder axis of the specimen. The specimen used was prepared in the laboratory and the pressure of the cell is 1 atm. Figure 10 (a) shows the original scanned image. Figure 10 (b) shows the locally smoothed image. In these images, the light part shows the area where CT-values are high and higher density area and the dark part shows the area where CT-values are low and lower density area. Figure 11 shows the change of smoothed CT-value distribution according to time in the scanned image. The figure

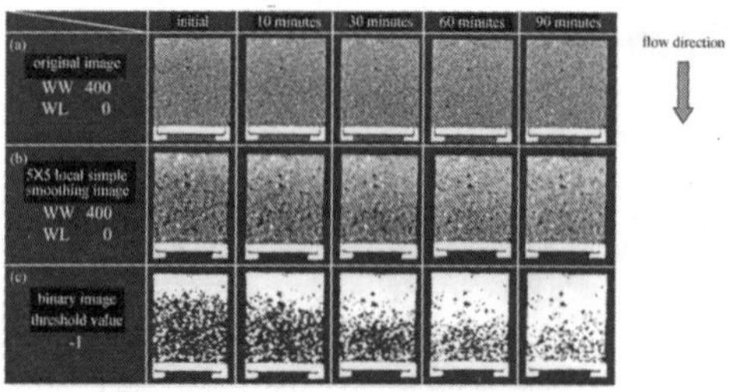

Figure 10. Images of CT during the permeability test.

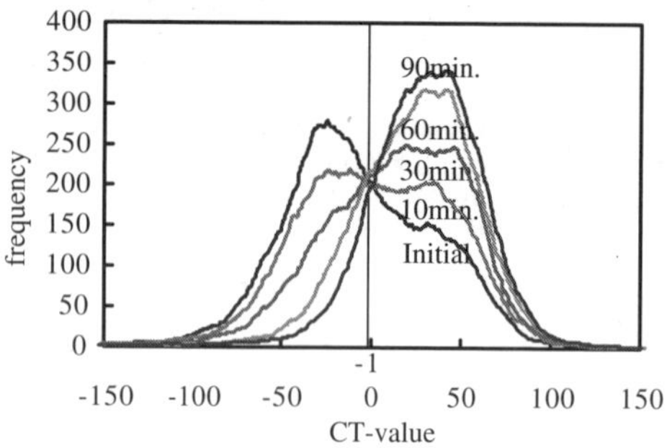

Figure 11. Histogram of CT values.

shows that intensity of CT-values smaller than 0 decrease with time and larger than 0 increase. Average CT-value increase with time. The density will increase in accordance with compression of air void and water seepage as the density change shown in 3. Because the void by air foam will be compressed and be saturated by water with water absorption.

According to the result of figure 11, the threshold value is selected where the intensity of the CT-value start to increase. Figure 10 (c) shows the binary image according to the threshold. From figure 10 (c), we can separate the area where water entered and visualize front line of the water entrance. Figure 10 (c) shows that the area of the white part increase with time and the front of white part moves to the capped end with time. Figure 10 (c) also shows that black area remains in the white part and it shows that water never entered to larger voids.

To speculate the seepage front, here define the ratio of seepage. The ratio of seepage is defined as the ratio of the white area to the diameter of the specimen for each distance from the entrance end. Here, we try to calculate the seepage velocity from the seepage ratio. In this calculation, the white areas are considered to be water and the volume of the water in the specimen is estimated from the white area. The income velocity of the water is calculated by the change of included water with time. Figure 12 shows the change of the expanding velocity of absorbed zone according to

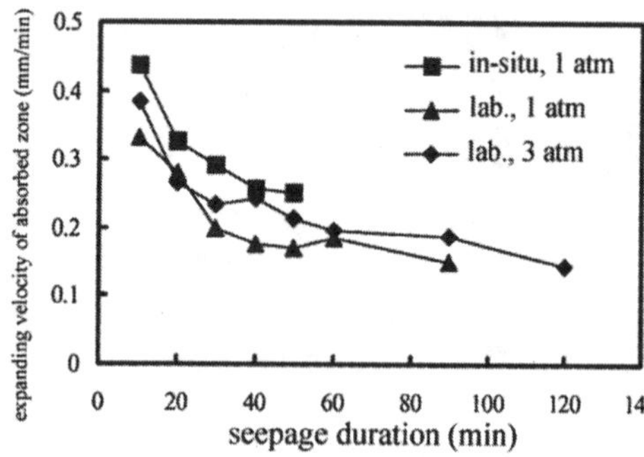

Figure 12. Absorbed zone expanding velocity change according to duration.

elapsed time. From this figure, expanding velocity decrease with time but it goes to be constant after long time. The coefficient of permeability is estimated from the final expanding velocity and the ingredient of water pressure. The coefficient of permeability calculated by the assumption is about 10-6 cm/s. The range of it is suit to that measured by the permeability experiment mentioned in 2.

5 CONCLUSION

In this paper, we discussed the permeability of new geo-material by mixing clay and cement and air foam. We have the hypothesis that the air void included in the material can be considered impermeable compressible media, and the coefficient of permeability of the cemented clay part of LWS is the same as the coefficient of permeability of cement treated clay. By X-ray scanner, we visualize the permeance mechanism, and the hypothesis is almost correct.

REFERENCES

Kikuchi, Y., and Yoshino, H. 1998. Permeability of light-weight soil made of dredged slurry mixed with air foam, *Report of Port and Harbour Research Institute*, 37(1): 33–56. (in Japanese)

Kobayashi, M., Mizukami, J., and Tsuchida, T. 1990. Determination of the horizontal coefficient of consolidation c_h, *Report of Port and Harbour Research Institute*, 29(2): 63–83. (in Japanese)

Terashi, M., Tanaka, H., Mitsumoto, T., Honda, S., and Ohhashi, T. 1983. Fundamental properties of lime and cement treated Soils (3rd Report), *Report of the Port and Harbour Research Institute*, 22(1): 69–96. (in Japanese)

Verruijt, A. 1969. Elastic storage of aquifers, *Flow through porous media*: Chapter 8, Academic Press.

Otani, J., Mukunoki, T., Nagatome, T., Kikuchi, Y., and Sato, T. 2001. Characterization of seepage and drying on light weight soil with air foam using X-ray CT method, *Journal of Geotechnical Engineering*, JSCE, No. 701/III-58: 293–302. (in Japanese)

X-ray CT for Geomaterials; Soils, Concrete, Rocks – Otani & Obara (eds.)
© 2004 Swets & Zeitlinger. Lisse, ISBN 90 5809 666 1

Shear banding in plane strain compression of Beaucaire Marl studied through post-mortem X-ray micro tomography

S. Marello, N. Lenoir, G. Viggiani, P. Bésuelle & J. Desrues
Laboratoire 3S, UJF-INPG-CNRS, Grenoble, France

M. Di Michiel
European Synchrotron Radiation Facility, Grenoble, France

ABSTRACT: Failure of geomaterials is commonly associated with the *localization of deformation* in zones of intense shearing, such as shear bands and fractures. In fine-grained, stiff soils and soft rocks, both shear bands and cracks form and possibly interact. Typically, a *process zone* exists at the tip of the propagating crack, where the material experiences damage and mechanical degradation. Getting experimental data is in this case a formidable task, because the regions of localization have a characteristic finite dimension which is in the order of some tens of microns, that is clearly inaccessible by means of conventional measurement techniques. In this paper, we present results obtained using X-ray micro tomography to evaluate shear banding in fine-grained stiff clays. Small cylindrical specimens (20 mm in diameter) were extracted from samples of Beaucaire Marl previously tested in plane strain compression tests at Laboratoire 3S. Using synchrotron radiation as the X-ray source, in combination with a suitable X-ray detector, allows for a high spatial resolution of density field (10 to 20 μm). The paper presents and discusses a selection of experimental results on the patterns of localization as observed in plane strain compression of Beaucaire Marl along with the related, micro tomography based measurements.

1 INTRODUCTION

Strain localization, the concentration of deformation into narrow zones of intense shearing, is a phenomenon commonly observed in virtually all geomaterials, including rocks, soils and concrete. The body of literature on the modeling of localization in geomaterials has been growing rapidly, especially during the last two decades, see for example Vardoulakis & Sulem (1995). Various experimental studies have also been carried out which have provided a number of important data on the onset and subsequent propagation of strain localization in a soil specimen subjected to shear (*e.g.*, Saada *et al.* (1994), Finno *et al.* (1997), Desrues & Viggiani (2003) – to quote but a few; more references are quoted therein). A wide range of experimental techniques have been applied over the years, which include optical and electronic microscopy, radiographic analysis, ultrasonic and acoustic techniques, multiple stress and strain local measurements, stereophotogrammetry and image analysis to name but a few. The challenge here, and the possible reason why so many different techniques have been used is the fact that one wants to measure deformations in a region the size of which, upon strain localization, reduces abruptly and dramatically, say from the scale of the specimen to the shear band scale. Measuring deformations throughout a test, that is: prior to, at, and after the onset of strain localization is then a formidable task, which can only be accomplished by using field measurements. In fact, when strains are (highly) localized, strain variables cannot be derived from boundary measurements of displacements.

A large experimental program was recently carried out in Grenoble, with the objective of investigating and providing insight into the phenomenon of shear banding in saturated stiff clayey soils. Undisturbed specimens of a natural stiff clay (Beaucaire Marl) were tested in plane strain conditions, under both drained and undrained conditions. Image correlation methods, including False Relief Stereophotogrammetry (FRS) and Particle Image Velocimetry (PIV), were extensively used to capture non-homogeneous deformation throughout a test. Local measurement of pore water pressure was also made, which greatly enhances the ability to capture the onset of strain localization during a test. Some time after the test, small cylindrical specimens (20 mm in diameter) were extracted from the samples, and then X-ray scanned using synchrotron radiation at the ESRF in Grenoble. The high spatial resolution achieved allowed to observe the regions of localization at the level of 10 to 20 μm.

The experimental apparatus, testing procedures and results are described in detail in a forthcoming paper by Viggiani *et al.* (2003). The focus of the present paper is rather on the *post-mortem* micro tomographic observation of strain localization in Beaucaire Marl. The results of a few selected plane strain tests are presented first, and the main findings are discussed concerning occurrence and progression of strain localization. The technical details of this application of X-ray micro tomography are then briefly given, and finally a number of observations are presented on the patterns of strain localization as obtained by micro tomography.

2 RESULTS FROM PLANE STRAIN TESTS

2.1 *Experimental apparatus*

The experiments on Beaucaire marl were performed in the plane strain compression apparatus at the Laboratoire 3S of Grenoble. Within this device, a 35 mm thick prismatic specimen, surrounded by a latex membrane, is mounted between two rigid walls inducing plane strain conditions (Fig. 1). The initial height and width of the specimen (in the plane of deformation) were 170 mm and 80 mm, respectively. The side walls are glass plates which allow photographs to be taken of the in-plane deformation of a specimen during the test. The bottom and top loading platens house porous stones connected to drainage lines. The top platen is free to slide horizontally in the plane of deformation, which allows free lateral displacement of the upper portion of the specimen when a shear band forms due to deviatoric loading. All surfaces in contact with the specimen are lubricated with silicone grease to minimize friction. A large cell, filled with silicone oil, surrounds the specimen allowing to apply a confining pressure. Strain-controlled axial loading is applied through a screw jack which rests on top of the device.

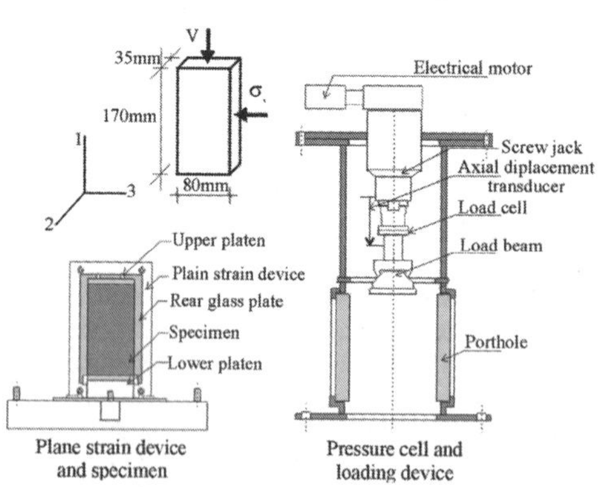

Figure 1. Schematic diagram of the plane strain apparatus.

An LVDT measures vertical displacement of the top platen, while the axial load is measured by an internal load cell at the top. Cell pressure is supplied by a compressor, and monitored by a pressure transducer, while the traditional self-compensating mercury control is used to apply a back pressure to the pore water. Global volume change is monitored with an LVDT measuring the drop in mercury level in the upper cylinder, whereas pore pressure is monitored by two miniature pore pressure probes which are mounted on the sides of the specimen subjected to confining pressure, at mid-height.

2.2 *Material tested and experimental program*

The material tested for this study (Beaucaire Marl) is a sedimentary soil which has been extensively studied in Grenoble over the last fifteen years. It comes from a natural deposit located at Beaucaire, in Southern France, which was deposited in a shallow marine environment during the Pliocene age. Beaucaire marl can be considered as a stiff clayey soil – or a soft clayey rock: in either case, it clearly falls into the category of hard soils-soft rocks. The soil is a CL clay according to the Unified Soil Classification System. The clay content is about 30%, and the calcium carbonate content can be as high as 30%. The specific gravity G_s is equal to 2.73. Microscopic observation did not reveal any evidence of pre-existing microcracks. The natural material is heavily overconsolidated and quite stiff, its natural water content ranging from 23 to 25%, which should be compared to a liquid limit and a plasticity index in the range 40–45% and 21–25%, respectively. The vertical yield stress from 1D compression tests is about 2 MPa, and its uniaxial compressive strength averages 0.9 MPa.

A total of 16 plane strain tests were performed on Beaucaire Marl from approximately isotropic stress conditions, after back pressure saturation and consolidation (or swelling). Shearing was performed under displacement control with a rate of applied displacement of 0.004 mm/min, which corresponds to a nominal axial strain rate of 0.14%/hour for a 170 mm high specimen. Both drained and undrained tests were carried out, starting from values of initial mean effective stress p'_0 in the range of 50 to 600 kPa. Note that all specimens had a degree of saturation close to 100% before testing.

2.3 *Observed response*

Both contractive and dilative behaviors were obtained in the experiments, depending on the initial value of mean effective stress. Results from just one test are presented in detail here, which is typical of a dilative behavior.

The results of drained test MBSM07 are shown in Figure 2. Figure 2a shows the axial load versus global axial strain, $\varepsilon_a = -\ln(H/H_0)$, where H_0 and H are the initial and current height of the specimen, respectively. The load monotonically increases until a peak is attained at approximately 2.5% strain, whereupon it sharply drops and levels off. Two minor load drops can also be observed at 1.0% and 4.0% axial strain, in the pre- and post-peak regime, respectively. Figure 2b shows the evolution of volumetric strain, $\varepsilon_v = -\ln(V/V_0)$, where V_0 and V are the initial and current volume of the specimen, respectively. The specimen compresses until 2.3% axial strain, shortly prior to the peak of axial load, and dilates thereafter. The rate of (global) dilatancy is quite high while the load is dropping, whereas it gets much smaller starting from 2.9% axial strain, when the load levels off.

Although test MBSM07 was performed under drained conditions, *i.e.* with free draining boundaries, recall that pore water pressure was measured throughout the test at the mid-height of the specimen. Figure 2c shows the difference Δu between the pore pressures measured by the two internal probes. Essentially the same pore pressure (equal to the back pressure) was measured at the two probes all throughout the test, except for a series of distinct jumps. Two of them occurred at 1.0% and 4.0% axial strain, whereas a more complex response was observed in between 2.4 and 2.9% axial strain, including a sequence of rapid increases and reductions of Δu. Remarkably, all these pressure jumps take place exactly at the points of the test when a load peak followed by a sharp reduction is observed. This is far to be a "coincidence", and was actually observed in every single test (under both nominally drained and undrained conditions). Pore pressure non-uniformities and the development of shear banding were found to be closely interacting phenomena, as thoroughly discussed by Viggiani *et al.* (2003), and previously suggested by Viggiani *et al.* (1994).

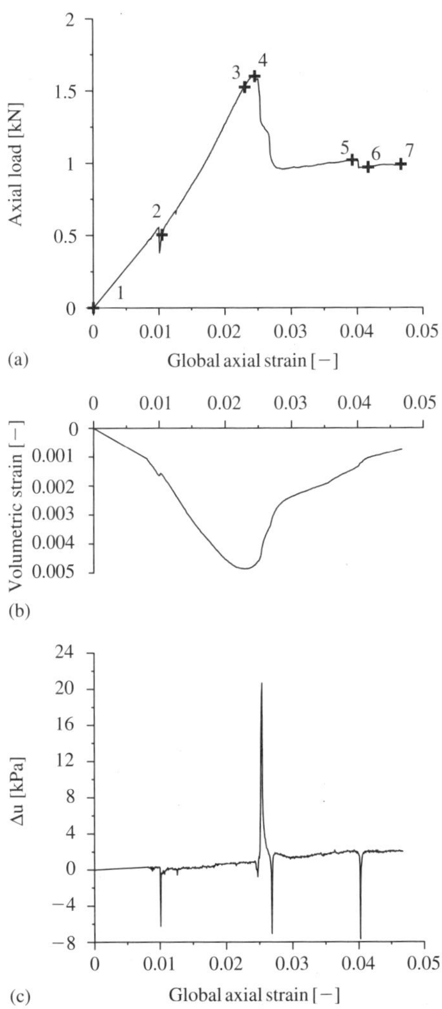

Figure 2. Response obtained in test MBSM07: (a) axial load *vs.* axial strain, (b) volumetric strain *vs.* axial strain, (c) difference in pore water pressure *vs.* axial strain.

2.4 *Patterns of shear banding*

Together with the measurement of boundary forces and deformations, FRS and PIV techniques were used to capture non-homogeneous deformation throughout a test. A thorough description of FRS, including principles, technical details, and accuracy, is given by Desrues and Viggiani (2003). As for the use of PIV for measuring plane strain fields, see for example Vacher *et al.* (1999). In essence, both methods are based on the analysis of successive pairs of (either analog or digital) photographs of the side of a specimen deforming under load. They allow for directly measuring (incremental) deformations and determining strain fields throughout the test.

The progression of strain localization as observed through stereo-comparison of the photographs taken during test MBSM07 is shown in Figure 3. For each photographic increment, the figure shows stereophotogrammetry-based fields of (incremental) shear strain $\varepsilon_s = (\varepsilon_1 - \varepsilon_3)/2$ and volumetric strain $\varepsilon_v = (\varepsilon_1 + \varepsilon_3)$, where ε_1 and ε_3 are the major and minor eigenvalues of the strain tensor, respectively. The size of the symbols is proportional to the value of the relevant quantity (note that symbol scale is different for each increment). As far as volumetric strain is concerned, square symbols are for dilatancy and hexagons for contractancy. The photographs numbers are noted on the relevant curve of axial load *vs.* global axial strain, see Figure 2a.

While no localization of strain is observed before photo 4, at the load peak, a shear band forms in the upper part of the specimen in the photographic increment 4–5. Such a band intersects the top platen and is reflected into another shear band in the "conjugate" direction (*i.e.*, the two directions are almost symmetrically reflected about the vertical). In the last two

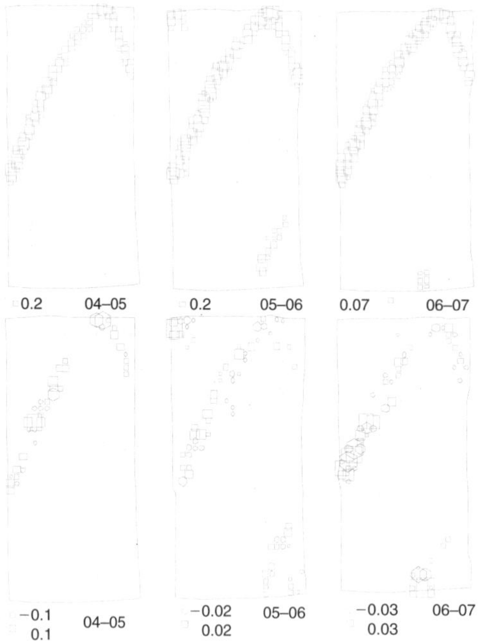

Figure 3. Test MBSM07: stereophotogrammetry-based incremental fields of shear strain intensity (top row) and volumetric strain (bottom row).

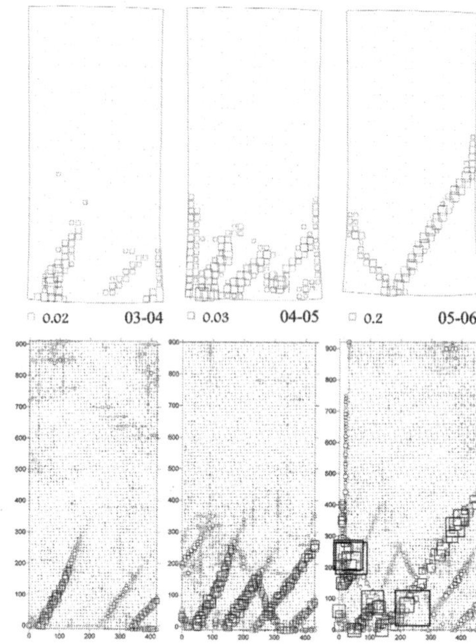

Figure 4. Test MBLL15: incremental fields of shear strain intensity based on FRS (top row) and PIV (bottom row).

increments (5–6 and 6–7), another band forms in the lower portion of the specimen. Volumetric strains are localized in the same bands as the shear strains, thus essentially confirming the general picture. Note that although the post-peak behavior is (globally) dilative in test MBSM07, stereophotogrammetry-based incremental strains indicate that both contractive and dilative behaviors are exhibited inside the localized regions.

It is important to stress that shear bands consistently occurred in all plane strain tests performed on Beaucaire Marl (for both contractive and dilative global responses). However, the patterns of shear localization can vary from one test to another. One further example is given in Figure 4, which shows the progression of strain localization as observed in drained test MBLL15. Around the axial load peak, multiple parallel zones of strain localization first form in the lower portion of the specimen. Several distinct parallel and conjugate shear bands then appear and develop as deformation progresses during the test.

The example shown in Figure 4 illustrates that the "single band" mechanism was not the only observed pattern of strain localization. In general, various patterns of localization were observed, including parallel and crossing shear bands, as well as temporary, or "non-persistent" modes of localization, that is, localized regions which form during the test and eventually "disappear". Band reflection at either the upper or the lower plate was observed in the majority of the tests.

3 POST-MORTEM MICRO TOMOGRAPHY

3.1 *Objectives of the experimental program*

The picture emerging from Figures 3 and 4 is that, at least based on the observation of one side of a deforming specimen, multiple zones of strain localization emerge and propagate during a test. In fact, it is likely that both shear bands (*weak* discontinuities, *i.e.*, discontinuities of the strain field) and cracks (*strong* discontinuities, *i.e.*, discontinuities of the displacement field) form and possibly interact in the course of deformation. It has been suggested by some authors (*e.g.*, Tillard-Ngan *et al.* 1993, Scavia *et al.* 1997) that in stiff clays and soft clayey rocks, the propagation of a strong discontinuity is typically preceded by shear strain localization; in other words, shear strain concentration takes place first, and then a fissure originates at the edge and subsequently propagates in the direction along which the strain previously concentrated. However, it is well known that in laboratory tests on fine-grained geomaterials the "bands" of localization deformation have a width in the order of some tens of microns (*e.g.*, Morgenstern & Tchalenko 1967), which makes it impossible to discriminate between a shear band and a crack propagating in shear, at the macro scale. Moreover, recall that in this experimental program the photographs were taken through a latex membrane, which follows the specimen deformation and inevitably *smears* any possible tangential displacement jump into a region of shear strain concentration.

To shed light on these crack-like propagation phenomena, it was decided to extract from the tested biaxial samples of Beaucaire Marl a number of small specimens for further analysis at the micro scale. X-ray micro tomography was selected as a suitable tool to evaluate cracking and shear banding, especially in order to investigate the features of the *process zone* which possibly exists at the tip of the propagating localized region. On the one hand, X-ray tomography allows to observe cracks in clayey soils (*e.g.*, Otani *et al.* 2000). On the other hand, geomaterials are characterized by a strong deviatoric-volumetric coupling (dilatancy and contractancy), *i.e.*, they experience volume changes when submitted to shear. This means that a shear band can be detected very clearly through tomography as a region of local density variation (*e.g.*, Desrues *et al.* 1996).

A total of fifteen cylindrical specimens were cut from the tested biaxial samples of Beaucaire Marl, with their axis orthogonal to the plane of deformation, see Figure 5. The final diameter of the cylinder, obtained using a lathe, is 20 mm, while the cylinder height equals the thickness of the biaxial sample (35 mm). Each cylinder was X-ray scanned at the high energy beam line ID15 at the European Synchrotron Radiation Facility (ESRF) in Grenoble, France. Only one tomographic section was made for each cylinder, because the patterns of deformation are in principle the same throughout the width of a specimen tested in plane strain.

3.2 *Technical details of X-ray micro tomography*

The typical set up for high resolution X-ray tomography includes a simple projection geometry with a high resolution imaging detector and a highly collimated beam, such as a synchrotron radiation source. In this study, the X-ray (white) beam is generated by an 11 poles wiggler and filtered to remove low energy photons in order to avoid beam hardening artifacts. The clay specimen sits on a rotation stage so that it can be viewed from the many different angles required for tomographic data collection. The X-ray energy used here ranges from about 50 to 70 keV. The scintillator is a Gadox fluorescent screen which transforms the X-rays into visible light. A 2048 by 2048 CCD Frelon camera captures the raw digital images. The pixel resolution of the system is essentially defined by the optics adopted. A 1X objective was used for the scans described here, which produced images with 14 μm pixels and a 28 mm field of view. The thickness of a tomographic section of the specimen is dictated by the width of the X-ray beam

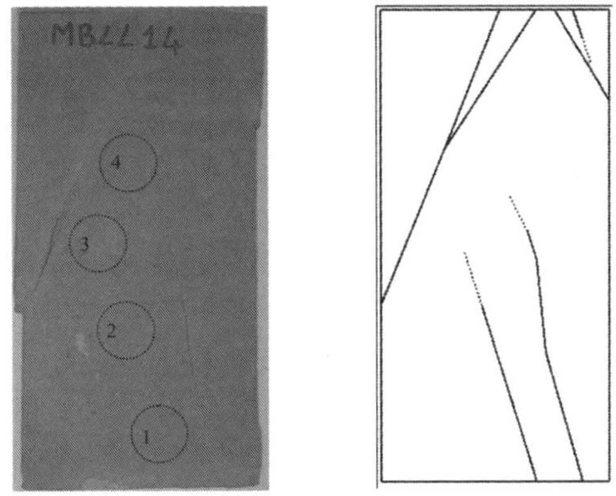

Figure 5. Biaxial sample MBLL14 after test: zones of localization (schematic) and location of cylindrical specimens for *post-mortem* X-ray tomography.

crossing the specimen. In this work, the section is 3 mm thick, which corresponds to 128 rows on the CCD camera. The complete scan of a section was obtained by taking 1200 radiographies at different equally spaced angles covering a range of 180° with an exposure time of 0.08 s for each one. It takes approximately 3.5 min to scan a section.

3.3 *Discussion of selected results*

Figures 6 and 7 show the tomographic slices obtained for the two specimens 1 and 4, both cut from sample MBLL14 (their actual location is shown in Fig. 5). Specimen 1 completely contained a visible zone of strain localization, whereas specimen 4 was cut from a portion of the sample which appears, at the macro scale, at or ahead the tip of the propagating band – based on visual inspection of the side of the sample after the test, as well as the strain field measured through FRS and PIV.

The scan in Figure 6 clearly reveals a fairly straight region of localization, which appears much darker than the rest of the specimen. Indeed, in this case it can be definitely referred to as a *crack* rather than a dilating shear band. In fact, this band is as black (*i.e.*, it has the same density) as the reference environment (air) all around the clay specimen. However, it is possible that the crack opened up to a certain extent while cutting and handling the specimen for tomography. Most importantly, it is also likely that crack opening, or even the crack itself, occurred as a result of soil *drying* (after the test), rather than during plane strain shearing. Recall that the marl was tested saturated, while tomography was performed several months later on a completely dry material. Whatever its origin (shearing, or drying, or both), the region of localization is quite narrow, with a larger crack aperture in the central part of the specimen.

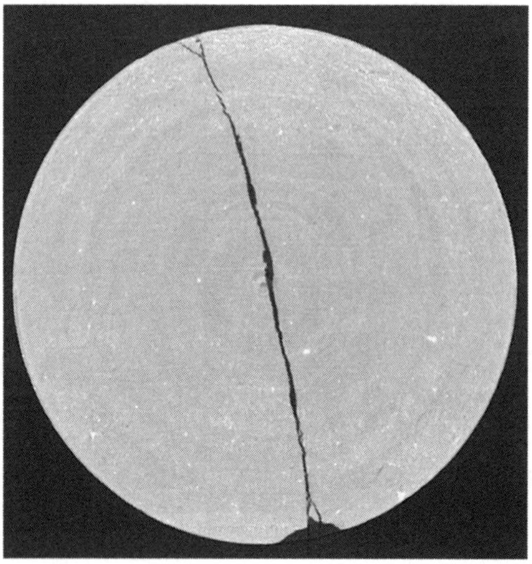

Figure 6. X-ray scan of specimen 1 from test MBLL14 (location shown in Fig. 5).

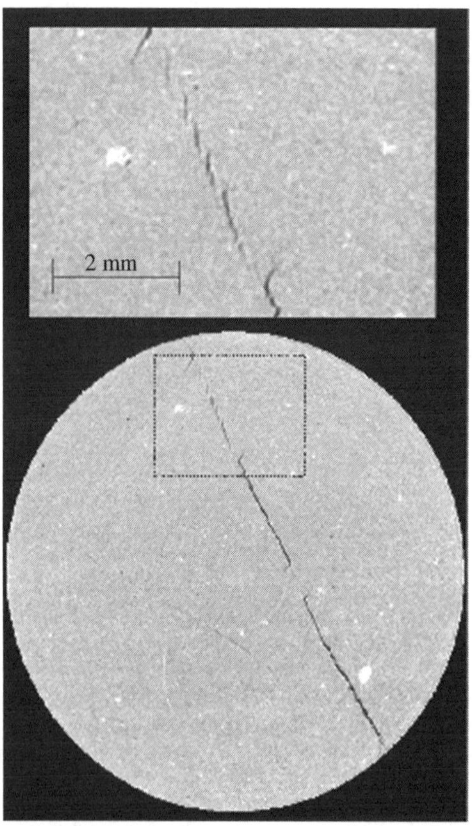

Figure 7. X-ray scan of specimen 4 from test MBLL14 (location shown in Fig. 5).

The most striking observation that can be made from the X-ray scan in Figure 6 is that there is no gradual change of soil density from the zone of localization to the zones of the specimen far from the crack. In other words, no density gradient can be observed (within the resolution of the method) on the two sides of the crack. This finding is in contrast with the commonly accepted notion of a shear band as a zone of localized dilatancy which attracts pore fluid from the surrounding soil. If this was the case, one would measure, across the band, a density profile similar, for example, to the water content profile reported by Henkel (1956). A number of thin sections from the scanned specimens are currently in preparation for SEM micro structural observation, which will shed further light on this particular feature. In any case, the results of both this study and a parallel program on the same material using *in-situ* X-ray tomography (Lenoir *et al.* 2003), indicate that localization in Beaucaire Marl is absolutely *sharp* in space.

Finally, it is worth to note that the location and inclination of the band as obtained from the tomographic image are consistent with what was observable on the side of the specimen (recall that all scans refer to specimen mid height). This observation, which applies to all the scanned specimens, has the important implication that the test conditions in the biaxial apparatus were actually plane strain, which in turn means that the strain fields obtained from the photographs of the specimen side are fully representative of specimen deformation (as already shown by Desrues (1984) for biaxial tests on sand).

In an area which macroscopically appears as the end region of a propagating zone of localization (specimen 4, see Fig. 5), tomography reveals quite a complex pattern, as shown in Figure 7. A straight crack is still visible as in Figure 6, yet its aperture is less, and the crack itself is not continuous in space. Moreover, ahead of the crack tip, a distinct series of *en echelon* inclined fractures can be detected, which together form a macroscopic band that is aligned with the main crack (see zoom in Fig. 7).

The picture emerging from Figures 6 and 7 is that of a single crack macroscopically propagating in shear, with a *process zone* ahead of its tip, where the material experiences localized damage and mechanical degradation. However, such a picture is possibly oversimplified: in some cases, even well behind its tip, the global shear zone comprises well-defined crack linear sections separated by zones of apparently sound material, see for example the scan in Figure 8. Moreover, in most of the scanned specimens, the shear zone (at the macro level) was found to correspond, at the micro level, to extremely thin (approximately 40 μm) bands of *denser* material, see Figures 9 through 11. The location and inclination of these denser bands (lighter areas in the tomographic images) are always consistent with those observed on the side of the specimen, both for simple

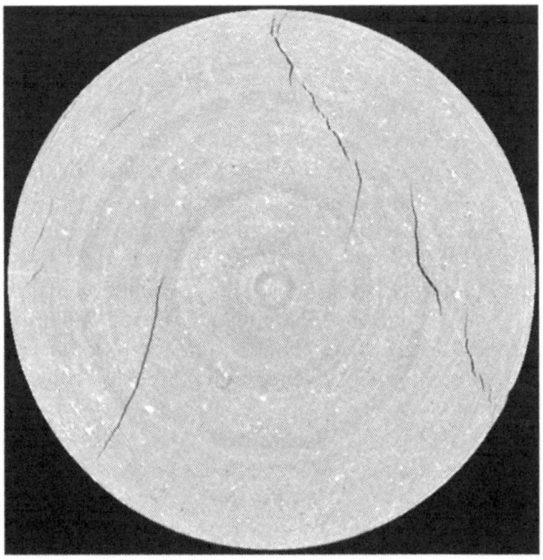

Figure 8. X-ray scan from test MBLL16.

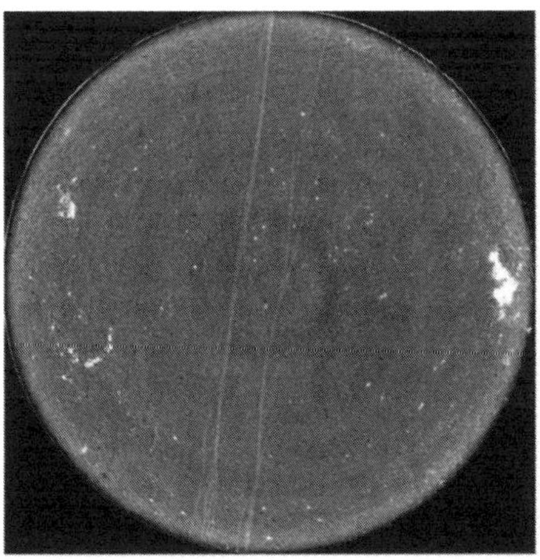

Figure 9. X-ray scan from test MBLL03.

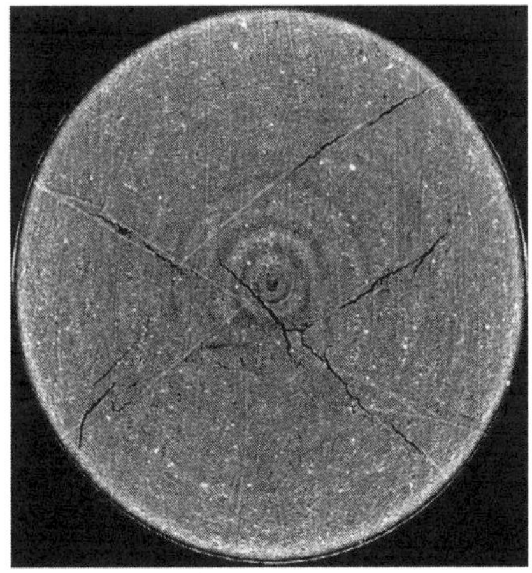

Figure 10. X-ray scan from test MBSM08.

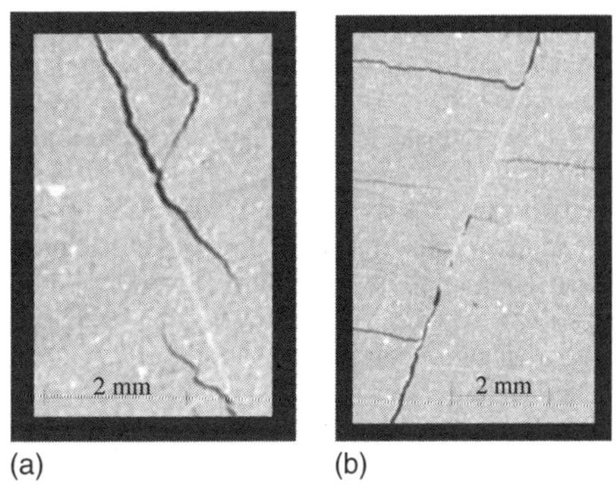

Figure 11. X-ray scans (zoom) from test MBSM03 (left), and test MBLL16 (right).

(Fig. 9) and definitely more complex patterns of localization (Fig. 10). The denser bands are often (but not always) combined with cracks, typically collinear with the bands (see Figs 10 and 11a). As stated above in the paper, it is likely that these cracks formed and opened up as a result of soil drying after the test, rather than during shearing. Actually, it is conceivable that the denser bands themselves are partially due to soil drying. More precisely, one may imagine that a shear band formed upon shearing, and then drying (after the test) made the soil inside the band become denser than the soil outside. In fact, it is well known that in a shear zone, the original fabric of a clayey material is progressively reoriented so that the platy clay minerals become aligned to the shear direction (*e.g.*, Morgenstern & Tchalenko 1967, Petley *et al.* 1993). Such a structure is definitely different from the original fabric prevailing outside the shear band. Upon soil drying, the plate-to-plate fabric inside the band allows the soil to reach much higher densities than outside. Although the above conjecture is still to be confirmed (through direct SEM micro structural observation), this implies that *post-mortem* tomography does not allow to conclude whether a shear band in Beaucaire Marl, for a given mean stress level, is dilative or rather contractive.

Recall that the tests were performed on a natural, geological material. Beaucaire Marl may contain natural imperfections and non-uniformities which are not visible by simple visual observation. Besides characterizing shear banding and cracking, X-ray tomography may assist in the detection of those material non-uniformities. As an example, the scan in Figure 11b shows a number of lighter (denser) thin bands, which are parallel to each other and sub-perpendicular to the axial direction. These bands correspond to the natural bedding of the natural clay deposit at Beaucaire. Interestingly, cracks are also observed to form along these non-uniformities.

4 CONCLUSIONS

Failure of geomaterials is commonly associated with the localization of deformation in zones of intense shearing, such as shear bands and fractures. In fine-grained, stiff soils and soft rocks, both shear bands and cracks form and possibly interact. Typically, a process zone may exist at the tip of a propagating crack, where the material experiences damage and mechanical degradation. Getting experimental data is in this case a formidable task, because the regions of localization have a characteristic finite dimension which is in the order of some tens of microns, that is clearly inaccessible by means of conventional measurement techniques.

In this study, the use of X-ray micro tomography provided a deep insight into the phenomenon and allowed for a number of detailed observations of shear bands and cracks. Within the resolution of the method, it can be concluded that, in the direction perpendicular to the shear zone, localization in Beaucaire Marl occurs *sharply* in space, with essentially no density changes on the two sides of a shear zone. This is also confirmed based on the results of a parallel program on the same material using in-situ tomography. However, a process zone is sometimes observable ahead of the tip of a propagating region of localization.

Because the tomographic study was carried out several months after the tests, it is not possible to assess whether the local behavior of the soil inside a zone of localization is contractive or dilative. The next, essential step of this study (which is already in progress) will include the SEM observation of a number of thin sections from the scanned specimens. Direct micro structural observation of soil fabric inside a band will allow to confirm the conjectures made concerning the volumetric behavior in a shear zone. Moreover, micro structure observation of a process zone will shed further light on the physical mechanisms associated to localized deformation in stiff fine-grained geomaterials.

ACKNOWLEDGEMENTS

This X-ray scanning program was made possible by the ESRF, which is gratefully acknowledged. The cylindrical specimens of Beaucaire Marl were obtained at the Politecnico di Torino by R. Maniscalco, to whom the authors extend their thanks. The contribution of M. Gerardo, who performed the PIV measurements, is also gratefully acknowledged.

REFERENCES

Desrues, J. 1984. *La localisation de la déformation dans les matériaux granulaires*. Thèse de Doctorat es Science, USMG & INPG, Grenoble, France.

Desrues, J., Chambon, R., Mokni, M. & Mazerolle, F. 1996. Void ratio evolution inside shear bands in triaxial sand specimens studied by computed tomography. *Géotechnique* 46: 529–546.

Desrues, J. & Viggiani, G. 2003. Strain localization in sand: an overview of the experimental results obtained in Grenoble using stereophotogrammetry. *Intern. Journal for Numerical and Analytical Methods in Geomechanics* (in print).

Finno, R.J., Harris, W.W., Mooney, M.A. & Viggiani, G. 1997. Shear bands in plane strain compression of loose sand. *Géotechnique* 47: 149–165.

Henkel, D.J. 1956. Discussion: Earth movement affecting LTE railway in deep cutting east of Uxbridge. *Proc. ICE*, Part II, 5: 320–323.

Lenoir, N., Marello, S., Viggiani, G., Bésuelle, P., Desrues, J. & Di Michiel, M. 2003. X-ray micro tomography characterization of strain localization upon deviatoric loading of saturated fine-grained stiff soils. This conference

Morgenstern, M.R. & Tchalenko, J.S. 1967. Microscopic structures in kaolin subjected to direct shear. *Géotechnique* 37: 309–327.

Otani, J., Mukunoki, T. & Obara, Y. 2000. Application of X-ray CT method for characterization of failure in soils. *Soils and Foundations* 40: 111–118.

Petley, D., Jones, M., Fan, C., Stafford, C., Leddra, M. & Kageson-Loe, N. 1993. Deformation and fabric changes in weak fine-grained rocks during high pressure consolidation and shear. *Proc. International Symposium on Hard Soils and Soft Rocks*, 1: 761–768.

Saada, A.S., Bianchini, G. & Liang, L. 1994. Cracks, bifurcation and shear bands propagation in saturated clay. *Géotechnique* 44: 35–64.

Scavia, C., Viggiani, G., Castelli, M. & Desrues, J. 1997. *An experimental and numerical study of shear fracture propagation in rock*. In A. Asaoka, T. Adachi & F. Oka (eds), *Deformation and Progressive Failure in Geomechanics, Proc. IS-Nagoya '97*: 175–180. Pergamon.

Tillard-Ngan, D., Desrues, J., Raynaud, S. & Mazerolle, F. 1993. Strain localisation in Beaucaire *marl. Proc. International Symposium on Hard Soils and Soft Rocks*, 2: 1679–1686.

Vacher P., Dumoulin, S., Morestin, F. & Mguil-Touchai, S. 1999. Bidimensional strain measurement using digital images. *Proc. Instn. Mech. Engrs.*, 213, Part C: 811–817.

Vardoulakis, I. & Sulem, J. 1995. *Bifurcation Analysis in Geomechanics*. Glasgow: Blackie Academic & Professional.

Viggiani, G., Marello, S., Lenti, L. and Desrues, J. 2003. Shear bands in plane strain compression of stiff clay (in preparation).

Viggiani, G., Finno, R.J. & Harris, W.W. 1994. Experimental observations of strain localisation in plane strain compression of a stiff clay. In R. Chambon, J. Desrues & I. Vardoulakis (eds), *Localisation and Bifurcation Theory for Soils and Rocks*: 189–198. Rotterdam: Balkema.

X-ray CT for Geomaterials; Soils, Concrete, Rocks – Otani & Obara (eds.)
© 2004 Swets & Zeitlinger. Lisse, ISBN 90 5809 666 1

X-ray micro tomography characterization of strain localization upon deviatoric loading of saturated fine-grained stiff soils

N. Lenoir
ANDRA & Laboratoire Sols, Solides, Structures, Grenoble, France

S. Marello, G. Viggiani, P. Bésuelle & J. Desrues
Laboratoire Sols, Solides, Structures, CNRS-UJF-INPG, Grenoble, France

M. Di Michiel
European Synchrotron Radiation Facility, Grenoble, France

ABSTRACT: The paper presents a few selected results of a unique experimental testing program recently carried out at the European Synchrotron Radiation Facility (ESRF) in Grenoble, France, where X-ray micro tomography has been used to evaluate the onset and evolution of shear banding in a fine-grained stiff soil under deviatoric loading. In the experiments, small specimens (20 mm in diameter, 40 mm high) of a saturated natural material called Beaucaire marl were loaded under displacement control in triaxial compression, using a custom-built triaxial system designed specifically for this program. An X-ray beam of 50–60 keV was used, with a resolution of 14 μm. A white X-ray beam was selected in order to have enough flux to perform very fast tomographic scans during a test. *In-situ* tomography allowed detailed observations of strain localization in a specimen at different deviatoric load levels.

1 BACKGROUND AND MOTIVATIONS

Strain localization, the concentration of deformation into narrow zones of intense shearing, is a phenomenon commonly observed in virtually all geomaterials, including rocks, soils and concrete. The body of literature on the modeling of localization in geomaterials has been growing rapidly, especially during the last two decades, see for example Vardoulakis & Sulem (1995). Various experimental studies have also been carried out which have provided a number of important data on the onset and subsequent propagation of strain localization in a soil specimen subjected to shear. Experimental investigations represent indeed an essential ingredient for improving the understanding of the mechanics and physics of shear banding.

The challenge here is the fact that one wants to measure deformations in a region the size of which, upon strain localization, reduces abruptly and dramatically, say from the scale of the specimen to the shear band scale. Measuring deformations throughout a test, that is: prior to, at, and after the onset of strain localization is then a formidable task, which can only be accomplished by using field measurements. In this respect, X-ray tomography provides interesting experimental possibilities, see Desrues (2003). However, the multiphase nature of soils makes it quite difficult to properly run a soil test within a typical X-ray tomography set up, especially if one intends to perform *in-situ* tomography, *i.e.*, to load the specimen and to scan it in the same setting and at the same time.

To our knowledge, there is only one study where this was fully achieved (Otani *et al.* 2002), whereas in other previous applications of X-ray tomography for studying shear banding in soils and rocks either the compression test and the scanning were not conducted simultaneously (*e.g.*, Raynaud *et al.* 1989, Desrues *et al.* 1996, Otani *et al.* 2000, Alshibli 2000), or no control of effective stress was implemented (*e.g.*, Vinegard *et al.* 1991, Kawakata *et al.* 1999, Tillard-Ngan 1992).

It should be noted that all the above experimental studies have been performed with conventional Computed Tomography (CT) systems used in medical and industrial applications. The present study makes use of a much more powerful source of X-rays, provided by the synchrotron radiation. In this way, it is possible to achieve both a high resolution and fast scanning, due to the high photon flux. On the one hand, high resolution is needed because shear bands may be extremely thin in fine-grained materials (clays, marls and clayey rocks). As a matter of fact, the few available tomographic images of shear zones in fine-grained geomaterials obtained so far (Otani *et al.* 2000, Tillard-Ngan 1992, Hicher *et al.* 1994) appear relatively unsatisfactory. On the other hand, fast scanning is crucial for *in-situ* tomography, due to possible time effects on the material behavior (stress relaxation).

This paper presents a few selected results from a recent, unique experimental testing program where synchrotron radiation micro tomography has been used for the first time to evaluate the onset and evolution of localized deformation in a saturated fine-grained stiff soil under deviatoric loading. A brief description of X-ray micro tomography is first given in Section 2. Section 3 describes the loading system which was specifically designed to be placed in the X-ray beam (*in-situ* tomography) and to meet in the mean time all the requirements for standard testing of saturated soils. The characteristics of the tested material as well as the experimental procedures are also detailed to some extent. A few results are presented and discussed in Sections 3 and 4, and finally some conclusions are drawn in Section 5.

2 X-RAY MICRO TOMOGRAPHY

X-ray absorption tomography essentially consists in recording radiographies of a specimen at different angular positions and then reconstructing a 3-D image of the internal structure of the specimen from the spatial distribution of the linear attenuation coefficient within the specimen. High resolution X-ray tomography (micro tomography) methods have been developed over the last two decades, their typical set up including a simple projection geometry with a high resolution imaging detector and a highly collimated beam, such as a synchrotron radiation source. The system used in this research allows performing micro tomography of a specimen under load (*in-situ*), using a specifically built load frame that could be placed in the X-ray beam.

The experiments were carried out at the high energy beam line ID15 at the European Synchrotron Radiation Facility (ESRF) in Grenoble, France. In fact, the work presented in this paper is one of the first applications of fast micro tomography at ID15. Previous applications concerned the study of sintering processes of metallic powders (Lame *et al.* 2003). The set up is schematically shown in Figure 1, see also the photograph in Figure 2. The X-ray white beam (1) is generated by an 11 poles wiggler and filtered to remove low energy photons in order to avoid beam hardening artifacts. A fast shutter is used to get short exposure times. The triaxial loading system (3) sits on a translation and rotation stage (2) so that it can be viewed, at different elevations, from the many different angles required for tomographic data collection. The X-ray energy used here ranges from about 50 to 70 keV, allowing the X-rays to go through the two 5 mm thick Plexiglas cell walls, the confining fluid, and the 20 mm diameter clay specimen. The scintillator is a Gadox fluorescent screen which transforms the X-rays into visible light. A 2048 by 2048 CCD Frelon camera (4) captures the raw digital images. The pixel resolution of the system

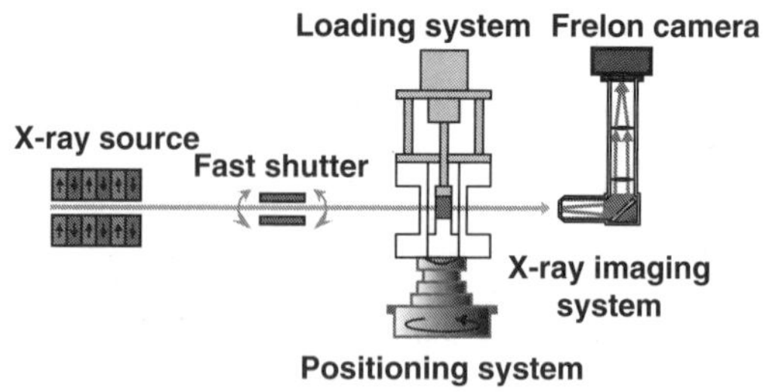

Figure 1. Experimental set up for micro tomography used at ESRF beam line ID15.

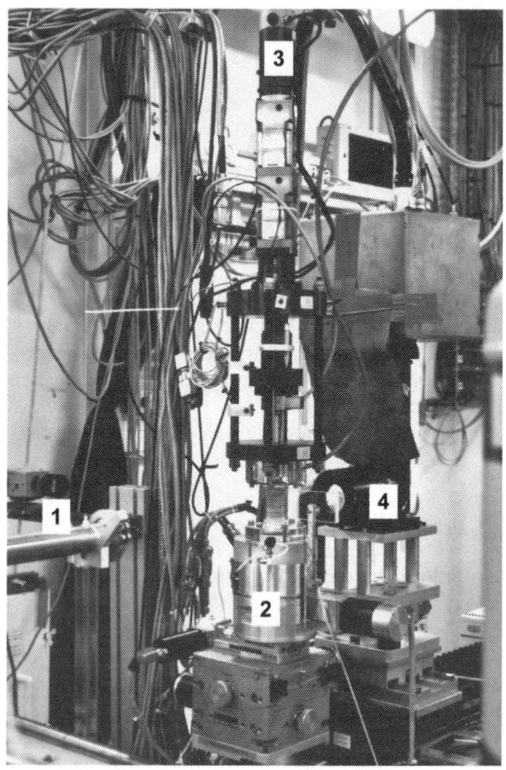

Figure 2. Experimental set up, including X-ray source (1), positioning system (2), loading system (3) and X-ray imaging system (4).

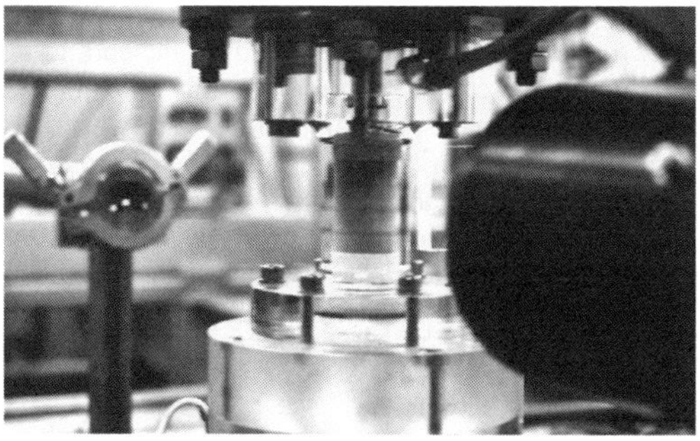

Figure 3. Detail of the triaxial cell.

is essentially defined by the optics adopted. A 1X objective was used for the scans described here, which produced images with 14 μm pixel and a 28 mm field of view. The thickness of a tomographic section of the specimen is dictated by the width of the X-ray beam crossing the specimen. In this work, each section is 1.75 mm thick, which corresponds to 128 rows on the CCD camera ("slices", hereafter). The complete scan of a section was obtained by taking 1200 radiographies at different equally spaced angles covering a range of 180° with an exposure time of 0.08 s for each one. Each section could be scanned in approximately 3.5 min, this value being dictated by the shutter opening/closing time, exposure time, and the read out time.

2.1 *Experimental apparatus*

The apparatus includes a small triaxial cell and a loading device designed specifically for this program. The triaxial apparatus is practically the same as a conventional triaxial testing system, except for its much smaller size and the shape of the confining cell, which was designed to be as transparent as possible to the X-rays (see Figure 3). The soil specimen is a cylinder with height twice the diameter (40 and 20 mm, respectively). The top and bottom rigid platens are enlarged and lubricated to minimize friction at the ends of the specimen. The specimen is enclosed in a thin latex sleeve sealed to the top and bottom platens; the sleeve acts both as a flexible membrane and as a seal to separate pore fluid pressures, u, and total stresses, σ. The sealed specimen is placed in a de-aired water-filled cell, which can sustain up to 1 MPa. The bottom platen houses an 8 mm diameter, high air-entry-value-pressure porous stone connected to the drainage line passing through the base of the cell to pore pressure and volume change measuring equipment. A frictionless ram passes through the top of the cell and allows applying a stress deviator q. The contact between the ram and the top rigid platen is such that the latter is allowed to rotate. The specimen is subjected to a mean total stress p and mean effective stress $p' = p - u$. The axial strain, ε_a, is obtained by measuring the ram displacement using a LVDT.

The axial load and hence the deviator stress is applied in a displacement-controlled manner using a motor-driven screw actuator. The loading system was designed specifically for this program (in cooperation with CSP – Composants et Systèmes de Précision) and can be placed in the X-ray beam line without interfering with the tomographic scans. It is quite compact and light (less than 30 kg), which is important since it directly sits on the translation and rotation stage during the experiment. The system has a maximum loading capacity of 7.5 kN, and allows to move the ram at a constant rate in the range of 1 to 100 μm/min. It is worth noting that while in a conventional system the tensile reaction force is carried by a loading frame, in this case it is carried by the cell walls, which therefore are subjected to traction in the axial direction. This allows a clear path, free of any obstacle (apart from the cell walls), for the X-ray beam within the region to be scanned. X-ray absorption through the apparatus must be small, so the walls of the cell have to be as thin as possible. The solution adopted was to reduce the thickness of the walls to a value of 5 mm only where needed, *i.e.* in the central region of the cell. The output signals of all transducers (for axial load, cell pressure, pore fluid pressure, and axial strain) are conditioned by a 16 bit process interface unit which is linked to a laptop computer, which also controls the loading actuator. The experiments are remotely controlled from a control cabin, because the shield room, the so-called experimental hutch, is obviously inaccessible when the shutter is open.

2.2 *Material tested*

The material tested for this study (Beaucaire Marl) is a sedimentary soil which has been extensively studied at the Laboratoire 3S in Grenoble over the last fifteen years. It comes from a natural deposit located at Beaucaire, in Southern France, which was deposited in a shallow marine environment during the Pliocene age. The material can be considered as a stiff clayey soil – or a soft clayey rock: in either case, it clearly falls into the category of hard soils-soft rocks. According to the Unified Soil Classification system, Beaucaire Marl is a clayey silt, with about 60% in weight of the solid particles having an equivalent diameter in the range 2–60 μm and 30% less than 2 μm. The calcium carbonate content can be as high as 34%, and the specific gravity of the solids is equal to 2.75. Microscopic observation did not reveal any evidence of pre-existing microcracks. The natural material is heavily overconsolidated and quite stiff, its natural water content ranging from 16 to 21%, which should be compared to a liquid limit and a plasticity index in the range 38–41% and 21–25%, respectively. The vertical yield stress from

1D compression tests is about 2 MPa, and its uniaxial compressive strength averages 0.9 MPa. The permeability of Beaucaire Marl is in the order of 10^{-9} m/s. The "intact" specimens for the experimental program described in this paper were obtained using a diamond wire saw which minimizes material disturbance during preparation.

2.3 *Test procedure and testing program*

For each test, an isotropic consolidation phase preceded the actual triaxial compression (deviatoric) phase. A back pressure of about 200 kPa was applied to the pore water. Opening the drainage lines allowed consolidation (or swelling, depending on the final value of mean effective stress). Each specimen was in an isotropic state of effective stress, $p'_0 = (p - u_0)$, at the end of consolidation (swelling), which took from 6 to 12 hours on average. Volume changes were recorded during consolidation. In addition, three complete tomographic sections of the specimen were taken before and at the end of the consolidation phase of each experiment. The subsequent phase of deviatoric loading was performed under displacement control, by advancing the loading ram at a rate of 3 μm/min, which corresponds to a nominal axial strain rate of 0.45%/hour for a 40 mm specimen height. The ram displacement was stopped at different levels of axial strain, *i.e.*, at those points of the test when a tomographic scan of the specimen was required. The specimen was scanned while the axial strain was held constant, which unavoidably causes some amount of axial load relaxation during scanning. However, the scanning operations were fast enough (40 to 120 minutes, depending on the number of scanned sections) for this relaxation to be relatively small. A total of five tests were performed, under either drained or undrained conditions. Table 1 summarizes the experimental program and lists the values of mean effective stress p'_0 at the end of isotropic consolidation. All specimens had a degree of saturation close to 100% before testing.

Table 1. Summary of tests.

Tests	XU01	XD02	XD03	XU04	XD05
p'_0 (kPa)	130	150	600	600	600

3 SELECTED RESULTS

Results from only two experiments are presented herein as examples of the responses observed on Beaucaire Marl in undrained (test XU01, see Figure 4a) and drained (test XD02, see Figure 4b) conditions. Deviator stress is computed by dividing the force in the loading ram by the current cross-sectional area of the specimen. Axial strain is computed as $\varepsilon_a = -ln(H/H_0)$, where H_0 and H are the initial and current height of the specimen, respectively. Similarly, $\varepsilon_v = -ln(V/V_0)$, where V_0 and V are the initial and current volume of the specimen, respectively. All stresses and strains are positive in compression.

The four small unloading-reloading branches on the q vs. ε_a curves correspond to the points of the test (1 to 4) when the ram was stopped and several cross sections of the specimen were scanned. It appears that, thanks to the fast scanning, stress relaxation during scans was small in both tests.

In test XU01 (Figure 4a), the deviator stress monotonically increases until approximately 0.014 axial strain whereupon it decreases sharply. At about 0.024 axial strain, the deviator stress essentially levels off. Increasing positive excess pore pressures (that is, a contractive behavior) are measured until approximately

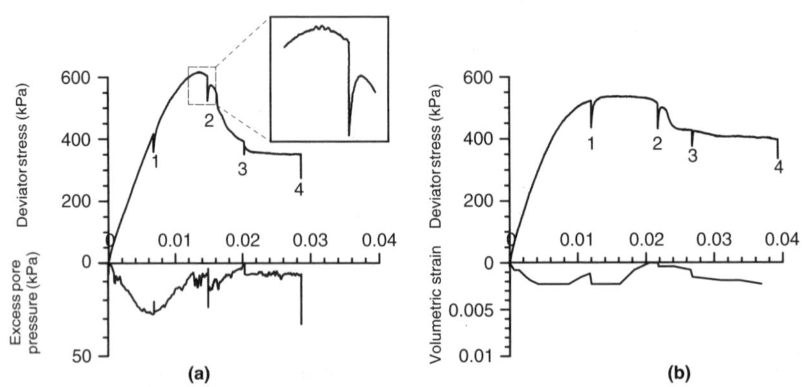

Figure 4. Evolution of deviator stress, q, and excess pore pressure, Δu vs. axial strain ε_a for the undrained test XU01 (a); evolution of deviator stress, q, and volumetric strain, ε_v vs. axial strain ε_a for the drained test XD02 (b).

0.006 axial strain whereupon a dilative response is observed. Shortly prior to the peak of deviator stress, excess pore pressure stops decreasing and eventually attains an essentially (positive) value. Note that around the peak of deviator stress, measured pore pressure shows some fluctuation, which interestingly corresponds to a similar response of the deviator stress (see zoom in Figure 4a).

In test XD02, the deviator stress first increases, reaches a plateau and then drops at an axial strain of approximately 0.021. Afterwards, the deviator stress essentially levels off. The global volumetric response is initially contractive, then dilative before an essentially zero slope is finally attained as the deviator stress levels off. A short interval of more pronounced dilative behavior occurs just before the drop of deviator stress.

A single shear band could be clearly observed in both specimens XU01 and XD02 at the end of the test (Figure 5). A closer inspection of the specimens actually reveals that in test XU02 the band is fairly planar throughout the specimen, whereas in test XD01 it shows major deviations from a plane in the upper portion of the specimen.

A series of cross-sectional slices from test XU01 are shown in Figure 6, at two different elevations, z, from the base of the specimen. Images from two scans are shown in the figure, which were both performed in the post-peak portion of the test, the former just before the deviator stress plateau and the latter at the end of the test (scans 3 and 4 in Figure 4a, respectively). While no evidence of strain localization was observed in scans 1 and 2 (not shown herein), in scan 3 (left column in Figure 6) the reconstructed tomographic slices at both elevations indicate that the specimen is undergoing localized deformation. At about 20 mm elevation, a curved, non continuous crack can be clearly identified (darker indicates lower mass density and black indicates no solid matter). While the aperture of the open portions of the crack is only a few pixels (or a few tens of microns), it is quite difficult to characterize the regions linking these open portions. In fact, it is not even possible to assess whether these zones are very thin (less than one pixel) cracks or rather dilating shear bands. On the right, close to the specimen boundary, the region of localization seems to split into two distinct branches, as shown by the zoom (magnification by 4) on the left bottom of Figure 6. These two branches can be interpreted as two dilating shear bands, a few pixels thick. At about 30 mm elevation, two distinct cracks of localization are visible which apparently are not connected to each other. However, a closer look at the tomographic slice indicates that the two cracks in fact belong to a unique region of localization, corresponding to the same region which was identified at the lower elevation. The zoom (magnification by 5) on the left top of the figure suggests a few pixels wide dilating (darker) shear band rather than a crack.

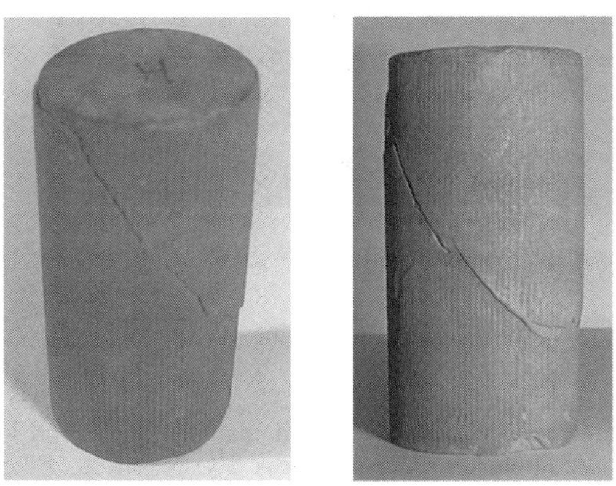

XU01 XU02

Figure 5. Photographs of specimens at the end of the tests.

The slices obtained in scan 4, shown on the right column in Figure 6, illustrate the subsequent evolution of localized deformation in specimen XU01. Two important features can be pointed out. First, it appears that wherever an open crack existed already at scan 3, its aperture definitely increased from scan 3 to scan 4. Second, and possibly more strikingly, the comparison of scan 3 and scan 4 indicates that in some cases dilating shear bands evolved to cracks in the course of deformation. This is clearly illustrated by the zooms at both elevations.

Figure 7 shows some cross-sectional slices of specimen XD02, at two elevations and two different scans. As in Figure 6, both scans were taken in the post-peak portion of the test (noted as 3 and 4 in Figure 4b). Scan 3 (left column) reveals two interacting regions of localized deformation in the middle section of the specimen. A region of localization appears also at a higher elevation, although it is less discernible. Once again, it is difficult to assess to what extent such regions can be considered as cracks or rather as dilating shear bands. In some cases, they have a thickness which is in the order of the system resolution or less. The left zoom (magnification by 5) shows that there are portions of the zone of localization which appear as slightly less dense (darker) bands, two or three pixels wide (see for example the right lower portion of the corresponding zoom). At the end of the test (scan 4, right column), localization is clearly visible also in the top section of the specimen. In the middle section, the regions of localization appear as non continuous cracks, see right zoom in the figure. Overall, this observed pattern of localization evolution is relatively complex. Some clear features to point out include the presence of more than just one shear zone, a curved shape, and a varying degree (in time and space) of crack opening.

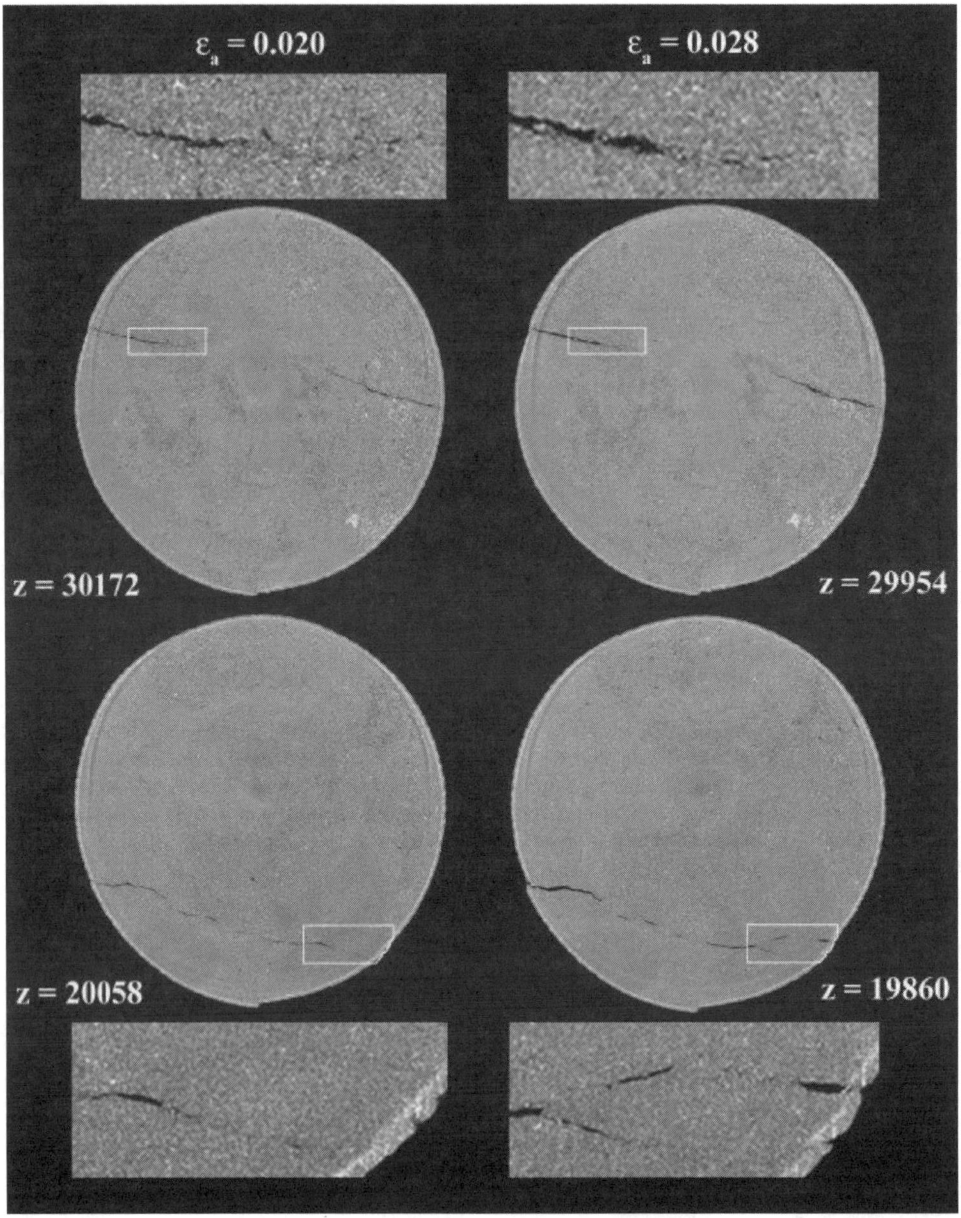

Figure 6. 2-D reconstructed cross-sectional slices of specimen XU01 (slice elevation is given in μm).

4 DISCUSSION

In both tests XU01 and XD02 no evidence of strain localization could be observed right after the peak deviator stress, that is, the first tomographic image showing localized deformation in the specimen was obtained only in the post-peak part of the test. This finding does not agree with the generally accepted idea that in triaxial compression of stiff clays the peak deviator stress coincides with the full development of a shear band (*e.g.*, Burland 1990, Viggiani *et al.* 1993). However, it was also found that pore water pressure fluctuates around the peak deviator stress of the undrained test, which may suggest that strains begin to localize already at the peak. In fact, that pore pressure non-uniformities represent an effective indicator

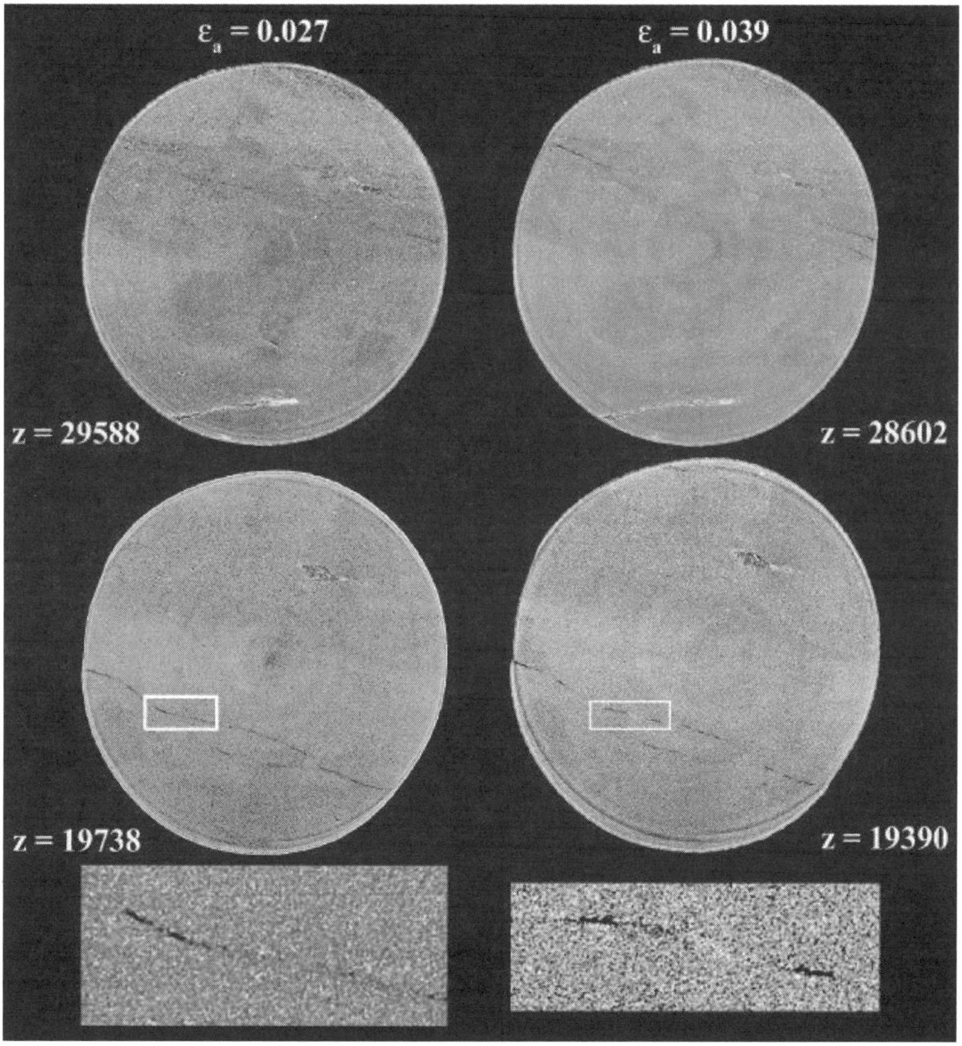

Figure 7. 2-D reconstructed cross-sectional slices of specimen XD02 (slice elevation is given in μm).

of the development of shear banding was first suggested by Viggiani *et al.* (1993, 1994) and recently confirmed by Viggiani *et al.* (2003b). If this was the case, then it should be concluded that, due to the system resolution used in the present study, tomography failed in revealing the early stages of strain localization.

Figures 6 and 7 illustrate that the pattern of localization observed through X-ray micro tomography during triaxial loading of Beaucaire Marl was quite complex. Both dilating shear *bands* (which are visible in tomography as bands of localized dilatancy) and *cracks* were observed to form and to interact in the course of deformation. In some cases, shear strain concentration took place first, and then a crack originated at the edge and subsequently propagated in the direction along which the strain previously concentrated. However, it should kept in mind that these regions of localization are in any case extremely thin (in the order of some tens of microns), which often makes it difficult to discriminate between a dilating shear band and a crack propagating in shear.

The most striking observation that can be made from the X-ray scans in Figures 6 and 7 is that there is no gradual change of soil density from the zone of localization to the zones of the specimen far from the crack. In other words, no density gradient can be observed (within the resolution of the method) on the two sides of the zone of localization. This indicates that, whatever its nature (crack or dilating shear band), localization in Beaucaire Marl is absolutely *sharp* in space. A number of thin sections from the tested specimens are currently in preparation for SEM micro structural observation, which will shed further light on this particular feature.

The tomographic images show that, at a given stage of the deformation process, the region of localization itself can be quite non-uniform, and that the dilatancy inside the band (or the aperture of the crack, in case of a strong discontinuity) is typically higher close to the specimen lateral boundaries than in the core of specimen. It is worth noting that this was also recently observed for sandstone (Bésuelle 2003).

What tomography does not necessarily bring out is a clear picture of why localization took place precisely where it did. In particular, there does not appear to be any evidence of zones of strain localization emerging from inclusions or other "defects" in the natural material (such as, for example, the white streak visible in the upper slices in Figure 7). Rather, strain localization appears in material that visually seems to be quite sound.

A final remark which can be done is that, besides illustrating how strain localization progressed in the specimen, micro tomography also allowed to directly evaluate the effects of specimen preparation. The images in Figures 6 and 7 indicate that wire saw cutting "damages" the specimen, in that it increases the soil density all around. However, this is only a skin effect (the affected thickness is less than 0.3 mm, which implies that, despite their relatively small size, the tested specimens can be fairly considered as "undisturbed").

5 CONCLUSIONS

This experimental program used synchrotron radiation micro tomography to evaluate the onset and evolution of localized deformation in a saturated fine-grained stiff soil under deviatoric loading. Recently used for studying damage evolution in mortars (Landis *et al.* 2003), *in-situ* synchrotron radiation micro tomography is used here for the first time for saturated geomaterials. A loading system was specifically designed to be placed in the X-ray beam and to meet in the mean time all the standard requirements for testing a saturated soil specimen (separate control and measurement of total stress and pore pressure; control of drainage into, or out of, the specimen; lateral confinement).

The unique combination of using synchrotron radiation and *in-situ* (under load) tomography allowed a number of detailed and interesting observations of strain localization in Beaucaire Marl at different deviatoric load levels. Most of these observations would have just not been possible without such a combination of powerful tools. However, X-ray micro tomography does not provide complete answers to every possible question. Among the items which deserve further investigation is the occurrence of localized deformation associated with a globally ductile response. As an example, one can mention test XD05, for which no evidence of localization was found up to the strain levels attained (6% axial strain), see Viggiani *et al.* (2003a). This finding should be contrasted with previous experiments on a similar clay (Tillard-Ngan 1992), where contracting bands were observed, through *post-mortem* X-ray CT, in a test performed at 250 kPa up to axial stain of 25%. This suggests that in the ductile regime, localization may only occur at a much later stage of deformation.

REFERENCES

Alshibli, K.A., Sture, S., Costes, N.C., Franck, M.L., Lankton, M.R., Batiste, S.N. & Swanson, R.A. 2000. Assessment of localized deformation in sand using X-ray computed tomography. *Geotechnical Testing Journal* 23: 274–299.

Bésuelle, P. 2003. X-ray CT observations of strain localization and failure in two porous sandstones. This conference.

Burland, J.B. 1990. On the compressibility and shear strength of natural clays. *Géotechnique* 40: 327–378.

Desrues, J. 2003. Tracking strain localization in geomaterials using computerized tomography. This conference.

Desrues, J., Chambon, R., Mokni, M., Mazerolle F. 1996. Void ratio evolution inside shear bands in triaxial sand specimens studied by computed tomography. *Géotechnique* 46: 529–546.

Hicher, P.Y., Wahyudi, H. & Tessier, D. 1994. Microstructural analysis of strain localisation in clay. *Computers & Geotechnics* 16: 205–222.

Kawakata, H., Cho, A., Kiyama, T., Yanagidani, T., Kusunose K. & Shimada, M. 1999. Three-dimensional observations of faulting process in Westerly granite under uniaxial and triaxial conditions by X-ray CT scan, *Tectonophysics* 313: 293–305.

Lame, O., Bellet, D., Di Michiel, M. & Bouvard, D. 2003. In situ microtomography investigation of metal powder compacts during sintering, *Nuclear Instruments and Methods in Physics Research* B 200: 287–294.

Landis, E.N., Nagy, E.N. & Keane, D.T. 2003. Microstructure and fracture in three dimensions. *Engineering Fracture Mechanics* 70: 911–925.

Marello, S., Lenoir, N., Viggiani, G., Bésuelle, P., Desrues, J. & Di Michiel, M. 2003. Shear banding in plane strain compression of Beaucaire Marl studied through post-mortem X-ray micro tomography. This conference.

Otani, J., Mukunoki, T. & Obara, Y. 2000. Application of X-ray CT method for characterization of failure in soils. *Soils and Foundations* 40: 111–118.

Otani, J., Mukunoki, T. & Obara, Y. 2002. Characterization of failure in sand under triaxial compression using an industrial X-ray scanner. *Int. J. of Physical Modelling in Geotechnics* 1: 15–22.

Raynaud, S., Fabre, D., Mazerolle, F., Géraud, Y. & Latière, H.J. 1989. Analysis of the internal structure of rocks and characterization of mechanical deformation by a non-destructive method: X-ray tomodensitometry. *Tectonophysics* 159: 149–159.

Tillard-Ngan, D. 1992. Étude de la rupture dans les géomatériaux cohésifs. Application à la marne de Beaucaire, *Ph.D. Thesis, Grenoble* (in French).

Vardoulakis, I. & Sulem, J. 1995. *Bifurcation Analysis in Geomechanics*, Glasgow: Blackie Academic & Professional.

Viggiani, G., Finno, R.J. & Harris, W.W. 1994. Experimental observations of strain localisation in plane strain compression of a stiff clay. In R. Chambon *et al.* (eds), *Localisation and Bifurcation Theory for Soils and Rocks*, Balkema, 189–198.

Viggiani, G., Lenoir, N., Bésuelle, P., Di Michiel, M., Marello, S., Desrues, J. & Kretzschmer, M. 2003. X-ray micro tomography for studying localized deformation in fine-grained geomaterials under triaxial compression. *C.R. Mécanique, Académie des Sciences, Paris* (submitted).

Viggiani, G., Marello, S., Lenti, L. & Desrues, J. 2003b. Shear bands in plane strain compression of stiff clay, in preparation.

Viggiani, G., Rampello, S. & Georgiannou, V.N. 1993. Experimental analysis of localisation phenomena in triaxial tests on stiff clays. *Proc. Int. Symp. on Hard Soils and Soft Rocks*, Balkema (1): 849–856.

Vinegar, H.J., De Waal, J.A. & Wellington, S.L. 1991. CT studies of brittle failure in Castlegate sandstone. *Int. J. of Rock Mechanics and Mining Sciences* 28: 441–448.

X-ray CT for Geomaterials; Soils, Concrete, Rocks – Otani & Obara (eds.)
© 2004 Swets & Zeitlinger. Lisse, ISBN 90 5809 666 1

Computed tomography-characterized strain localization in granular materials

K.A. Alshibli
Louisiana State University and Southern University, Baton Rouge, Louisiana, USA

S. Sture, S.N. Batiste & M. Lankton
University of Colorado at Boulder, Boulder, Colorado, USA

ABSTRACT: The authors have conducted an extensive study utilizing computed tomography to characterize the internal structure/fabric and to track the onset and propagation of shear bands in granular materials subjected to uniaxial loading. This paper presents a description of the three CT systems used in the investigation along with examples of CT results. The sand specimens bulge uniformly at the post-peak stress level and develop complex multiple symmetrical radial shear bands at higher axial strain levels. The CT technique has demonstrated good ability to detect specimens' inhomogeneities and localization patterns, and to quantify void ratio variation within sand specimens.

1 INTRODUCTION

Computed Tomography (CT) has emerged as a powerful non-destructive density mapping technique in the last two decades. The first applications of tomography were in radio astronomy (Bracewell 1956), and now it is widely used in medical imaging, seismology, petroleum engineering, acoustic imaging, soil science, powder industry, etc. (e.g. Coshell *et al.* 1994, Amos *et al.* 1996, Denison and Carlson 1997, Denison *et al.* 1997, Phillips and Lannutti 1997). Steude *et al.* (1994) presented a bibliographic listing of research conducted to determine soils physical properties using x-ray computed tomography. Recently, CT has been successfully used to characterize the internal structure and to describe the failure modes of soil specimens (e.g. Desrues *et al.* 1996, Otani *et al.* 2000, Alshibli *et al.* 2000).

The authors have applied CT to assess the homogeneity and to track the onset and propagation of shear bands in F-75 Ottawa quartz sand and glass beads. Three separate CT scanning systems were used between 1997 and 2003. This paper will document a description of the CT systems that were used in the research, including scanning conditions, and example results. The research is sponsored by the National Aeronautics and Space Administration (NASA) and is aimed at studying the strength and deformation properties, as well as liquefaction phenomena of granular materials at very low effective stresses.

2 CT EXPERIMENTS

2.1 *LANL CT Facility*

The first set of scans were performed at Los Alamos National Laboratory (LANL), Los Alamos, New Mexico, USA. The device is classified as a second generation CT system. It comprises a 450 KeV x-ray source and a 32-element array of detectors. The specimens were scanned by a 400 keV, 2.15 mA electron beam stopped by a thick tungsten target. Thus a bremsstrahlung energy distribution of x-rays was created. 1024 × 1024 16-bit pixel images were aquired. The spatial calibration of the images was about 0.197 mm which is smaller than the mean particle size (0.22 mm) of Ottawa sand. CT analysis was performed on three flight specimens (F1-specimens tested during the NASA STS-79 mission in a microgravity environment (μg) in September of 1996, Sture *et al.* 1998) and two additional terrestrially tested specimens. One specimen was not compressed (U-Specimen) but prepared at the same density, which serves as a reference for the specimens' internal fabric condition before compression, while the other specimen was tested in a terrestrial laboratory (1-G specimen) at 1.30 kPa effective confining pressure. Herein, flight specimens are denoted as F1-05 (Flight 1, 0.05 kPa confining pressure specimen), F1-52 (Flight 1, 0.52 kPa confining pressure specimen), and F1-130 (Flight 1, 1.30 kPa confining pressure specimen). The CT scans were collected at 1 mm-spaced "slices" along the height of each F1 specimen (z-direction) and 5 mm spacing on the U-Specimen. It took approximately one hour to acquire data for each slice (Alshibli *et al.* 2000).

The sand specimens measured 75 mm in diameter and 150 mm in height before compression and were contained in special test cells (Fig. 1, see Alshibli *et al.* 1996 for more information about the experimental apparatus description). In preparation for scanning, the LANL specimens were first stabilized by injecting a very low viscosity epoxy into the pore space. They were then removed from the cells and directly exposed to x-rays during scanning. The epoxy-filled pore spaces had a significant effect on the data, discussed below.

2.2 *KSC CT Facility*

The second set of scans was performed at the Industrial Computed Tomography System (ICTS) of NASA/Kennedy Space Center (KSC), Cape Canaveral, Florida, USA. The ICTS scanner is model CITA-201, manufactured by Scientific Measurement Systems, Inc, classified as a second-generation CT system. A Cobalt-60 gamma ray source was used, with an energy level of approximately 1.25 MeV and source spot size of 2.5 mm. The source aperture was set at 36 degrees by 4 mm high. The 125 detector apertures were set at 2 mm wide by 4 mm high, which samples from approximately a 2-mm thick CT data region. The data object acquisition circle was 600 mm at 1581.85 mm from the source. Ray spacing data acquisition was every 0.5 mm. Second generation data acquisition was used, with time per datum of 0.2 seconds, thus taking approximately 1 hour to acquire data per complete slice. Slices were computed at 1 mm intervals over the height of each specimen. Data was returned in the form of arrays ranging from 250 × 250 to 300 × 300, with a length calibration of 0.387 mm/voxel. The CTN were scaled in the range of 0 to 0.25. For further information related to the system, readers are referred to Engel (1998).

A total of 15 triaxial sand specimens were scanned at KSC: the three F1 and one 1-G specimens also scanned at the LANL facility; 6 specimens tests aboard the NASA STS-89 Space Shuttle mission; and 5 ground specimens. The 11 previously unscanned specimens were examined while still located inside the cells. Four test cells were placed on the CT scanner stage and were scanned simultaneously, which was made possible due to the high energy level of the gamma ray source.

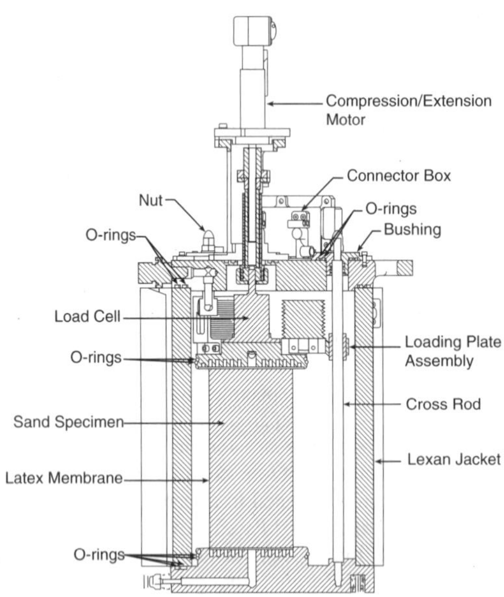

Figure 1. Cross section of the sand triaxial test cell.

2.3 *MSFC CT Facility*

The third set of scans was performed using the CT system of the NASA/Marshall Space Flight Center (MSFC) in Huntsville, Alabama, USA. The CT scanner is a third generation system called FlashCT manufactured by HYTEC Inc., Los Alamos, New Mexico, USA. It incorporates an amorphous Silicone (a-Si) flat panel detector (Fig. 2) that can accommodate objects with a projected area up to 304.8 mm × 406.4 mm (12 × 16 in). The detector resolution is 0.127 mm.

Second generation industrial CT systems use a line-detector array and therefore can only scan a thin slice (~1 mm thick) along the object axis. Then, the object is moved vertically to scan the next slice until the entire object is covered. The flat-panel detector

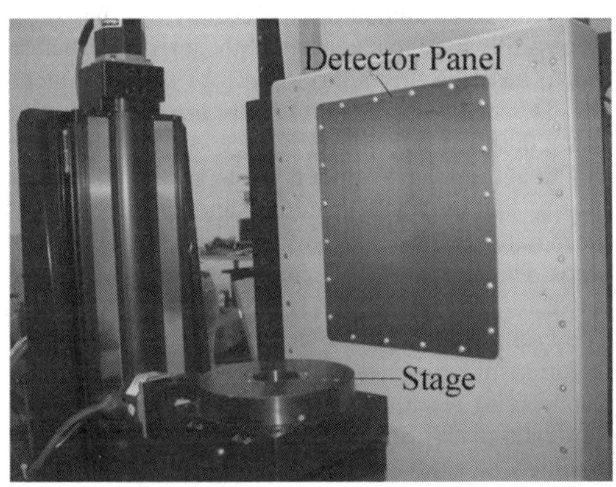

Figure 2. Photo of MSFC detector panel array and stage.

technology of the FlashCT system eliminates the need for time-consuming individual line scans associated with other types of industrial CT systems. It utilizes the concept of "volume tomography" where the entire specimen area is projected onto the CT detector and the x-rays attenuation is collected simultaneously. Then the specimen is rotated to acquire the data for the next area. This reduces the scanning time by a factor of 100.

The MSFC CT system was used to scan specimens composed of glass beads. Cylindrical specimens which measured 71 mm (2.8 in) in diameter by 142 mm (5.6 in) in height were tested under conventional triaxial compression (CTC) conditions. Uniform spherical glass beads with average particle size of 1.55–1.85 mm and void ratio of ~0.600 were used to prepare the specimens and vacuum was used to apply confinement. Specimens were prepared and scanned first before compression. Then, they were subjected to quasi-static axial compression under a constant displacement rate until peak strength was reached (at ~4% nominal axial strain), the compression was paused, and the specimen was scanned. The procedure was repeated for 12% and 21% axial strains. It took approximately 30 minutes for each scan which consisted of about 1400 slices.

3 CALIBRATION OF CT DATA

Aside from qualitative observation, the CT data were intended for measuring both internal structure geometry and density (or void ratio). Calibration has been performed on LANL and KSC data, but has not yet been performed on the MSFC data.

In the CT scans, the shape of an interface between two materials is examined and the modulation as a function of line pairs per millimeter (lpm) is derived. The CT number across an edge (called the edge response function, or ERF) is recorded and the slope of the ERF (point spread function, PSF) is calculated point-wise. A Fourier transform of the PSF is then calculated to find the modulation transfer function, or MTF, which indicates modulation as a function of distance, or lpm. This affects both length and density measurements.

For the LANL specimens, the interface between the acrylic end platen and air was examined and it was determined that data shows 50% modulation at 0.55 line pair per millimeter (lpm), and 10% at 0.96 lpm. This may be interpreted as objects separated by 0.91 mm can be identified with 50% modulation, and objects 0.52 mm apart can be identified with 10% modulation. This affects data interpretation both in length and void ratio measurements. Minimum resolution is 3 voxels (0.52 mm/0.197 mm/voxel = 2.6 voxel) at 10% modulation. This equates to 2.7 grain diameters at 10% modulation, or 4.5 grain size diameters at 50% modulation.

For the scans performed at the KSC facility, an aluminum phantom was used to measure spatial resolution. The medical phantom data indicates 50% modulation at 0.275 lpm, and 10% at 0.53 lpm. Objects separated by 1.8 mm (8 grain diameters) can be identified with 50% modulation, and objects 0.94 mm apart (5.3 grain diameters) can be identified with 10% modulation. Minimum resolution is 3 voxels at 10% modulation.

Calibration of density was performed using ASTM Guidelines (ASTM-E1935, 1997). A linear relation (Fig. 3) between the CT numbers (CTN) provided in the scans and their individual attenuation coefficients (Ca) [cm^{-1}], retrieved from National Institute of Standards and Technology (NIST) (Hubbell and Seltzer 1997), was calculated.

No independent calibration standards were scanned with the LANL specimens. Though not ideal, the acrylic end platens were used as standards. The only other data collected were the specimens themselves; the bulk density data for all five specimens and the end platens could be used to calibrate the data. A large uncertainty is present due to the epoxy stabilization. The mass coefficient of attenuation of the epoxy is not certain due to the propiretary nature of the epoxy. Secondly, cutting into a stabilized specimen reveals small air bubbles, mostly along shear bands. This is not too surprising, as this has been previously reported (Oda *et al.* 1997) and given the single-fill process of impregnating a specimen.

To perform density calibration of the KSC scans, water and Lexan available in scans of the triaxial test cells, were used as standards. An aluminum standard (the medical phantom) was scanned and the data provided by KSC, but was not used due to its high density in comparison with the granular material of interest. The calibration was checked against the bulk density of all specimens. A standard deviation of the

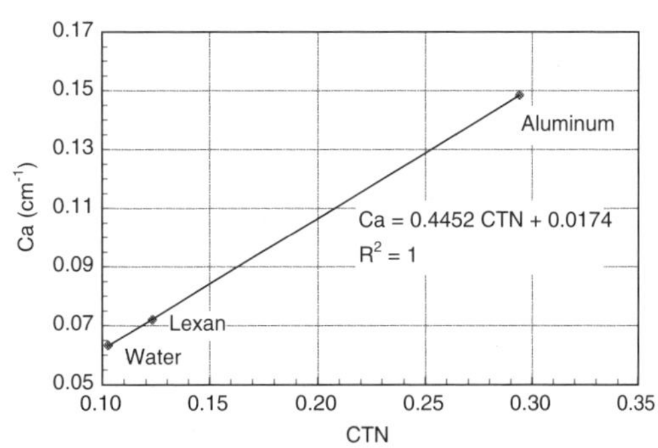

Figure 3. Relationship between CT numbers and coefficients of attenuation for KSC scans.

void ratio error was 0.033. For applying this calibration to granular material, which has a narrow range of possible void ratios, the calibration lacks desired precision: the standard deviation is equivalent to 10.3% relative density. Even though the standard deviation appears fairly high, the different structure types within the specimen have large void ratio differences, allowing a reasonable analysis. However, this indicates the need for higher resolution when a narrow density band is being considered.

For the density scans, relations between coefficient of attenuation and porosity (both sand-air and sand-epoxy) were found, as the resolution was not sufficient to identify individual sand particles.

4 RESULTS

Image processing software was used in order to extract 2- and 3-D images of the CT scans. First, qualitative assessments of data were made. Figure 4 shows typical 3-D renderings of one of the analyzed sand specimens. Darker areas represent less dense material due to dilatancy effects along sheared zones. The shearing behavior was characterized by the development of two major conical surfaces and multiple secondary symmetrical shear bands, which expanded outward in the radial and axial directions. The development of the new shear bands may have caused the observed continuous increase of the specimens volume change. Desrues *et al.* (1996) observed similar failure patterns in CTC specimens tested at 60 kPa confining pressure using the CT technique. These CT images confirm Desrues *et al.* (1996) findings and present results for specimens tested at much lower confining pressures.

The CT scans on the μg experiments could not reveal information about the development and progress of the shear bands as the scans were performed following compression. To further investigate when shear bands will develop and how they progress, five specimens were prepared with similar densities and were tested at 1.30 kPa confining pressure in a terrestrial laboratory. As shown in Figure 5, the principal stress ratio versus axial strain, and volumetric strain versus axial strain responses for these experiments are very similar. Figure 6 shows two orthogonal axial sections and two cross sections taken at one third and two third of the specimen's height. Generally, one would expect that shear band (s) would develop at or very near the peak principal stress level. However, the CT scan for the KSC5 experiment (Fig. 6), which was taken at 4.6% axial strain show no evidence of shear bands and the specimen had deformed uniformly. Then, the first shear conical surface accompanied by secondary shear bands developed between 4.6% and 9.2% axial strains (KSC9 in Fig. 6). As the test

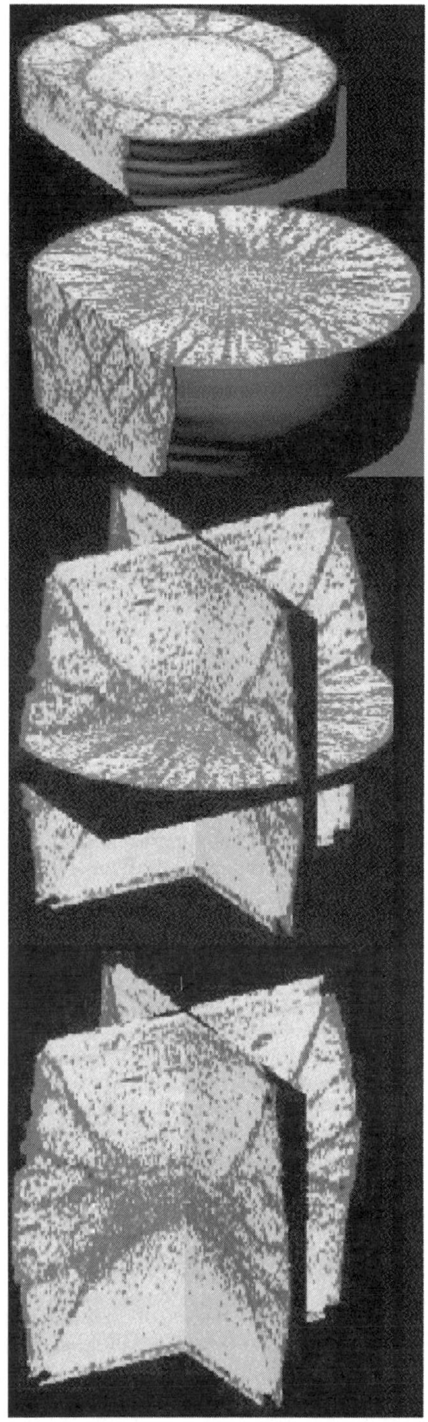

Figure 4. Typical CT 3D renderings of a sand experiment tested under μg environment taken at 25% axial strain (scanned at LANL CT facility).

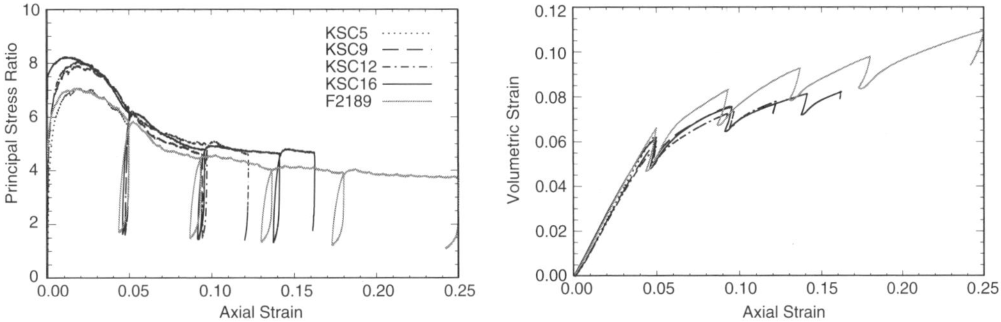

Figure 5. Principal stress ratio versus axial strain and volumetric strain versus axial strain for the scans shown in Figure 6.

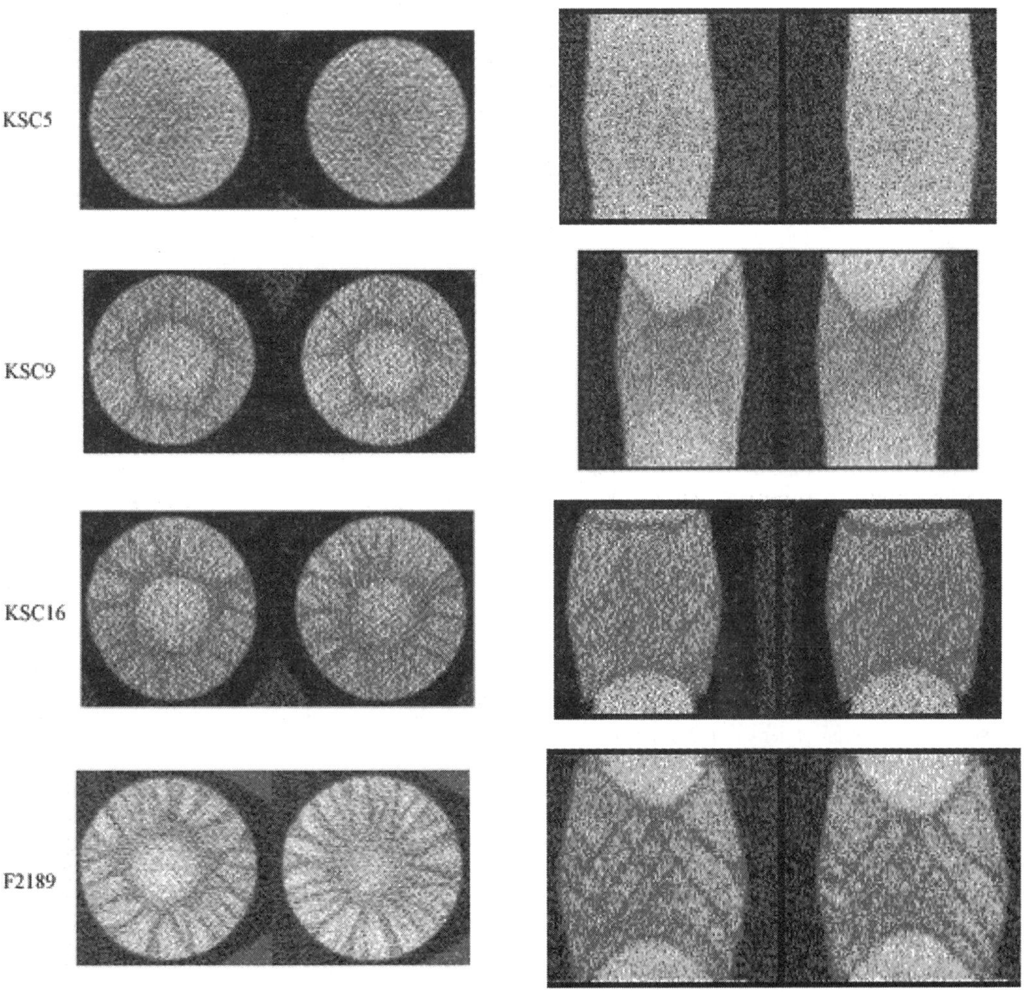

Figure 6. The progress of deformations in sand at 4.6% nominal axial strain, ε_a (KSC5), ε_a 9.2% (KSC9), $\varepsilon_a = 16\%$ (KSC16), and $\varepsilon_a = 25\%$ (F2189). Scans were taken at KSC CT facility.

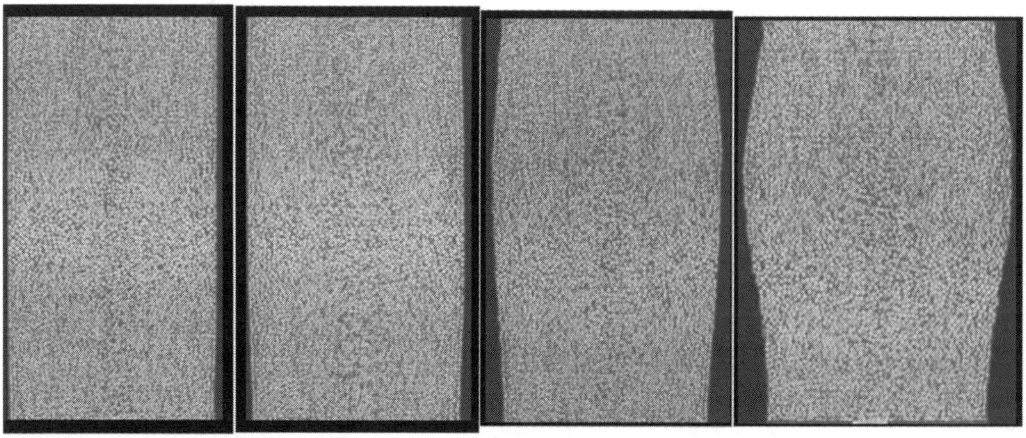

(a) $\varepsilon_a = 0$ (b) $\varepsilon_a = 4\%$ (c) $\varepsilon_a = 12\%$ (d) $\varepsilon_a = 12$

Figure 7. The progress of deformations in a specimen composed of glass beads. Scans were performed at MSFC CT facility.

proceeded more shear bands developed, which were bounded by two main conical surfaces, that were affected by the two end plates. The continuous volumetric increase (dilation) of the specimens is due to continuous development of shear bands. However, the dilation rate at the residual stress level is about 1/4th of the dilation before 4.6% axial strain.

In addition to qualitative assessments, a vigorous quantitative analysis was performed. Regional density, structural distribution, and shear band characteristics including orientation, width, and void ratio, were measured. The epoxy-embedded specimens were very useful for qualitative assessment, but due to the air bubbles in the epoxy, good quantitative analysis is difficult: therefore the quantitative analysis described below was performed on non-embedded specimens.

Examining regional density through statistical analysis of both individual slices and the entire specimen show specimens tested to low axial strain have undergone global volume change but remain overall homogeneous. As compression increases however, the standard deviation of density increases, indicating non-homogeneity. Density profiles show a decrease in density in the central portions of compressed specimens. This analysis indicates general dilatancy behavior. One may first suspect that the central increase in the density profile of a fully compressed specimen was result of a concentration of shear bands in the central region of the specimen. However, as the same shape is present prior to shear banding, the continued role of the entire specimen in diffuse dilation post-bifurcation is apparent. The shear bands are not the only active portion of a triaxial specimen after their formation.

Shear band features were examined as well. Orientation was measured through a combination of manual and programmed steps. Bands were chosen one at a time by marking points on the shear band with a unique value which could be located analytically, as well as visually checked on screen output. Once a band was marked over numerous cross-sections, the locations of the points were then calculated, and the equation for the plane was found using a least-squares fit. Using the equation for the plane, the angle with the horizontal was calculated. This orientation was then used in corrections of shear band thickness measurements. As the CT data was presented in cartesian coordinates aligned with the vertical axis, shear bands were most easily accessed by examining them along a horizontal (or vertical) plane, at an angle to the shear band. A 10-voxel wide averaged shear band profile generated through a program involving hand-identification of profile location. Width of the profiled band was then identified and angle and slice thickness corrections were applied. The same profile was also used to measure shear band density, again considering the influence of slice thickness and orientation on density. Rather than making corrections, density was measured only in a thin band along the center of the profile, where only shear band data (free from edge effects) was represented.

The CT analysis of specimens composed of glass beads at the MSFC CT facility (Fig. 7) revealed no evidence of shear bands as compared to the case of the sand specimens. Continuous compression resulted in the development chains of voids throughout the specimens with more bulging in the middle part of the specimens. This might be attributed to using uniform spherical particles (beads) with the same surface properties. Further experiments are underway to investigate this issue.

5 CONCLUSIONS

CT has demonstrated good ability to detect specimens' inhomogeneities and localization patterns, and has been successfully used to quantify void ratio variations within sand specimens. Compared to destructive methods, this non-destructive technique provides a highly efficient way of visualizing and measuring internal structures in the specimens. While the resolution of the systems used is not sufficient to see interactions at the level of individual grains, even complex patterns of shear bands can be identified and evaluated.

ACKNOWLEDGEMENTS

The authors gratefully acknowledge the financial support provided by NASA/George C. Marshall Space Flight Center under contracts NAS8-38779 and NAS8-01042. Thanks are also due to Martin Jones and David Stupin of LANL, Peter Engel of NASA/KSC and Ron Beshears of NASA/MSFC for help in performing the CT scans.

REFERENCES

Alshibli, K.A., Costes, N. & Porter, R. 1996. Mechanics of Granular Materials. *Space Processing of Materials, International Symposium on Optical Science, Engineering, and Instrumentation,* SPIE-The International Society for Optical Engineering, Denver, CO, 2809, 8/1996, 303–310.

Alshibli, K.A., Sture, S., Costes, N.C., Frank, M., Lankton, M. Batiste, S. & Swanson, R. 2000. Assessment of Localized Deformations in Sand Using X-ray Computed Tomography. *ASTM Geotechnical Testing Journal*, 23(3): 274–299.

Amos, C.L., Sutherland, T.F., Radzijewski, B. & Doucette, M. 1996. A Rapid Technique to Determine Bulk Density of Fine-grained Sediments by X-ray Computed Tomography. *Journal of Sedimentary Research*, 66(5): 1023–1039.

Batiste, S. 2001. "An Investigation of Deformations in Granular Material Using Computed Tomography." Diss., University of Colorado at Boulder, CO.

Bracewell, R.N. 1956. Strip Integration in Radio Astronomy. *Australian Journal of Physics*, 9: 198–217.

Bossi, R.H., Friddel, K.D. & Lowrey, A.R. 1990. Computed Tomography in *Non-Destructive Testing of Fibre-Reinforced Plastic Composites*, J. Summerscales (Editor), Elsevier Applied Science, NY, 2: 201–252.

Coshell, L., McIver, R.G. & Chang, R. 1994. X-Ray Computed Tomography of Australian Oil Shales: Non-Destructive Visualization and Density Determination. *Fuel*, 73(8): 1317–1321.

Denison, C., Carlson, W.D. & Ketcham, R.A. 1997. Three-dimensional Quantitative Texture Analysis of Metamorphic Rocks Using High-Resolution Computed X-ray Tomography: Part I. Methods and Techniques. *Journal of Metamorphic Geology*, 15(1): 29–44.

Denison, C. & Carlson, W.D. 1997. Three-dimensional Quantitative Texture Analysis of Metamorphic Rocks Using High-Resolution Computed X-ray Tomography: Part II. Application to Natural Materials. *Journal of Metamorphic Geology*, 15(1): 45–57.

Desrues, J., Chambon, R., Mokni, M. & Mazerolle, F. 1996. Void Ratio Evolution Inside Shear Bands in Triaxial Sand Specimens studied by Computed Tomography. *Geotechnique,* 46(3): 529–546.

Engel, P. 1998. NASA/KSC Industrial Computed Tomography (CT) System. Unpublished Report.

Hubbell, J.H. & Seltzer, S.M. 1996. Tables of X-Ray Mass Attenuation Coefficients & Mass Energy-Absorption Coefficients. (http://physics.nist.gov/PhysRefData/XrayMassCoef/cover.html).

Oda, M., Iwashita, K. & Kazama, H. 1997. Micro-Structure Developed in Shear Bands of Dense Granular Soils and Its Computer Simulation-Mechanism of Dilatancy and Failure. *IUTAM Symposium on Mechanics of Granular and Porous Materials,* N.A. Fleck and A.C.F. Cocks (eds), pp. 353–364.

Otani, J., Mukunoki, T. & Obara, Y. 2000. Application of X-ray CT Method for Characterization of Failure in Soils. *Soils & Foundations*, 40(2): 111–118.

Phillips, D.H. & Lannutti, J.J. 1997. Measuring Physical Density with X-ray Computed Tomography. *NDT & E International*, 30(6): 339–350.

Steude, J.S., Hopkins, F. & Anders, J.E. 1994. Industrial X-ray Computed Tomography Applied to Soil Research. *Tomography of Soil-Water-Root Processes, Soil Science Society of America Special Publication*, 36: 29–41.

Sture, S., Costes, N., Batiste, S., Lankton, M., Alshibli, K., Jeremic, B., Swanson, R. & Frank, M. 1998. Mechanics of Granular Materials at Low Effective Stresses. *ASCE, Journal of Aerospace Engineering*, 11(3): 67–72.

X-ray CT for Geomaterials; Soils, Concrete, Rocks – Otani & Obara (eds.)
© 2004 Swets & Zeitlinger. Lisse, ISBN 90 5809 666 1

Correlation between air permeability and biodegradation in hydrocarbon-contaminated soil columns studied by X-ray CT

M.C. Alfaro
University of Manitoba, Winnipeg, Manitoba, Canada

R.C.K. Wong
University of Calgary, Calgary, Alberta, Canada

ABSTRACT: This paper presents a study on the correlation between air permeability and biodegradation in hydrocarbon-contaminated soil columns with the aid of X-ray computer tomography (CT) scan data. The study was undertaken as part of a laboratory experiment to determine the rate of biodegradation of hydrocarbon in the soil using bioventing technique. The experiment consisted of unsaturated soil columns that were contaminated with 2% crude oil by weight. Each soil column was purged with breathing quality air. Off-gas samples for each column were analyzed using gas chromatograph (GC) in order to determine CO_2 production rates. Air permeability tests on these columns were also conducted in an attempt to correlate them with the biodegradation rate of hydrocarbon. Difficulties arose in interpreting the relationships between the biodegradation rate and air permeability. So it was decided to use X-ray CT scan data to assist in interpreting air permeability and biodegradation measurements. It was found that soil columns with higher percentage below average CT number have higher permeability. This implies that higher percentage of pore volume above the average pore volume of the entire column resulted in higher permeability. It was also found that more uniform soil columns have higher permeability compared to less uniform soil columns. The amount of bioremediation is inversely proportional to the air permeability, such that low biodegradation in the hydrocarbon-contaminated soil columns is associated with high air permeability.

1 INTRODUCTION

An experimental study was undertaken to determine the rate of biodegradation of hydrocarbon in the soil under cold temperature (5°C). The experimental design consisted of 14 soil columns, 12 of which were contaminated with 2% crude oil by weight. Each soil column was purged with breathing quality air at a flow rate of 4 ml/min. Off-gas samples for each column were analyzed using gas chromatograph (GC) in order to determine CO_2 production rates. Details of the test setup (shown in Figure 1) and procedures can be found in Gibb (1999). As part of Gibb's study, air permeability tests on unsaturated soil columns were conducted. In these tests, an ultra-low pressure transducer was connected to measure the pressure drop between the inlet and outlet of each column. A flow of about 4 ml/min was used for each column. After the columns were connected to the transducer, an interval of 15 minutes was allowed for stabilization before reading was taken. The readings were then converted into pressure head of water. After a series of calculations, this data was converted into air permeability.

The results of air permeability tests are summarized in Table 1. As will be discussed later in the paper, no clear correlation exists between the biodegradation rate and air permeability. To assist in interpreting the results of air permeability and biodegradation measurements, it was decided to use CT scan data.

2 ANALYSIS OF CT MEASUREMENT

2.1 *Brief description of CT measurement*

Computer tomography (CT) is a non-destructive analysis that produces an image of the internal structure of a material by reconstruction of attenuation coefficients of X-rays passing through the body. As X-rays pass through the object, some are absorbed, some are scattered, and some are transmitted. The radiation transmitted through the object is measured by detectors and referred to as attenuation data. Attenuation is a measure of the reduction in X-ray intensity that results from absorption and scattering by the object. The attenuation data is summed over the many different angles from which it was collected using a computer in a method called reconstruction. Reconstruction essentially builds the CT image from the data collected and represents a cross-section of the object. This image contains a matrix of pixels (picture element). Each pixel represents a specific computer tomograph number (χ). The computer tomograph number in turn represents the average X-ray attenuation within a volume element, often referred to as a voxel. The size of the voxel is limited by the thickness of the X-ray beam and by the instrument resolution. The volume of a voxel in the present study is $0.75 \times 0.75 \times 3\,\text{mm}^3$. The type of CT scanner used is the General Electric Model Hi Speed CT/i. The settings were: 120 kV (KVP), 150 mA (X-ray tube current), 0.8 sec full rotation scan, and 25 cm FOV (field of view).

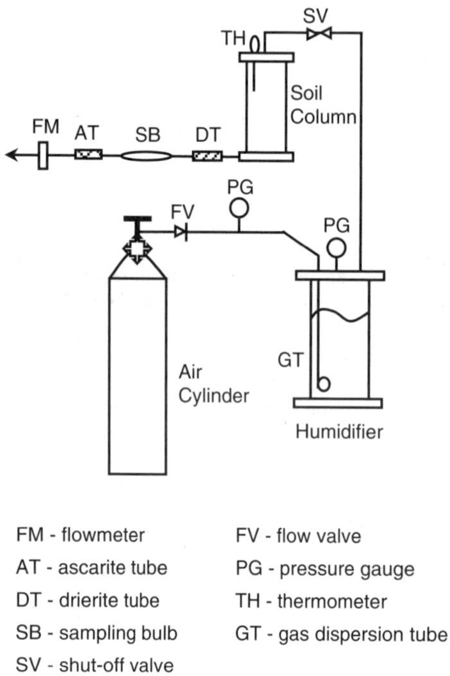

Figure 1. Experimental setup for bioventing test (after Gibb 1999).

Table 1. Air permeability and biodegradation test results (after Gibb 1999).

Column number	Sample symbol	Air permeability (μ^2)	Oil degraded (g)
AN-2	MIC1	3.339	0.3
AN-3	NSC1	2.003	7.0
AN-4	CC1	0.639	2.7
AN-5	T1	0.577	10.2
AN-6	T2	3.339	7.1
AN-7	T3	0.601	10.1
AN-8	T4	3.005	7.1
AN-9	CC2	0.578	2.5
AN-10	NSC2	0.859	7.6
AN-11	MIC2	3.005	0.5
AN-12	T5	0.939	8.6
AN-13	AC1	0.612	11.0
AN-14	AC2	0.637	10.8

Note: $\mu^2 = 10^{-8}\,\text{cm}^2$

Relationship between X-ray attenuation coefficient, μ and CT number, χ is established by the following equation:

$$\chi = \frac{\mu - \mu_{water}}{\mu_{water}} k \tag{1}$$

where k is the scaling factor either 500 or 1000; μ and μ_w are the attenuation coefficients of the material and water, respectively. Bossi et al. (1990) have shown that the measurement of attenuation from CT is predominantly proportional to the local electron density of the material under consideration. If the material has uniform chemical composition, the measurement is proportional to the local mass density of the object. In effect, CT scanner measures density as a CT number. Each pixel of a scanned image represents the average density of a voxel at (x, y) cross-section location. The interpretation and analysis of CT scan data depends on the composition of the volume scanned. Selected applications of CT imaging technique in experimental geotechnics are given in Alfaro and Wong (2001).

For the case of two-phase geotechnical materials (i.e., solid-air or solid-water system), the average CT number can be defined using mixture theory (Wong and Wibowo 2000):

$$\chi_{sa}(x,y) = \chi_a \phi(x,y) + \chi_s [1 - \phi(x,y)] \tag{2}$$

$$\chi_{sw}(x,y) = \chi_w \phi(x,y) + \chi_s [1 - \phi(x,y)] \tag{3}$$

where χ_a, χ_w, and χ_s are CT numbers of air, water and solid, respectively. The calibrated value of χ_a is -1000 while that of χ_w is 0. The values of $\chi_{sa}(x, y)$ and $\chi_{sw}(x, y)$ are the average CT numbers for solid-air and solid-water at (x, y) location, respectively. The value of the porosity $\phi(x, y)$, which is defined as the volume of void divided by the volume of a voxel, represents the local porosity at each (x, y) location that can be determined by combining Equations (2) and (3):

$$\phi(x,y) = \frac{\chi_{sw}(x,y) - \chi_{sa}(x,y)}{\chi_w - \chi_a} \tag{4}$$

For the case of three-phase geotechnical materials (i.e., solid-air-water system), the average CT number at location (x, y) is given as:

$$\chi(x,y) = \chi_a \phi(x,y) S_a + \chi_w \phi(x,y) S_w + \chi_a \phi(x,y) + \chi_s [1 - \phi(x,y)] \quad (5)$$

where S_a is the air saturation ($S_a = \phi(1 - S_w)$); S_w is the water saturation, and χ is the CT number for the scanned voxel. Recall that crude oil accounts only for 2% by weight, so it was not considered as another phase in the system.

Combining Equations (2), (3), and (5), the air saturation at any (x,y) location can be estimated from:

$$S_a(x,y) = \frac{\chi_{sw}(x,y) - \chi(x,y)}{\chi_{sw}(x,y) - \chi_{sa}(x,y)} \quad (6)$$

It can be seen that the estimation of spatial distributions of porosity and air saturation requires determination of CT scan data for $S_w = 0$ and 100%.

2.2 *Raw data and filtering*

The raw CT scan data was converted to a raster image using a computer code written in C++. The code allowed for a variety of mapping scales in creating the pictures so that various ranges of CT numbers could be enhanced in the image. The CT scan data was then filtered to eliminate all CT numbers that were not representative of the soil sample. Since the cell was cylindrical in shape and the data was in the form of a matrix, there was a lot of air surrounding the column that was included within each slice. This background CT number was filtered out using a computer code that takes all of the numbers in the matrix below the specified number and replaces them with another user specified number. Since the soil was held in a plexi-glass cylinder, the CT numbers corresponding to the container had to be filtered out as well.

The CT scan data collected for all thirteen soil columns have been converted to an image form. Figure 2 shows the CT scan images of two of the soil columns with 9 CT images (9 slices for each column). Slice 1 was taken near the top, Slice 9 was taken near the bottom, and the rest were taken at equal intervals along the column. Not all of the columns have the same constitution. Some have soil uniformly distributed whereas others have cracks running through the cross-section. However, the presence of cracks alone did not necessarily resulted to higher air permeability because these cracks were generally discontinuous all throughout the length of the columns.

2.3 *Methods of analysis*

Three different methods of analysis were used in order to find a correlation between air permeability and CT numbers. The first method used was to take the filtered arrays and do a basic statistical analysis of the data, finding the average CT number and standard deviation. To do this, another C++ computer code was written which created a file that could be viewed with any spreadsheet program. The results are summarized in Table 2. The distribution of the average CT number from each slice along the column length is shown in Figure 3. As can be seen in this figure, the average CT number for each slice is in the range of 550 to 650,

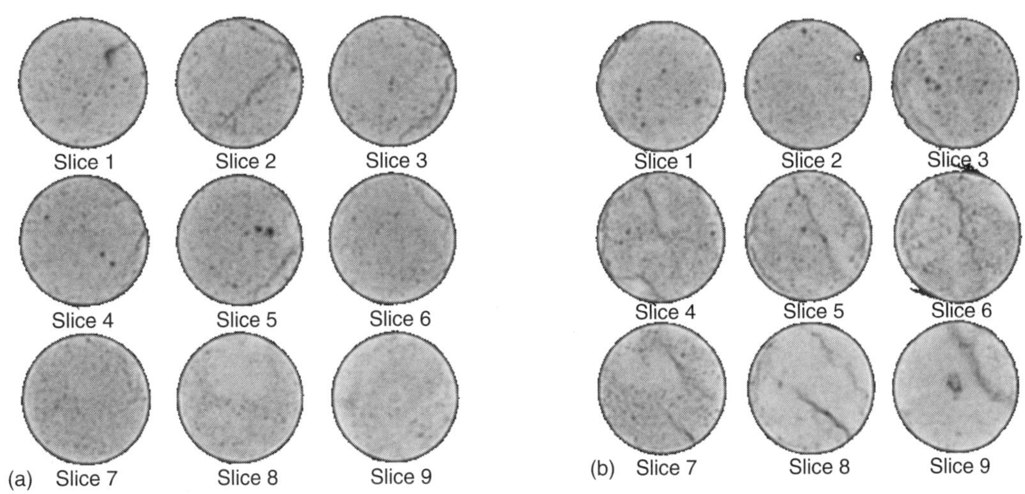

Figure 2. CT scan images of hydrocarbon-contaminated soil columns: (a) AN-4 and (b) AN-9.

except for two outliers. Also, the average CT number generally increases as one goes along the column length from top to bottom. This indicates that the soil was more compacted near the bottom of the column, due in part to the experimental setup wherein the columns were positioned vertically. Consequently, the weight of the soil allowed more compression in the bottom than in the top.

The second method that was used to analyze the data was to look at the percentage of each cross-section that was below the average CT number for that soil column. This was done by taking the average CT number from Table 2 and running the data through a program, again in C++, to count all numbers per slice that were below the average. The total count per slice was then divided by the circular area of each sample after the data was filtered to find the percentage of the cross-sectional area below the average. The averages used for soil columns were the ones shown in Table 2.

The third method used was to look at the percentage of CT numbers below the estimated maximum void ratio, which corresponds to a CT number of 530. The data was analyzed in the same way as previously described except that the number 530 was substituted for the average CT number.

After looking at each column slice by slice, it was thought that the average percentage for each sample would be useful for analysis. The percentage below average and percentage below 530 numbers were averaged to produce one number per soil column. The results of the calculations using these methods of analysis are shown in Table 3. As can be seen in this

Table 2. Average CT number and standard deviation.

Column number	Average CT number	Standard deviation
AN-2	568.457	66.085
AN-3	610.895	99.642
AN-4	605.237	108.791
AN-5	597.337	101.197
AN-6	613.309	90.416
AN-7	602.812	107.697
AN-8	595.047	103.015
AN-9	617.383	115.199
AN-10	603.898	100.191
AN-11	565.492	74.930
AN-12	607.605	101.119
AN-13	597.269	127.252
AN-14	635.451	101.522

Table 3. Average percentages for below average and below 530.

Column number	Below average	Below 530
AN-2	41.703	9.460
AN-3	36.221	10.799
AN-4	31.441	9.586
AN-5	31.918	12.005
AN-6	36.652	8.266
AN-7	29.682	11.150
AN-8	34.172	11.932
AN-9	33.410	10.095
AN-10	36.064	11.158
AN-11	36.191	10.202
AN-12	30.475	11.376
AN-13	26.055	15.706
AN-14	29.069	10.521

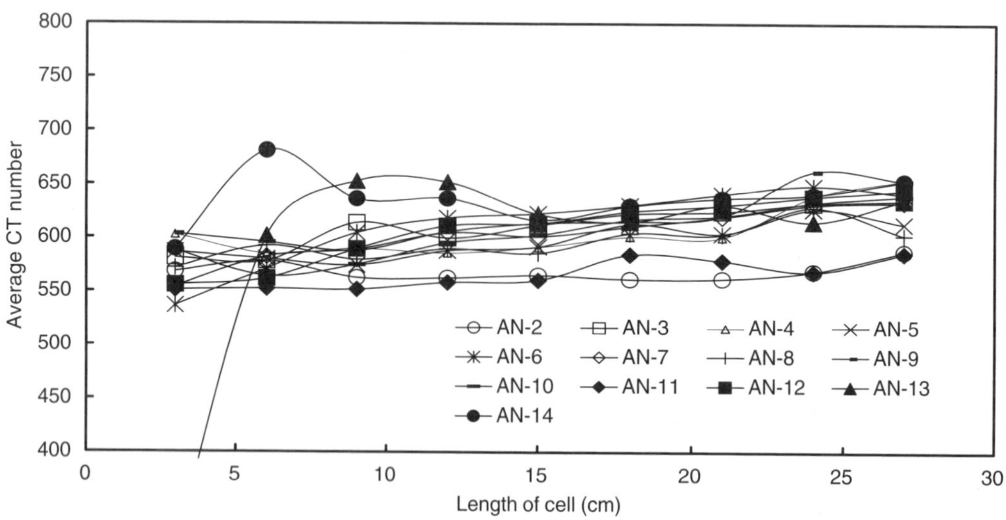

Figure 3. Average CT number versus column length.

table, there does not seem to be clear relationship between the average percentage below average and the average percentage below 530.

3 CORRELATION BETWEEN AIR PERMEABILITY AND CT SCAN DATA

The next step in analyzing the CT scan data was to find a correlation between the air permeability and the CT numbers. To do this, the air permeability was plotted against: 1) the average CT number, 2) the standard deviation, 3) the average percentage below average, and 4) the average percentage below 530. These figures are shown respectively in Figures 4 to 7. As can be seen from these figures, the air permeability only seems to have a good correlation with the standard deviation (Figure 5) and with the average percentage below average (Figure 6). Figure 5 shows that soil columns with lower standard deviation in CT numbers have higher permeability in comparison to those with higher standard deviation. This means that more uniform soil columns have higher permeability compared to the less uniform soil columns. In Figure 6, soil columns with higher percentage below average CT numbers have higher air permeability. This implies that higher percentage of pore volume above the average pore volume of the entire column (larger permeable zones) resulted in higher air permeability.

4 CORRELATION BETWEEN BIODEGRADATION AND AIR PERMEABILITY

A correlation can also be found with the permeability of air and the amount of oil degraded. To find this correlation we looked at the soil columns that correspond to sample symbols labeled T1 to T5, as shown in Table 1. These five soil columns were tested with similar initial condition, namely at a temperature of 5°C. Of these soil columns, AN-6 and AN-8 (Symbols T2 and T4, respectively) had low biodegradation while soil columns AN-5, AN-7 and AN-12 (Symbols T1, T3 and T5, respectively) had higher biodegradation. Table 1 also shows that AN-6 and AN-8 had higher air permeability than AN-5, AN-7 and AN-12 by about an order of magnitude. Thus the amount of biodegradation and the permeability of air in the soil columns are inversely proportional, so that low bioremediation is associated with high air permeability. This can be explained with the aid of the CT scan data.

Soil columns AN-6 and AN-8, which have higher air permeability, are characterized by larger permeable zones as demonstrated by soil columns with higher percentage above average CT number. This resulted in lower resistance of air moving through the soil column. On the other hand, soil columns AN-5, AN-7 and AN-12 have lower air permeability with smaller permeable zones. According to Gibb (1999), soil columns that have low resistance to air flow

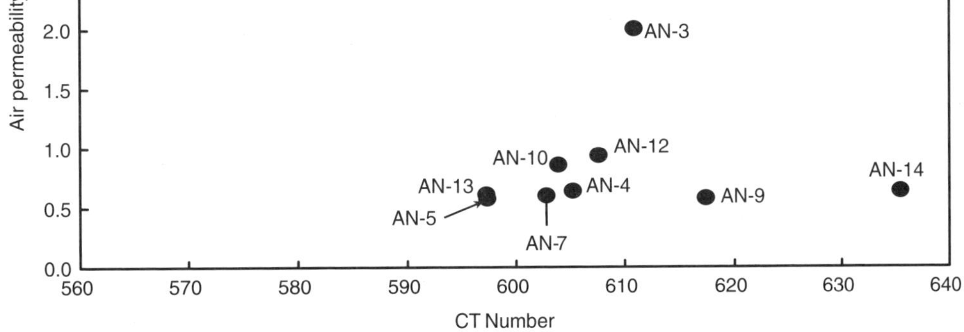

Figure 4. Air permeability versus average CT number.

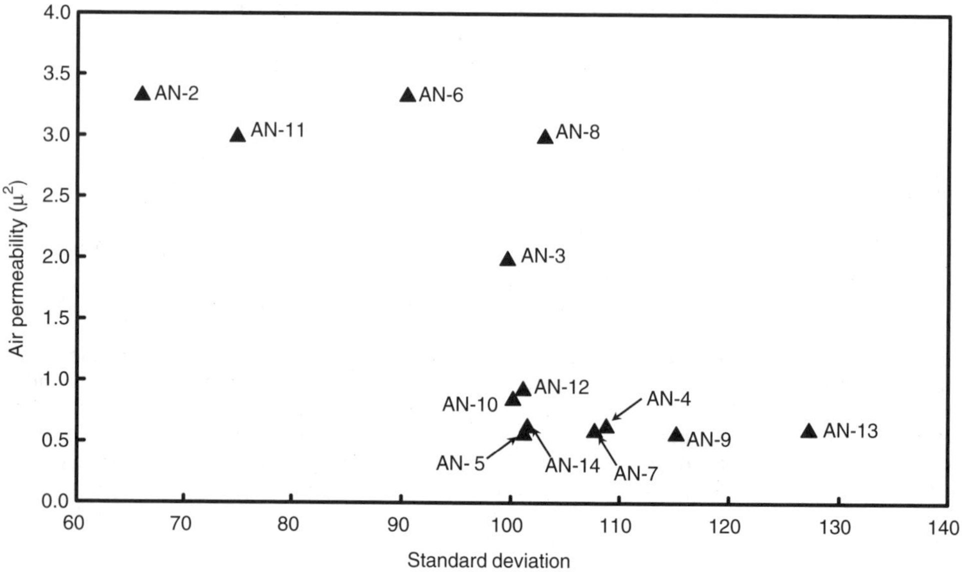

Figure 5. Air permeability versus standard deviation of CT number.

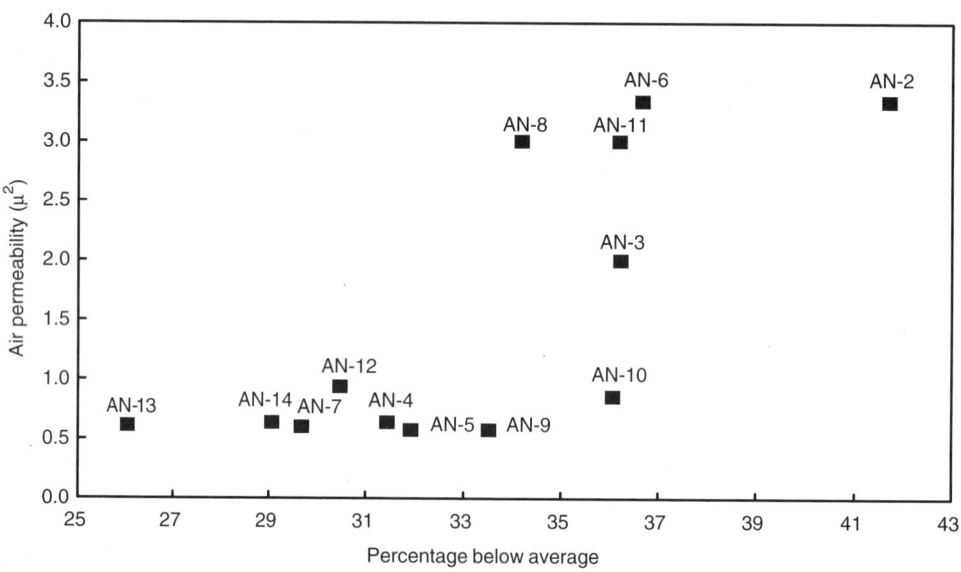

Figure 6. Air permeability versus percentage below average CT number.

(higher air permeability) could have resulted in pockets of low (or minimal) O_2 concentrations, which would have a negative effect on oil degradation. Although columns with larger permeable zones also correspond to columns that are more uniform, the relative uniformity of the soil columns did not suggest an even diffuse pattern of the O_2 throughout the columns. An even diffusion of air to water saturated zones would ensure few localized areas of O_2 limitations and become directly related to higher biodegradation. Note that the breathing quality air that was purged through the soil column comprised of about 20% of

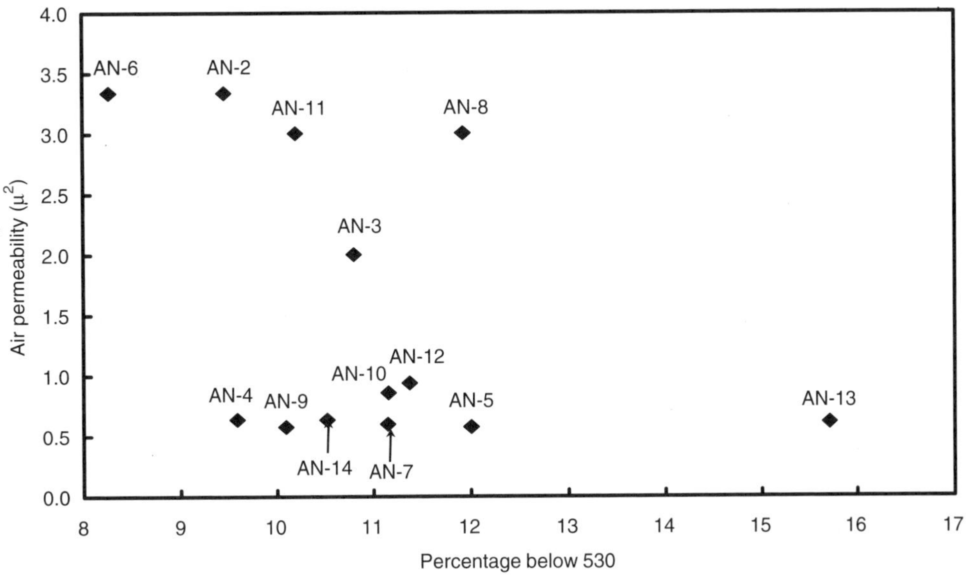

Figure 7. Air permeability versus percentage below CT number = 530.

O_2. The degradation of oil in the soil column is very much dependent to the availability of O_2 in the soil system for stimulation of hydrocarbon contaminant metabolism in aerobic indigenous organisms (Dupont 1993).

5 CONCLUSIONS

This study has demonstrated how the CT data could be used to assist in interpreting the results of air permeability and biodegradation measurements. The CT images of two of the soil columns show that there could be channeling inside the columns due to cracks. However, the presence of fractures alone did not necessarily resulted to higher air permeability. It was found that air permeability only have good correlation with the percentage below average. This implies that the higher percentage of pore volume above the average pore volume of the entire column resulted in higher permeability. It was also found that the more uniform soil columns have higher permeability compared to the less uniform soil columns. The amount of bioremediation is inversely proportional to the air permeability, such that low biodegradation in the hydrocarbon-contaminated soil columns is associated with high air permeability.

ACKNOWLEDGEMENT

This study was funded by the Natural Sciences and Engineering Research Council (NSERC) of Canada. Angela Gibb carried out the laboratory bioventing experiment and Mona Maini helped in writing computer codes for the analysis of CT scan data.

REFERENCES

Alfaro, M.C. and Wong, R.C.K. 2001. Some applications of computerized tomography (CT) in experimental geotechnics. *Proc. 15th International Conference in Soil Mechanics and Geotechnical Engineering*, Istanbul, Turkey, Vol. 1, pp. 337–342.

Bossi, R.H., Friddel, K.D. and Lowrey, A.R. 1990. Computed tomography. *Non-Destructive Testing of Fibre-Reinforced Plastic Composites*. Elsevier Applied Science, New York.

Dupont, R.R. 1993. Fundamentals of bioventing applied to fuel contaminated sites. *Environmental Progress* 12(1): 45–53.

Gibb, A. 1999. *Bioremediation of crude oil in cold climates*. MSc. thesis, University of Calgary, Alberta, Canada.

Wong, R.C.K. and Wibowo, R. 2000. Tomographic evaluation of air and water flow patterns in soil column. *Geotechnical Testing Journal* 23(4): 413–422.

X-ray CT for Geomaterials; Soils, Concrete, Rocks – Otani & Obara (eds.)
© 2004 Swets & Zeitlinger. Lisse, ISBN 90 5809 666 1

Characterization of soil cutting with flat blade in sand by using X-ray CT method

T. Kobayashi, R. Fukagawa & K. Tamoi
Department of Civil Engineering, Ritsumeikan University, Shiga, Japan

J. Otani
Department of Civil and Environmental Engineering, Kumamoto University, Kumamoto, Japan

ABSTRACT: This paper deals with the visualization of failure mechanisms for soil cutting with a blade by means of X-ray CT method. The model tests of soil cuttings using a simple flat blade were performed in air-dried sand. The failure mechanisms were scanned at every 1.0 mm thickness in the vertical direction of the soil chamber and reconstructed into 2-D and 3-D images. As a result, configurations of slip surface generated in the model ground could be clarified. This will facilitate a reasonable modeling of the soil cutting resistance under 3-D conditions.

1 INTRODUCTION

For the purpose of rational design of earth-moving machines, for a long time a lot of studies on soil-tool interactions have been attempted. Specifically, the soil cutting problem, which is one of the main processes of earth-moving work, has been undertaken as an important subject in the field of Terramechanics.

In order to evaluate the soil cutting resistance acting on a cutting blade, passive earth pressure theory based on soil mechanics has been applied as a conventional rule. However, according to circumstances, it is reported that this theoretical approach may not be valid. When dealing with soil cutting by a narrow cutting bit in particular, some researchers indicated that the actual resistance exceeds the theoretical value derived under the condition of plane-strain. It is considered that this is due to disregarding the effects of failure regions three dimensionally generated aside from the flank of the bit.

As matters now stand, treatment of the 3-D failure mechanism is not yet clearly understood owing to lack of information on the actual failure mechanism. In this study, model tests using a flat simple cutting bit were performed on Toyoura sand and then, the failure mechanisms in the ground were visualized by using an X-ray computed tomography (CT) scanner.

The X-ray CT method has been used as a medical diagnostic method. But recently, this method has been adopted as a nondestructive method for engineering purposes. Using this technique, not only 2-D cross sectional images but also 3-D images of the failure mechanism can be obtain by investigating the changes of density in the soil specimen when the materials deform with dilatancy.

2 X-RAY CT METHOD

2.1 *Principle of X-ray CT method*

When X-rays penetrate a substance, the energy level declines in connection with the density and the penetration thickness of the substance. The difference (or change) in density can be examined by irradiating X-rays and measuring the intensity of the beams that penetrate through. Hence, it is possible to spatially evaluate the positions and/or size of the shear band (slip surface) by visualizing the changes in density of the materials using the effect of dilatancy that accompanies shearing deformation.

As shown in Fig. 1, X-ray intensity, $t(s, \omega)$ which is attenuated after penetrating a specimen is expressed by the following equation:

$$i(s,\omega)=i_0 \exp\left\{-\int_{L_{s,\omega}} f(x,y)dt\right\} \tag{1}$$

where, i_0: incident intensity of X-ray, s, ω: variables which represent translational, rotational scanning, t: rectangular coordinate against the s-axis. Here, $f(x, y)$

called "coefficient of absorption" expressed in the right side of the equation (1) is the spatial distribution that ought to be obtained hereafter. Now, the value of $p(s, \omega)$ known as 'projection' which can be actually acquired by X-ray CT scanning is defined as follows:

$$p(s,\omega) = \ln \frac{i_0}{i(s,\omega)} = \int_{L_{s,\omega}} f(x,y)dt \quad (2)$$

In order to calculate the distribution of the coefficient of absorption, $f(x, y)$ from the projection data measured, mathematical techniques have long been established. Recently, with advances in computer technology, many innovative algorithms were developed. In the X-ray CT scanner system used in this study, $f(x, y)$ is obtained by the Filtered Back-Projection Method (e.g. Kak and Slaney, 1987) as a reconstruction method of images.

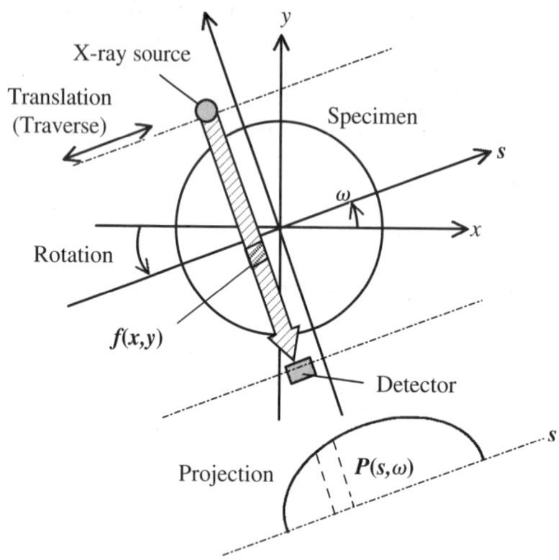

Figure 1. Principle of X-ray CT method.

2.2 *CT value*

In general, an image consists of the smallest elements called "the Pixel". The coefficient of absorption at each pixel is converted into a CT value which is defined by the following equation:

$$\text{CT value} = \frac{\mu_t - \mu_w}{\mu_w} k \quad (3)$$

where μ_t: coefficient of absorption at the scanning point, μ_w: coefficient of absorption with respect to water, k: proportionality constant, which is fixed at a value of 1000.

Accordingly, the CT value for water is 0, whereas air has a value of −1000 because the coefficient of absorption with respect to air is given as 0. As mentioned above, the coefficient of absorption is proportional to the density of the spacemen. Therefore, the CT value defined by equation (3) is also considered to be proportional to the density.

The CT value provides a monochrome image with 256 tones of light and shade through the image processing; light gray or white color signifies a region comparatively distinguished for high CT values (high density), while gray shades or black regions signify low CT values (low density).

2.3 *X-ray CT scanner system*

The X-ray CT scanner system used in this study is the same type as that used by Otani, et al (2000, 2002). In this apparatus, the collimated X-ray is penetrated by rotating and translating the specimen table as shown in Fig. 2. The specifications of this X-ray scanner are shown in Table 1.

Cross sectional images of the CT values are obtained by assembling the detected data, followed by reconstruction using an image processing device by

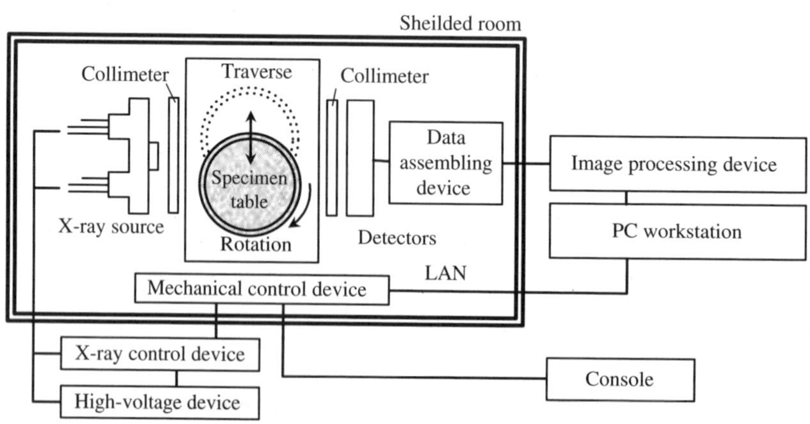

Figure 2. Schematic view of X-ray CT scanner system.

Table 1. Specification of X-ray scanner (Toscaner-23200 min TOSHIBA Corp.).

Scan type	Traverse/Rotation
Power of X-ray	300 kV/200 kV
Number of detectors	176 channels
Maximum size of specimen	D: 400 mm, H: 600 mm
X-ray beam	0.5 mm, 1 mm, 2 mm
Spatial resolution	0.2 mm (diameter of hole) for 20 mm thickness of steel

means of the Filtered Back-Projection Method. Fur-thermore, three dimensional (3-D) images can be constructed by compiling those cross sectional images with computer software.

3 TEST PROCEDURE

Fig. 3 shows the outline of the test apparatus. In this study, Toyoura standard sand was used for the model ground under an air-dried condition. The model ground specimens were prepared in an acrylic cylinder of 130 mm inner diameter in consideration of the X-ray penetrability and the applicability of reconstructing of the images. Here, the initial relative densities of the ground specimens were prepared to be 40% (loose) and 80% (dense), under the situations of cutting blades being initially stuck into the ground. The cutting blade is made of acrylic and it is 40 mm in width, 5.0 mm in thickness with a 40 deg. angle of relief. During the soil cutting process the cutting bits were kept moving at a constant cutting depth of 40 mm performed using two rake angles; 90 deg. (for dense sand) and 60 deg. (for dense and loose sand). The test conditions are summarized in Table 2.

A series of the tests were carried out as follows: The test specimen was set on the specimen table, after which preliminary CT scanning was demonstrated in order to check the states of the initial soil distribution. Subsequently, the cutting bit was started to move horizontally along a guide rail attached to the cylinder and then stopped and fixed when a sign was seen showing a slip surface had developed in the ground surface. The scanning was carried out at every 1.0 mm thickness in the vertical direction of the chamber.

4 RESULTS AND DISCUSSIONS

4.1 *Cross sectional images*

Fig. 4 shows the cross sectional images which were obtained at every 10 mm interval with respect to excavation depth from $z = 0$ to 40 mm. An arrow displayed in the upper row of Fig. 4(a) indicates the direction of the cutting and rectangular area of black color seen in

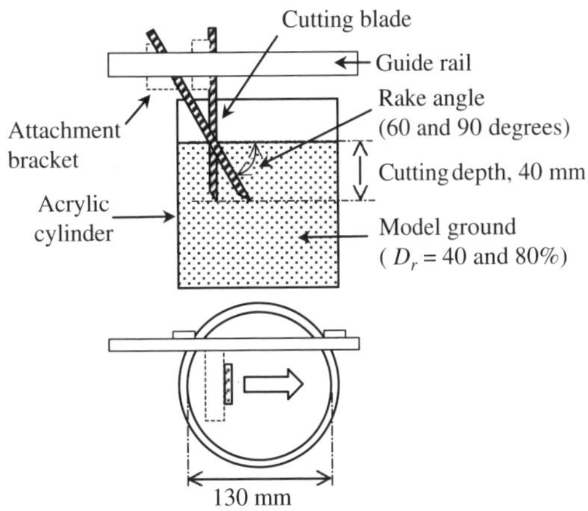

Figure 3. Outline of model test apparatus.

Table 2. Model test conditions.

Test case	Relative density (%)	Rake angle (deg.)	Traveling distance (mm)
Case 1	80	90	8.5
Case 2	80	60	7.0
Case 3	30	60	13.0

the center of the images represents a section of the cutting blade. As mentioned above, the dark region in the images represents an area of low density while the region of high density is represented by light color. In addition, the threshold CT value was unified in all cases. Therefore, in the case of loosely packed ground shown in Fig. 4(c), the images are darkly reflected compared with the cases of densely one.

Conspicuous regions suggesting disturbance or unevenness in the ground were not observed from the results of preliminary CT scanning. Therefore, it can be said that the gray or black-colored zones that appeared in front of the cutting bit imply sections of shear bands (slip surface).

Fig. 4(a) shows the result of soil cutting using a cutting blade with a rake angle of 90 deg. in a densely packed ground (Case 1). From these images, it could be observed that the section of the slip surface becomes curved (shear band), and the failure region enclosed by the shear band is enlarged as the ground surface is approached. Moreover, CT value of the interior region enclosed by shear bands seems to be lower than that of shear bands by comparing the colorings, implying that the sands deform as a one clod of soil and the shear failure took place on a boundary surface between the soil clod and its circumference.

Fig. 4(b) shows the result of soil cutting using a cutting blade with a rake angle of 60 deg. in a densely

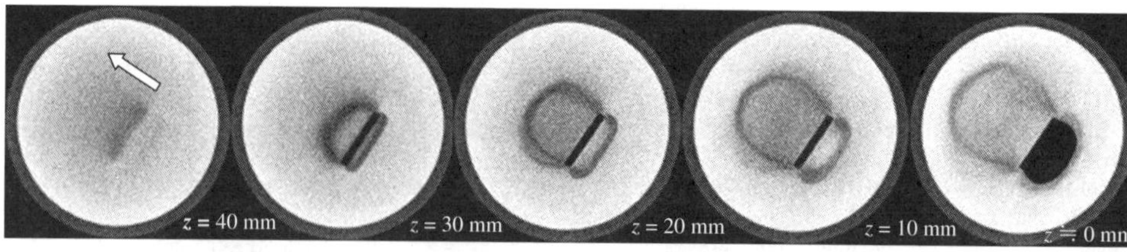

(a) Case 1 (Relative density: 80%, Rake angle: 90 deg., Traveling distance; 8.5 mm)

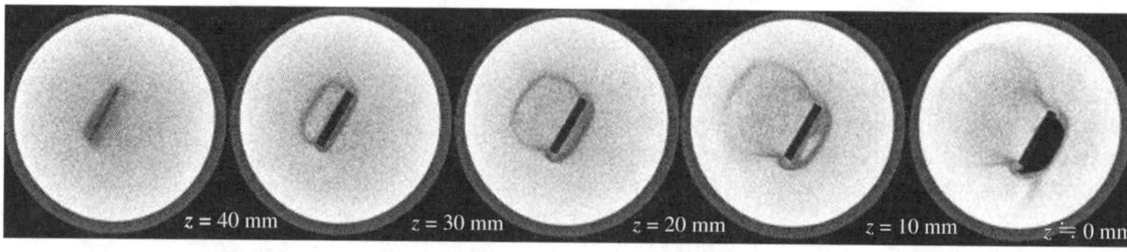

(b) Case 2 (Relative density: 80%, Rake angle: 60 deg., Traveling distance; 7.0 mm)

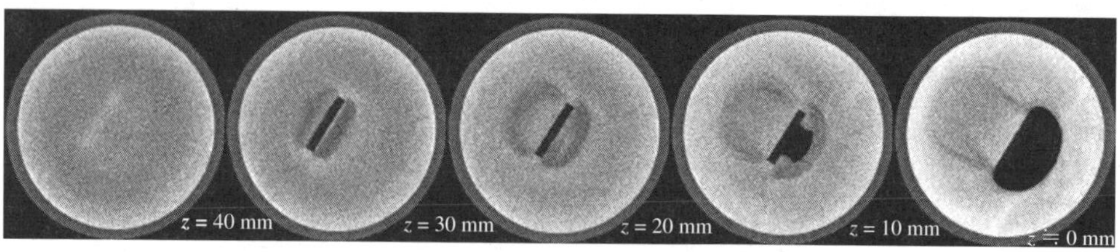

(c) Case 3 (Relative density: 30%, Rake angle: 60 deg., Traveling distance; 13.0 mm)

Figure 4. Cross sectional images of CT value.

packed ground (Case 2). The images obtained in this case are similar to those of Case 1, however, comparing them with Case 1, as can be seen in the images of z = 0 and 10 mm, angles of the direction of shear band from the excavation direction at the edge of the cutting bit seem to become wider than that of Case 1.

When the model ground is loose, as shown in Fig. 4(c), a distinct shear band is not so clear in comparison to the densely packed grounds. Ordinarily, it is expected that compression would occur in loose sand. However, we observed expansion which was represented by the regions slightly darker than the circumference in front of the cutting bit.

4.2 *3-D images*

Fig. 5 shows three dimensional (3-D) images which were obtained by reconstructing the X-ray CT cross sectional images. It should be noted that, in these images, the brightness of color tone, indicating the CT value, is expressed inversely against the cross sectional images mentioned above. Coloring was set under the condition of the same threshold CT value in all cases in order to make a relative comparison of the failure mechanism. The images, from left to right, were described as viewed from a horizontal and vertical direction as well as from two different slanting upper viewpoints. With the exception of one on the extreme right on each row, the cutting bits were moved leftward in all images.

Fig. 5(a) shows the result of Case 1. From these images, a three dimensional configuration of the failure mechanism was clarified when the ground is densely packed. The configuration of 3-D image reconstructed here is considered to be exceedingly helpful in assuming a failure mechanism on the limit equilibrium analysis, etc. for reasonable modeling of the soil cutting mechanism.

From Fig. 5(b), it can be observed that a region of whitish color, generated from the tip and the edges of the cutting bit, vanishes into the ground. Furthermore, the 3-D failure mechanism such as the one shown in Fig. 5(a) cannot be seen in this case. However, it can be seen in CT cross sectional images shown in Fig. 4(b) that shear bands were generated even at shallow domain of the ground although it was not so clear compared to Fig. 4(a), implying that the slip actually occurred but the density change with dilatancy (volume expansion) was relatively small on the slip surface.

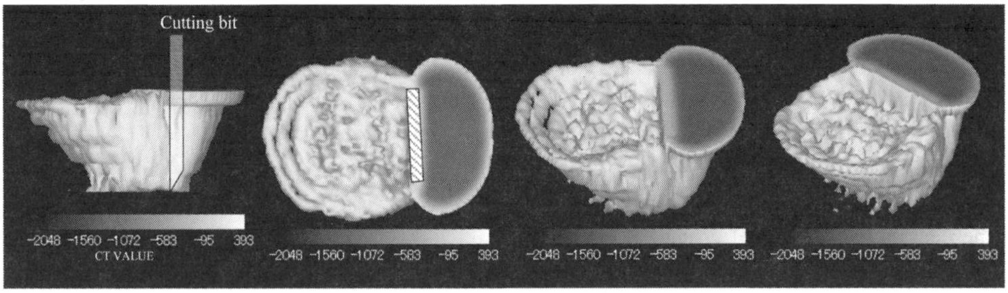

(a) Case 1 (Relative density: 80%, Rake angle: 90 deg., Traveling distance; 8.5 mm)

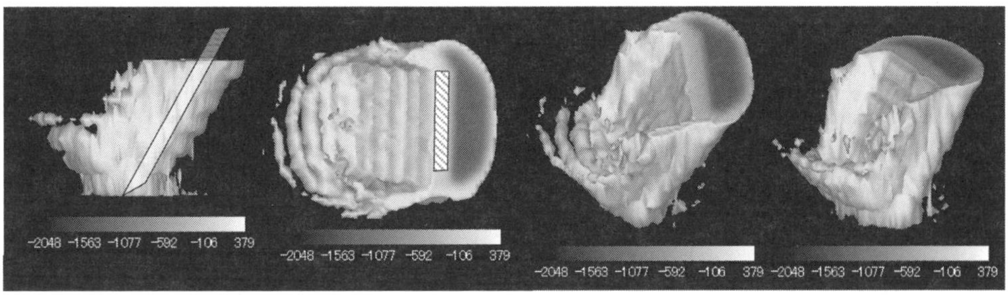

(b) Case 2 (Relative density: 80%, Rake angle: 60 deg., Traveling distance; 7.0 mm)

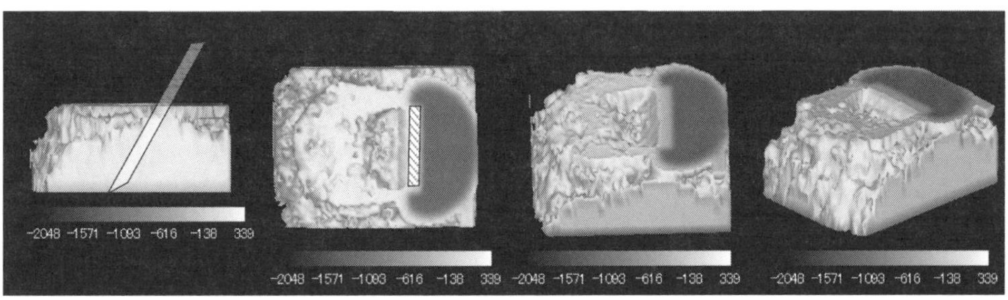

(c) Case 3 (Relative density: 30%, Rake angle: 90 deg., Traveling distance; 13.0 mm)

Figure 5. 3-D images.

Fig. 5(c) shows the result of a loosely packed model ground. In this figure, the initial state of the whole ground density was previously so low that it was not so easy to distinguish the regions where the density changes took place. However, as well as the CT cross sectional images shown in Fig. 4(c), it seems that compression in front of the cutting bit never occurred. But expansion, which was not expected to occur during soil cutting of loose sand, was observed with the exception for the region right in front of the cutting blade.

Owing to the 3-D image reconstructions under the condition of the same threshold CT value for all cases, the failure mechanism of Case 1 could be visualized clearly, whereas those of Case 2 and 3 were difficult to evaluate. In this paper, though examples of those 3-D images were presented as they were and only given a simple comparative and qualitative discussion, yet quantitative evaluation of the nature of what the CT value means is expected hereafter by further devises of image processing analysis including precise determination of the threshold CT value.

5 CONCLUSIONS

An X-ray CT scan technique was applied for the purpose of investigating the three dimensional soil cutting by a simple narrow cutting blade in sand. The conclusions drawn from this study are summarized as follows:

1) Using the X-ray CT scan technique, cross sectional images of the soil cutting mechanism could be

observed as shown in Fig. 4 without any destruction of the model ground.

2) When the ground is densely packed, the angle of the direction of shear band from the cutting direction at the edge of the cutting bit seems to become wider as the rake angle of the cutting blade decrease.
3) The 3-D image of failure mechanism could be well reconstructed in case with the rake angle of 90 deg. in the densely packed model ground as shown in Fig. 5. In this case, it seems that the inside of the failure surface deforms as a one clod of soil.

ACKNOWLEDGEMENT

The system of X-ray CT scanner used in this study is a property of the Department of Civil and Environmental Engineering, Kumamoto University, Japan. We would like to express our sincere gratitude to Mr. A. Ezoe, Mr. J. Sano and Mr. T. Kakita for their cooperation with this research.

REFERENCES

Kak, A. C. and Slaney, M. 1987, *Principles of Computed Tomographic Imaging*. IEEE Press.

Otani, J. Mukunoki, T. and Obara, Y. 2000, Application of X-ray CT method for characterization of failure in soils. *Soils and Foundations*, 40, No. 2: 111–118.

Otani, J. Mukunoki, T. and Kikuchi, Y. 2002, Visualization for engineering property of in-situ light weight soils with air foams. *Soils and Foundations*, 42, No. 3: 93–105.

X-ray CT for Geomaterials; Soils, Concrete, Rocks – Otani & Obara (eds.)

Visualization of 3-D failure patterns of ground due to lateral pile loadings

K.D. Pham & J. Sano
Graduate School of Science and Technology, Kumamoto University, Kumamoto, Japan

J. Otani
Department of Civil and Environmental Engineering, Kumamoto University, Kumamoto, Japan

A. Ezoe
Geo Engineering Division, Fudo Construction, Tokyo, Japan

ABSTRACT: The objective of this paper is to visualize 3-D failure patterns of ground due to lateral pile loadings using X-ray CT method. Here, an apparatus of model loading test has been developed and a series of model loading tests was conducted using this apparatus in the system of X-ray CT scanner. Then, CT scanning was done for model ground during the process of lateral loadings at the pile top. Not only cross sectional images for the ground but also 3-D images were reconstructed. Besides, proper methods of image processing analysis were used for this visualization. And the failure patterns of the ground under lateral pile loadings and lateral bearing capacity mechanism of pile foundation were visualized. Finally, quantitative discussion was done and the effectiveness of X-ray CT scanner was confirmed based on all the results in this study.

1 INTRODUCTION

Lateral bearing capacity of pile foundation is one of the most important factors for any kinds of structural design. In general, the ground failure due to lateral pile loading is complicated because the behavior of compression and that of stress relaxation around the pile shaft take place. As far as design method for lateral pile loading is concerned, there is a pioneer work by Broms (Broms et al. 1964 and Broms et al. 1972). This is the method to obtain ultimate lateral resistance of pile categorized by its bending stiffness, length of pile and ground stiffness after discussing the failure patterns of pile-soil interaction due to lateral loadings. However, it is considered that this method was developed with the purpose of conventional design calculation and it was not proposed based on the real failure patterns due to lateral pile loadings. As far as the future prospect of such pile foundation design is concerned, it is worthwhile to investigate more precise behavior of ground failure.

In the meantime, an X-ray CT scanner has become a useful tool even for geotechnical engineering as a non-destructive testing method. And authors have done some researches on the application study of this X-ray CT scanner in geotechnical engineering (Otani et al. 2000 and Otani et al. 2002). The results of CT scanning can be realized as the change of the density in the material and this apparatus produces visual images not only in cross section but also the ones in three dimension.

The purpose of this paper is to visualize three dimensional (3-D) failure patterns of the ground due to lateral pile loadings using industrial X-ray CT scanner and then, 3-D lateral bearing capacity mechanism of pile foundation is discussed based on the results of CT scanning. The data and discussion are based on an experiment, which is concerned on the application of lateral loadings at the top to a long vertical pile. After that, the soil box is scanned at several loading steps and a number of cross sectional images of the pile-soil behavior in each step are obtained. From those cross sectional images, 3-D images are reconstructed by using image processing analysis. Based on all the results, the change of material density is observed and 3-D lateral bearing capacity mechanism of pile foundation is visualized with its quantitative discussion.

2 PILE LOADING TEST AND RESULTS

2.1 *Material property*

The soil used in this test was Toyoura sand with properties shown in Table 1. The property of model pile is shown in Table 2.

2.2 *Test apparatus*

Figure 1 shows total testing apparatus for pile loading test with measurement equipments. Soil box was made by PVC with the size of 350 mm height and 125 mm inner diameter with 5 mm thickness. Model ground was made using multiple sieves (425 μm + 2 mm × 2) and the relative density was around 87.0 to 91.0%. Model pile was fixed at the bottom of the soil box and total length of the pile in the ground was 320 mm. The pile loading was applied at the top by dead load (weights) using a string with steel frame as seen in this figure. It is noted that this steel frame was taken out of this apparatus when the CT scanning was conducted because there should be no obstacles around the soil box where X-ray attenuates. And in order to obtain the distribution of bending moment, total number of 18 strain gauges was installed on the model pile as shown in Figure 1. All the measurements were operated using personal computer.

2.3 *Test procedure*

The pile loading test and CT scanning were conducted as a series of consecutive tests. Following is the process of this test:

1. The model ground was made in the steel frame;
2. The load was applied step by step until 88.3 N with 9.81 N step and strain on the pile was measured by the gauges;
3. CT scanning was conduced at the loading levels of initial, f = 29.4 N, f = 58.9 N and f = 88.3 N;
4. As shown in Figure 2, the area of CT scanning was the depth of 15 mm under the ground surface to the total depth of 70 mm and;
5. Total number of cross sections for scanning was 8 for every 10 mm thickness. Only for the case of loading step, f = 88.3 N, the total number of 70 slices was scanned with every 1 mm thickness in order to obtain the results of high accuracy of 3-D reconstruction images.

It is noted here that a special treatment for rebound of pile displacement during CT scanning was conducted using screws as shown in Figure 3. It is considered from this treatment that the stress condition in the ground during pile loading can be sustained without any disturbances.

Table 1. Soil property of Toyoura sand.

Maximum dry density (t/m^3)	1.64
Minimum dry density (t/m^3)	1.33
Specific gravity	2.64
Relative density (%)	87–91

Table 2. Property of model pile.

Length of pile (mm)	375
Length of pile in soil (mm)	320
Cross sectional dimension (mm)	30 × 3 (square)
Material	Aluminum

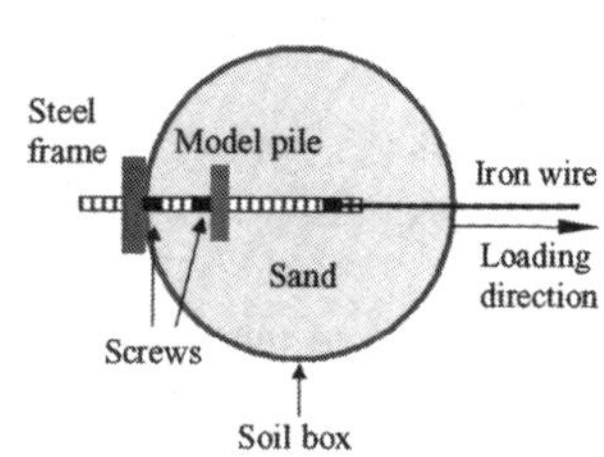

Figure 2. Fixing the pile top displacement and loading direction.

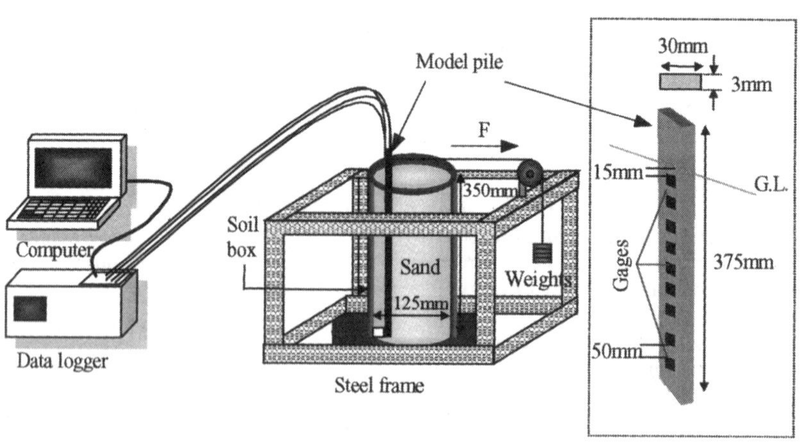

Figure 1. Testing apparatus.

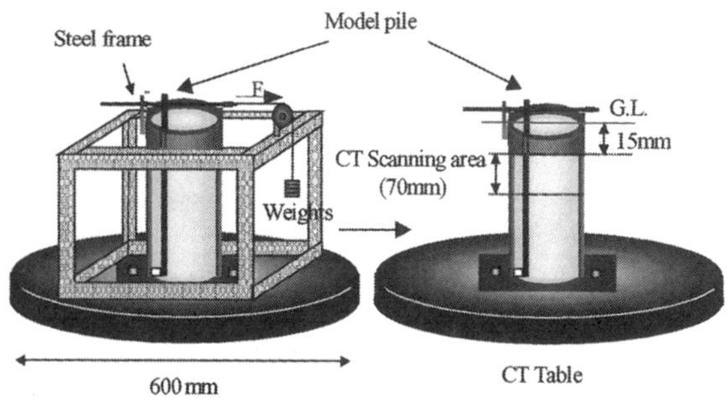

Figure 3. Procedures before scanning.

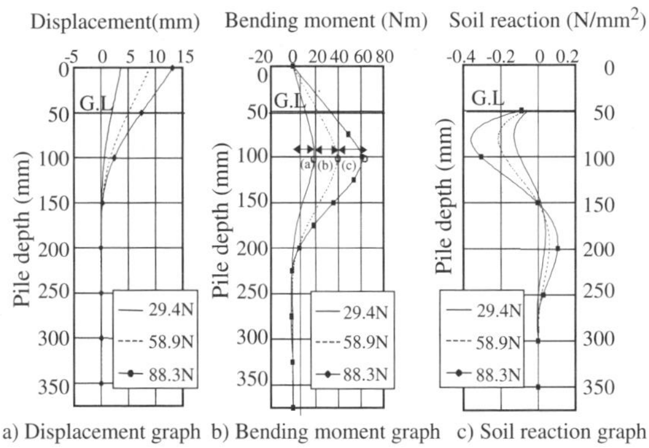

Figure 4. Displacement, bending moment and soil reaction versus pile depth curves.

2.4 *Results and discussion*

Figure 4 shows the results of strain gauges, which are the distributions of pile displacement and those of moment and soil reaction. Those were calculated by the distribution of strain along the pile. In the figure of moment distributions, (a), (b) and (c) show the increment values of the moment among two adjacent loading steps and it is realized that these values are slightly increased with increasing pile loading. It is convinced that the results of pile loading test here in this study show the same tendency as the one for previous researches on pile loading test. Therefore, it may be said that the behavior in this test should be reliable.

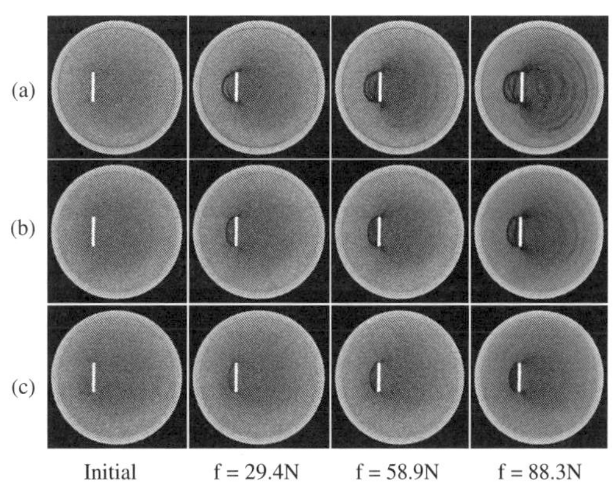

Figure 5. Cross sectional images.

3 CT SCANNING

3.1 *CT image*

Figure 5 shows cross sectional images for several loading steps (initial, f = 29.4 N, f = 58.9 N and f = 88.3 N) with three different heights of the pile. These depths were (a) 15 mm, (b) 35 mm, and (c) 55 mm from the ground surface, respectively. It can be realized that the area of strain localization, which shows the area of black color in the image, appears towards the direction of applied loading and these are extended as the pile loading is increased. It is also observed that the size of this localization becomes smaller as the depth of the ground increases. Figure 6 shows the relationship between the ground displacement at the surface by the calculation from strain gauges and that of CT scanning. As easily realized, both values

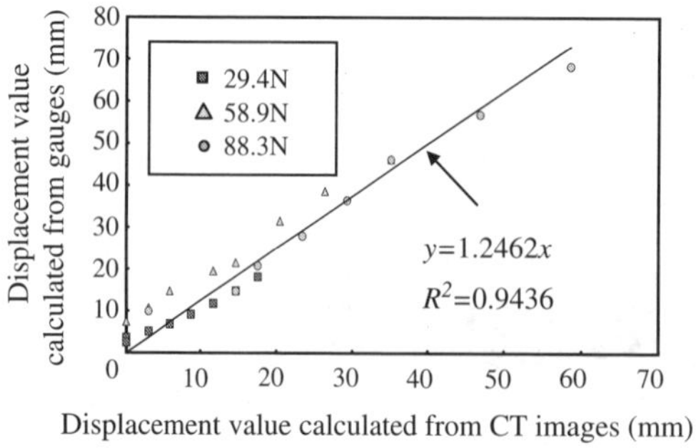

Figure 6. Comparison between ground displacement values calculated from CT images and gauges.

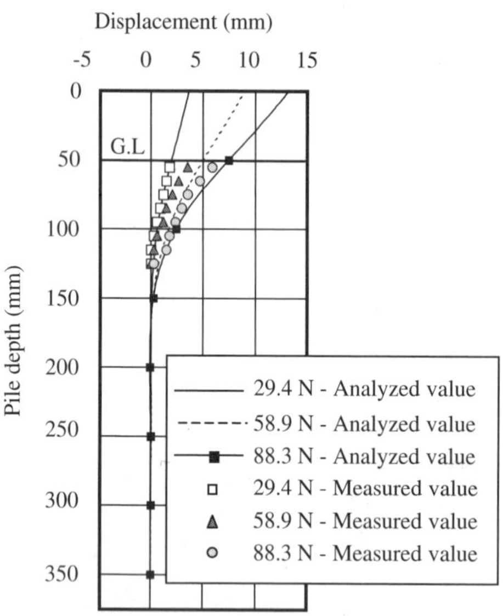

Figure 7. Comparison between ground displacement values calculated from CT images and gauges along pile depth.

are fairy close under statistical consideration. Figure 7 shows these comparisons on the distributions along the pile shaft. These results convince that the results from CT scanning can be used in the quantitative discussion.

3.2 *Visualization of failure patterns*

Figure 8 shows 3-D reconstruction images through soil box including pile at the area from 15 mm to 70 mm from the ground surface for the case of f = 88.3 N. There are two images which are two different directions and a smoothing technique was used for these images. Here, the relative low density area or strain localization in the ground is presented by the difference of darkness in the image. It is considered that this strain localization is the area of failure surface.

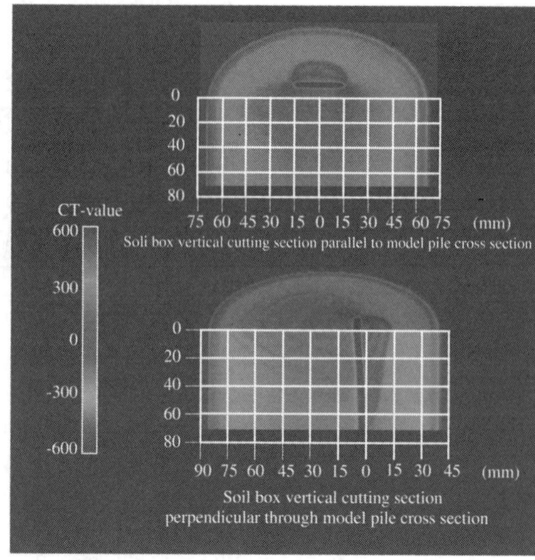

Figure 8. 3-D reconstructed images for 88.3 N loading condition.

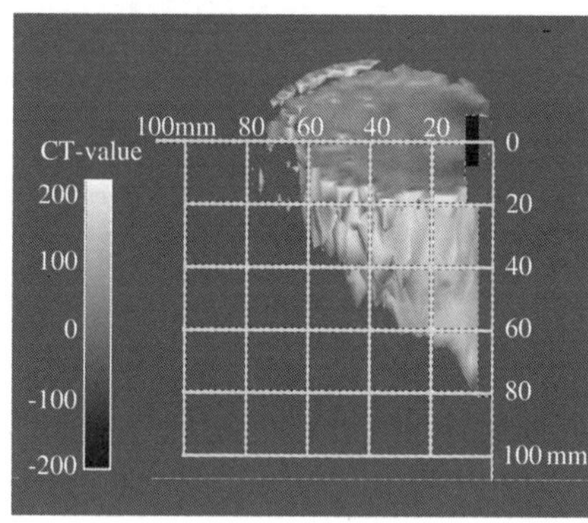

Figure 9. 3-D extraction image of soil failure pattern.

As seen in the figure, there is a large number of this area. It reaches the edge of soil box according to applied loading direction. The size of this area tends to decrease along the pile depth. It can be said that this localization area is the area of soil resistance against lateral pile loading and can be used for the calculation of lateral bearing capacity using limit analysis. Figure 9 shows a 3-D extraction image which the relatively low density area is extracted from original CT image. As easily realized from this figure, the failure zone due to lateral pile loading can be obtained in three dimension and the shape of this failure zone is that of cone.

3.2 *Quantitative discussion*

Although the soil failure pattern was visualized and characterized based on CT images in both 2-D and 3-D,

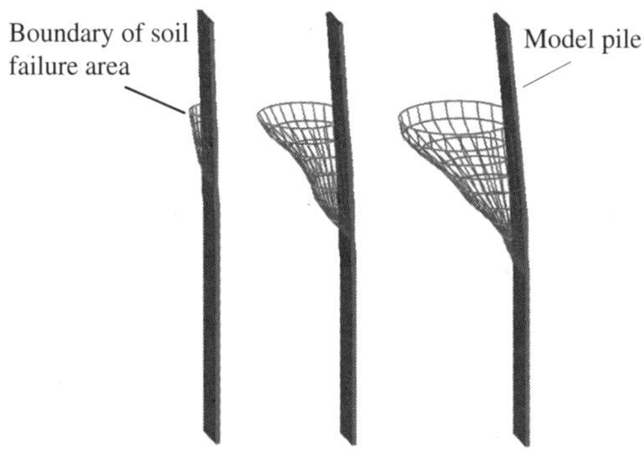

Figure 10. 3-D images of soil failure mechanism.

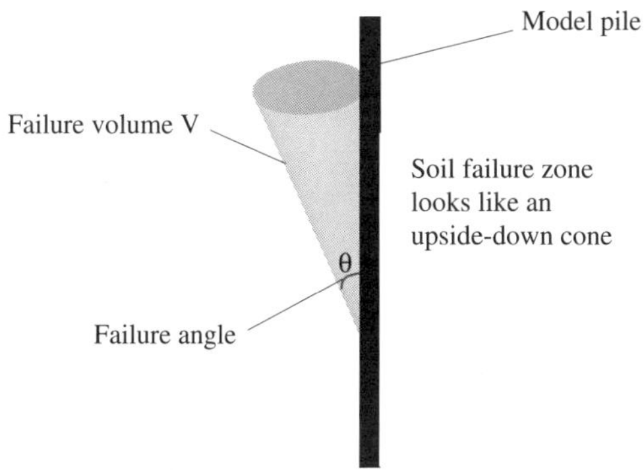

Figure 11. Assumption of typical 3-D shape of soil failure zone.

more quantitative discussion is indispensable. Figure 10 shows the total failure zone at three different loading steps (f = 29.4 N, f = 58.9 N and f = 88.3 N). It is noted that these images included the displacement of pile. Here, the thinning technique which is one of the technique in image processing analysis was used for obtaining failure zone with the assumption of ellipse shape in each cross section. It is realized that when the lateral loading is increased, this failure zone is enlarged. And it is interesting to note that the angle of this failure zone becomes larger as the increase of pile loading.

In order to discuss more details of this progress, the changes of volume and angle of failure zone, which is shown in Figure 11, were calculated with the increase of pile loading. Figure 12 shows the change of the failure angle against the increase of pile loading while Figure 13 shows the same change for the volume of failure zone. It is easy to realize from these results that both values are increased as the increase of pile loading but the increment of this change becomes smaller at some large loading steps. This means that there are some

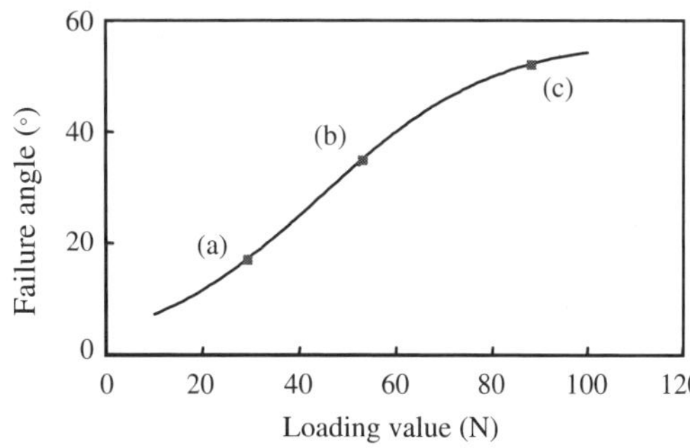

Figure 12. Failure angle versus loading value curve.

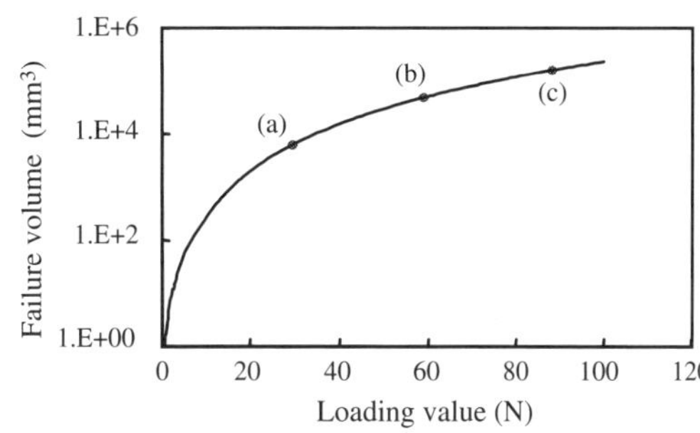

Figure 13. Failure volume versus loading value curve.

ultimate values for this angle and volume. Therefore, it may be concluded that there is an ultimate failure stage for lateral bearing capacity of pile foundation.

4 CONCLUSIONS

Failure patterns of ground due to lateral pile loading were precisely observed using X-ray CT scanner. And not only visualization of the failure patterns but also its quantitative discussion were performed without any destruction in three dimension. The conclusions drawn from this study are shown as follows:

1. The failure patterns for the ground due to lateral pile loading are well visualized using X-ray CT scanner.
2. The failure of the ground due to lateral pile loading is the type of progressive one and the failure zone is extended as the increase of pile loading.
3. The size of failure zone is decreased as the increase of ground depth along the pile and the shape of this failure zone is that of cone in three dimension.
4. The volume and angle of failure zone against lateral pile loading are increased as the increase of pile loading but there exist ultimate values at some loading stages.

Finally, it is the first time that the failure patterns of the ground due to lateral pile loading were obtained in three dimension without any destruction using industrial X-ray CT scanner. In this sense, it is confirmed that this special apparatus could be a power tool even in the field of geotechnical engineering.

REFERENCES

Broms, B.B. 1964. Lateral Resistance of Piles in Cohesionless Soils, *Proc. ASCE* 90, SM, 3: 27–63.

Broms, B.B. 1972. Stability of Flexible Structures (Pile and pile Groups), *Proc. of 5th European Conf. S.M.F.E.*, 2: 239–269.

Otani, J., Mukunoki, T. and Obara, Y. 2000. Application of X-ray CT method for characterization of failure in soils, *Soils and Foundations*, 40(2): 111–118.

Otani, J., Mukunoki, T. and Kikuchi, Y. 2002. Visualization for engineering property of in-situ light weight soils with air foams, *Soils and Foundations*, 42(3): 93–105.

X-ray CT for Geomaterials; Soils, Concrete, Rocks – Otani & Obara (eds.)
© 2004 Swets & Zeitlinger. Lisse, ISBN 90 5809 666 1

Visualization of the mechanism of tunnel face failure

H. Nagatani
Geotechnical Engineering Group, Kajima Technical Research Institute, Tokyo, Japan

J. Otani & D. Takano
Department of Civil and Environmental Engineering, Kumamoto University, Kumamoto, Japan

ABSTRACT: A number of experimental studies have been done regarding the mechanism of tunnel face failure. Most of the studies are based on the observation of failure mechanisms using experimental models of two- or three-dimensional planes, and the three-dimensional behavior of face failure is not well studied yet. The authors have investigated the failure zone behind a face quantitatively by using X-ray computed tomography (CT) to visualize face failure on a three-dimensional basis through a tunnel pull-out model test. As a result, failure zone development at the time of face failure could be described elaborately. The quantitative findings include that arching effect occurs when the overburden ratio is 2D (two time the outer diameter of the pull-out core) or more and that the volume of the failure zone behind the face is independent of the overburden ratio.

1 INTRODUCTION

In the mountain tunneling and shield tunneling methods, tunnel faces become very unstable due to stress release caused by excavation. When a face loses its stress balance, a slip surface occurs in the ground behind the face, leading to a local failure or a large-scale failure that extends up to the ground surface as shown in Figure 1. Some information is needed to evaluate the stability of the face: the failure strength corresponding to the weight of the entire slide mass at the critical state of failure, resistance on the face, and shear resistance on the slip surface. In a typical design approach, face stability is evaluated based on the slip surface behind the face, which may be estimated by a logarithmic spiral, and a loosening zone caused by arching effect above the slip surface. This approach evaluates the failure zone two-dimensionally, which is actually three-dimensional in shape. Because of the three-dimensional nature of shear resistance on the slip surface, the conventional approach may lead to overestimation of the failure strength of the face.

In this study, a face failure is simulated by pulling out a tunnel model set in a model ground. The ground is then investigated by X-ray computed tomography (CT) to visualize the failure zone on a three-dimensional basis and elucidate the mechanism of face failure. Also, the effect of overburden and pull-out length on the failure zone is evaluated quantitatively.

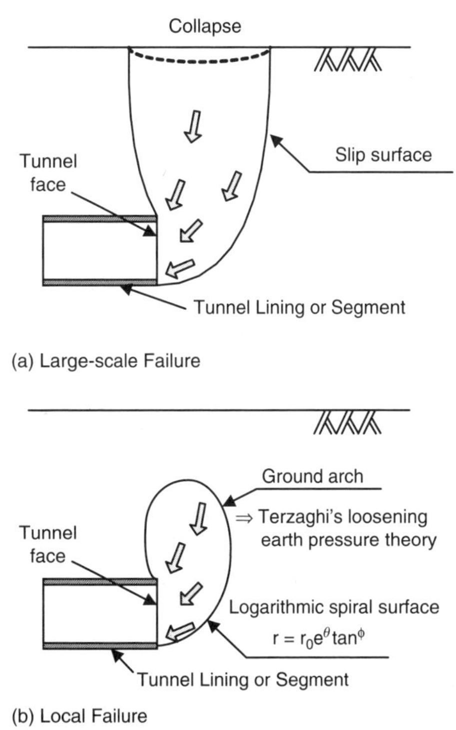

Figure 1. Tunnel face failure.

2 OUTLINE OF TEST

2.1 *Test setup*

The setup of the tunnel pull-out model test using X-ray CT is shown in Figure 2. The cylindrical soil tank has an outer diameter of 150 mm and an inner diameter of 125 mm. The ground model can be as high as 200 mm. The tunnel model consists of a pipe, which has an outer diameter of 20 mm, and a pull-out core, which has an outer diameter of 13 mm. The center of the tunnel model is set at a height of 100 mm from the bottom of the cylindrical soil tank, with the tunnel model extruding 20 mm from the tank side. By sealing the top of the soil tank and placing a water bag on the ground surface, a surcharge by air pressure can be provided.

2.2 *Test method*

The test procedure is shown in Figure 3. Dry Toyoura sand was used as the ground model material, and a relative density of 85% was achieved by the free-fall method using multiple sieves. After preparing the soil, the cylindrical soil tank was set for the tunnel pull-out model test system and the core part was pulled out. The tank was then removed and set on a turntable in an X-ray CT booth for investigation. CT images were taken at a 1-mm pitch from the tunnel bottom. The detected data are assembled and the cross sectional images are reconstructed using an image data processing device by means of the filtered back-projection method. By using all these cross sectional images around the circumference of the specimen, three-dimensional image can be also reconstructed.

2.3 *Test conditions*

The cases and the conditions of the test are shown in Table 1. With the outer diameter of the pull-out core (13 mm) being 1D, the conditions of the basic case are an overburden ratio of 4D, a pull-out length of 1 mm, and a pull-out rate of 0.1 mm/sec. Four different cases, including a pull-out length of 10 mm and overburdens of 1D, 2D, and 4D, were investigated.

3 TEST RESULTS

3.1 *Visualization of the mechanism of face failure*

When confirming face stability by a tunnel pull-out model test, a typical practice is to simulate the critical state of face failure by pulling out the tunnel by 10% of the face height. In the present test, therefore, the core part was pulled out by 1 mm to loosen the face and evaluate the critical state of failure. Overburden was set to 4D so that sufficient arching effect would occur in the soil at the time of face failure. Cross-sectional CT images are shown in Figure 4. The vertical-section image indicates that a slightly arced slip line is developed behind the face and a failure zone (loosening zone) caused by arching effect, which is typically

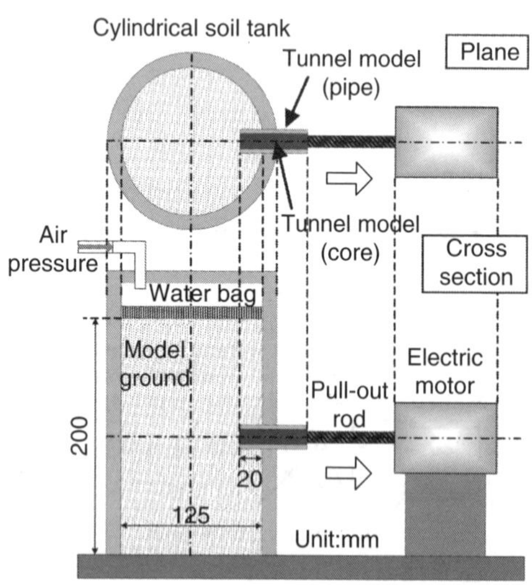

Figure 2. Tunnel pull-out model test system.

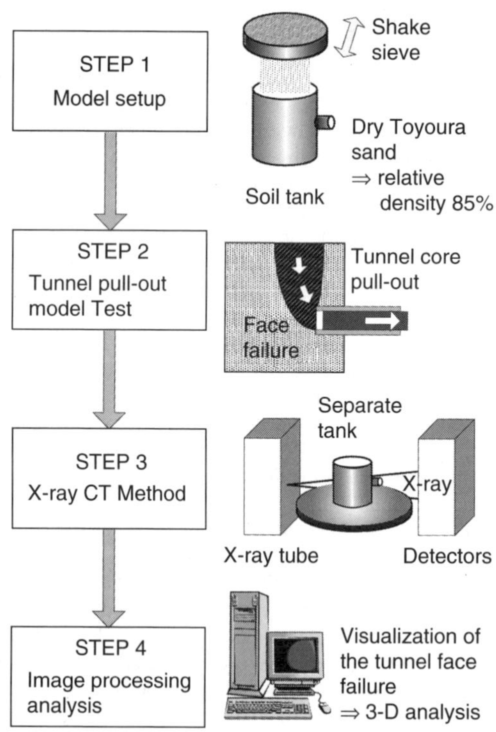

Figure 3. Experimental procedure.

observed in trap door tests, is present above the level of tunnel roof. The horizontal-section images indicate that the semicircular slip line that extends behind the face becomes elliptic above the level of tunnel crown and gets smaller upward. This corresponds to the failure zone described in Figure 1, indicating that this zone is well recognized three-dimensionally in the present study. Figure 5 shows the failure zone extracted from the sectional CT images and processed three-dimensionally. The figure depicts how the failure zone extends from the face.

The mechanism of large-scale face failure is discussed next. A large-scale failure in the tunnel was modeled by increasing the pull-out length to 10 mm with an overburden ratio of 4D. Cross-sectional CT images are shown in Figure 6, and a three-dimensional image of the failure zone is given in Figure 7. As seen from the vertical-section and three-dimensional images, the failure zone extends nearly up to the ground surface and is closed near the surface because of the arching effect. The horizontal-section images indicate that the failure zone near the tunnel crown is elliptic as

Table 1. Test cases.

Test case	Overburden ratio	Overburden length (mm)	Pull-out length (mm)	Pull-out ratio (mm/sec)	Remark
①	4D	52	1	0.1	Critical state model
②	4D	52	10	0.1	Large-scale failure model
③	2D	26	1	0.1	Critical state model (Effect of overburden)
④	1D	13	1	0.1	

* 1D: Tunnel core outer diameter 13 mm

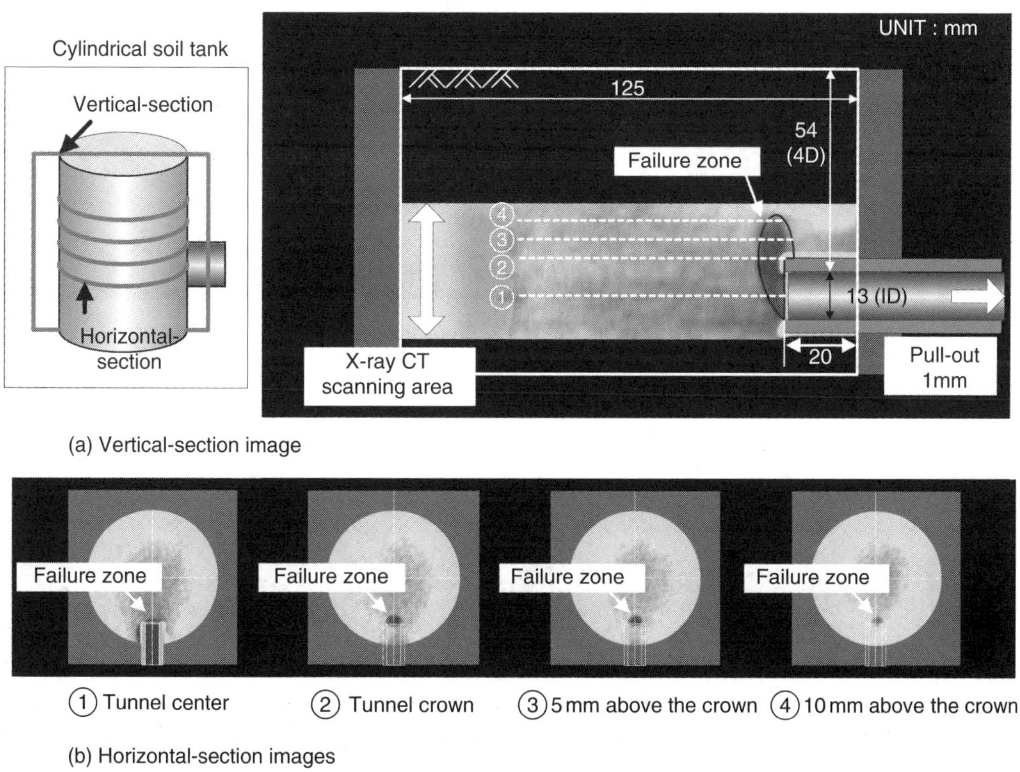

Figure 4. Cross sectional images (CASE1: Critical state model).

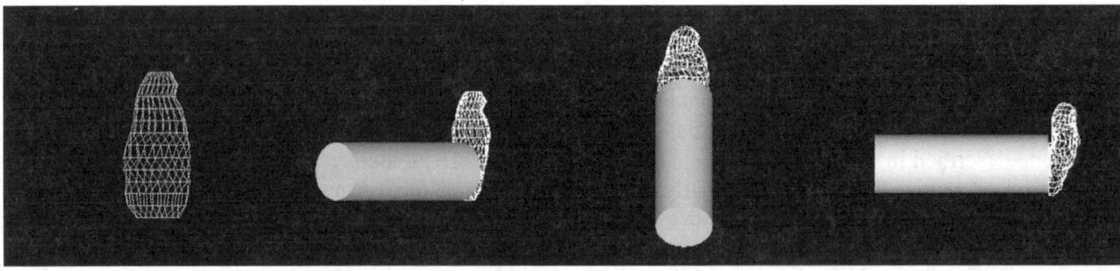

Figure 5. Three-dimensional wire-frame images (CASE1: Critical state model).

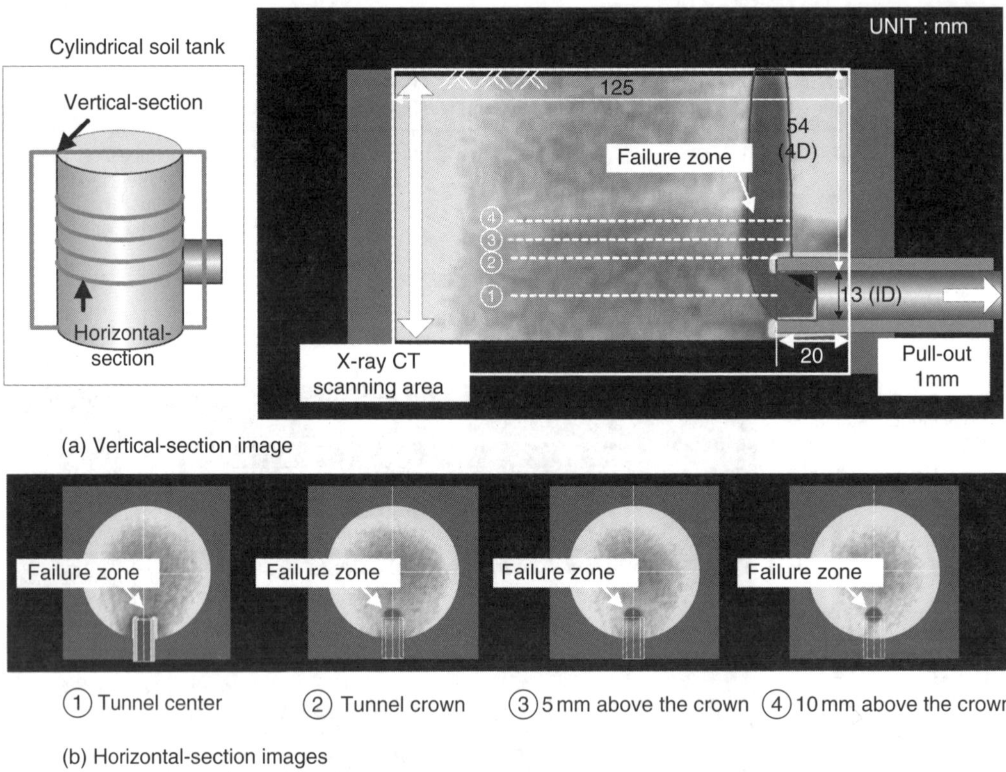

Figure 6. Cross sectional images (CASE2: Large-scale failure model).

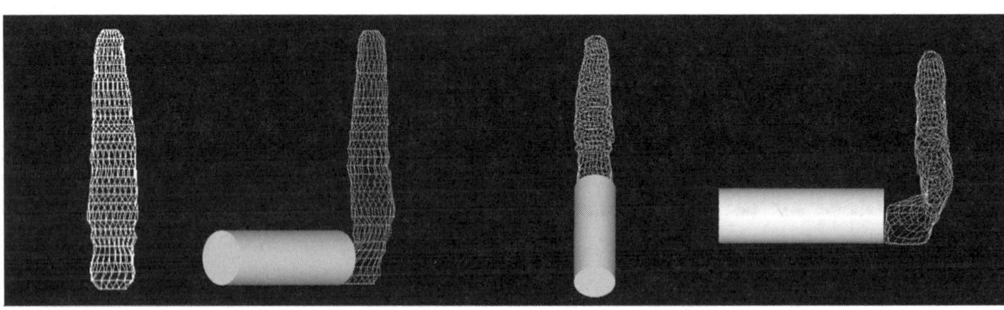

Figure 7. Three-dimensional wire-frame images (CASE2: Large-scale failure model).

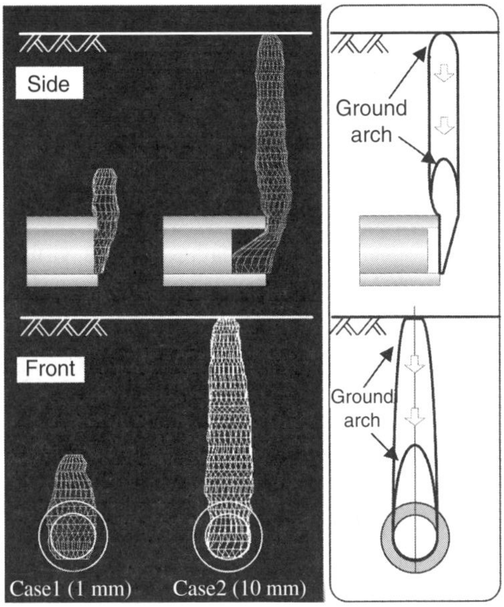

Figure 8. Comparison between CASE1 and CASE2.

is the case with the critical-state model with a pull-out length of 1 mm and that the zone extends upward while maintaining the elliptic shape.

Based on the above test results, the slip surface behind the face and the failure zone extending upward are compared for the critical state and the large-scale failure in Figure 8, which shows three-dimensional wire-frame images. The slip surface generated behind the face does not change much between the critical state and the large-scale failure. The failure zone, on the other hand, extends straightly upward from the critical state to the large-scale failure.

3.2 *Effect of overburden on arching*

As shown by the X-ray CT images, a failure zone (loosening zone) is generated by arching effect when there is a sufficient overburden at the time of face failure. Although depending on soil conditions, it is generally said that arching occurs when overburden exceeds 1D or 2D. The effect of overburden on arching is discussed by comparing the failure zones corresponding to the overburden ratios of 1D, 2D, and 4D. The three-dimensional wire-frame images are shown in Figures 9.

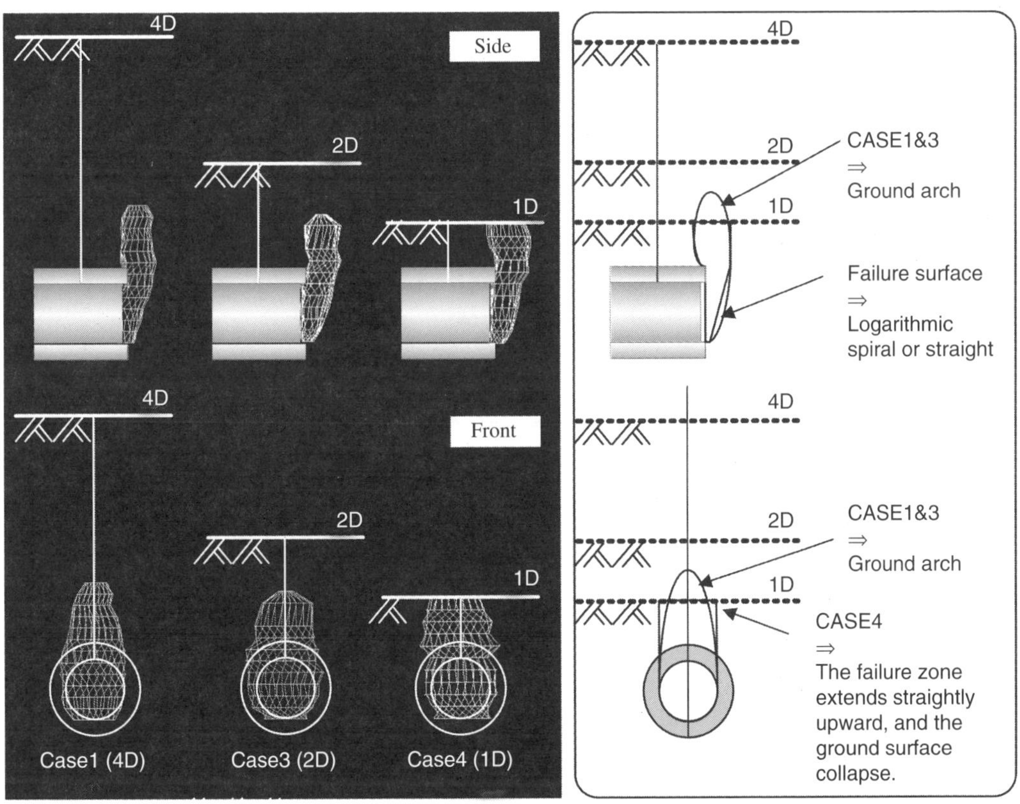

Figure 9. Comparison between CASE1, CASE3 and CASE4.

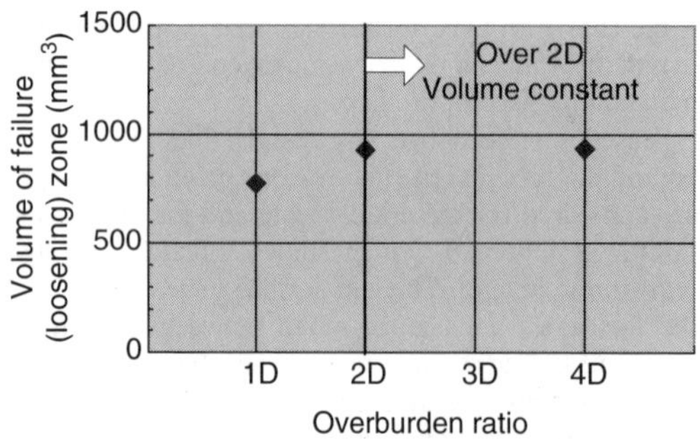

Figure 10. Volume of failure (loosening) zone.

In the side view images, arching is not observed in the case of 1D because the failure zone extends straightly upward to the ground surface, but the failure zone is closed in the cases of 2D and 4D because of the arching effect. This suggests that arching effect occurs at an overburden ratio of 2D or more. In this case, the slip surface generated behind the face is not affected by overburden, and the shape and the volume of the failure zone do not depend much on overburden.

From the above results, the volume of failure zone behind the face was calculated for each overburden ratio, as plotted in Figure 10. The volumes are nearly the same in 2D and 4D, but smaller in 1D because the failure zone did not reaches the ground surface. In the present test, an overburden ratio of 2D or more is sufficient to cause arching, and the shape of failure zone is not affected by overburden. It should be noted, however, that dry sand without viscosity was used in the model ground. A similar test using a cohesive soil material is therefore required to make a general discussion.

4 CONCLUSIONS

The mechanism of face failure was visually investigated on a three-dimensional basis in this study through a tunnel pull-out model test using X-ray CT. Also, the volume of failure zone associated with face failure was evaluated quantitatively. The findings are summarized as follows:

- The mechanism of face failure can be visually investigated three-dimensionally by the test method used in this study.
- A semicircular slip surface is generated behind the face, and the failure zone extends straightly upward with an elliptic sectional shape above the tunnel.
- Arching effect occurs at an overburden ratio of 2D or more. The shape and the volume of the failure zone do not depend much on overburden.
- When a large-scale failure is caused by a pull-out length of 10 mm, a failure zone develops along a slip surface similar to that observed in the critical state.

The authors intend to further study the mechanism of face failure on a three-dimensional basis, with such attempts as load measurements on a face, application of surcharge on a ground model, and use of cohesive soil as a soil material.

REFERENCES

Otani, J., Hironaka, J. and Mukunoki, T. 2003. Visualization of Failure Patterns under Vertically Loaded Pile Foundation Using X-ray CT Method, 12th ASIAN Regional Conference on soil mechanics and Geotechnical Engineering.

Concrete and related materials

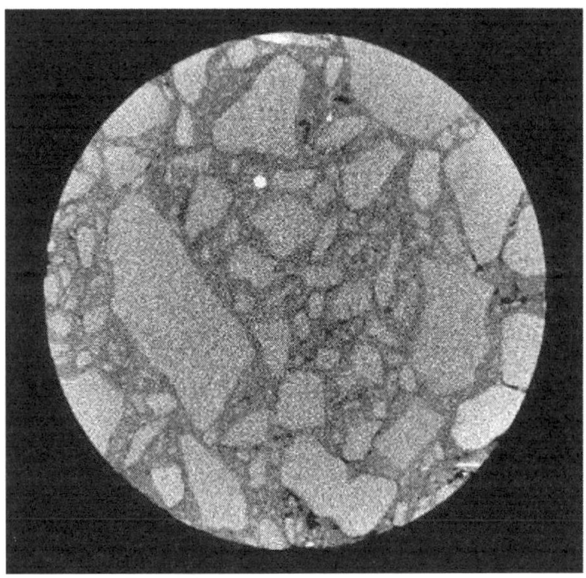

X-ray CT for Geomaterials; Soils, Concrete, Rocks – Otani & Obara (eds.)

A consideration on the durability of fiber-cement-stabilized mud produced from construction sludge

H. Takahashi, F. Maruhashi & Y. Suto
Graduate School of Environmental Studies, Tohoku University, Sendai, Japan

M. Mori
MORI Institute for Environmental Technology Co.,Ltd., Shinjo, Japan

K. Kumakura
Yachiyo Engineering Co.,Ltd., Tokyo, Japan

M. Ohtani
Tokyo Soil Research Co.,Ltd., Tokyo, Japan

T. Ishii
Mogami Area General Branch Administration, Shinjo, Japan

ABSTRACT: In this study, the durability of the fiber-cement-stabilized mud produced from construction sludge was investigated. In order to use the modified soils as lightweight landfill materials, the durability is very important. Therefore, repeated cycle tests of drying and wetting were carried out. It was found that the durability of fiber-cement-stabilized mud is higher than that of cement-stabilized mud. It is often said that the durability depends on the generation of the crack in the drying process. In order to investigate the relationship between generation of the crack and the ability to hold the water in the mud, the inside of the mud was visualized by using X-ray CT equipment. However, a clear difference was not observed in both fiber-cement-stabilized mud and cement-stabilized mud. From this result, it can be considered that the ability to hold the water in the mud is not related to the durability and the fiber in the mud restrains the generation of the crack.

1 INTRODUCTION

Construction sludge is the typical high water-content mud and is produced more than 10 million ton per year from the construction sites in Japan. However, the recycling rate of the construction sludge is extremely low. Therefore, we have already developed a new recycling system of high water-content mud by using the paper debris and polymer (Bon Terrain Method) in order to increase the recycling rate of the construction sludge (Mori et al., 2003, Takahashi et al., 2003). By using this system, 200–500% water content mud has been modified to the landfill materials by approximately 20 minutes mixing process. The modified soils have several features and one of the features of the modified soils is lightweight. The fields where lightweight landfill materials are effectively applied will be as follows:

1) *The large scale reclaimed works*
   Generally, a large amount of soils are used in the reclaimed works. In result, the ground sinkage easily occurs because of the consolidation by the heavy soils. Therefore, utilization of lightweight landfill materials is tried in the upper layer of reclaimed land to decrease the rate of ground sinkage. However, it costs much to make lightweight landfill materials. If the lightweight landfill materials are produced inexpensively from the construction sludge, cost saving will be significant and recycling rate of the construction sludge will increase largely.
2) *A tree-planting on rooftop to prevent heat island*
   It is often said that a tree-planting on the rooftop is useful to prevent heat island. In order to plant the

rooftop with small trees, the soils have to be carried from the ground to the rooftop. In this case, if the soils are light, the construction will be easy. And easy construction means that large cost saving is possible.

3) *Measures works for landslides*
There are many hazardous areas of landslides in Japan. If the heavy soils in the hazardous areas of landslides are replaced by the lightweight landfill materials, the possibility of landslides will be extremely reduced.

In order to use the modified soils as landfill materials, it is very important to know the durability of the modified soils. However, the characteristics of the durability of modified soils produced by BonTerrain method is not made clear yet.

Therefore, the objective of this study is to investigate the durability of modified soils through repeated cycle tests of drying and wetting, and to examine the mechanism of failure by X-ray CT equipment.

2 REPEATED CYCLE TESTS OF DRYING AND WETTING

High-water content mud, such as construction sludge, is in the state which soil particles are distributing in the water. Therefore, by carrying out solidification processing with cement, they can be recycled as landfill materials, and some processing methods have been already proposed. The modified soils produced by the conventional methods are generally called the cement-stabilized mud. However, usually the failure strain of the cement-stabilized mud in the unconfined compression test is much smaller that that of the ordinary soils. This means that quality improvement is not enough for the cement-stabilized mud. In result, the cement-stabilized mud has plentifully the cases of not being suitable for the use as landfill material. For example, Mr. Murata (2002) reported that the adhesion strength of the cement-stabilized mud is extremely small, and they are easily broken at very small stain if the external force acts on the cement-stabilized mud. That is, although the conventional methods are comparatively easy to process, the cement-stabilized mud shows strength properties like concretes or rocks. Therefore, a rigid difference arises between the circumference foundation and new landfill materials by using the cement-stabilized mud. Consequently, in case of an earthquake, the generation of a crack or excessive earth pressure will be a big problem. As mentioned above, in order to produce the high quality modified mud, we have already developed a new recycling method of high-water content mud by using paper debris and polymer. The modified soils produced by this new method are called fiber-cement-stabilized mud. In this method, as paper debris absorb the great portion of water, it is not necessary to add a lot of cement to the high-water content mud. Furthermore, since the new method uses only a few amounts of polymer to produce the fiber-cement-stabilized mud, it leads to sharp reduction of processing costs. Moreover, since the fiber is included inside the modified mud, the strength of stickness of the fiber-cement-stabilized mud is much larger than that of the cement-stabilized mud (Mori et al., 2003).

By the way, in order to reuse the modified soils as landfill materials, it is very important to know the durability of the modified soils. Repeated cycle tests of drying and wetting have been already conducted for the cement-stabilized mud, and the durability of the cement-stabilized mud was already investigated (Ogawa et al., 1996). According to the previous works, it was found that the crack produced in the cement-stabilized mud in the contraction process reached the deep inside, and a massive collapse was observed with increasing the cycle numbers of the tests. Furthermore, it is also reported that the unconfined compressive strength of the cement-stabilized mud decreased with increasing the cycle numbers of the tests. Therefore, the previous researches suggested that in the actual construction works, the cement-stabilized mud have to be covered by the ordinary soils so that the cement-stabilized mud may not be exposed in the circumstance. On the other hand, the durability of the fiber-cement-stabilized mud is not made clear as yet. Therefore, in order to examine the durability of the fiber-cement-stabilized mud, repeated cycle tests of drying and wetting were carried out based on the conventional test method.

Figure 1 shows the flowchart of making specimen of the fiber-cement-stabilized mud. Silt and clay were mixed by the weight ratio of 40:60, and the imitation mud was made by adding the water. The amount of water was adjusted so that the water content ratio becomes 105% and 150%. In creation of the cement-stabilized mud, desired cement was mixed to this imitation mud, and then the specimens were made by using the cement-stabilized mud and the standard mold of 50 mm diameter × 100 mm height, and they were cured for 28 days. In creation of the fiber-cement-stabilized mud, paper debris, polymer and chemical flocculants were mixed with the imitation mud. The addition rate of paper debris, polymer and chemical flocculants were 65 kg/m^3, 1.2 kg/m^3 and 8.6 kg/m^3, respectively. The next, the cement was mixed. The addition rate of cement was the same as the cement-stabilized mud. Then, the specimens were made by using the fiber-cement-stabilized mud and the standard mold of 50 mm diameter × 100 mm height, and they were cured for 28 days. After the specimens were made, repeated cycle tests of drying and wetting were carried out. In this experiment, 1 cycle consists of submersion for one day at 20 degrees and drying for two days at 40 degrees. The observation of the surface of the specimens was conducted after each cycle is over, and the unconfined compression test was performed after the 2nd, 6th and 10th cycle is over in order to measure the unconfined compressive strength of the specimens.

Figure 2 sows the relationship between the cycle number and the unconfined compressive strength in the repeated cycle tests of drying and wetting. As for the cement-stabilized mud, it was possible to carry out the unconfined compression test and to measure the strength until the 2nd cycle. However, the deterioration was significant and it was impossible to continue the unconfined compression test after the 2nd cycle because all specimens were broken by the terrible deterioration. This result shows the same tendency as the one reported by the previous researchers. On the other hand, the unconfined compressive strength of the fiber-cement-stabilized mud showed approximately the constant value irrespective of the increase in the cycle number. The value of the unconfined compressive strength of the fiber-cement-stabilized mud after the 10th cycle was almost the same as the initial unconfined compressive strength, and the deterioration was not observed. We have already confirmed that the ability of the water holding of the fiber-cement-stabilized mud is much better than that of other soils (Mori et al., 2001). That is, it is considered that the fiber-cement-stabilized mud holds much water inside, consequently a contraction crack cannot be generated easily. Therefore, we tried to observe the inside of the specimens after drying process and submersion process by using X-ray CT equipment.

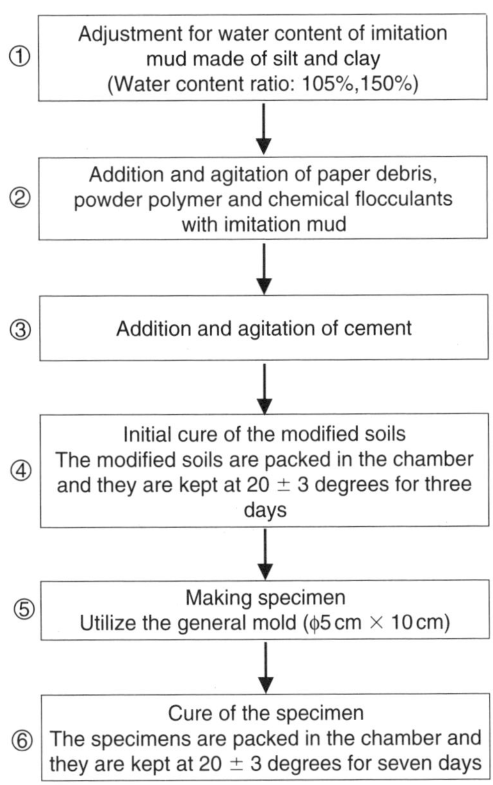

Figure 1. Flowchart of making specimen of fiber-cement stabilized mud.

3 OBSERVATION OF INSIDE THE MODIFIED SOILS BY X-RAY CT EQUIPMENT

Observation was carried out by using the X-ray CT equipment installed in Kumamoto University. Figure 3 shows the outline of the System. The X-ray bulb, 300 kV/2 mA, and the detectors of 176 in number are fixed in a horizontal plane, and they can be moved

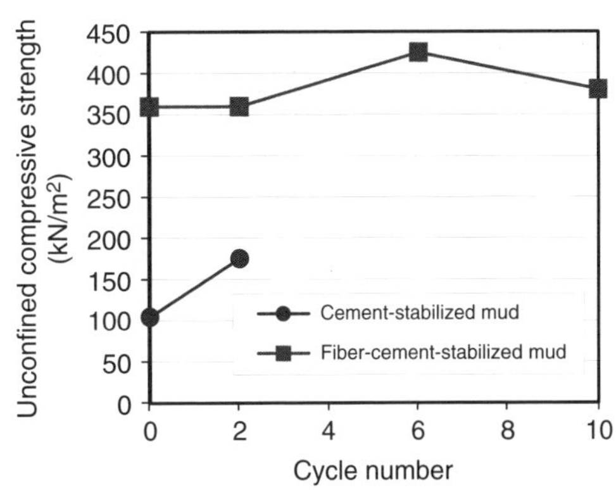

Figure 2. Relationship between the cycle number and unconfined compressive strength in the repeated cycle tests of drying and wetting.

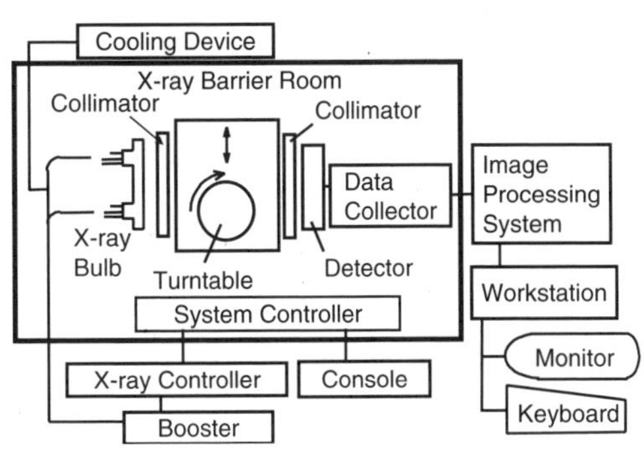

Figure 3. Outline of X-ray CT equipment.

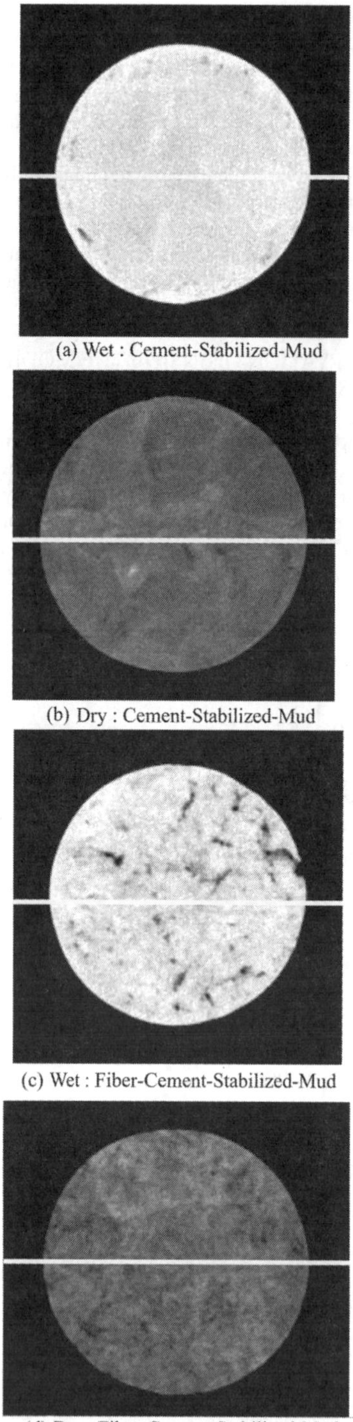

(a) Wet : Cement-Stabilized-Mud

(b) Dry : Cement-Stabilized-Mud

(c) Wet : Fiber-Cement-Stabilized-Mud

(d) Dry : Fiber-Cement-Stabilized-Mud

Figure 4. Images of cross section of the specimen measured by X-ray CT equipment.

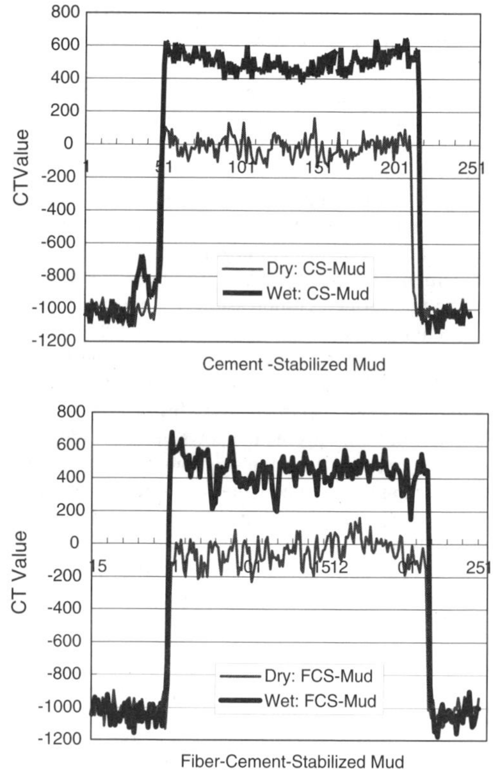

Figure 5. Profiles of CT values along the straight line in Figure 4.

together in the vertical direction, with a specified interval. The specimens are set on the turn table for traversing and rotation, of which the axis is vertical. By the detectors, a few attenuation profiles is recorded for each incidence.

Figure 4 shows the image of cross section of the specimen, which was measured by the X-ray CT equipment. Figures 4(a), (b), (c) and (d) show the images of the cement-stabilized mud and the fiber- cement-stabilized mud, respectively. In the image taken by X-ray CT equipment, a portion with high density becomes white and a portion with low density becomes black. Therefore, Figures (a) and (c) show the images after the submersion process, and Figure (b) and (d) show the images after drying process. A clear difference is not observed in these two images.

Figure 5 shows the profile of CT values along the straight line in Figure 4. The differences of CT values of drying and submersion for the cement-stabilized mud and fiber-cement-stabilized mud are 514 and 503, respectively, and both values are almost the same. Therefore, it is inferred that both mud takes the water inside in the submersion process and they are dried perfectly in the drying process. That is, it is considered

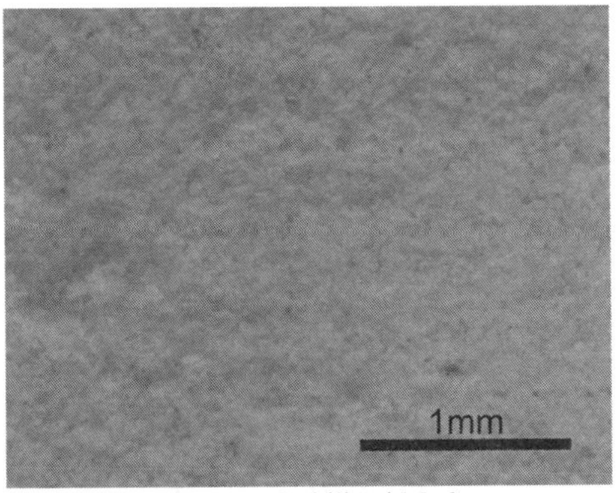

Cement-Stabilized Mud

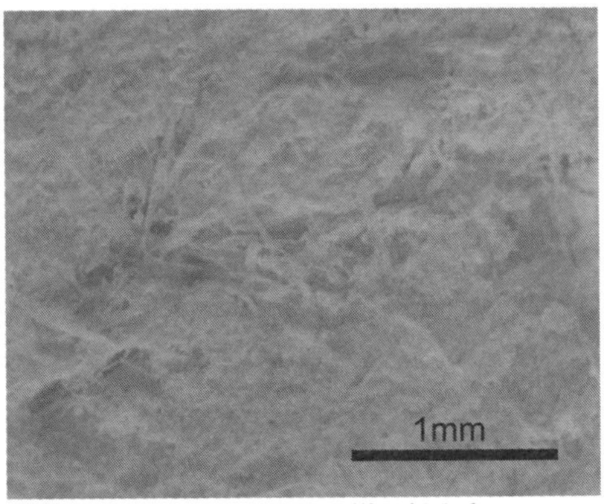

Fiber-Cement-Stabilized Mud

Figure 6. Photographs of the surface of the cement-stabilized mud and the fiber-cement-stabilized mud taken by the optical microscope.

that the reason why the cement-stabilized mud deteriorate and the fiber-cement-stabilized mud do not deteriorate is related to the structure of the mixtures containing the fiber. It is concluded that the excelling in the water holding property of the fiber-cement-stabilized mud is not related to the deterioration of the soils. Therefore, the observation of the specimen by using the microscope was carried out.

4 OBSERVATION OF THE SURFACE OF THE MODIFIED SOILS BY MICROSCOPE

Figure 6 shows the photographs of the surface of the cement-stabilized mud and the fiber-cement-stabilized mud taken by the optical microscope. Moreover, the thin sections were made by using the cement-stabilized mud, and the fiber-cement-stabilized mud. Figure 7 shows the photographs of the thin sections taken by using the polarization microscope. In this figure,

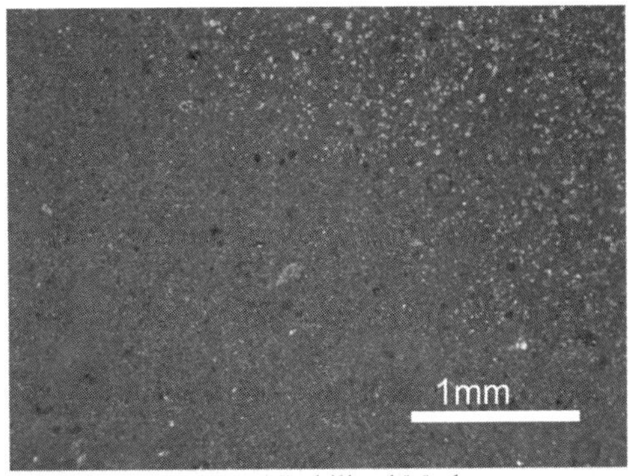

Cement-Stabilized Mud

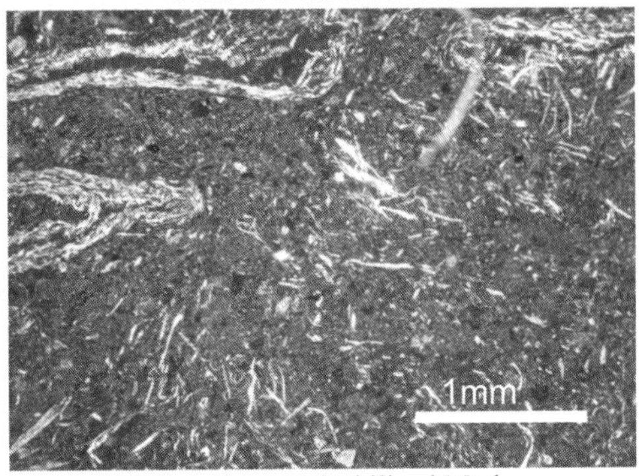

Fiber-Cement-Stabilized Mud

Figure 7. Photographs of the thin sections of the cement-stabilized mud and fiber-cement-stabilized mud taken by using the polarization microscope.

white and black parts correspond to the fiber and soils, respectively.

It can be seen from these figures that the fiber was not observed in the cement-stabilized mud and soil particles are connected each other by only adhesive force between soil particles. On the other hand, it can be seen that the fiber-cement-stabilized mud form the complicated structure which the soil particles and fiber are intertwined. According to the previous researches, it can be considered that once the contraction crack is generated, the water will enter the inside from the crack. Furthermore, the contraction crack will grow according to the drying process, and soils will be soon destroyed. It is considered that the fiber-cement-stabilized mud do not deteriorate easily since the soil particles were hard to be separated each other and the generation of the crack was restrained because of the complicated structure of the fibers and soil particles.

5 CONCLUSIONS

Repeated cycle tests of drying and wetting were carried out by using the cement-stabilized mud and the fiber-cement-stabilized mud, and then the durability of the modified soils was experimentally investigated. It was confirmed that the cement-stabilized mud deteriorated with increasing the cycle number. This result was not inconsistent with the result obtained by the previous researches. On the other hands, it was confirmed that the fiber-cement-stabilized mud did not deteriorate even if the cycle number increased. In order to explore the reason why the fiber-cement-stabilized mud show high durability, the observation of the inside and the surface of specimens by using X-ray CT equipment and the microscope was carried out. It was confirmed that the reason why the fiber-cement-stabilized mud did not deteriorate was not the high water holding property. It was inferred that the fiber-cement-stabilized mud form the complicated structure which the soil particles and fibers are intertwined and this complicated structure restrain the deteriorate of the soils.

REFERENCES

Mori M., Ishikawa S., Ousaka A., Kanari H., Kataoka I., Horii K. & Tamazaki J. 2001 Recycling System of High-Content Mud by Paper Debris and Polymer System Modifier, Proc. of Japan Society for Multiphase Flow Annual Meeting 2001, pp.135–138.

Mori M., Takahashi H., Ousaka A., Horii K., I Kataoka, Ishi T. & Kotani K. 2003 A Proposal of New Recycling System of High-Water Content Mud by using Paper Debris and Polymer and Strength Property of Recycled Soils, J. of the Mining and Materials Processing Institute of Japan, Vol.119, No.4–5, pp.155–160.

Murata O. 2002 Ryudokashoridokouhou, J. of the Japan Society of Civil Engineering, Vol.87, April, pp.25–28.

Ogawa S., Sugiyama M., Yokoyama K. & Yamamoto H. 1996 An Attempt of Effective Use of Construction Sludge(Part 9) – Slaking Properties, Proc. of the 31th Japan National Conference on Soil Mechanics and Foundation Engineering, pp.2227–2228.

Takahashi H., Mori M., Horii K., Ousaka A., Kotani K. & Naganuma T. 2003 A New Utilization System of Lightweight Landfill Materials Produced from High-Water Content Mud, Proc. of 4th ASME/JSME Joint Fluids Engineering Conference (CD-ROM).

X-ray CT for Geomaterials; Soils, Concrete, Rocks – Otani & Obara (eds.)
 ISBN 90 5809 666 1

Estimation of structural characteristics of RCD by an X-ray CT method

T. Temmyo & Y. Murakami
Hazama Co. Ltd., Tokyo, Japan

T. Tsutsumi
The Tokyo Electric Power Co. Inc., Tokyo, Japan

Y. Obara
Kumamoto University, Kumamoto, Japan

ABSTRACT: The RCC (Roller Compacted Concrete) method for concrete structures is widely adopted in the world. At the same time, the RCD (Roller Compacted Dam-concrete) method is uniquely developed for constructing concrete gravity dam in Japan. Since the RCD has less viscosity, it is necessary to pay especially attention to the segregation of coarse aggregate. Then, the cores drilled from an embankment are usually used to check the segregation of the materials and the effect of vibrating compaction by cutting cores. In this paper, in order to examine the segregation of materials and the condition of compaction non-destructively and quantitatively, an X-ray CT method is suggested. Then applying the method to the core drilled from an embankment, it is shown that the distribution of coarse aggregates and voids within the core are clarified, and that the X-ray CT method is effective for estimating structural characteristics of concrete.

1 INTRODUCTION

Shimajigawa dam with a height of 89 m constructed in 1978, which major portion was constructed using the RCC (Roller Compacted Concrete) method, is known as the first dam in the world (Matsumoto et al. 1981). After that, many new technologies were developed to construct concrete gravity dam. One of them is RCD (Roller Compacted Dam-concrete) method. The RCD method is uniquely developed from the RCC method, utilizing seismic, hydraulic and topographic features of ground in Japan.

Main operation in the RCD method, which is almost the same as that in the RCC method, is the spread of concrete with dry consistency by bulldozer and the compaction of it by vibration roller. An embankment is constructed with the executing thickness of one lift of 1m, using the RCD having coarse aggregate with a maximum size of 150 mm.

The important factors required for quality of dam concrete are strength, density, durability, etc. In order to ensure these factors, the concrete must be mixed uniformly and kept homogeneous condition during spread by bulldozer and compaction by vibration roller. Therefore, a special attention should be paid not to be occurred concrete segregation during dump track transportation, since the RCD has less viscosity than conventional dam concrete.

In general, the cores drilled from an embankment are used to check the segregation of the materials and the effect of vibrating compaction by observing core surface, cutting core and so on. However, the time and cost for investigation by this method are consumed very much. An X-ray CT (Computed Tomography) method is also an applicable technology which makes it possible to evaluate structural characteristics not only on the surface of a drilled core but also within it. This technology is convenience for visualizing fracture within rock and soils non-destructively and quantitatively (Ito et al. 2001, Otani et al. 2002).

In this paper, in order to examine the segregation of materials and the condition of compaction non-destructively and quantitatively, an X-ray CT method is suggested. Firstly, the materials and mix proportion of the RCD used in constructing an embankment are described, as well as the system and the specification of an X-ray CT scanner used in this research. Secondly, the procedure of the method is described. Then applying the method to the core drilled from the embankment, it is shown that the distribution of coarse aggregate and void with depth and the existence of bleeding near the boundary of lifts are clarified, and

Table 1. Physical property of aggregate.

Item		Density (SSD)	Water absorption	Bulk density	Solid content	FM (fineness modulus)
Test method		JISA1109 (2002), JISA1110 (2002)	JISA1109, 1110	JISA1104	JISA1104	JISA1102
Unit		(g/cm^3)	(%)	(t/m^3)	(%)	
Coarse aggregate						
G1	150–80 mm	2.68	0.15	1.47	55.1	9.94
G2	80–40 mm	2.68	0.33	1.57	58.7	8.45
G3	40–20 mm	2.68	0.56	1.57	58.9	7.89
G4	20–5 mm	2.67	0.44	1.53	57.5	6.72
Fine aggregate						
S	5–0 mm	2.65	1.47	1.69	64.7	2.63

Table 2. Mix proportion of RCD.

				Unit content (kg/m^3)								
								Coarse aggregate				
Max. size of coarse aggregate (mm)	Vibrating compaction value (sec)	Water–cement ratio, W/(C + F) (%)	Fine percent, s/a (%)	Water, W	Cement, C	Fly ash, F	Fine aggregate, S, 0–5 mm	G1, 150–80 mm	G2, 80–40 mm	G3, 40–20 mm	G4, 20–5 mm	AE reducer Ad
150	15	95	32	95	70	30	724	389	389	389	388	(C + F) × 0.25%

that the X-ray CT method is effective for estimating structural characteristics of concrete.

2 MATERIALS AND MIX PROPORTION OF RCD

The cementitious material for the RCD used in constructing test embankment consists of moderate cement (density 3.21 g/cm^3) and fly ash (density 2.14 g/cm^3). The replacement rate from cement to fly ash is 30%. Fine sandstone is used for coarse aggregate with a maximum size of 150 mm and 4th categories. The physical properties of the aggregate are shown in Table 1.

The mix proportion of the RCD for the embankment is summarized in Table 2. The cementitious material content is only 100 kg/m^3. This value of mix proportion is extremely small, comparing with the RCD commonly used in Japan.

The embankment is constructed under the condition that the thickness of one lift is 1 m. One lift is stratified by five layers. Each layer is spread by a bulldozer with a weight of 15 ton. The vibration roller with a weight of 10 ton having a vibrating force of 23 ton is used for compaction of the RCD. The times of compaction by vibration roller are two cases, namely 16 times and 12 times.

3 X-RAY CT METHOD

3.1 *X-ray CT scanner*

The system of the X-ray CT scanner used here is TOSCANER-23200 min shown in Figure 1, developed for an industrial use by the Toshiba Corporation. The collimated X-ray is penetrated from all the circumference of a specimen by rotating and traversing the turntable. The detected data are assembled and the cross sectional images are reconstructed using the image processing system by means of the filtered back-projection method, and the image is displayed on display of engineering workstation. By using all these cross sectional images around the circumference of the specimen, the three dimensional images can be reconstructed. The specification of the X-ray CT scanner is given in Table 3. The medical CT scanners are most commonly equipped with a 140 kV X-ray tube, while the industrial model here is equipped with a 400 kV X-ray tube, that the capacity of scanning for the industrial use is much higher than that of medical one.

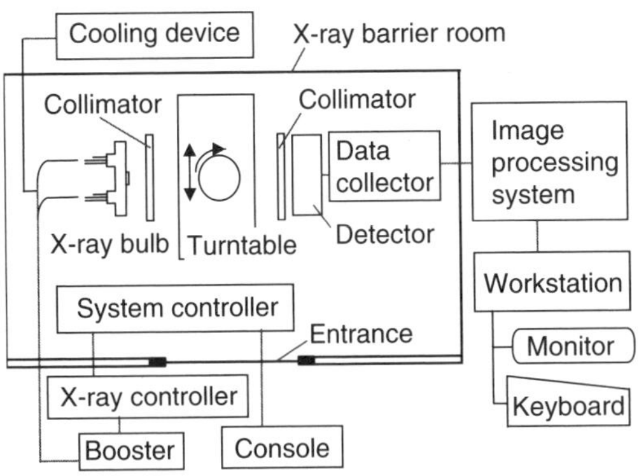

Figure 1. Composition of the X-ray CT scanner.

Table 3. Specification of X-ray CT scanner.

Scan type	Traverse/rotation
Power of X-ray	300 kV/400 kV
Number of detectors	176 channels
Maximum size of specimen	40 cm in diameter, 60 cm in height
Thickness of X-ray beam	0. 5 mm, 1 mm, 2 mm
Spatial solution	0. 2 mm (diameter of hole) for steel bar of 20 mm diameter

The cylinder specimen of drilled core is ø20 cm by 100 cm. Specimen A with a compaction times of 16 and Specimen B with a compaction times of 12 are cut into 50 cm in length. The X-ray CT image is taken at every 2 cm. The total number of sections is 50 in each specimen. The cutting and scanning method of the drilled core is shown in Figure 2.

3.2 *CT value*

The image by the X-ray CT scanner consists of 512 by 512 pixels and the CT value defined by the following formula is given to each pixel. In this research, the size of each pixel is 0.293 mm by 0.293 mm.

$$\text{CT value} = \frac{\mu_t - \mu_w}{\mu_w} K \tag{1}$$

where μ_t : Linear absorption coefficient of X-ray at scanning point
μ_w : Linear absorption coefficient of X-ray for water
K : Constant for projection

Here, it is noted that constant K is fixed to the value of 1000. Thus, the CT value of air is -1000 because

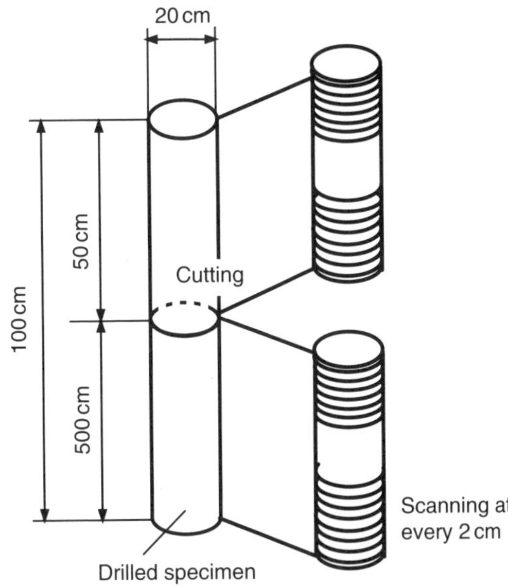

Figure 2. Drilled core and scanning.

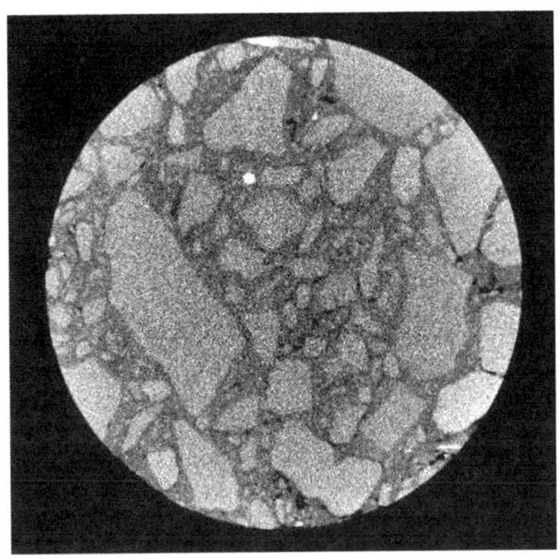

Figure 3. Cross sectional gray-level image of Specimen A.

the linear absorption coefficient for air is almost zero, and then the CT value of water is 0.

The CT images are presented with shaded gray or black color for low CT value and light gray or white color for high CT value. The total number of levels on these colors is 256, as gray-level image. An example of cross sectional gray-level image of Specimen A is shown in Figure 3. The white color portion is the specimen and its surrounding black portion is air. The

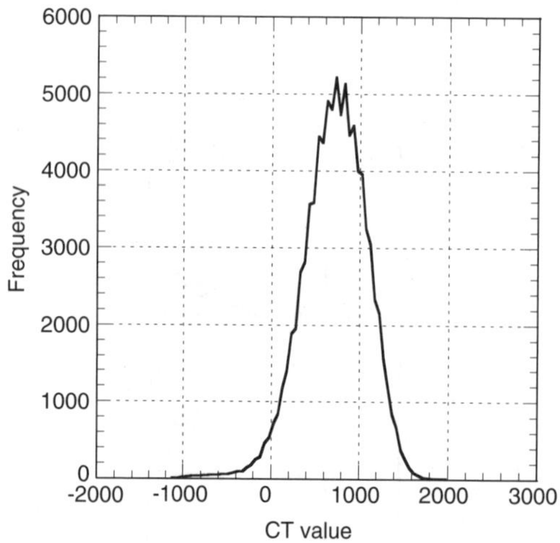

Figure 4. Distribution of CT value of cross sectional image.

inner light gray portion is coarse aggregate, dark gray portion is mortar and black portion is voids. Thus, they can be distinguished visually on the image.

4 BINARIZATION OF COARSE AGGREGATE AND OTHERS OF IMAGE

The Figure 4 shows the frequency distribution of CT value of Figure 3. The lateral axis represents the CT value and the longitudinal axis is the frequency. The distribution shows normal distribution and does not indicate any particular characteristic for aggregate, mortar and void. The similar phenomenon is found in all cross sectional images.

In order to distinguish aggregate, mortar and void and to analyze the characteristics of their distribution within the specimens, the binarization of coarse aggregate and remains is performed in the original image as Figure 3. However, the boundary between aggregate and mortar is not so clear in the data of CT value. Therefore, it is difficult for the binarization to use existing software, and then a manual processing is adopted for the binarization as the following.

Firstly, the boundary between aggregate and mortar in X-ray CT image is emphasized by an image processing software, so that the boundary becomes more clear. A tracing paper is superposed on the printed image, and then the boundary is drawn by marker pen by person. The drawn diagram is shown in Figure 5. Secondly, the data of diagram is stored to the computer with a scanner. Finally, painting the inner portion enclosed by the boundary black color, the binary image is obtained as shown in Figure 6.

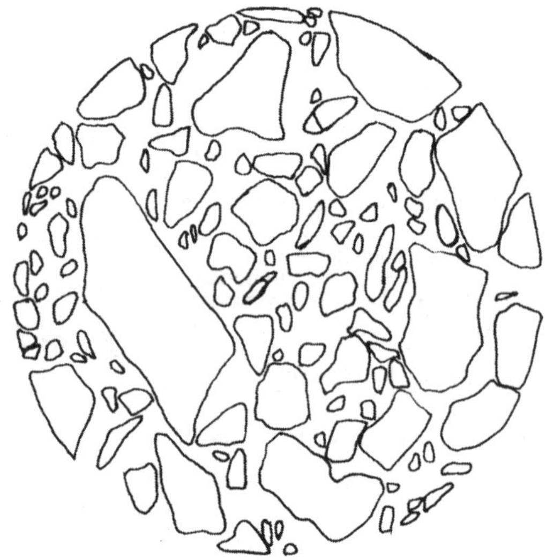

Figure 5. Image of traced boundary between aggregate and mortar.

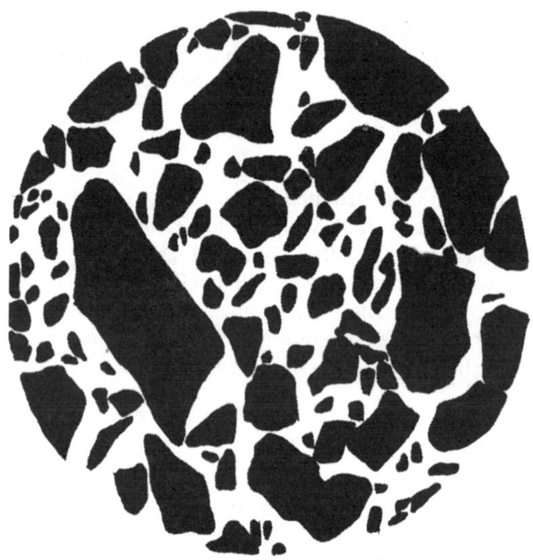

Figure 6. Binary image by manual processing.

5 ESTIMATION OF STRUCTURAL CHARACTERISTICS OF RCD

5.1 *Distribution of coarse aggregate*

The black portions represent the coarse aggregate in Figure 6. Therefore, the ratio of area of black portions to whole cross sectional area of the specimen is considered to be a ratio of coarse aggregate contained

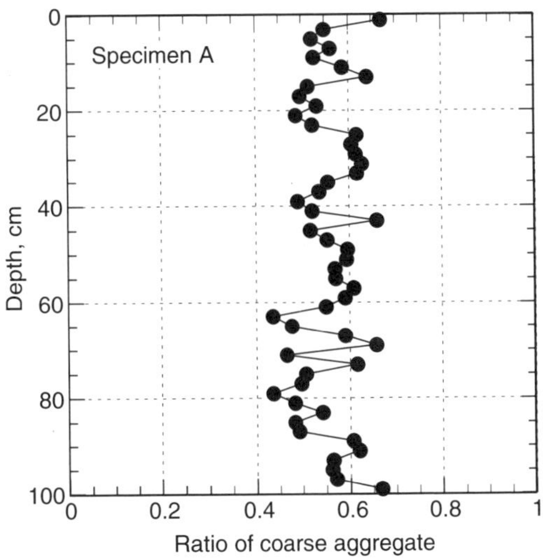

Figure 7. Distribution of ratio of coarse aggregate with depth in Specimen A.

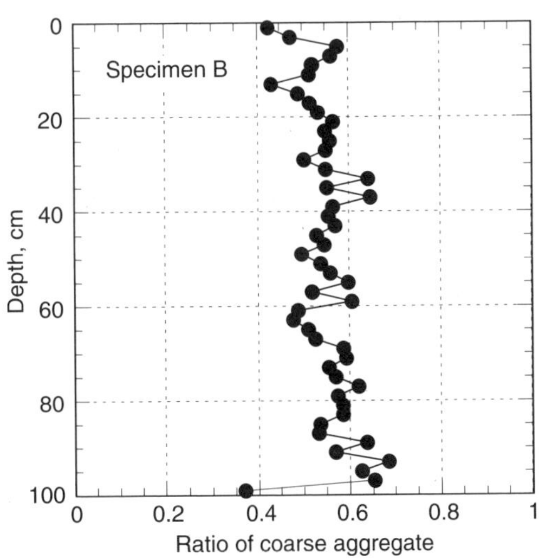

Figure 8. Distribution of ratio of coarse aggregate with depth in Specimen B.

in a cross section. Then, this ratio is defined as the ratio of coarse aggregate. The ratio of coarse aggregate is calculated in all cross sectional binary images obtained by the manual processing.

The relations between the ratio of coarse aggregate and the depth of the both specimens are shown in Figures 7 and 8 respectively. It is found that the ratio of coarse aggregate for the upper part on the embankment is slightly smaller than that for the lower part in

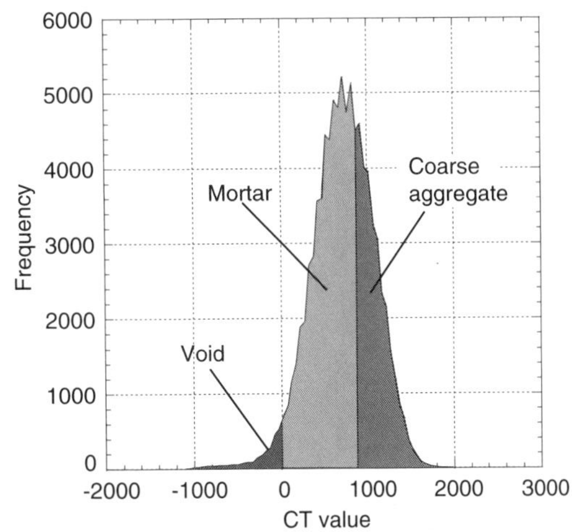

Figure 9. Classification of CT value into coarse aggregate, mortar and void.

Specimen B. However, the ratio of coarse aggregate of both specimens is considered to be uniformly distributed with depth. This means that the spread by a bulldozer and compaction by a vibration roller in RCD method is uniformly carried out without the segregation and the concentration of coarse aggregate. The theoretical volume ratio estimated from mix proportion is 59%. On the other hand, the average values of the area ratio of coarse aggregate for Specimen A and B are 56% and 55% respectively. These values, which are estimated as area ratio in a cross section, indicate approximately 93~95% of the theoretical ones. Therefore, it is concluded that the manual binarization and the area ratio of aggregate in cross section is available for estimating the ratio of aggregate in practice.

5.2 *Distribution of void*

The CT value of coarse aggregate is higher than that of mortar, because that the density of coarse aggregate is higher than that of mortar. Therefore, the CT value of coarse aggregate is distributed in the relatively higher region of CT value of the frequency distribution as shown in Figure 4. The CT values except those of aggregate are due to mortar and voids. Furthermore, since the inside of void is considered to be air, the CT value of it is defined less than zero.

Then, the frequency distribution of CT value is classified into void, mortal and aggregate as shown in Figure 9. The area of void is obtained by integrating the distribution function in the range of less than zero of CT value. The whole area of the frequency distribution is also calculated. Therefore, the ratio of void

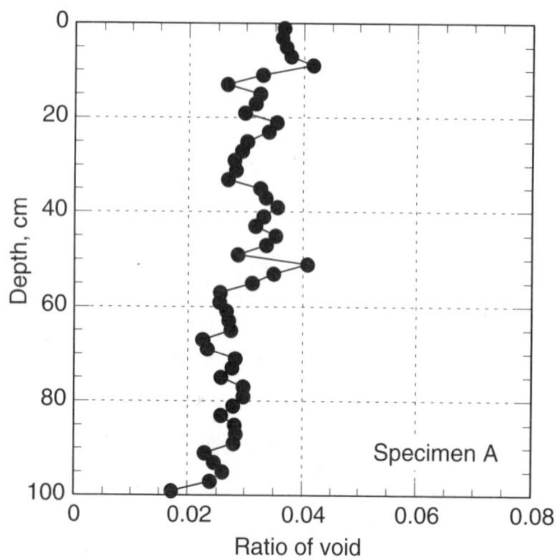

Figure 10. Distribution of ratio of void in Specimen A.

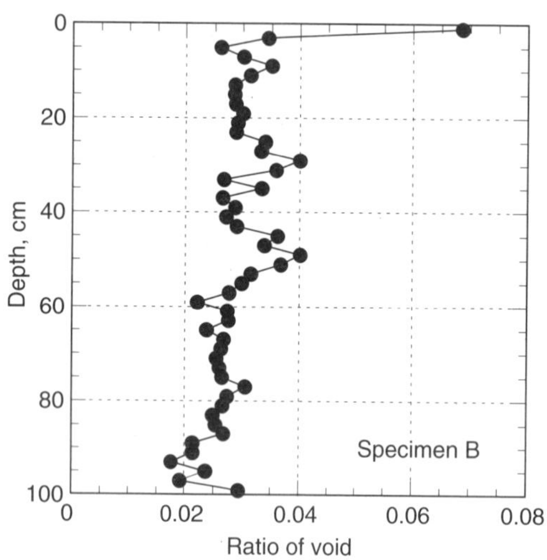

Figure 11. Distribution of ratio of void in Specimen B.

is defined as ratio of area of void to the total area of the frequency distribution. On the other hand, since the ratio of coarse aggregate is known, the area of this ratio is occupied in the whole area of the frequency distribution from higher CT value. The remains except the areas of aggregate and void represent the mortal portion.

The distributions of the ratio of void for both specimens are shown in Figures 10 and 11 respectively. The results show that the ratio of void of both specimens indicates 2~4% and 3% in average despite of difference in compaction times.

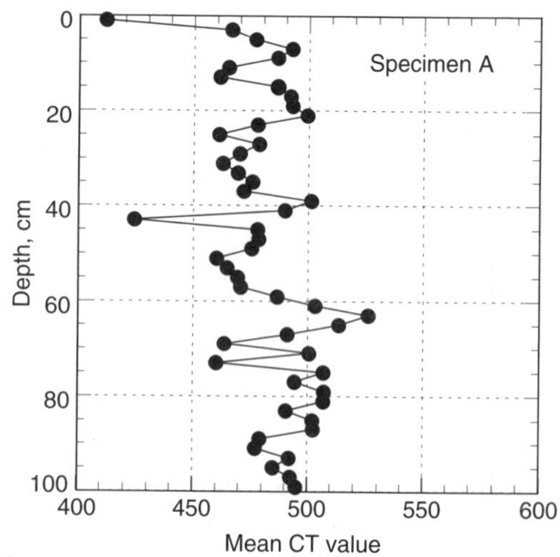

Figure 12. Distribution of mean CT value for the mortal portion in Specimen A.

The porosity, which is estimated by the conventional method, is 0.5%. The ratio of void estimated by the X-ray CT method is larger than that by the conventional one, because that the CT value of void is defined less than zero.

Furthermore, the ratio of void decreases with increasing the depth. It is considered that the voids move from lower part to the upper part during compaction by a vibration roller. As the results, the concrete at lower part is relatively compacted. In addition, though the value of the ratio of void is estimated slightly larger than its actual one, this tendency in the distribution of porosity is considered to be qualitatively the same in practice.

5.3 *Distribution of CT value for mortar portions*

The frequency distribution of CT value is classified as shown in Figure 9. Therefore, the mean CT value of mortar portion in each cross sectional image can be estimated. The mean CT values of both specimens are shown in Figures 12 and 13 respectively. In Specimen A, though the CT value is scattered, the mean CT value in the upper part is lower than that in the lower part. Considering that CT value is proportional to the density, the mortar has lower density in the upper part and higher one in the lower part. From this result, the bleeding may occur near upper part in Specimen A. On the other hand, in Specimen B, the mean CT values are scattered uniformly between 450 and 500, and then the change in value dependent on the depth of specimen can not be seen. This means that the RCD was mixed uniformly and kept homogeneous condition during spread and compaction for embankment.

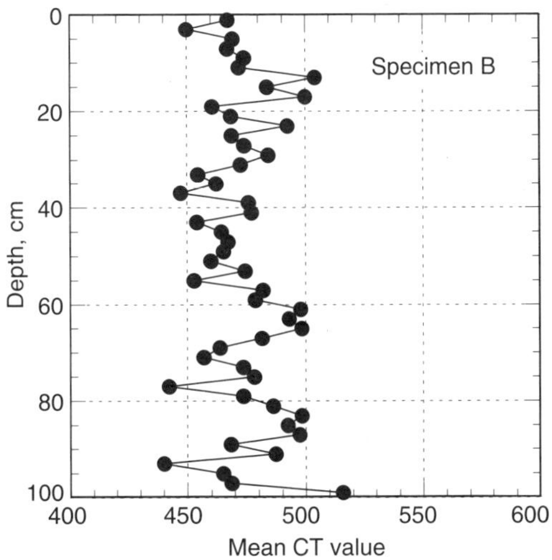

Figure 13. Distribution of mean CT value for the mortal portion in Specimen B.

6 CONCLUSIONS

In order to examine the segregation of materials and the condition of compaction non-destructively and quantitatively, an X-ray CT method is suggested. Then applying the method to the core drilled from an embankment, the distribution characteristics of coarse aggregate and void within the core were made clear.

The obtained results are summarized as follows:

(1) The ratio of coarse aggregate of two specimens is uniformly distributed with depth. It is concluded that the spread by a bulldozer and compaction by a vibration roller in RCD method is uniformly carried out without the segregation and the concentration of coarse aggregate.

(2) The ratio of void of two specimens is estimated from the frequency distribution of CT value in the cross sectional image. It is clarified that the ratio of void indicates 2~4% and 3% in average despite of difference in compaction times.

(3) The mean CT value of mortar portion in each cross sectional image is estimated from the frequency distribution of CT value. Then the distribution of mean CT value with depth is analyzed. It is clear that the bleeding may occur near the boundary of lifts, and that the change in mean CT value dependent on depth can not be seen.

(4) Putting these results together, the X-ray CT method is effective for estimating structural characteristics of concrete non-destructively and quantitatively.

The water–cement ratio can be estimated by the X-ray CT method, utilizing the facts that the water–cement ratio is in proportion to the bulk density of concrete and that the bulk density is also in proportion to the CT value. The estimated results of water–cement ratio will be shown in another paper.

REFERENCES

Matsumoto, N. and T. Sakata. Construction of Shimaji-gawa Dam. In: *Large Dam*, 96: 26–46, 1981.

Ito, F., F. Nakahara, R. Kawano, S.S. Kang and Y. Obara. Visualization of failure in a pull-out test of cable bolts using X-ray CT. In: *Construction and Building Materials*, 15: 263–270, 2001.

Otani, J., T. Mukunoki and Y. Obara. Characterization of failure in sand under triaxial compression using an industrial X-ray CT scanner, In: *Int. J. of Physical Modelling in Geotechnics,* 1: 15–22, 2002.

X-ray CT for Geomaterials; Soils, Concrete, Rocks – Otani & Obara (eds.)
© 2004 Swets & Zeitlinger. Lisse, ISBN 90 5809 666 1

Evaluation of 3-D orientation factor of steel fiber by X-ray CT

K. Baba & T. Ito
Expressway Research Institute, Japan Highway Public Corporation, Japan

I. Yoshitake & K. Nakagawa
Department of Civil & Environmental Engineering, Yamaguchi University, Japan

ABSTRACT: The present study proposes an estimation method for steel fiber arrangement with three dimensions. In the proposed method, an orientation factor of fiber reinforced concrete is evaluated by using X-ray CT and numerical analysis. The proposed method can estimate accurately the orientation factor of fiber with relatively small cubic specimen. This paper represents fundamental theory of the estimation method and utilization for design of lining concrete with steel fiber.

1 INTRODUCTION

Most of concrete structure has generally been constructed as RC structure; some of those structures have troubles of concrete exfoliation due to corrosion of reinforcing bar. On the other hand, a tunnel lining is usually constructed as plain concrete without reinforcing bar. Tunnel has rarely no accident of exfoliation due to corroded reinforcement. However, such tunnel has actually been cracked and deformed by some causes. Such tunnel has caused recently some accidents by concrete exfoliation, i.e. to damage a passing automobile.

When cracks occurred in concrete lining are linked in three dimensions, the possibility of exfoliation of concrete mass are higher. A mass of concrete falling from lining of road tunnel is extremely danger for passing driver. The road administrator must keep the safety traffic condition without concrete exfoliation.

Fiber reinforced concrete is an effective plan for deterrent of exfoliation (Kito et al. 1996). To employ fiber reinforced concrete as tunnel lining can reduce the accident of concrete exfoliation. Concrete lining using fiber reinforcement may become required more and more.

Here, fibers in tunnel lining must be arranged with various directions for the higher effectiveness. Orientation factor is often used for evaluation of fiber arrangement. In the present situation, 2 kind of method are generally employed in order to estimate an orientation factor. One method is to determine from number of fiber in the cutting area of concrete. Another method is to determine from a projective picture of fiber by using X-ray CT. However, each evaluation method is based on fiber arrangement in cross section of concrete, i.e. two-dimensional evaluation. The evaluation method for three-dimensional arrangement has not been established even now. The orientation factor with three dimensions is generally estimated from layer of fiber arrangements of many thin plates by cutting.

The objective of the present study is to evaluate steel fiber arrangement in concrete appropriately. As a tool for appropriate evaluation, the present study proposes an estimation method for steel fiber arrangement with three dimensions. In the proposed method, an orientation factor of fiber reinforced concrete is evaluated by using X-ray CT and numerical analysis. The proposed method can estimate accurately the orientation factor of fiber with relatively small cubic specimen. This paper represents fundamental theory of the estimation method and utilization for design of lining concrete with steel fiber.

2 ORIENTATION FACTOR OF FIBER IN CONCRETE

An orientation factor is often employed for evaluation of the arrangement of fiber in concrete. The orientation factor in a direction is defined as ratio of projective length with the direction and total length of fiber (Kobayashi 1981). Figure 1 presents the definition of orientation factor. When only one fiber is embedded in concrete, the orientation factor with fiber direction is "1.0" and that of other direction is defined as "0" (see Figure 1).

There are two methods for obtaining the orientation factor of fiber in concrete. One method is to count the number of fiber in a cutting section. This method is based on an assumption that the fiber density is constant in every cross section. In many cases, the assumption is not appropriate and the method cannot usually give a real orientation factor.

Another method is to employ the projective picture by X-ray CT. An object of the method is limited in steel fiber that can be cleared by projective picture. The projective picture of steel fiber in sliced concrete represents the projective fiber length of cross-angle; the orientation factor can be evaluated by using the trigonometric function and true length of fiber (see Figure 2).

The state of evaluation method by X-ray CT is applied in two-dimensional sliced concrete, thus a lot of specimen is needed in order to obtain the appropriate orientation factor. For obtaining the orientation factor of steel fiber directly, this study presents three-dimensional evaluation method by using X-ray CT and image analysis. The present method can simply obtain the orientation factor with various directions.

3 ESTIMATION METHOD OF FIBER ARRANGEMENT BY X-RAY CT

3.1 *Detail of X-ray CT*

The present study employed X-ray system shown in Figure 3 for scanning the fiber arrangement in concrete. The employed system was FCR system (*Fuji Computed Radiography*), which the voltage of this apparatus was 100 kV. As summarized in Table 1, the size of focus was 2 × 2 millimeter and the distance was 800 millimeter. Thus, the photographic images on FCR film were extended to 120 percent of the real size approximately.

The film in this system differed from usual X-ray film, it was special film called as "Imaging Plate". In

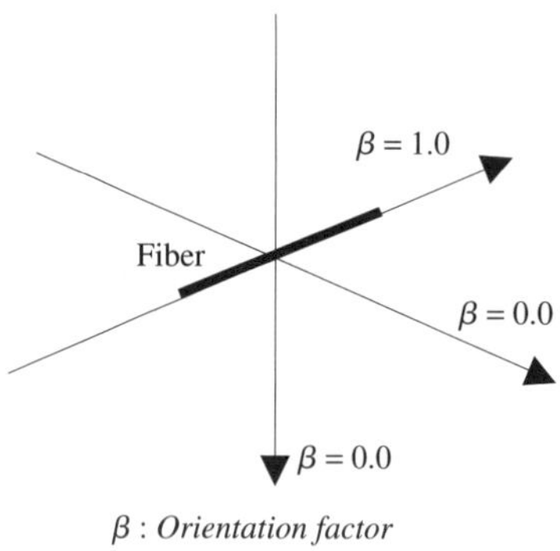

Figure 1. Definition of orientation factor.

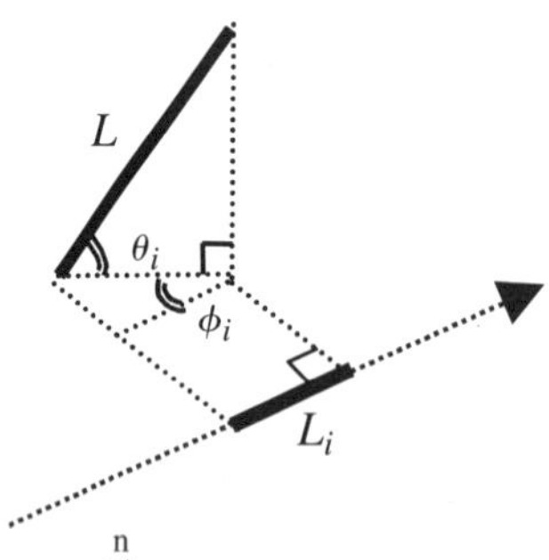

$$\beta = \frac{\sum_{i=1}^{n} L \cdot \cos\theta_i \cdot \cos\phi_i}{n \cdot L}$$

Figure 2. Fiber in the rectangular coordinates.

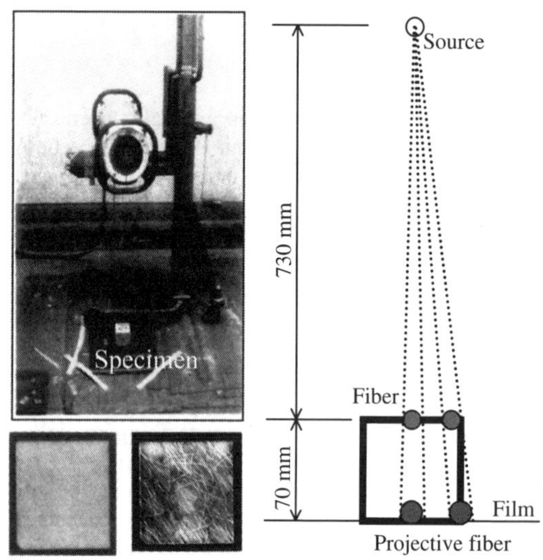

Figure 3. X-ray CT system.

Table 1. Definition of orientation factor.

Voltage	100 kV
Focus size	2 × 2 mm
Exposure time	0.3 minute (18 seconds)
Film	Imaging plate
Paper	Pb 0.1 or Pb 0.03 #
Distance	800 mm

Number means the thickness of leaden foil (mm).

order to decrease the scatter-ray, the paper for this system consisted of the leaden foil on each surface. The exposure times were commonly 0.3 minute (18 seconds).

3.2 *Measurement method*

A cubic specimen with 70-millimeter length is cut from cylinder concrete by using a diamond cutter. The 3 directional faces of cubic specimen are irradiated X-ray, a projective length of steel fiber are measured.

The cubic specimen after X-ray CT are measured the size and mass, are ground by using a concrete crusher. Steel fibers in crushed concrete are collected by magnet; and the weight of fibers are measured in order to obtain a quantity of the including fiber.

3.3 *Image analysis*

By applying the X-ray CT for steel fiber reinforced concrete, the picture of fiber is nearly black. Conversely, mortar matrix or coarse aggregate are pale color. The present study employed a boundary value in 256 colors in order to divide the fiber from other materials. The boundary color as value was decided respectively in every projective picture.

Here, the length of steel-fiber employed is known, and the slant of fiber can be evaluated from the projective length. Namely, an orientation factor in a direction is obtained by summing the fiber component.

The digital picture of fiber can be evaluated with accuracy of 0.25 millimeter per a pixel. The size is regarded as sufficient accuracy for distinguishing fiber.

4 FUNDAMENTAL EXPERIMENT

4.1 *Purpose of fundamental experiment*

The present study aimed at new evaluation method for fiber arrangement, especially the orientation factor with 3-dimension. Projective image of fibers in concrete are piled up in case of thick specimen. To the contrary, usual test using thin specimen has little such trouble. Additionally, the projective picture of fiber near the edge tends to become large so that the distance between a light source and fibers in concrete are not constant. The tendency is more remarkable with thicker specimen.

The fundamental experiment was conducted in order to investigate such influences of 3-dimensional evaluation method.

4.2 *Specimens*

Figure 4 illustrates the model specimens of fiber reinforced concrete. One model is definite line with 5 fibers, and the other model is definite cross-formed with 10 fibers. Each model has fibers formed in a row on a plain of specimen.

All specimens were cube with 70 × 70 × 70 millimeter. The depth of fibers from the top-surface were 10, 20, 30 millimeters as shown in Figure 4. By irradiating X-ray to 6 surfaces of these specimens, the influence of fiber depth of 10 ~ 60 millimeter were investigated.

Embedded fibers has diameter of 0.8 millimeter and length of 60 millimeter, each edge of the fiber has hooks for reinforcement of bond.

The specimen was made of mortar in order to eliminate the influence of coarse aggregate. The mix proportion was decided from the actual concrete of tunnel lining.

4.3 *Ratio of projected fiber area*

A theoretical fiber area is defined from the product of fiber diameter, length and number. Ratio of projected fiber area is obtained by dividing the area of fibers in the projective filter against the theoretical fiber area. The ratio presents the existence percentage of projective fiber area on the cross face to X-ray direction.

Tables 2 and 3 give the experimental results of the ratio of projected fiber area. Here, the theoretical ratio took account of the size change due to the distance from light source; it doesn't always indicate a constant ratio.

Based on the distance effect, a measurement ratio of fiber area are ought to become larger than theoretical ratio. The measurement ratios, however,

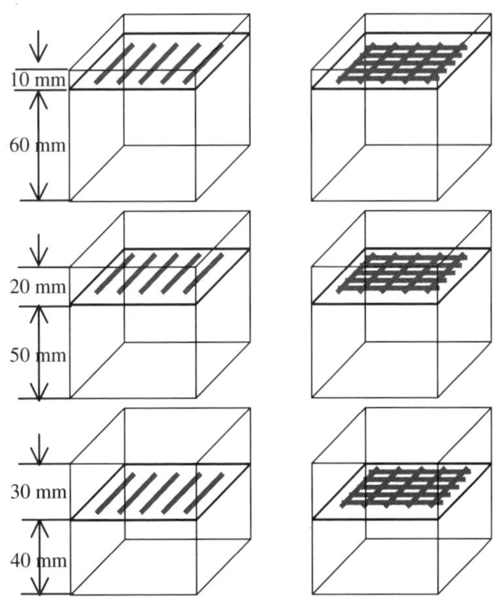

Figure 4. Specimen for fundamental experiment.

were smaller than theoretical ratio; the average measurement ratio actually represented 75.6 percent.

Figure 5 shows the change of ratio of projective fiber area. This figure indicates that the depth of fiber little influences on the consistency between measurements and theoretical value.

These differences between measurement and theory must be due to the criterion to distinguish the color of fiber. Conversely, projective-area loss due to overlap of fiber are small influence on the accuracy than the treatment of criterion. To sum up the fundamental experiment, the projective fiber area tends to become smaller than theoretical value, and its decreases are approximately 75 percent.

5 ORIENTATION FACTOR

5.1 *Estimation of orientation factor*

This paper presents an estimation method for orientation factor of steel fiber by using the ratio of projective fiber area. Here, target fibers are round bar with circle of cross-section; another evaluation is needed in case of fiber with oval section.

The area for image analysis is 50 × 50 millimeter in center of the SFRC specimen. In order to eliminate an influence by edge of specimen, the present method targets the center of specimen without perimeter of 10 millimeter. Thus, a decrease coefficient of the fiber volume of 70-millimeter cube is required so that the target area is different in both estimations. A following equation gives the decreased volume of fiber.

$$V'_{sf} = \frac{W_{sf}}{\rho_s} \times \frac{S_{center} \cdot H_x}{V_{specimen}} = \frac{W_{sf}}{7.85} \times \frac{5 \cdot 5 \cdot 7}{7 \cdot 7 \cdot 7} \qquad (1)$$

where, V'_{sf}: decreased volume of fiber, W_{sf}: measured weight of fiber.

When every fiber is oriented with a cross direction to evaluated section, the ratio of fiber area (S_{sf}) are obtained from the following equations.

$$N = \frac{4 \cdot V'_{sf}}{\pi \cdot D_{sf}^{\,2} \cdot L_{sf}} \qquad (2)$$

$$S_{sf} = \frac{N \cdot D_{sf} \cdot L_{sf}}{25} \times 100 \qquad (3)$$

where, N: number of fiber in 5 × 5 cm, D_{sf}: diameter of fiber (cm), L_{sf}: length of fiber (cm).

As above mentioned, X-ray CT has tend to become smaller 75 percent approximately than real area. An orientation factor can be evaluated by using ratio of fiber area as shown in next equation.

$$OF_x = S_x / (S_{sf} \times 0.75) \qquad (4)$$

where, OF_x: orientation factor of x direction, S_x: fiber-area ratio of x direction, which estimated from previous chapter.

Table 2. Ratio of projected fiber area (liner-form).

Depth (mm)	10	20	30	40	50	60
Measure (%)	5.3	4.7	4.8	5.0	4.2	7.8
Theory (%)	6.4	6.7	6.4	6.4	6.7	8.0
M/T (%)	83	70	75	80	63	98

Table 3. Ratio of projected fiber area (cross-form).

Depth (mm)	10	20	30	40	50	60
Measure (%)	11.9	10.9	10.1	10.8	10.1	12.7
Theory (%)	16.0	14.6	12.8	15.8	15.2	16.0
M/T (%)	74	75	79	68	66	79

Measure: Measurement ratio of fiber area.
Theory: Theoretical ratio of fiber area.

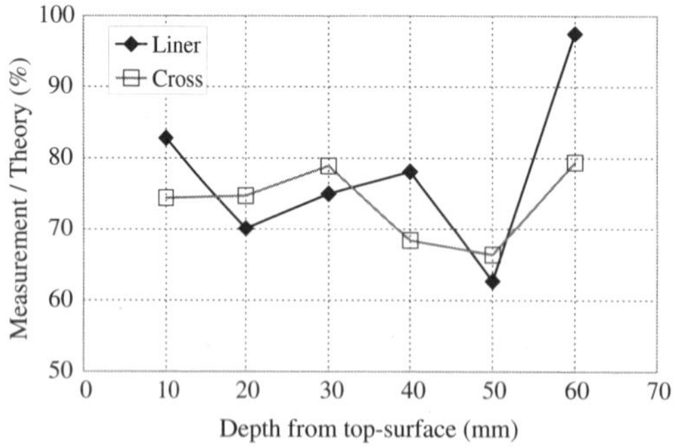

Figure 5. Consistency between depth of fiber and ratio of projective fiber area.

5.2 *Verification experiment for proposed method*

5.2.1 *Specimen*

In order to verify the application of proposed method, the experiment was conducted by using specimens whose orientation factors were known. The specimens are shown in Figure 6. Specimen 1 was fibers located a center section with Y-direction (Case 1). Specimen 2 had fibers inclined against specimen 1 (Case 2). Specimen 3 was Y-directional fibers embedded with 3 levels (Case 3). Specimen 4 had fibers inclined against specimen 3 (Case 4). Every specimen had 9 fibers, which were steel fiber with diameter of 0.6 millimeter and length of 30 millimeter.

5.2.2 *Evaluation results*

An example of photograph by X-ray CT is illustrated in Figure 7. Figure 7 represents the fiber arrangement with 3 directions in the test of case 4.

The orientation factor of each direction was calculated from such projective photograph of fiber. Table 4 gives the orientation factor of each direction of all specimens.

The orientation factor with Z-direction must become zero from the definition of orientation factor. However, the orientation factor with Z-direction was not zero, it actually indicated the value from 0.8 to 1.2. This tendency was due to the image analysis for distinguishing the steel fiber in the concrete specimen. As explained in Figure 8, we cannot evaluate the difference between the continuous cross-sections or liner placement of fiber by using the image analysis. The evaluation by image analysis includes the error due to dealing with the projective area of fiber. However, actual fibers are embedded complexly in the concrete,

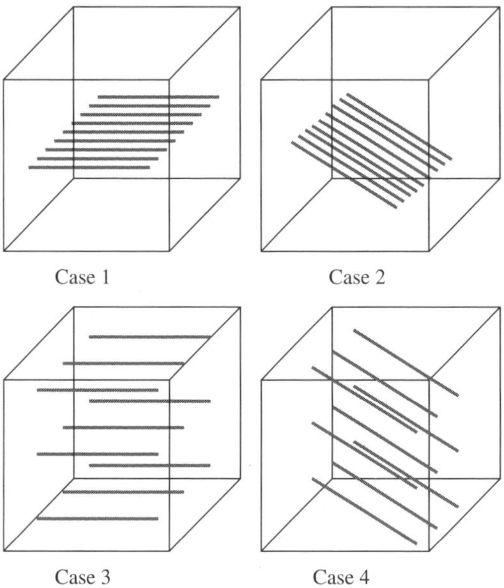

Figure 6. Specimens for verification experiment.

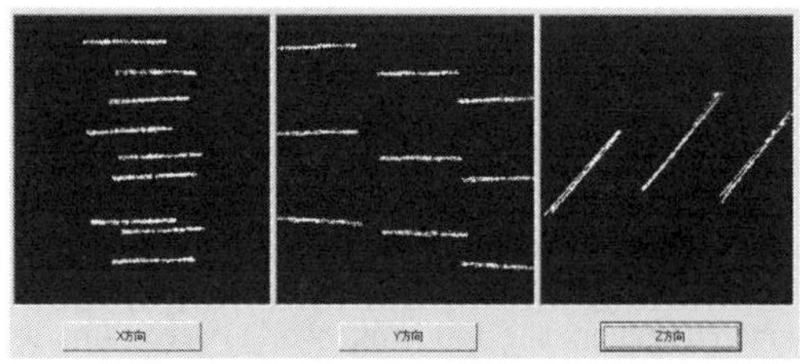

Figure 7. Fiber arrangement (Case 4).

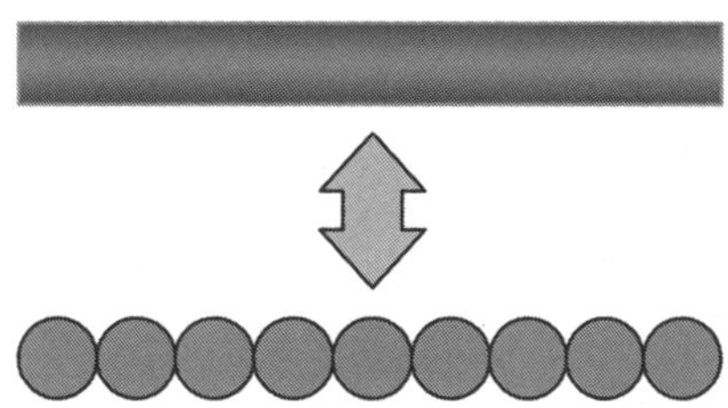

Figure 8. Error factor from continuous cross-sections of fiber.

Table 4. Comparison of orientation factor in the verification experiment.

	Specification of fiber						Orientation factor	
	Diameter (cm)	Length (cm)	Volume (cm^3)	Direction	Percentage of fiber area (measured)	Ratio of projected area	Measurement	Theory
Case 1	0.06	3.0	0.0085	X	4.4	0.905	0.100	0.000
	0.06	3.0	0.0085	Y	0.3	0.062	0.966	1.000
	0.06	3.0	0.0085	Z	0.8	0.165	0.898	0.000
Case 2	0.06	3.0	0.0085	X	3.4	0.700	0.105	0.707
	0.06	3.0	0.0085	Y	3.0	0.617	0.422	0.707
	0.06	3.0	0.0085	Z	1.0	0.206	0.900	0.000
Case 3	0.06	3.0	0.0085	X	5.0	1.029	0.100	0.000
	0.06	3.0	0.0085	Y	0.3	0.062	0.980	1.000
	0.06	3.0	0.0085	Z	1.6	0.329	0.836	0.000
Case 4	0.06	3.0	0.0085	X	3.3	0.679	0.310	0.707
	0.06	3.0	0.0085	Y	2.9	0.597	0.505	0.707
	0.06	3.0	0.0085	Z	1.7	0.350	0.806	0.000

it rarely influences on the accuracy of estimation. The orientation factor with X or Y directions generally indicated the value in according to the definition. From the verification experiment, it was found that the proposed evaluation method has relatively higher accuracy in spite of including the factor of the error.

6 INVESTIGATION OF ORIENTATION FACTOR IN TUNNEL LINING CONCRETE

The actual condition of fiber-arrangement was investigated in tunnel lining with steel fiber reinforced concrete. Here, the employed fiber in the tunnel was different from the fiber shown in previous chapter, which steel fiber with diameter of 0.55 millimeter and length of 35 millimeter.

Firstly, cylinder specimens were cored from the concrete lining with various directions. The specimen for X-ray CT was made from the core specimen by concrete cutter. The following works were same as above explained.

The projected picture of steel fiber was shown in Figure 9. This figure presents the fiber arrangement complexly in every direction, and the reinforcing effect by steel fiber was confirmed in actual tunnel concrete.

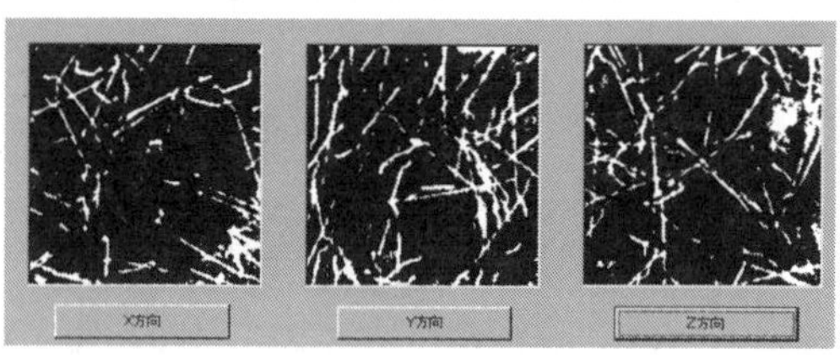

Figure 9. Fiber arrangement in tunnel lining.

The orientation factor in actual concrete was calculated by proposed method. The evaluation results were given in Table 5. The orientation factor without prejudice are in range of 0.4~0.5 approximately, i.e. steel fibers are dispersed sufficiently. From the results shown in Table 5, it was confirmed that orientation factors in actual concrete structure were in the range of general value. In other words, the proposed method can evaluate appropriately the orientation factor of steel fiber. It may regard the proposed method as an effective tool for evaluating the fiber arrangement.

7 SUMMARY

The present paper focused on the arrangement of steel fiber in concrete. In order to quantify the fiber arrangement, the evaluation by orientation factor under 3 dimensions was proposed. Additionally, fundamental experiment was conducted for verification of proposed method. The conclusions of this study are summarized as follows:

(1) The evaluation method, which can estimate an orientation factor of steel fiber under 3 dimensions, was proposed. The proposed method consist of X-ray CT and Image analysis, thick specimen is employed for evaluation.
(2) The proposed method had been extended from usual technique by using the sliced concrete; it can directly estimate the several condition of embedded fiber more appropriate than the usual method.
(3) From the fundamental experiments, the characteristics of proposed method were investigated. The obtained characteristics indicated that loss of projected area of fiber were little influence on the accuracy for estimation. The criterion of numeric color had more influence on the evaluation of fiber area.

Table 5. Orientation factor in tunnel lining concrete.

	Specification of fiber							
	Diameter (cm)	Length (cm)	Volume (cm^3)	Direction	Number of fibers	Percentage of fiber area	Ratio of projected area	Orientation factor
Specimen A	0.055	3.50	0.0083	X	68	22.8	0.863	0.504
	0.055	3.50	0.0083	Y	69	19.5	0.772	0.635
	0.055	3.50	0.0083	Z	69	20.9	0.811	0.585
Specimen B	0.055	3.50	0.0083	X	36	13.1	0.879	0.476
	0.055	3.50	0.0083	Y	37	8.80	0.660	0.751
	0.055	3.50	0.0083	Z	37	13.3	0.889	0.457
Specimen C	0.055	3.50	0.0083	X	38	10.4	0.749	0.662
	0.055	3.50	0.0083	Y	38	13.9	0.924	0.382
	0.055	3.50	0.0083	Z	37	10.7	0.765	0.645
Specimen D	0.055	3.50	0.0083	X	33	14.1	0.834	0.552
	0.055	3.50	0.0083	Y	33	13.1	0.781	0.624
	0.055	3.50	0.0083	Z	34	14.1	0.834	0.552

(4) The orientation factor was generally adapted for definition. The proposed method has relatively higher accuracy in spite of including the factor of the error.
(5) The orientation factors of steel fiber in tunnel lining were investigated by the proposed method. The proposed method had been able to evaluate appropriately the orientation factor even in 3-dimensional field.

ACKNOWLEDGEMENTS

This study was carried out for establishment of the design of SFRC for tunnel lining in Japan Highway. This study had been supported from many staff of JHRI and other organizations. The authors would like to thank to Mr. K. Asano and Mr. K. Takahashi (Hachiyo Consultant Co. Ltd.) for their supports.

REFERENCES

Kito Makoto et al (1996). Design for Tunnel Linings which Involve Property of Steel Fiber Reinforced Concrete, Journal of Geotechnical Engineering, JSCE. (in Japanese)

Kobayashi Kazusuke ed. (1981). Fiber Reinforced Concrete – properties and application. (in Japanese)

Non-Destructive Inspection corporation, FCR manual.

X-ray CT for Geomaterials; Soils, Concrete, Rocks – Otani & Obara (eds.)

Quality control of the cement concrete by filling of the fine sand to void

A. Hirata, K. Hirata & H. Okamura
Sojo University, Kumamoto, Japan

M. Beppu & W. Inakazu
Kumamoto Keisya Kogyo Corp., Kumamoto, Japan

ABSTRACT: A technique to control the quality of the cement concrete by filling up the void in concrete with the fine sand is discussed. X-ray CT images show the segregation of the distributed sand particle. Mixing of different distributed sands and gravel remarkably changes the concrete characteristic. A mortal is workable and high of strength in case of low void ratio. But, a concrete does not show such simple relation for the large gravel is mainly occupied in concrete. It is better that the size distribution of the aggregate is not uniform and continuous.

1 INTRODUCTION

The demand of crushed sand and macadam is being extended by exhaustion and extraction restrictions of natural aggregate. In Japan, in 1979 and afterwards, production of a macadam and a crushed sand exceeds the quantity of production of a natural gravel and sand, and it has continued till present. As of 2000, 60% of 730 million-ton total aggregate quantity of production as aggregate used for cement concrete is the macadam and the crushed sand, and the remainder is a natural gravel and sand. Moreover, the crushed sand was presumed to be about 40 million-ton, and occupies 18% in the total fine aggregate (METI, 2000). Thus, although the quantity of production of macadam and crushed sand is increasing steadily, the growth is not remarkable for the moment. It is mentioned that production of macadam and crushed sand becomes high cost as the reason compared with natural material and workability of fresh concrete is scarce in fluidity (JSCE, 2002).

Although it is thought that production of Japanese natural aggregate continues for a while, it is estimated that production of natural resources decreases in the long run, considering that decrease of natural resources and the correspondence to an environmental problem became severe. The rock of materials is an inexhaustible supply although the environmental problem is the same even if it makes it in case of macadam and crushed sand. When it does so, reduction of the production cost of macadam and crushed sand and a quality improvement are important subjects for securing stable supply of the concrete which are main industrial materials. The development of the production machine of macadam and crushed sand is also tried for solving these subjects. However, if the quality improvement of the concrete itself which used macadam and crushed sand as aggregate is possible, it is not necessary to make the quality improvement of aggregate.

When past research is investigated from such a viewpoint, there is an example which blended mineral fine powder with concrete, and tried the quality improvement of concrete. It is reported that the compressive strength of concrete increases about 20% by 10–15% addition of the mineral fine powder which does not produce a hydration reaction. This is interpreted as it being for making the conditions which a hydration reaction tends to promote while a fine mineral particle enters between cement particles and disperses a cement particle. Moreover, if it mixes with a spherical particle with the smooth surfaces, such as a fly ash, fluidity can improve, and the amount of water added to concrete can be reduced as a result. When the particle size distribution of aggregate was optimized instead of making the quality improvement of aggregate itself, the quality improvement of concrete will be realizable highly.

2 AGGREGATE TO BE USED IN THIS STUDY

The material of fine aggregate used for research is granite ordinarily produced in northern part of Kyushu Island. The granite is well weathered. It is less necessary to apply artificial crush power for usage as a fine

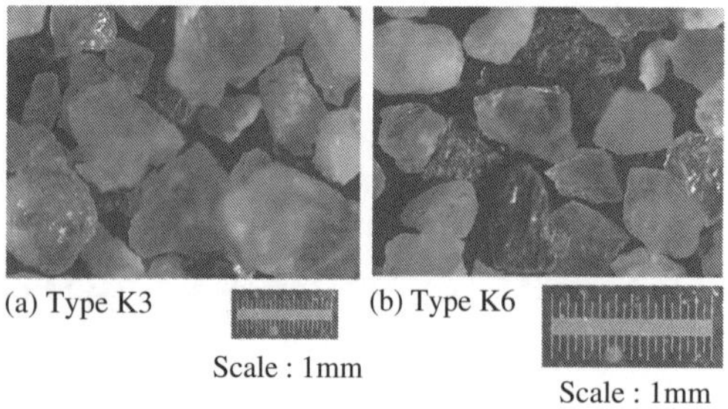

Figure 1. Photographs of fine aggregate used in this research.

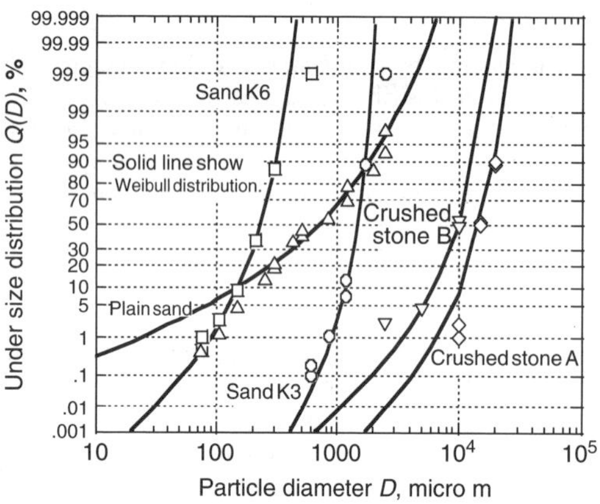

Figure 2. Particle size distribution as material of concrete in this study. It used 3 type sands for fine aggregate and 2 types crushed stone as mixture for coarse aggregate.

aggregate. However, in order to remove a part for clay, washing in cold water is required. Figure 1 shows two type fine sands after crushing, washing and passing through a sieve. Figure 1(a) is named Type K3, and (b) is Type K6. Except that diameter differ, both show similar form and all are massive to be sharp at corner. Both are produced in response to particle size control from the sand called plain sand. These size distributions are shown in Figure 2. The mean diameter of 50% particle size of K3 is 1.3 mm, and that of K6 is 0.22 mm. The diameter of 50% particle of K3 is about 6 times of K6. Each of both shows the narrow particle size distribution.

Amphibolites widely adopted as aggregate for concretes on the western part of Japan is used for coarse aggregate. Amphibolite is crushed and the crushed stones are classified into a size of 15 to 20 mm and a size of 5 to 15 mm. We call Type A macadam with a size of 15 to 20 mm, and call Type B macadam with a size of 5 to 15 mm. It is mixed by the same weight ratio and the macadam of two types is used as coarse aggregate for concretes. Figure 3 is a photograph of the mixed macadam. The appearance of the coarse aggregates is presenting a massive shape which has a sharp corner like the fine aggregates to use for concrete. The solid curves of Figure 2 approximate with Weibull distribution function about each material. Every material is generally in agreement with Weibull distribution.

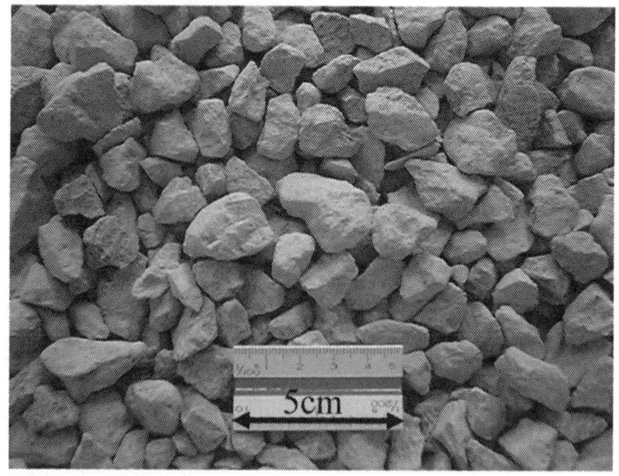

Figure 3. Photograph of coarse aggregate.

3 QUALITY OF MORTAR

3.1 *Void change by combination of sand*

The sand of Type K3 and Type K6 is mixed, and a container with fixed capacity is filled up by the mixture sand. The capacity of the container is 700 cm^3. Since the density of sand is 2.57 g/cm^3, if the mass of sand in the container are measured, a void volume in a container can be calculated. Void ratio is defined as the rate of void to the capacity of a container, and this is expressed as R_V. When the rate of Type K6 to the mass of mixed sand is set to R_{K6}, the relation between R_V and R_{K6} will be shown as Figure 4. Open circles are measurements. Solid curve is a fitting curve and the function form is given as a secondary function of R_{K6}. The result shows that void becomes the minimum, if sand with a different particle size distribution is mixed at same rate. Since bulk density becomes the largest when void decreases most, the filling density of fine aggregate will be in the largest state.

3.2 *Segregation*

The mixed state of the sand of Type K3 and Type K6 is checked in X-ray CT image analysis. The cylinder case made from a plastic with a diameter of 100 mm and a height of 200 mm was prepared so that the pass through of X-rays might not be blocked. The case was filled up by the mixed sand, adding vibration to it.

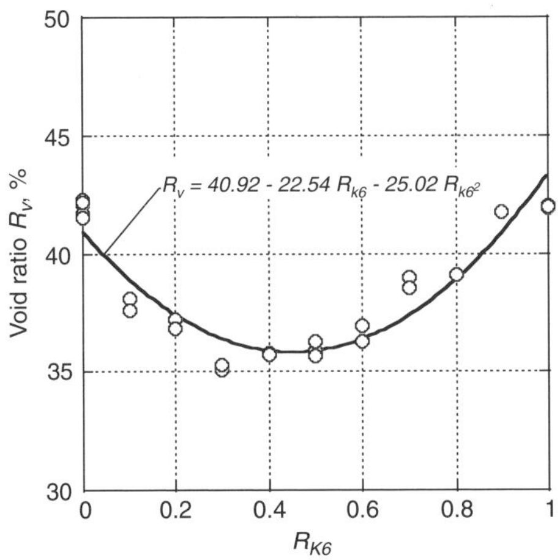

Figure 4. Change of void ratio by two type sand mixture.

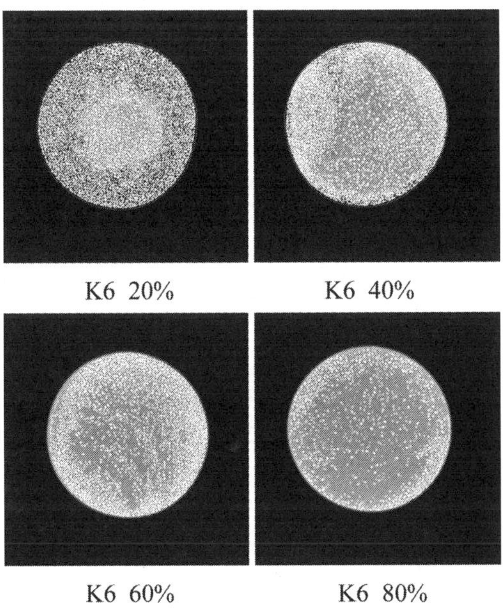

Figure 5. X-ray CT images of mixed sand of Type K3 and Type K6.

The weight rate of K6 was changed by a unit of 20% to mixed sand, and X-ray CT images of six sections was performed. An imaging section is a central section of the height of the case. Figure 5 is the X-ray CT images of the packing sand in the plastic case. The surface thickness of the case is 0.5 mm, so it can not distinguish clearly. Incidentally, Figure 6 is an X-ray CT image at the time of being filled up only with K3 (K6 0%) and K6 (K6 100%) before mixture. Moreover,

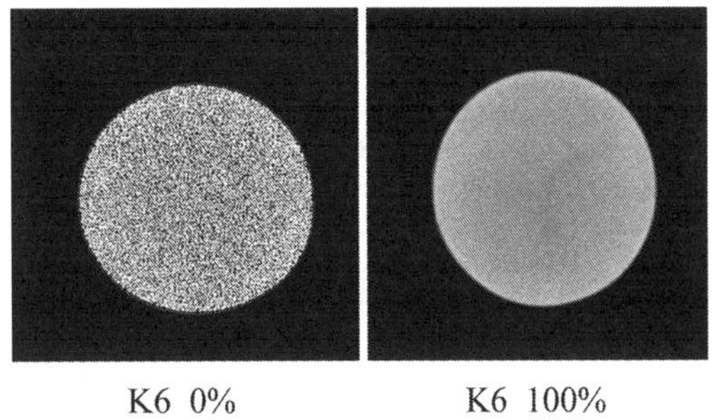

Figure 6. Sand Type K3 and Type K6 before mixture.

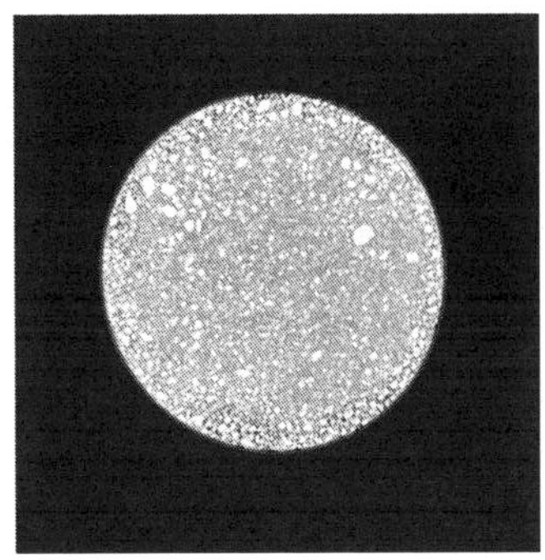

Figure 7. X-ray CT image of plain sand.

X-ray CT image at the time of being filled up with Plain sand for comparison was also performed as shown in Figure 7.

In filling of a particle with an equal particle size distribution, it is homogeneous as shown in Figure 6. Although a difference is in the X-ray CT image itself since the sizes of the particle itself differ, both may think that the inside of a section is almost homogeneous. Although not shown by an image, the X-ray CT image to photo in a different section was also completely the same result.

However, a mixture of two types of sand did not become homogeneous by any cases, and segregation was remarkable. The difference between sizes, density, forms, resilience, etc. become a cause of segregation, and it is thought that it is in the stable state in when each particle is distributed in segregation. But, when a particle position is fixed by the hydration reaction of cement and the resistance to external force is expected, segregation causes variation in strength. Therefore, segregation of aggregates in concrete is not desirable. In fact, a segregation phenomenon is not observed if the X-ray CT image of Plain sand actually used for concrete is seen. This is considered to be because for it to be continuously distributed from a large particle to a small particle in Plain sand.

3.3 *Fluidity of fresh mortar*

The fluidity of mortar investigated being influenced by the difference in a particle size distribution of sand. The mortar which changed R_{K6} by a unit of 10% was built, and the fluidity of fresh mortar before initial setting was investigated. At this time, mix proportion of mortar is completely the same except the sand which changed R_{K6}. A slump corn is filled up with mortar and fluidity is evaluated from the change of the mortar height when removing a slump corn. Figure 8 is the result of slump test. Solid circles show the measurement and a broken line is fitting curve of measurements. The fluidity of mortar is so large that the slump measured value S_L is large. When R_{K6} is about 0.3, the fluidity becomes the largest, and even if R_{K6} becomes large from it and it becomes small, fluidity falls. When considering the moving of a set of a granular object, it has suggested that there is the optimal particle size distribution between particles.

If the cement used in construction of concrete is fixed, an economical efficiency does not change, and if it does not change the quantity of water simultaneously, its concrete strength is also fixed. It can be said that it has good workable nature in concrete, if fluidity is large at this time.

3.4 *Uniaxial strength and bulk density*

The compression strength of the mortar accompanying change of R_{K6} becomes like Figure 9. Open circles show measurement and solid line is a fitting curve of maximum measurements at each R_{K6}. Compression strength becomes the maximum when R_{K6} is 0.45. Since void ratio is also the minimum in the 0.5 of R_{K6}, bulk density becomes the maximum at the same of R_{K6}. If R_{K6} will become close to 0.5, the bulk density and compression strength become the maximum. The relationship is shown in Figure 10. If the filling bulk density of thin aggregate becomes large, the compression strength will also increase proportionally as a result. Although both relations are expressed with the secondary curve which has a sharp curvature as shown with a broken line, you may consider that it has a straight line relation.

This relation is in agreement with the knowledge that the strength of concrete will become large if solid volume percentage is raised as well known from the

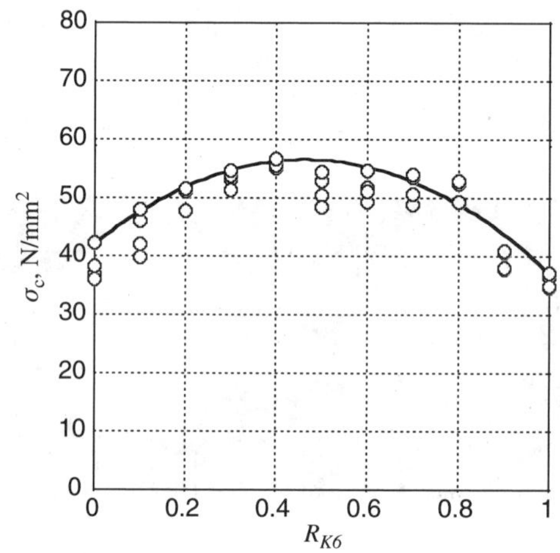

Figure 9. Uniaxial compression strength of the mixture sand of Type K3 and Type K6.

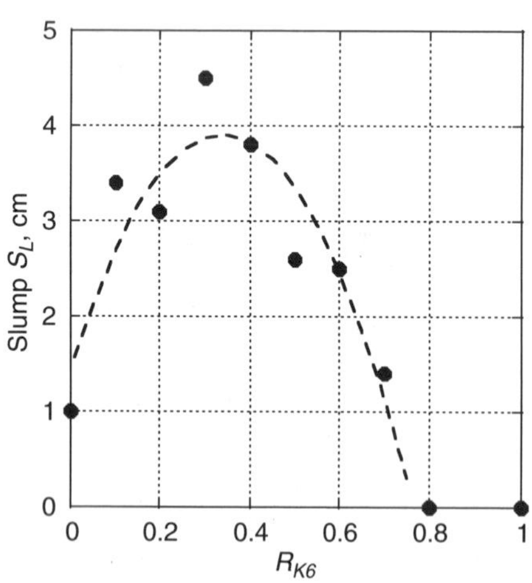

Figure 8. Result of slump test to Type K3 and Type K6 mixture sand.

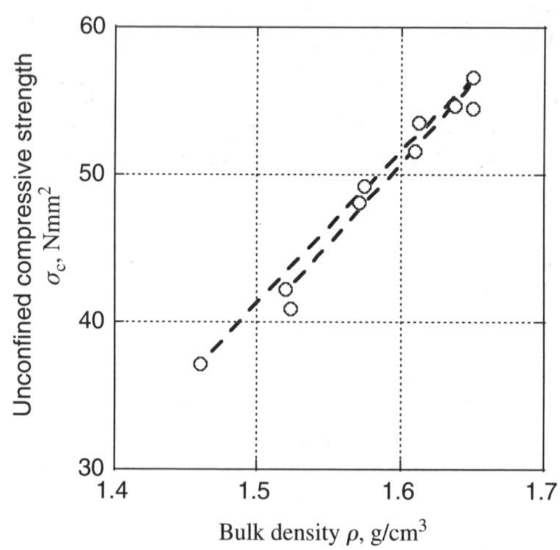

Figure 10. Relationship between unconfined compression strength and the bulk density of the mixture sand.

former, and it can economically save the amount of the cement used to concrete.

4 ADDITION OF COARSE AGGREGATE

4.1 *Coarse aggregate*

Since a coarse aggregate of large size is added in concrete, it is expected that concrete shows different character with mortar. As Figure 2 showed, the macadam used for coarse aggregate uses the macadam of two types with which particle size distributions differ, mixing it by a unit weight of 50%.

It checks that a filling condition changes with the mixed rates of the coarse aggregate to be used. Since the diameter of an average particle of Macadam B is smaller than Macadam A, it sets to R_B the weight ratio of Macadam B to the gross weight of mixed macadam. Measurement of bulk density and void ratio was shown as Figure 11 when it changes R_B by filling up a container. Bulk density became the maximum at the time of mixing both by a unit of 50% also by the case of the mixture of macadam which has a different particle size distribution. The lowest void ratio was shown at the time of $R_B = 0.5$. It turns out that it is mixed so that the macadam used for concrete may become the highest-density as a result.

4.2 *Fine aggregate*

The filling character of the usual sand used for concrete is examined. Since plain sand is used as fine aggregate for concretes, the conditions for carrying out high-density filling of this sand are investigated. plain sand is a particle size distribution as shown in Figure 12. Open circles are measurement, and solid curve shows a fitting line as a Weibull distribution. Although measured value is in agreement with a Weibull distribution in general, it separated from the Weibull distribution in 0.3 mm or less. Since the original material was washed in cold water in order to use it as fine aggregate, it is the reason that the fine particle 0.3 mm or less was spilt out.

This plain sand is divided into the larger sand than 1.2 mm and smaller sizes. Separation size is set to 0.6 mm and the same operation is performed. The separated sand is mixed and fine aggregate is made artificially. The weight ratio to the mixed sand of the sand which passed along the separation mesh is set to R_{US}. Figure 13 is change of bulk density of the mixed sand with which the case was filled up. Also in this case, maximum is shown in $R_{US} = 0.5$. With a natural thing, void ratio becomes the minimum at the time of $R_{US} = 0.5$. That is, the mixed sand of $R_{US} = 0.5$

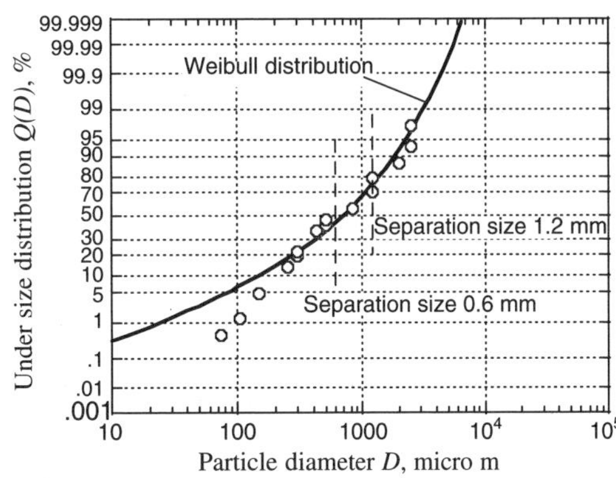

Figure 12. Particle size distribution of plain sand used to concrete usually. Separation size for making a sand to be high bulk density.

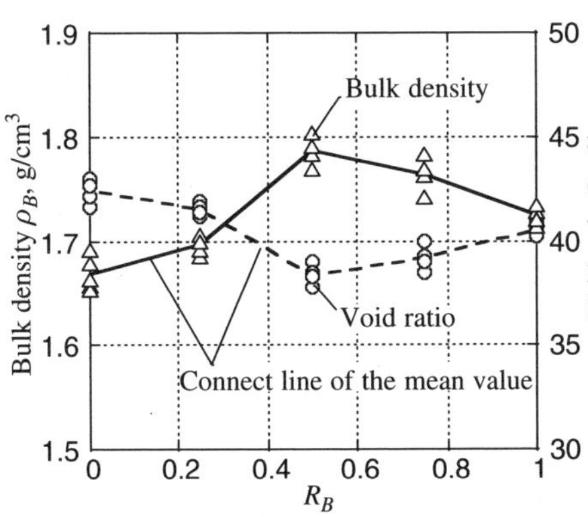

Figure 11. Change of bulk density and void ratio of mixed coarse aggregate.

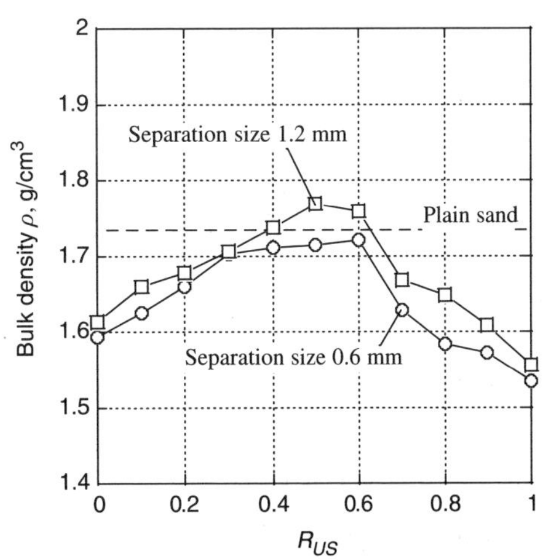

Figure 13. Change of bulk density by packing to a case artificially mixed sand of plain sand separation.

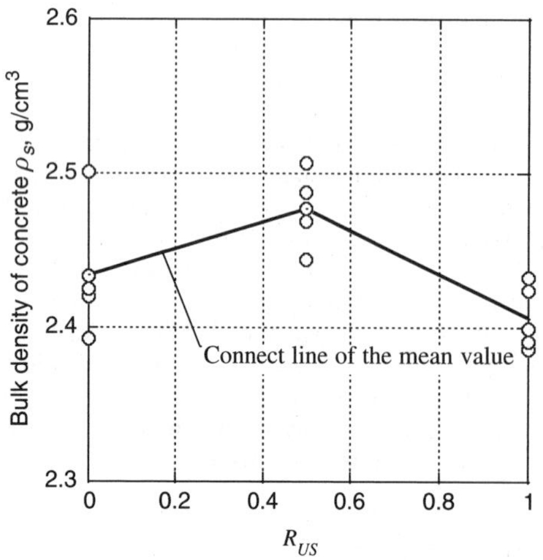

Figure 14. Bulk density of concrete test pieces with the fine aggregate change.

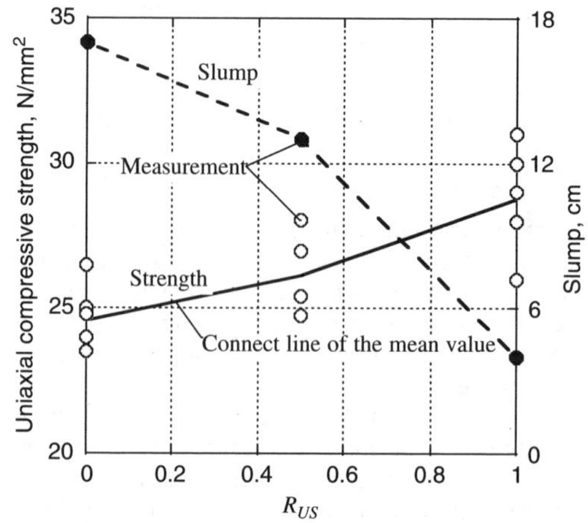

Figure 15. Fluidity and uniaxial compression strength with 3 types R_{US}.

becomes to fine aggregate with the highest filling density. Especially, when separation size is 1.2 mm, it has larger bulk density than the case where it is filled up with plain sand shown by broken straight line in Figure 13.

4.3 *Concrete with optimized fine and coarse aggregate*

About each of fine aggregate and coarse aggregate, since the particle size distribution which becomes the maximum filling density was determined, concrete was manufactured using this. It presupposed that mix proportion of the concrete to manufacture is the same as the usual concrete, and the weight ratio of fine aggregate and coarse aggregate was set to 4:5 following the mix proportion of the usual concrete. At this time, coarse aggregate was used as the mixed macadam of $R_B = 0.5$ so that filling density might become high most. Fine aggregate used the sand of three types of $R_{US} = 0$, $R_{US} = 0.5$, and $R_{US} = 1$. That is, the concrete into which only fine aggregate was changed was manufactured.

As the bulk density of test piece is shown in Figure 14, it shows highest density with the concrete of $R_{US} = 0.5$ as expected.

The result of a slump test and a compression strength test is shown in Figure 15. The fluidity of concrete is so high that R_{US} is small according to the slump test. In the state where large coarse aggregate is in very fine sand, fluidity becomes scarce. Conversely, fluidity becomes high when there is fine aggregate near the size of rough aggregate. When fine aggregate works as bearing of coarse aggregate, it can be said that the bearing effect of large size sand has high performance.

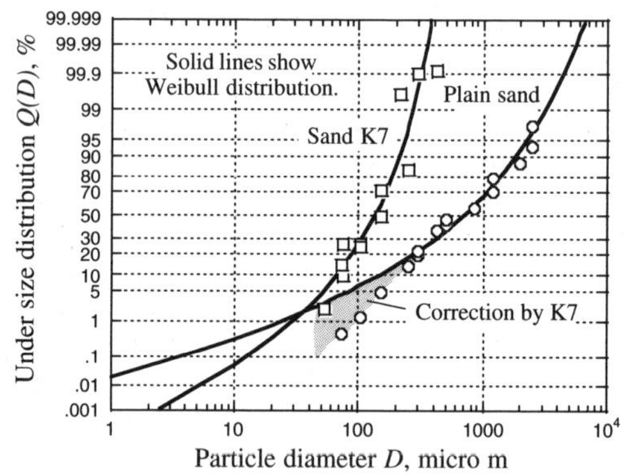

Figure 16. Particle size distribution of Type K7 for filling up a part for the particle size distribution of plain sand.

On the other hand, the compression strength of concrete becomes large, so that R_{US} is large. The strength of concrete becomes large, and fluidity falls, so that a fine aggregate will be fine, if it says about the particle size of fine aggregate. This relation is different from the result of the experiment in mortar. Addition of coarse aggregate has brought about this result. When the difference in the mass of aggregate, coarse aggregate and fine aggregate is too great, and there is the discontinuity of a particle size distribution, it is considered that the dynamic action more complicated than the case of mortar has appeared.

4.4 *Addition of very fine sand*

It is spilt out by the amount of 0.3 mm or less sand in order to wash in cold water in the production process

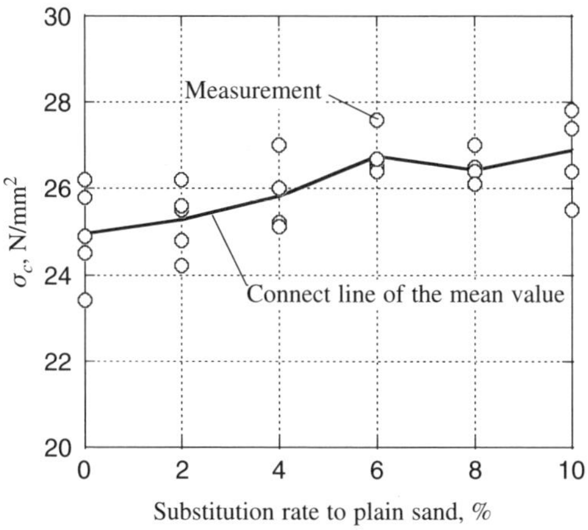

Figure 17. Change of compression strength by substitution of very fine sand instead of plain sand.

of fine aggregate. It considers filling up a part for this particle and bringing a particle size distribution close to a Weibull distribution as one of the views of control of a particle size distribution of aggregate. The sand of Type K7 shown in Figure 16 shows the particle size distribution with which the particle 0.3 mm or less which lacks in plain sand exactly is compensated. A part of plain sand was replaced by the sand of Type K7 in 0 to 10% of range, and a concrete used the sand as a fine aggregate the was made. The results of a slump test were about 5 cm with the rate of substitution of the sand of K7. The fluidity of the fresh concrete is uniform.

With the increase in the rate of substitution of K7 sand to plain sand, the compression strength increases and will be in a balanced state at the time of 6% or more of rate of substitution as shown in Figure 17.

5 CONCLUSIONS

By adjusting a particle size distribution of the aggregate used for concrete, the character, such as compression strength and fluidity, was controllable. In mixture of the granular object of a different particle size distribution, when equal mass was mixed, it turns out that filling density becomes high most. Although there is no reason for not necessarily having to follow a Weibull distribution, it is considered that the concrete with the particle size distribution which consists of various diameters of a particle keeps the character good.

REFERENCES

JSCE ed. 2002. *STANDARD SPECIFICATIONS FOR CONCRETE, STRUCTURES-2002, Materials and Construction*, Japan Society of Civil Engineers.

METI report. 2000. *Estimation Report of METI*, Ministry of Economy, Trade and Industry of Japan.

X-ray CT for Geomaterials; Soils, Concrete, Rocks – Otani & Obara (eds.)
© 2004 Swets & Zeitlinger. Lisse, ISBN 90 5809 666 1

Evolution of air voids in concrete specimen under uniaxial loading using X-ray computer tomography

R.C.K. Wong
University of Calgary, Calgary, Alberta, Canada

K.T. Chau
Hong Kong Polytechnic University, Hong Kong, China

ABSTRACT: Cylindrical concrete specimens were loaded uniaxially. Computer tomography scanning technique was used to examine the evolution of air voids inside the specimens at various loading states up to 85% of the ultimate compressive strength. There was an excellent correlation between the measured nonlinear stress–strain response of the concrete specimen and the total number of air voids generated inside the specimen. All air voids were grouped according to varying sizes. It was detected that each air void size group had its own characteristics in nucleation and growth. The air void initiation and growth were concentrated at air voids of small sizes with high population. The large-size air voids were fairly stable having a high fracture toughness resisting fracture propagation.

1 INTRODUCTION

Air entrainment is one of the important requirements for durability of concrete. It results in increased protection against frost action and de-icing salt deterioration. Freeze-thaw action induces cyclic changes in concrete length resulting in spalling, scaling, and cracking in concrete.

Air exists in concrete in various different forms: capillary voids, entrained air bubbles, entrapped air voids, and fractures (Mehtra and Monteiro 1991; pp. 29). In addition, there are other openings of submicroscopical dimensions or voids within particles of aggregate. Capillary voids represent the space not filled by the solid components of the hydrated cement paste. In well-hydrated, low water–cement ratio pastes, the capillary voids may range from 10 to 50 nm; in high water–cement ratio pastes, at early ages of hydration the capillary voids may be as large as 3 to 5 μm. Entrained air bubbles of 0.05 to 1 mm in diameter can be introduced in concrete by adding small amount of air-entraining agents. These spherical bubbles are well spaced in the hydrated cement paste to resist damage due to frost action. To ensure adequate frost protection, the spacing factor should not exceed 0.2 mm (Mindess and Young 1981; pp. 172). The spacing factor is defined as the average maximum distance from any point in the paste to the edge of a void. The smaller the spacing factor, the more durable the concrete. Large entrapped air voids of 1 to 4 mm can be formed during compaction and casting. Microcracks and fractures can be induced when the concrete is subjected to loading.

This paper aims at illustrating that computer tomography (CT) could be a viable, non-destructive method in estimating the air content of hardened concrete. The method offers a 3-D spatial scan of the entire concrete specimen. Continual scanning can be conducted to allow determination of the evolution of air voids under sustained loading. However, this indirect method requires calibration of CT scan data with results obtained from direct measurement methods. The accuracy of the method depends on the resolution of the CT scanner, limited by the size of the picture element.

2 EXPERIMENTAL TECHNIQUE

Cylindrical concrete specimens of 100 mm in diameter and 200 mm in length were cast. Table 1 summarizes the concrete mix proportions. The concrete was designed to have a 28-day compressive strength of 30 MPa. The specimens were cured in a moisture room for more than 12 months. Then, unconfined compression tests were conducted on three specimens to estimate the average ultimate strength. One specimen from each batch was examined using a computer tomography (CT) scanner. After the CT scanning, two sets of electrical resistance strain gauges were mounted on the specimen to monitor the axial strains under axial loading. The specimen was placed inside a high capacity loaded frame, and loaded to 50% of its estimated ultimate strength. Then, the specimen was dismounted from the loading frame, and CT scanned. The above procedures were repeated with the specimen loaded up to 85% of its estimated ultimate strength. Then, the specimen was loaded to failure.

Pressure (ASTM-C231) method was used to determine the average air content of freshly mixed concrete.

3 DATA COLLECTION

3.1 *Stress–strain responses in uniaxial compression tests*

Figure 1 shows the stress–strain response of the specimen loaded up to 50%, 85% of the estimated ultimate strength, and failure in uniaxial compression, respectively.

The specimen exhibited a linear stress–strain with a slope of 36 GPa when it was loaded up to 50% of the estimated ultimate strength. Upon unloading and reloading to 85%, the specimen showed some nonlinearity indicating occurrence of some inelastic deformation. Two strain gauges read different responses, that might be due to eccentric loading. The specimen failed at an ultimate compressive strength of 50 MPa, at an average axial strain of 2%. This ultimate strength value was higher than the designed one (30 MPa) because the concrete specimen was cured more than 28 days.

Table 1. Concrete mix proportions.

Cement (kg/m^3)	300
Water (kg/m^3)	195 (w/c = 0.65)
Sand (kg/m^3)	870
Aggregates (kg/m^3)	1085
Other admixture (kg/m^3)	nil

3.2 *Computer tomography (CT) scan data*

The CT scanner used in this study is General Electric Model Hi Speed CT/i. The settings were: 120 kV (KVP), 150 mA (X-ray tube current), 0.8 sec full rotation scan, and 25 cm FOV (field of view).

The resolution of each pixel is 0.25 mm by 0.25 mm by 3 mm. Figure 2 shows a CT image taken at the mid-section of the concrete specimen prior to uniaxial loading. The light areas represent dense solid aggregates. The dark spots are air voids. It appears that most air void sites were entrained in the sand–cement paste matrix.

4 RESULTS AND DISCUSSION

4.1 *Air content (void) estimation*

The pressure method (ASTM-C231) was used to determine the air content of the concrete specimen. The specimen had an air content of 4.2%. No air-entraining agent was added to the concrete mix.

It is obvious that the interpretation of the raw CT data is dependent on the values chosen for air content. In order to investigate the effect of the chosen parameters on the air content estimation, a sensitivity analysis

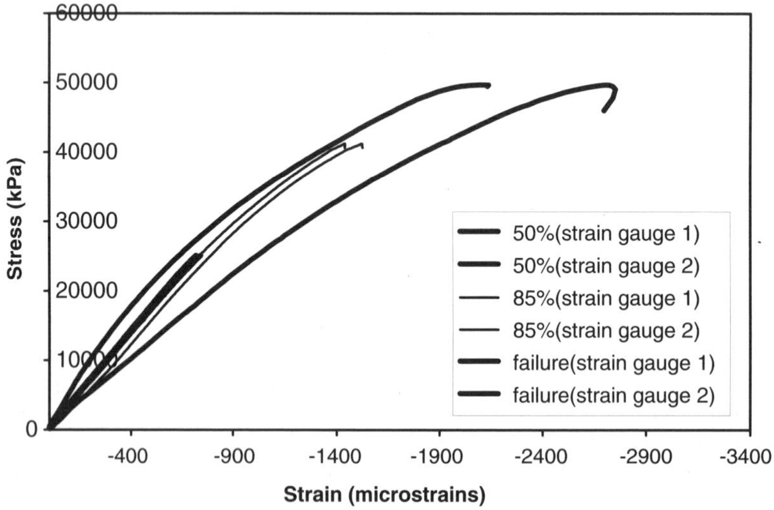

Figure 1. Stress–strain responses of the concrete specimen under uniaxial compression.

was conducted. The overall air content measured from the pressure method (ASTM-C231) was compared to those calibrated with CT data. Figure 3 presents the result of the sensitivity study. CT numbers of 1300 provides a good agreement between the CT and pressure measurement methods.

It is important to distinguish how the pressure and CT methods measure the air content of the concrete specimen. The pressure method determines the air content from the change in the volume of the freshly prepared concrete slurry due to a change in the applied pressure. This measured air content includes most collapsible air voids dispersed in the cement paste, but not the micro-pores in the aggregates. Since the CT method is based on the principle of density contrast, this method should detect any air void or space within the concrete. The pixel size used in this study was smaller than that of the spacing factor of the entrained air voids. Thus, the CT methods calibrated with the air content values determined from the pressure method should provide an estimation of the air content contributed mainly from the entrained and entrapped air voids. Micro-pores and capillary pores were too small to produce a sufficiently large density contrast shown by the CT pixel. The performance of the CT method would be improved if the pixel size was reduced.

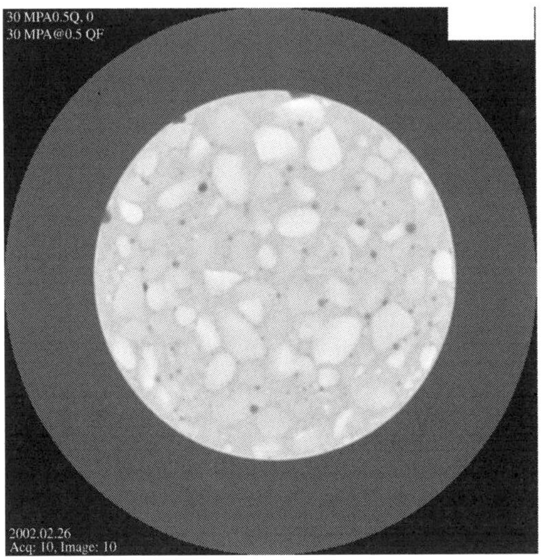

Figure 2. Computer tomography scan of concrete specimen.

4.2 *Evolution of air void under uniaxial loading*

Figure 4 shows the air content distribution along the specimen length under various stages of loading when the threshold CT number of 1300 was used. The detailed population of the air voids of varying pore sizes are presented in Figures 5 to 7 at three loading stages. The air voids were divided into 5 groups according to their sizes (Table 2). Several features are observed as follows:

- The air content is fairly uniformly distributed along the specimen length (Figure 4), except at two locations (slice numbers 1 and 46).
- The dominating air void group is in the range of 0.25–0.79 mm square (Table 2 and Figure 5). This group occupies about 53% of the total void frequency. This void size group affects not only the durability of the concrete but also the strength

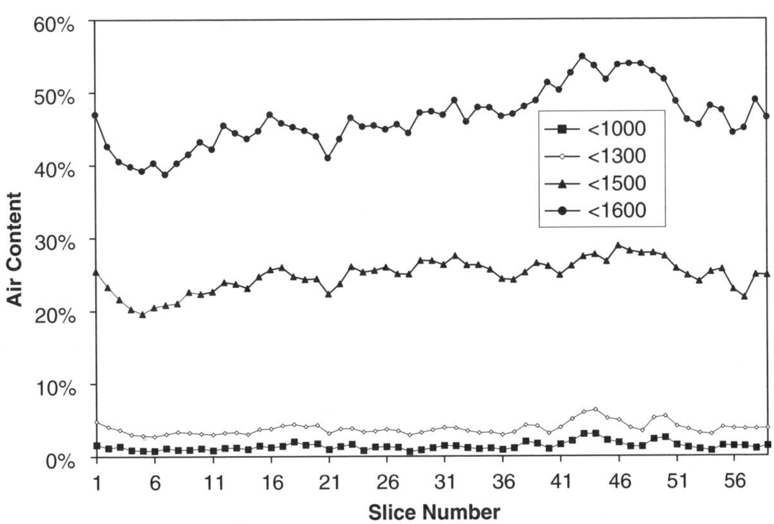

Figure 3. Sensitivity of threshold CT numbers on estimation of the air content of the concrete specimen.

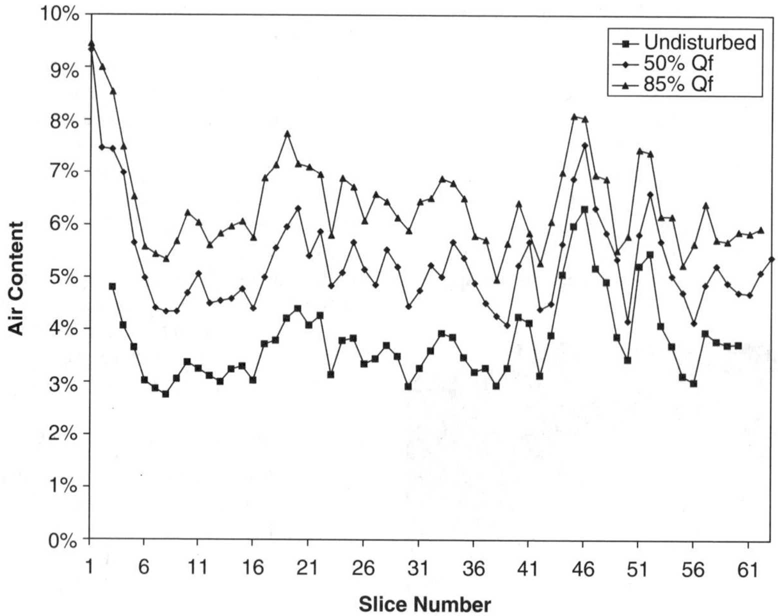

Figure 4. Air content distribution in the concrete specimen: (a) prior to loading, (b) loaded to 50% of the ultimate strength, (c) loaded to 85% of the ultimate strength.

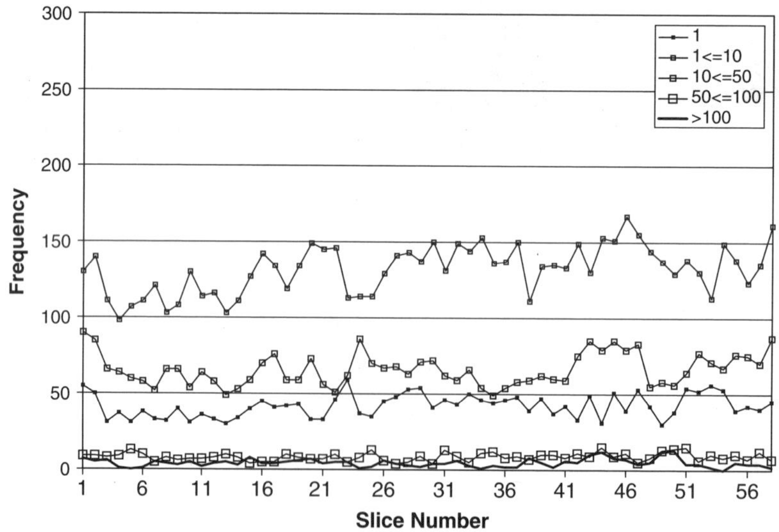

Figure 5. Air void population in the concrete specimen prior to loading.

(Mindness and Young 1981; pp. 179). The compressive strength of the concrete decreases with increasing air content. The durability factor increases to an optimum value with air content increasing from 1 to 7%, and starts to decrease thereafter.

- The increase rate in average air content at each slice is consistent up to 85% of loading (Figure 5). This homogenous behaviour implies that no localized deformation was induced due to the shear loading.

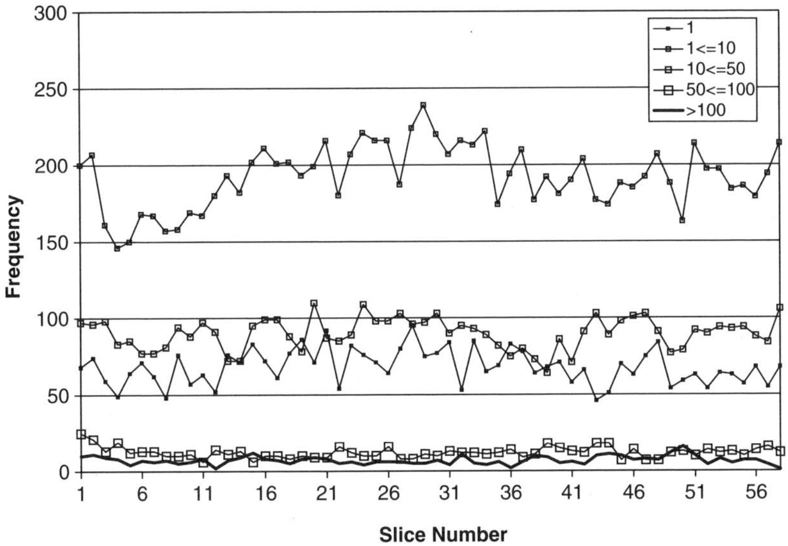

Figure 6. Air void population in the concrete specimen loaded to 50% of ultimate strength.

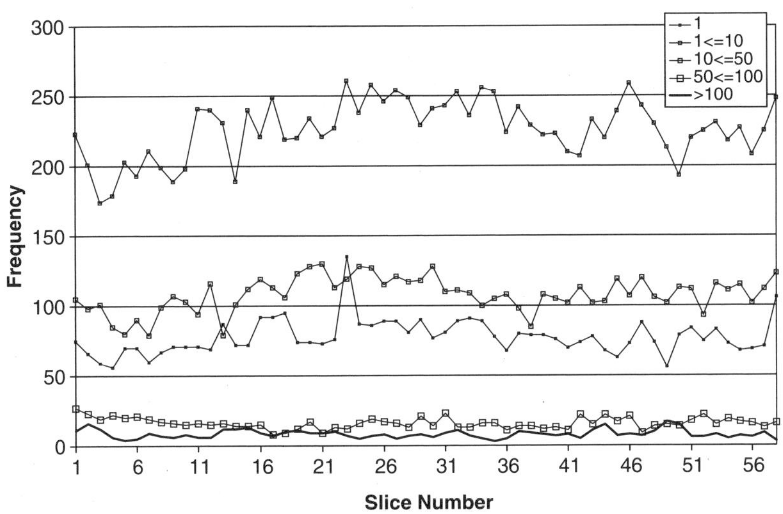

Figure 7. Air void population in the concrete specimen loaded to 85% of ultimate strength.

Table 2. Number of air voids detected at various loading states.

Pixels	Void size (mm^2)	Loaded state Initial	50%	85%
1	0.25	46	65	73
>1–10	>0.25–0.79	134	174	227
>10–50	>0.79–1.77	59	89	110
>50–100	>1.77–2.50	8	10	15
>100	>2.50	5	6	6

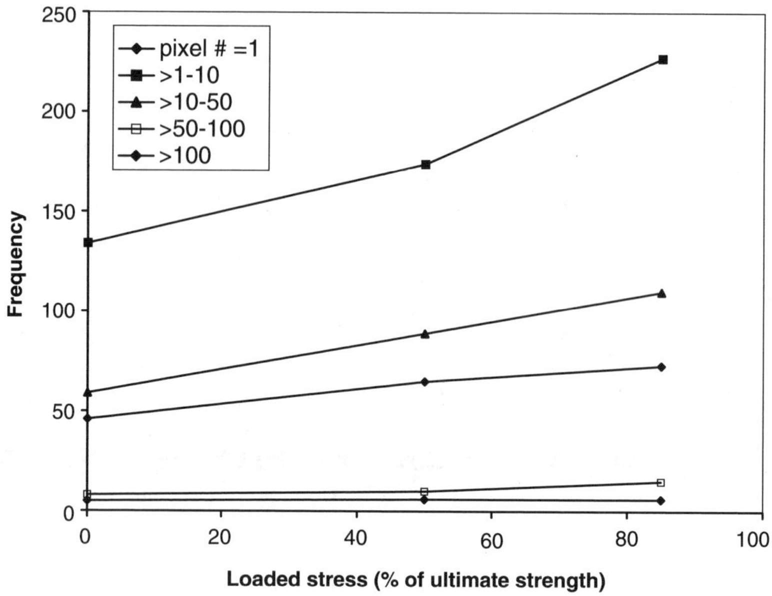

Figure 8. Frequency of air voids versus loaded stress.

- Each air void group has a different increase rate upon loading. The increase rate may be due to new nucleation or growth or micro-cracking. The air void group of 0.25–0.79 mm square has the highest increase rate (Figure 8) as compared to the other groups. In addition, the increase rate of this group becomes larger or nonlinear from 50% to 85% loading whereas the rates of other groups are constant. This nonlinear response explains the nonlinear stress–strain relation observed in the uniaxial loading. Total 92 and 87 new air voids of the smallest size were generated in the load increments from 0 to 50% and 50 to 85% of the ultimate load, respectively.

5 CONCLUDING REMARKS

The experimental findings of this research investigation have verified that computer tomography technique could be used as a non-destructive analytical tool to determine the spatial distribution of the air voids in hardened concrete specimen. Evolution of air voids in the normal strength (30-MPa) concrete under uniaxial compression loading were attributed from significant nucleation and growth in air voids. This finding implies that concrete under axial compression may reduce its durability and resistance against chemical diffusion and corrosion.

ACKNOWLEDGEMENT

This study was made possible under collaboration between University of Calgary and Hong Kong Polytechnic University (through Project G-T213). Financial supports from both universities are appreciated. Peter Thomson (on NSERC Post-Graduate Scholarship) and Alex Cheung (on NSERC Undergraduate Research Award) conducted part of CT data analysis.

REFERENCES

ASTM. Volume 04.02 Concrete and Aggregates. American Society for Testing and Materials 1998. (ASTM-C231)

Mehta, P.K. and Monteiro, P.J.M. 1991. Concrete: structure, properties, and materials. Prentice Hall, Englewood Cliffs, New Jersey, 548 pages.

Mindess, S. and Young, J.F. 1981. Concrete. Prentice Hall, Englewood Cliffs, New Jersey, 671 pages.

X-ray CT for Geomaterials; Soils, Concrete, Rocks – Otani & Obara (eds.)
© 2004 Swets & Zeitlinger. Lisse, ISBN 90 5809 666 1

Multiple-point statistics to generate pore space representations of sandstones

H. Okabe & M.J. Blunt
Department of Earth Science and Engineering, Imperial College London, UK

ABSTRACT: Multiple-point statistics based on two-dimensional (2D) thin-sections as training images to generate geologically realistic three-dimensional (3D) pore space representations has been validated using Fontainebleau and Berea sandstones. The method is borrowed from geostatistical techniques that use pixel-based representations to reproduce large-scale patterns. 2D thin-section images can provide multiple-point statistics, which describe the statistical relation between multiple spatial locations. Assuming that the particulate medium is isotropic, a 3D image can be generated that preserves typical patterns of the void space seen in the thin sections. We test the method on two sandstones for which 3D images from micro-CT scanning are available. We show that the use of multiple-point statistics better predicts the long-range connectivity of the structure, as measured by the local percolation probability, than standard two-point statistics methods. The proper selection of multiple-point statistics is a key issue and is discussed in detail.

1 INTRODUCTION

Transport properties such as relative permeability and capillary pressure functions define flow behavior in porous media. These functions critically depend on the geometry and topology of the pore space, the physical relationship between rock grains and the fluids, and the conditions imposed by the flow process. A quantitative prediction of petrophysical properties in disordered media, such as sedimentary rock, frequently employs representative microscopic models of the microstructure as input. It is necessary that proper pore structural information is supplied as input to predict fluid flow properties using network models (Blunt et al., 2002) or other approaches, such as the lattice-Boltzmann method (Chen et al., 1992).

The reconstruction of 3D porous media is of great interest in a wide variety of fields, including petroleum engineering, biology, and medicine. Several methods have been proposed to generate three-dimensional pore space images. A series of 2D sections can be combined to form a 3D image. However, this is a delicate and laborious operation limited by the impossibility of preparing cross sections with a spacing of less than about 10 μm (Dullien, 1992). Another approach is to use non-destructive X-ray computed microtomography (Spanne et al., 1994) to image the 3D pore space directly at resolutions of around a micron. However, this resolution is not sufficient to image the sub-micron size pores that are abundant in carbonates, which can only be imaged by 2D techniques such as SEM. In the absence of direct experimental 3D structural data, other reconstructions from readily available 2D microscopic images are the only viable alternative.

1.1 *Stochastic methods*

2D thin sections are, in contrast, often readily available at high resolution. Geometrical properties such as the porosity and the two-point correlation function can be measured from these sections and used to generate a 3D image with the same statistical properties. This has the advantage of being quite general, allowing a wide variety of porous media to be described (Adler et al., 1990; Quiblier, 1984). The most widely studied stochastic reconstruction is based on conditioning and truncation of Gaussian random fields, which generates a 3D binary image given its porosity and two-point autocorrelation function. These two constraints have been found to be insufficient to reproduce the microstructure of particulate media, such as grain or sphere packs (Hazlett, 1995; Levitz, 1998; Kainourgiakis et al., 2000). Including other morphological descriptors such as pore and solid phase chord distributions can improve the results (Talukdar et al., 2002). As we discuss below, the disadvantage is that the simulated pore space may ignore the long-range connectivity of the pore space (Biswal et al., 1999; Øren & Bakke, 2002; Øren & Bakke, 2003).

One alternative is to reconstruct the porous medium by modelling the geological process by which it was

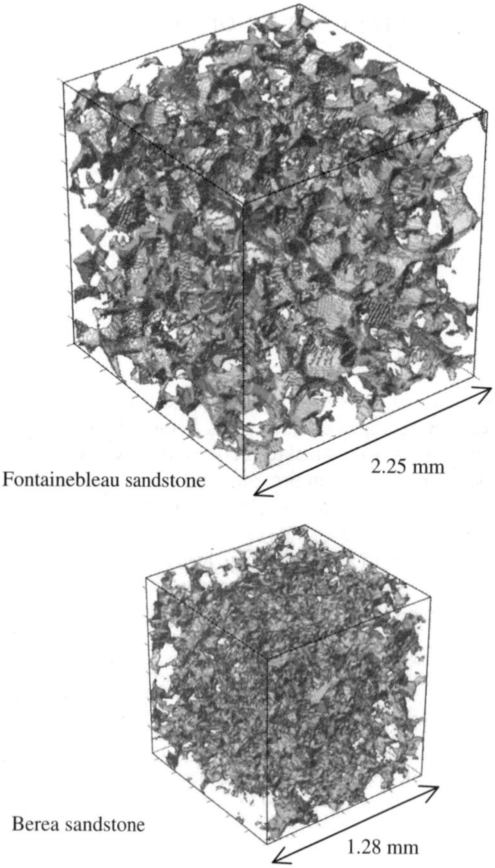

Figure 1. 3D pore space representations of a Fontainebleau sandstone (above) and a Berea sandstone (below). The pore space is shown in gray. These images were generated using micro-CT scanning with resolutions of approximately 7.5 μm (Fontainebleau) and 10 μm (Berea).

made (Bryant & Blunt, 1992; Coehlo et al., 1997; Bakke & Øren, 1997; Øren et al., 1998; Biswal et al., 1999; Pilotti, 2000; Øren & Bakke, 2002; Øren & Bakke, 2003).

1.2 *New methodology – multiple-point statistics*

While geological reconstruction overcomes the problem associated with statistical techniques, there are many systems for which a direct 3D representation of the pore space is very difficult or impossible to generate. Most carbonates with intra- and inter-granular porosity are good examples (Lucia, 1999). Moreover, it would be very complex to use a process-based reconstruction that mimics the geological history involving the sedimentation of irregular shapes, significant compaction and dissolution. In these cases it is necessary to find another approach to generate a pore space representation. One method is to use statistical techniques to produce a 3D image from 2D thin section analysis as mentioned before. Traditionally two-point statistics have been used to achieve this. However, as we have already said, these images often fail to reproduce the long-range connectivity of the pore space (Biswal et al., 1999; Øren & Bakke, 2002). Therefore, we will pursue a multiple-point statistical technique first introduced in geostatistics to represent connected geological bodies, such as sand channels, at the field scale. Conceptually our problem is similar – we need to generate pore spaces that have a high degree of interconnectivity. One key aspect of the work is the proper selection of the multiple-point statistics to reproduce satisfactory images. In this paper we will study mainly Fontainebleau sandstone since this rock has been characterized thoroughly by other means (Biswal et al., 1999).

2 METHODOLOGY

2.1 *The need for higher-order information*

Recent studies have cast doubt concerning the sufficiency of traditional spatial correlation functions in describing rock texture, especially in terms of the reproduction of the connectivity of the media (Hazlett, 1997; Biswal et al., 1999; Øren & Bakke, 2002). Traditional stochastic reconstructions, such as Gaussian random field and the simulated annealing method, are limited to the reproduction of low-order statistics inferred from readily available 2D images. Identification of low-order statistics is, however, not sufficient to reproduce connected long-range geometry, or patterns with characteristic shapes (e.g. pore spaces) for some cases. The reconstruction of such specific patterns calls for characterizing the spatial continuity at three or more locations at a time. Reproduction of multiple-point continuity in the structure is critical, not so much to produce geologically realistic images, but also to provide accurate flow predictions through the structure. A more realistic reconstruction can be obtained by using structural information beyond the two-point correlation. A straightforward way to reproduce a geologically realistic structure with specific shapes consists in generating patterns with shapes observed in a reference then distributing these patterns over the model.

In geostatistics, two approaches are traditionally used to build models for facies distributions at the field scale. Pixel-based techniques generate simulated realizations that honor the conditioning data and reproduce a given variogram that models the two-point spatial correlation. Since the variogram cannot take account of spatial continuity between more than two locations at a time, such pixel-based algorithms give poor representations.

In contrast, object-based techniques allow the reproduction of specific geometries. However, the conditioning data require iterative corrections, which can be time-consuming, and the efficiency of these techniques depends on the number and location of data.

Strebelle et al. (2001) pioneered a approach that combines the easy conditioning of pixel-based algorithms with the ability to reproduce patterns of object-based techniques without being too time and memory demanding. The complex geological structures expected to be present at the field scale are characterized by multiple-point statistics. Such multiple-point statistics can be read from training images. The multiple-point statistics inferred from the training images are then exported to the model, where they are anchored to the conditioning data using a pixel-based sequential simulation algorithm. Their algorithm was used to simulate a turbidite reservoir where flow is controlled by meandering channels. The final numerical models reproduced these channel patterns and honored all conditioning data. Caers (2001) also applied this method to a synthetic sand channel reservoir. He compared the realization generated by the multiple-point method with a traditional indicator method (Deutsch & Journel, 1998) using the exhaustive variogram of the training image as a model. The use of two-point statistics failed to reproduce the channeling behavior. The multiple-point method, which appeared to be practical, general, and fast, can be applied to our problem at the pore scale. We will make one major extension of the method. In the work of Strebelle et al. (2001) and Caers (2001), a 2D training image was used to generate a 2D statistical realization. In this paper we will generate a 3D image from 2D data.

2.2 *Multiple-point statistics method*

Multiple-point statistics cannot be inferred from sparse data; their inference requires a densely and regularly sampled training image describing the geometries expected to be exist in the real structure. For example, photographs of outcrops at the field scale and microscope images at the pore scale can be used as training images. The extraction of multiple-point statistics from the training image and their reproduction in a stochastic model consists of two steps: (1) borrowing multiple-point statistics from training images and (2) pattern reproduction.

The training image of Figure 2 is scanned using a template t composed of n_t locations $\mathbf{u}_\alpha$ and a central location $\mathbf{u}$:

$$u_\alpha = u + h_\alpha \quad \alpha = 1,\ldots,n_t \tag{1}$$

where the $\mathbf{h}_\alpha$ are the vectors describing the template. For instance, in Figure 3, $\mathbf{h}_\alpha$ are the 80 vectors of the square 9 × 9 template.

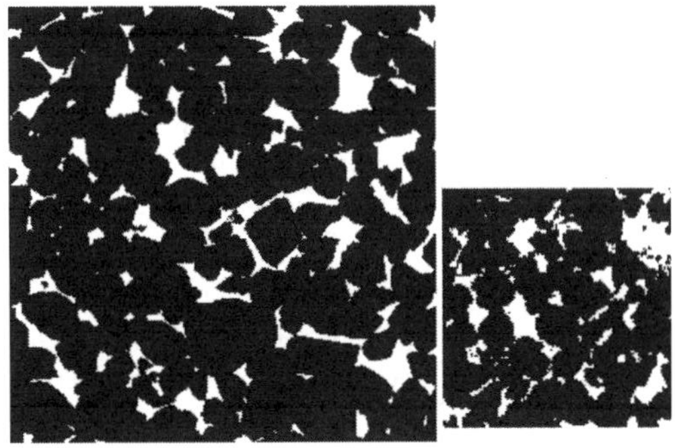

Figure 2. Thin-sections as training images. The pore space is shown white and the grain black. The left image is Fontainebleau sandstone with a porosity, $\phi = 0.1364$ (300^2 pixels). The right image is Berea sandstone with $\phi = 0.1773$ (128^2 pixels). Resolutions of images are 7.5 μm and 10 μm, respectively.

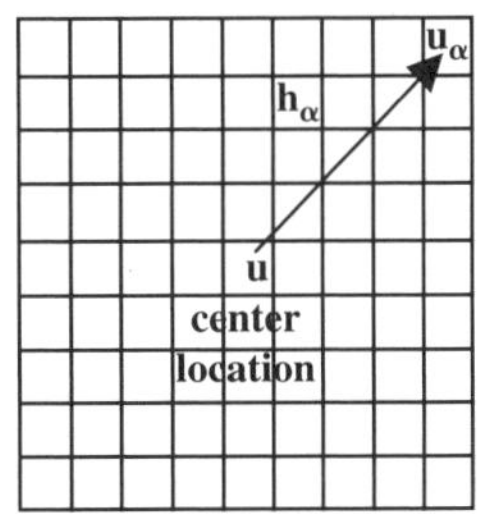

Figure 3. A 9 × 9 template to capture multiple-point statistics. The training image is scanned and each occurrence of any possible pattern of void space and grain is recorded.

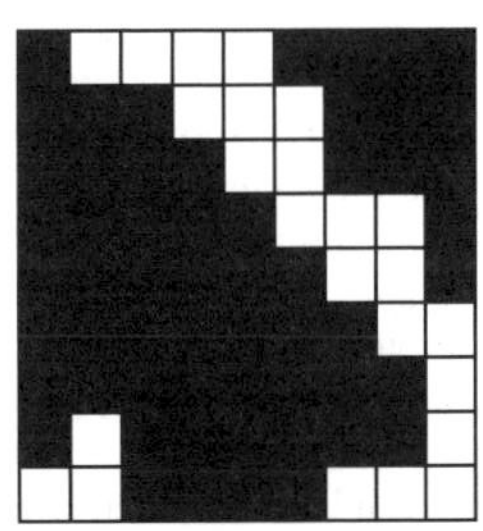

Figure 4. A data event (or a pattern) measured by 9 × 9 template. The frequency of every possible data event is found by scanning the template, Figure 3, over the training image.

The template is used to scan the training image and collect the data event at each location $\mathbf{u}$. The data event (or the pattern), for instance shown in Figure 4, is defined by

$$dev(u) = \{i(u); i(u + h_\alpha),\ \alpha = 1,\ldots,n_t\} \tag{2}$$

where $i(u)$ is the data value at the point within the template. Each point in the template has a number to identify the pattern and to store the pattern in memory. The set of all data events scanned from the training image results in a *training data set*

$$Set = \{dev(u_j),\ j = 1,...,N_t\} \tag{3}$$

where *Set* refers to the training data set constructed with template t. N_t is the number of different central locations of template t over the training image.

The selection of the template geometry is important and various template sizes n_t and geometries should be tried in order to reproduce better structures. In our modeling to reconstruct pore scale structures, binarized thin section images are used as training images that have only void or solid. A detailed discussion of the training image can be found in the Rock Sample section.

The multiple-point statistics are actually probabilities of occurrence of the data events. The probability of occurrence of any data event dev_n associated with the data template t can be inferred from the training image by counting the number $c(dev_n)$ of replicates of dev_n found in the training image. A replicate should have the same geometry and the same data values as dev_n. The multiple-point statistics can be identified to the proportion: $\Pr(dev_n) \approx c(dev_n)/N_n$ where N_n is the size of the pattern.

The key to this algorithm is the determination of local conditional probability distribution functions (cpdf). We need to evaluate the probability that the unknown attribute value $i(u)$ takes any of 2 possible states – void or solid – given n nearest data during the reproduction at any unsampled location $\mathbf{u}$. If multiple-point statistics are available, then the conditioning of $i(u)$ to the single global data event dev_n can be considered, and the conditional probability can be identified to the training proportion. The cpdf is inferred directly and consistently from the training image. The multiple-point statistics, the geometrical structures in other words, are borrowed directly from the training image.

This approach can be theoretically applied to a 3D field when 3D structural information is available. Since it is difficult or impossible to measure 3D sub-micron scale data as mentioned above, our only alternative is to use 2D images to measure multiple-point statistics. In our case, in order to generate 3D structure from 2D information, measured multiple-point statistics on one plane are rotated 90 degrees around each principal axis. In other words, measured statistics on the XY plane are transformed to the YZ and the XZ planes with an assumption of isotropy in orthogonal directions.

To borrow directly all required cpdf from a training image possibly leads to having excessive amounts of information. In a designated template t of n data variables, inference of a probability distribution function conditional to a data event dev_n requires that enough occurrences, which are dependent on the size of the training image, should be found. For our reconstruction, each of the 80 nodes in the data template (9×9 square shape) except a center point can take 2 states (void or solid). The total number of possible data events is thus 2^{80} which mean that only a relatively small number of cpdf can be actually inferred from the training image. To alleviate this problem, at each unsampled node, infer the local cpdf by scanning the training image with progressive reduction of the size n of the conditioning data event dev_n until a designated minimum number of replicates of dev_n are found. To minimize the repetitive process and the calculation time, each unsampled grid node is visited only once using a random path and each simulated value becomes a conditioning datum value. Needless to say, conditioning data are frozen at their data location and are used for the successive simulation. These cycles are iterated until all the grids are simulated. In order to avoid the repetitive scanning of the training image and to store multiple-point statistics effectively, a dynamic data structure called a search tree is used to store all training cpdf in advance.

In the presence of large-scale structures, the use of a single limited size template would not suffice to model the large-scale characteristics observed in the training image. A large template is necessary to reproduce large-scale structures. The template size can be theoretically expanded to match the largest structure in the training image. However, the template size is limited by memory limitations in the numerical simulation. Although the numerical modeling is always limited at certain points, an alternative approach can be introduced by a sort of multigrid simulation. Four different sized templates are used to scan the training image, resulting in four different data sets *Set* t_1, *Set* t_2, *Set* t_3 and *Set* t_4. Larger scale templates can simply be expanded from the small-scale template. In a multigrid system, a simulation is first performed on the coarsest grid. Once the coarse simulation is finished, the simulated values are assigned to the correct grid locations on the finer grid, and are used as conditioning data on the finer grid. When large-scale structures exist in the training image, this multigrid approach captures the large-scale multiple-point statistics effectively while requiring relatively little memory (Strebelle & Journel, 2001; Caers, 2001).

2.3 *Image processing – noise reduction and smoothing*

There is noise in 3D images generated from 2D data, due to the lack of statistical information, which is inevitable when stochastic methods are used. This unrealistic noise in the image can be reduced by image processing. Some researchers (Ioannidis et al., 1997; Liang et al., 1998) who use stochastic reconstruction have taken noise canceling as a post-processing step. For example, Liang et al. (1998) measured the fractions of non-percolating solid and void phases as 0.0008 and 0.012, respectively in their reconstructed structures. The non-percolating solid phases correspond to islands isolated inside the void phase. Since this is impossible in real porous media, they were changed to appear as void phase. We used the same process for noise canceling. This process may slightly increase the porosity of the reconstructed structure; however, Liang et al. confirmed the effect of changing structure was negligible by comparing the normalized two-point correlation function in the reference and the reconstruction. For our realizations (see later) only a very small fraction of isolated solid phase (around 0.0001) was changed to the void phase. In addition to this process, we use simple binary image processing to reduce noise in the void phase and smooth the boundary between void and solid. First we use a 3D dilation and erosion processes in a 3^3 cubic neighborhood pattern containing a total of 27 pixels (Serra, 1992). Although we can explore more effective operations for the simulated pore space representation, we have confirmed this simple operation reasonably smoothes the 3D image and reduces the noise. After dilation-erosion the image has a higher porosity than the original. We adjust the porosity by counting the number of neighbor pixels of the other phase in a 3^3 region and compare this number to some threshold value (coefficient value). The phase of the central pixel is changed if the count is exceeded (Russ, 1994). Classical erosion or dilation is this operation using a coefficient of zero. The coefficient value is chosen to result in the correct, original, value of porosity.

3 ROCK SAMPLE

3.1 *Experimental sample – Fontainebleau sandstone*

3D X-ray microtomographic images of sandstones are used as the experimental reference data and parts of training images for our method (Dunsmuir et al., 1991; Lindquist et al., 2000). These sandstones generally serve as a basis for many rock physics experiments because of its simplicity.

Fontainebleau sandstone consists of monocrystalline quartz grains that have been well rounded through transport for long periods before being deposited. The sample we studied had well sorted grains of around 200 μm in diameter. The sand was cemented by silica crystallizing around the grains (quartz overgrowths). Fontainebleau sandstone exhibits intergranular porosity ranging from 0.03 to roughly 0.3 depending on the degree of compaction and diagenesis. The porosity of the microtomographic image is 0.1355 compared to 0.1484 of the larger original core which has a permeability of 1.3D and a formation factor of 22.1.

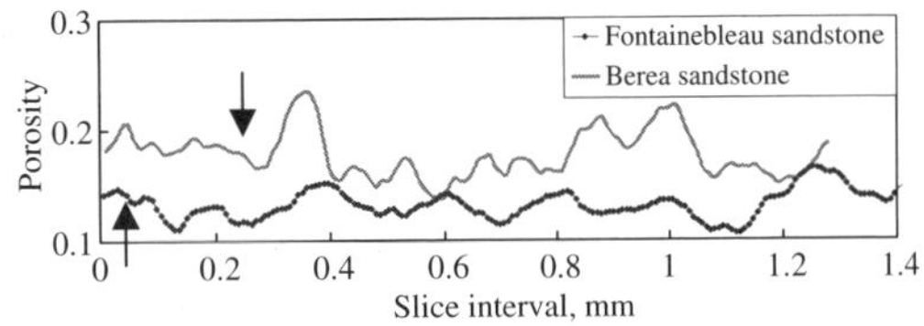

Figure 5. Porosity fluctuation within measured microstructures of sandstones. The average porosity = 0.1355, slice size = 2.25 × 2.25 mm^2, slice interval = 7.5 μm for a Fontainebleau sandstone. The average porosity = 0.1775, slice size = 1.28 × 1.28 mm^2, slice interval = 10.0 μm for a Berea sandstone. The arrows indicate the slices from which our training images were taken, which have porosity close to the average.

The more complex Berea sandstone sample with clays has a porosity of 0.1778 compared to 0.23 of the larger original core which has a permeability of 1.1D (Hazlett, 1995). The differences between the porosity of the original core and that of the microtomographic data are due to the heterogeneity of the sandstone, the difference in sample size and the resolution of the microtomography. The experimental sample is referred to as microCT in the following. 2D slices of the microCT images are shown in Figure 2.

3.2 *Selection of a 2D thin-section*

Porosity measured from a 2D slice fluctuates as shown in Figure 5. In order to reconstruct a 3D structure effectively from 2D cuts, representative 2D images should be selected in terms of porosity. We took the slices indicated in Figure 5 by arrows.

4 RESULTS

4.1 *Template selection*

This method has more flexibility than the traditional two-point correlation method because we can change the template used to generate multiple-point statistics as well as the training image. A key aspect of this research is the proper selection of the multiple-point statistics to produce satisfactory images. We used four different sized templates with the same 9 × 9 square shape, spanning 9 × 9, 18 × 18, 27 × 27 and 36 × 36 pixels. A larger template can capture large structures; however, it takes much more CPU time and introduces more noise if the training image does not provide sufficient statistics. We decided to use a 9 ×9 template after considering larger and smaller templates – this

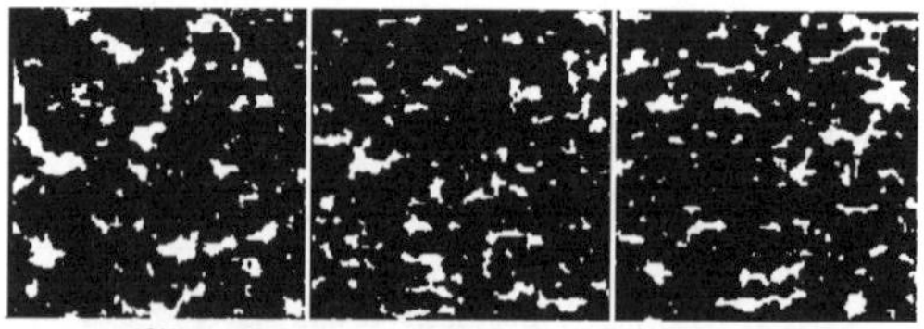

(f1) (f2) (f3)

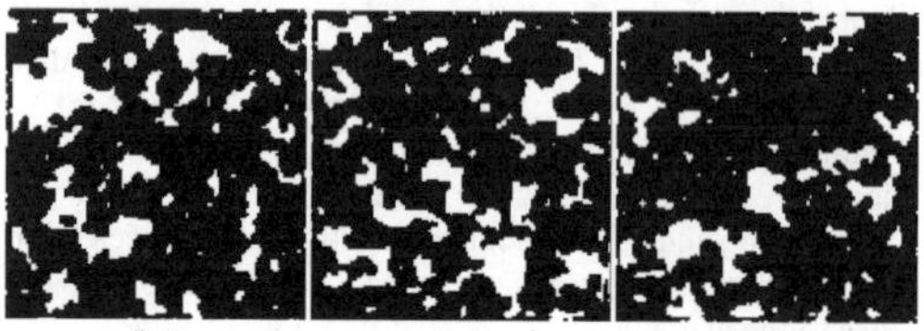

(b1) (b2) (b3)

Figure 6. 2D cuts through an unconditional 3D reconstruction of Fontainebleau sandstone (above, 200^3 pixels, 7.5 μm/pixel) and Berea sandstone (below, 128^3, 10 μm/pixel) with the slice porosities, ϕ indicated. (f1) XY plane (Z = 100, $\phi = 0.1356$), (f2) XZ plane (Y = 100, $\phi = 0.1110$), (f3) YZ plane (X = 100, $\phi = 0.1336$). (b1) XY plane (Z = 64, $\phi = 0.2051$), (b2) XZ plane (Y = 64, $\phi = 0.2045$), (b3) YZ plane (X = 64, $\phi = 0.1541$).

gave the optimum combination of CPU time, lack of noise and preservation of large features in the pore space.

4.2 *Unconditional 3D reconstruction*

Generating a 3D structure from 2D information is a challenging task. The training image and template were used and the multiple-point statistics in a 2D plane were rotated by 90 degrees around the principal axes in order to generate a 3D structure.

Figure 6 shows 2D cuts of 3D reconstructions of both sandstones without conditioning data. In order to suppress unrealistic noise and smooth the image, we applied post-processing as described in the Methodology section. We used the classical dilation and erosion, and then took additional erosion with a coefficient of 12 in order to adjust the porosity value. The noise is significantly reduced and characteristic structures of the void space are reasonably preserved after the processing. The porosity of each plane is decreased or increased slightly – however, it is not drastically changed.

4.3 *Conditional 3D reconstruction*

A part of the training image can also be used as conditioning data to generate a more realistic structure. Since more information is incorporated, a better reconstruction can be made. However, it is not always necessary because the amount of conditioning data from the training image is limited. For example, when

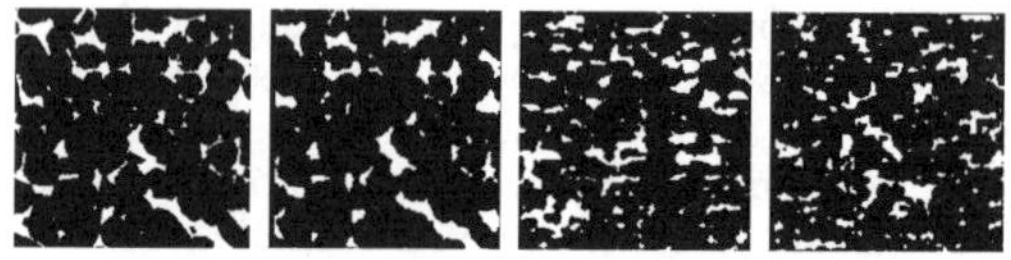

(f1) (f2) (f3) (f4)

Figure 7. 2D cuts for a conditional 3D reconstruction of Fontainebleau sandstone (200^3) after post-processing. (f1) XY plane (Z = 100, conditioning data, $\phi = 0.1376$). (f2) XY nearest conditioning plane (Z = 101, $\phi = 0.1347$). (f3) XZ plane (Y = 100, $\phi = 0.1525$). (f4) YZ plane (X = 100, $\phi = 0.1311$).

a 200^3 structure is generated with one plane as a constraint, the ratio of the number of conditioning data over that of total data points in the structure is 1/200, too small to make a significant difference to the quality of the final image. However, the constraints affect the reconstruction in the region near the conditioning data. Figure 7 shows a conditional 3D multiple-point reconstruction of Fontainebleau and its 2D slices after post-processing. This reconstruction took 37 hours CPU time with an Intel Xeon 1.7 GHz computer. Part of the 2D training image was used as conditioning data. It is evident from Figure 7 that near the conditioning data the quality of the image is good, and that typical pore shapes are more poorly reproduced away from the conditioning plane or in orthogonal directions. Isotropy is assumed in our reconstruction. However, more conditioning data such as several thin section images can be used as constraints and multi-orientation thin section images can provide more statistics when significant anisotropy is expected.

4.4 *Autocorrelation function and specific surface area*

The void-void autocorrelation function of the 3D microstructure is used in traditional two-point statistical reconstruction as one of the matching parameters. When the microstructure is defined by the binary phase function ($Z(r) = 1$ if r belongs to void space, $Z(r) = 0$ otherwise), the void-void autocorrelation function $R_Z(u)$ is defined by

$$\phi = \overline{Z(\vec{r})} \tag{4}$$

$$R_Z(\vec{u}) = \frac{\overline{[Z(\vec{r})-\phi][Z(\vec{r}+\vec{u})-\phi]}}{[\phi-\phi^2]} \tag{5}$$

where overbars denote statistical averages and u is a lag vector.

The autocorrelation functions of our sandstones are virtually identical in the three directions. Figure 8

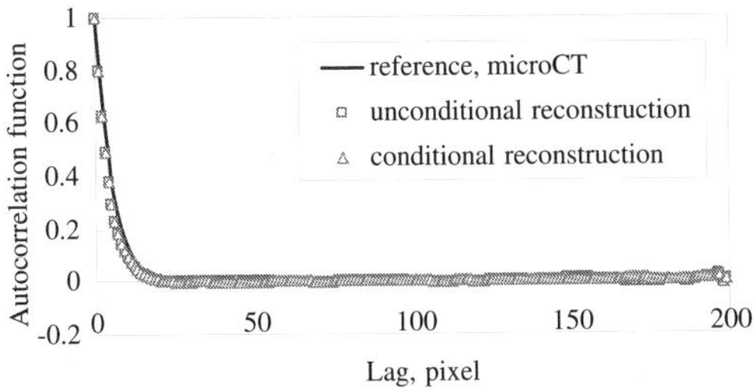

Figure 8. Void-void autocorrelation functions of Fontainebleau sandstone averaged over the three principal orthogonal axes. The results of the reconstructed structures after post-processing (unconditional: squares, conditional: triangles) are compared with that from the structure measured by microCT (line).

shows the autocorrelation functions of Fontainebleau sandstone averaged over three orthogonal directions compared to that measured on the reconstructed images. The agreement is excellent, demonstrating that the multiple-point statistical method preserves two-point statistics adequately. The autocorrelation functions of Berea sandstone are not shown here, but these are also identical.

When the reconstruction has same correlation function as the microstructure measured by microCT, both digitized 3D structures are expected to have same specific surface area defined by (Yeong & Torquato, 1998).

$$s = -6\left(\phi - \phi^2\right)\left.\frac{dR_z(u)}{du}\right|_{u=0} \tag{6}$$

The specific surface areas calculated from the measured microstructures are 0.122 for Fontainebleau, 0.188 for Berea, while the calculated average values for the reconstructed media are 0.145 and 0.191, respectively. The difference was due to noise in the images generated by the multiple-point reconstruction even after post-processing.

4.5 *Fraction of percolating cells in the reconstructed microstructure*

A key aspect of our reconstruction method is the possibility to reproduce long-range connectivity. Visual inspection of structures does not reveal the degree of connectivity. The traditional characteristics such as porosity, specific surface area and two-point correlation functions are also insufficient to distinguish different microstructures because they are all low-order information and relatively easy to reproduce. A quantitative characterization of the connectivity is provided by the local percolation probabilities or fraction of percolating cells (Biswal et al., 1998; 1999; Biswal & Hilfer, 1999; Manwart et al., 2000; Hilfer, 2002) defined by

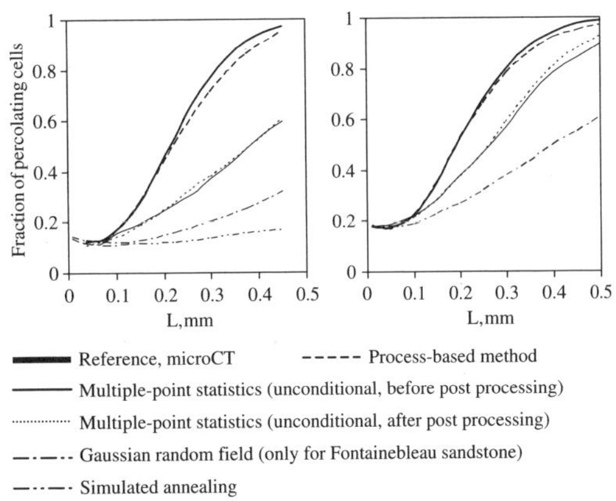

Figure 9. Fraction of percolating cells for images using different reconstruction methods. The left figure is for Fontainebleau and the right figure is for Berea. Notice that incorporating higher-order information in the reconstruction significantly improves the long-range connectivity of the pore space, although it still performs less well than process-based reconstruction methods. The data except multiple-point statistics and microCT are taken from (Biswal et al., 1999; Øren et al., 2003).

$$p_3(L) = \frac{1}{m}\sum_r \Lambda_3(r, L) \tag{7}$$

where m is the number of measurement and is an indicator of percolation.

$$\Lambda_3(r, L) = \begin{cases} 1 & \text{if } M(r, L) \text{ percolates 3 directions} \\ 0 & \text{otherwise} \end{cases} \tag{8}$$

A measurement cube $M(r, L)$ of sidelength L centered at position **r** is used to calculate the condition of continuous connectedness from one face to opposite face by percolation theory (Stauffer & Aharony, 1994). In 3D discretized media, 26 nearest neighbors are used to measure the pore connectedness. This property shows considerable difference between different reconstruction approaches. Figure 9 shows the reproduction of long-range connectivity by our method. The post-processing does not change the fraction of percolating cells. Although we show the result from one unconditional realization, the other two unconditional realizations and two conditional realizations gave essentially identical results. This figure also plots the fraction of percolating cells for Fontainebleau sandstone reconstructions using the Gaussian random field and simulated annealing, both which matched traditional low-order properties such as porosity and two-point correlation functions (Biswal et al., 1999). The results are also compared to process-based reconstruction by Øren et al.(1998). In Figure 9 the reference measured by microCT and the process-based method are similar but differ from those for samples generated using the Gaussian random field and simulated annealing. This figure shows that reconstruction methods based on the low-order correlation functions fail to reproduce the long-range connectivity of porous media, while the process-based method successfully reproduces the connectivity. Our multiple-point statistical method significantly improves the connectivity over two-point methods, although the pore space is still less well connected than the reference image.

5 CONCLUSIONS

A multiple-point statistics method using 2D thin sections to generate 3D pore-space representations of rocks has been validated in this paper. Fontainebleau and Berea sandstone were used for the study because their pore sizes are large enough to be captured by microtomography to provide reference datasets. Visual inspection of the images and the measurements of the fraction of percolating cells have confirmed the ability of the method to reproduce long-range connectivity, which is difficult to achieve using traditional two-point stochastic reconstructions.

ACKNOWLEDGEMENTS

The authors would like to express their gratitude to all the members of the Imperial College consortium on Pore-Scale Modeling (BHP, Enterprise Oil, Gaz de France, JNOC, PDVSA-Intevep, Schlumberger, Shell, Statoil, the U.K. Department of Trade and Industry and the EPSRC) for financial and technical support of our research. We thank David Stern (ExxonMobil) and Pål-Eric Øren (Statoil) for sharing the experimental data set with us.

REFERENCES

Adler, P.M., Jacquin, C.G. & Quiblier, J.A., 1990. Flow in Simulated Porous-Media. International Journal of Multiphase Flow, 16(4): 691–712.

Bakke, S. & Øren, P.E., 1997. 3-D pore-scale modelling of sandstones and flow simulations in the pore networks. SPE Journal, 2(2): 136–149.

Biswal, B. & Hilfer, R., 1999. Microstructure analysis of reconstructed porous media. Physica A, 266(1–4): 307–311.

Biswal, B., Manwart, C. & Hilfer, R., 1998. Three-dimensional local porosity analysis of porous media. Physica A, 255(3–4): 221–241.

Biswal, B., Manwart, C., Hilfer, R., Bakke, S. & Øren, P.E., 1999. Quantitative analysis of experimental and synthetic microstructures for sedimentary rock. Physica A, 273 (3–4): 452–475.

Blunt, M.J., Jackson, M.D., Piri, M. & Valvatne, P.H., 2002. Detailed physics, predictive capabilities and macroscopic consequences for pore-network models of multiphase flow. Advances in Water Resources, 25(8–12): 1069–1089.

Bryant, S. & Blunt, M., 1992. Prediction of Relative Permeability in Simple Porous-Media. Physical Review A, 46(4): 2004–2011.

Caers, J., 2001. Geostatistical reservoir modelling using statistical pattern recognition. Journal of Petroleum Science and Engineering, 29(3–4): 177–188.

Chen, S.Y., Wang, Z., Shan, X.W. & Doolen, G.D., 1992. Lattice Boltzmann Computational Fluid Dynamics in Three Dimensions. Journal of Statistical Physics, 68(3–4): 379–400.

Coehlo, D., Thovert, J.F. & Adler, P.M., 1997. Geometrical and transport properties of random packings of spheres and aspherical particles. Physical Review E, 55: 1959–1978.

Deutsch, C.V. & Journel, A.G., 1998. GSLIB: Geostatistical Software Library and User's Guide 2nd Edition. Oxford Univ. Press, Oxford.

Dullien, F.A.L., 1992. Porous Media: Fluid Transport and Pore Structure. Academic Press, San Diego.

Dunsmuir, J.H., Ferguson, S.R., D'Amico, K.L. & Stokes, J.P., 1991. X-ray microtomography. A new tool for the characterization of porous media, Paper SPE22860 proceedings of SPE Annual Technical Conference and Exhibition held in Dallas, Texas, October 6–9, 1991.

Hazlett, R.D., 1995. Simulation of Capillary-Dominated Displacements in Microtomographic Images of Reservoir Rocks. Transport in Porous Media, 20(1–2): 21–35.

Hazlett, R.D., 1997. Statistical characterization and stochastic modeling of pore networks in relation to fluid flow. Mathematical Geology, 29(6): 801–822.

Hilfer, R., 2002. Review on scale dependent characterization of the microstructure of porous media. Transport in Porous Media, 46(2–3): 373–390.

Ioannidis, M.A., Kwiecien, M.J. & Chatzis, I., 1997. Electrical conductivity and percolation aspects of statistically homogeneous porous media. Transport in Porous Media, 29(1): 61–83.

Kainourgiakis, M.E. et al., 2000. Structural and transport properties of alumina porous membranes from process-based and statistical reconstruction techniques. Journal of Colloid and Interface Science, 231(1): 158–167.

Levitz, P., 1998. Off-lattice reconstruction of porous media: critical evaluation, geometrical confinement and molecular transport. Advances in Colloid and Interface Science, 77: 71–106.

Liang, Z.R., Fernandes, C.P., Magnani, F.S. & Philippi, P.C., 1998. A reconstruction technique for three-dimensional porous media using image analysis and Fourier transforms. Journal of Petroleum Science and Engineering, 21(3–4): 273–283.

Lindquist, W.B., Venkatarangan, A., Dunsmuir, J. & Wong, T.F., 2000. Pore and throat size distributions measured from synchrotron X-ray tomographic images of Fontainebleau sandstones. Journal of Geophysical Research: Solid Earth, 105(B9): 21509–21527.

Lucia, F.J., 1999. Carbonate reservoir characterization. Springer, Berlin, Germany.

Manwart, C., Torquato, S. & Hilfer, R., 2000. Stochastic reconstruction of sandstones. Physical Review E, 62(1): 893–899.

Øren, P.E. & Bakke, S., 2002. Process based reconstruction of sandstones and prediction of transport properties. Transport in Porous Media, 46(2–3): 311–343.

Øren, P.E. & Bakke, S., 2003. Reconstruction of Berea sandstone and pore-scale modelling of wettability effects. Journal of Petroleum Science and Engineering, 39(3–4): 177–199.

Øren, P.E., Bakke, S. & Arntzen, O.J., 1998. Extending predictive capabilities to network models. SPE Journal, 3(4): 324–336.

Pilotti, M., 2000. Reconstruction of clastic porous media. Transport in Porous Media, 41(3): 359–364.

Quiblier, J.A., 1984. A New Three-Dimensional Modeling Technique for Studying Porous-Media. Journal of Colloid and Interface Science, 98(1): 84–102.

Russ, J.C., 1994. The image processing handbook, 2nd Edition. CRC Press, Boca Raton, Florida.

Serra, J., 1992. Image Analysis and Mathematical Morphology. Academic Press, New York.

Spanne, P. et al., 1994. Synchrotron Computed Microtomography of Porous-Media – Topology and Transports. Physical Review Letters, 73(14): 2001–2004.

Stauffer, D. & Aharony, A., 1994. Introduction to Percolation Theory, 2nd ed.

Strebelle, S. & Journel, A.G., 2001. Reservoir Modeling Using Multiple-Point Statistics. Paper SPE71324 proceedings of SPE Annual Technical Conference and Exhibition held in New Orleans, Louisiana, 30 September–3 October 2001.

Talukdar, M.S., Torsaeter, O. & Ioannidis, M.A., 2002. Stochastic reconstruction of particulate media from two-dimensional images. Journal of Colloid and Interface Science, 248(2): 419–428.

Yeong, C.L.Y. & Torquato, S., 1998. Reconstructing random media. Physical Review E, 57(1): 495–506.

X-ray CT for Geomaterials; Soils, Concrete, Rocks – Otani & Obara (eds.)
© 2004 Swets & Zeitlinger. Lisse, ISBN 90 5809 666 1

Fractal dimension analysis of shales using X-ray computer tomography

R.C.K. Wong
University of Calgary, Calgary, Alberta, Canada

M.C. Alfaro
University of Manitoba, Winnepeg, Manitoba, Canada

ABSTRACT: Shales are probably the most commonly encountered weak rocks on earth. However, there are many types of shales, depending on the fabric, structure, and composition. Quantification of shale type is of importance for engineering geology and geotechnical engineering. Standard geotechnical tests, such as index tests, sieve analysis, and XRD, are destructive methods. Computer tomography (CT) technique offers a viable non-destructive method providing information on the 3-D spatial distribution of the shale structure without sample retrieval. Fractal dimension analysis of the CT data of shale cores was proposed for classification shale types. Different types of cores (silty shale, clayey shale, and sandy silt) were used in this study.

1 INTRODUCTION

To understand the behaviour of any geomaterial, measurement of the geomaterial structure is essential. Geomaterial structure can be defined as the spatial arrangement of grain particles and pores. The configuration of grain particles and pores exerts a significant on the geomechanical properties of the materials. Most of engineering problems cannot be formulated and solved at the microscopic level due to the lack of information concerning the microscopic configuration of the interface boundaries between the grain particles and pores and at the grain contacts. In addition, such solution is usually, of no interest in practice. Thus, continuum model approach has been adopted in practical applications. Continuum models are built on the concept of representative elementary volume (REV). In addition, (REV) is always an important concern in laboratory testing, i.e., the minimum dimensions of the tested specimen yielding representative response of the tested material. This REV concept is introduced as a first step in passing from the microscopic level, at which we consider phenomena at every point within a phase, to the macroscopic level at which we associate with each point in space volume averaged quantities describing phenomena in its vicinity (Bear 1972).

Several researchers used fractal geometries to quantify soil structures (e.g., Bartoli et al. 1991; Brakensiek et al. 1992; Crawford et al. 1993). The fractal dimension (D) is the central concept of fractal geometry (Mandelbrot 1983). It is a real number calculated using a "box-counting method" to characterize irregular variations in a fractal object represented as a curve, surface or other configuration. The fractal D may have the potential to describe irregular spatial variations in soil structure.

Computer tomography (CT) scanning was used to quantify the internal structures of soil structures (e.g., Anderson et al. 1988; Wong 1999; Wong and Wibowo 2000). Anderson et al. (1990), Peyton et al. (1994), and Zeng et al. (1996) combined fractal dimension analysis and CT data to characterize soil structure. They showed that the CT data of soils were fractal. However, no study of REV using CT data was done. This paper demonstrates the use of fractal dimension analysis to estimate the size of REV for shale.

2 EXPERIMENTAL TECHNIQUE

2.1 *Samples*

The cores for this experimental study were recovered from a well (13-09-66-04) at a site near Cold Lake, Alberta, Canada. Core sampling was carried out using a conventional rotary core barrel of 89 mm inside diameter. Silty shale, clayey shale and locked

Table 1. Properties of tested samples.

Sample	Depth (m)	Porosity (%)	Plastic limit	Liquid limit	Clay content (%)	Fractal dimension
Locked sand	510	30	N/A	N/A	N/A	2.25
Silty shale	294	27	22	39	25	2.29
Clayey shale	294	27	26	110	55	2.33

sand cores were selected from three sections of 173–175 m, 199–201 m, and 490–492 m deep, respectively. Trimmed specimens of 89 mm in diameter and 90 mm in height was mounted inside a neoprene sleeve with two plastic end platens to prevent moisture loss. Table 1 summarizes some physical properties of the three tested samples. From the X-ray diffraction analysis, the dominant clay mineral is mixed-layer smectite-illite (about 75% smectite and 25% illite layers). There are some unmixed illite, chlorite, and kaolinite. The locked sand sample is composed of quartz mainly. The average grain diameter is about 0.170 mm. The grains are intocked at the contacts producing some apparent cohesion.

2.2 *Computer tomography (CT) scaning*

The CT scanner used in this study is General Electric Model Hi Speed CT/i. The settings were: 120 kV (KVP), 150 mA (X-ray tube current), 0.8 sec full rotation scan, and 25 cm FOV (field of view).

This study used a voxel size in the plane of a 3 mm slice was 0.25 mm by 0.25 mm. A 472 by 472 matrix of voxel data was obtained for each scan. To reduce beam-hardening effects around the edge of the core, a reduced size of 210 by 210 voxel matrix of data was used for fractal dimension analysis.

2.3 *Fractal dimension analysis*

An important property associated with fractal objects is "self-similarity". In a self-similar object, the entire object is composed of small copies of itself. Each of these small copies is made of even smaller copies. Thus, the fractal is a union of replicates at reduced scales. If a fractal is made up of N copies that are scaled by a reduced factor of L, and if the scaled copies do not overlap, then, the fractal dimension D is given by:

$$D = log[N(L)]/log(1/L) \tag{1}$$

"Box counting method" (BCM) was used in this study. This method involved counting the number of boxes required to cover the fractal object. Firstly, the minimum and maximum CT numbers were sorted from the data set of the cropped 210 by 210 voxel matrix for each CT scan. Then, the CT data of each set were scaled from 0 to 210. The scaled CT data formed a surface in a 3-D plot. In this plot, the horizontal x- and y-axes represent the locations of CT numbers whereas the vertical z-axis represents the scaled CT values. For 1-voxel side length box, there were 210^2 scaled CT data points in a 3-D space made up of 210^3 cubic boxes. For 2-voxel side length box, there were 105^3 cubic boxes. The number of boxes (N) required to cover the surface were counted. This process was repeated for a range of box side lengths (L). The fractal dimension was determined from Equation [1] or the slope of a plot of log[N(L)] versus log(1/L). Thus, D determined from this study is the surface fractal dimension.

3 RESULTS AND DISCUSSION

Figures 1 to 3 present plots of log[N(L)] versus log(L) for CT values obtained from the locked sand, silty shale, and clayey shale samples, respectively. In each plot was included the results of the linear regression analysis of the data set. For the three tested samples, the coefficient of regression increases when the data of voxel side length of less 1 mm were excluded. This illustrates that the samples are made of copies of "1-mm cubic boxes". Thus, the REV is 1-mm cube. For locked sand sample, the average grain diameter is 0.170 mm. A 1-mm cube contains about 6^3 or 216 grains. In an idealized cubic packing, the minimum number of grains in a REV is 8.

From Table 1 and Figures 1 to 3, the fractal dimension of the clayey shale sample ranks the highest, followed by silty shale and locked sand samples, respectively.

The fractal dimension D has been used for characterizing the roughness of object (Turcotte 1997). Surfaces having larger D appear rougher, or vary at a higher frequency. In this study, higher D infers the uniformity or homogeneity of the sample. Locked sand sample displays a more uniformity than the shale samples. This trend was also observed when the fractal dimension of each scan or slice was plotted against the sample length (Figure 4). The locked sample shows less variation along the sample length as compared to the other two shale samples.

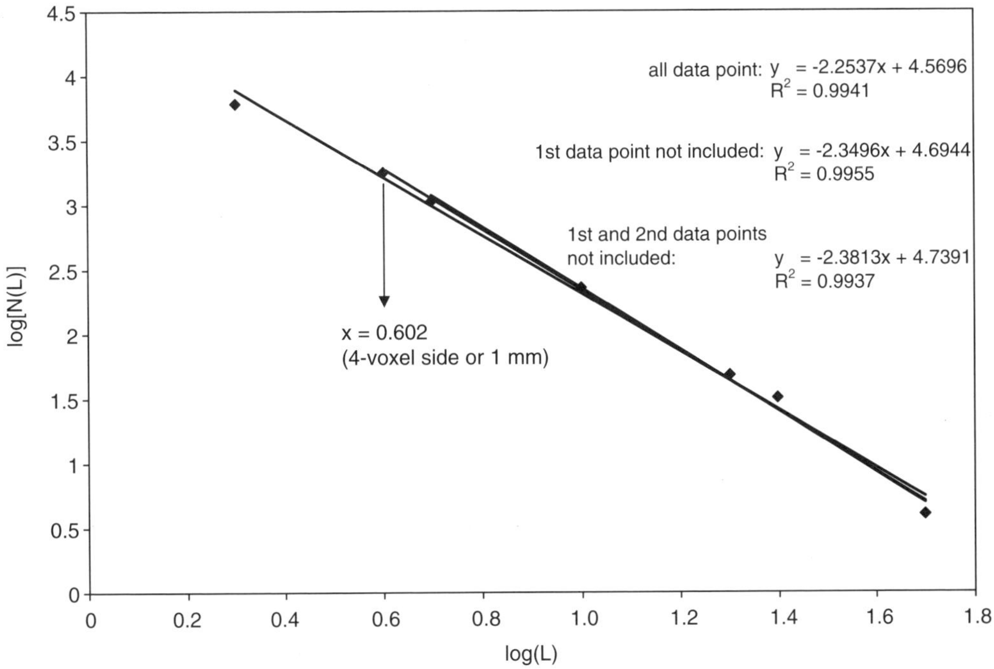

Figure 1. Fractal dimension analysis for locked sand.

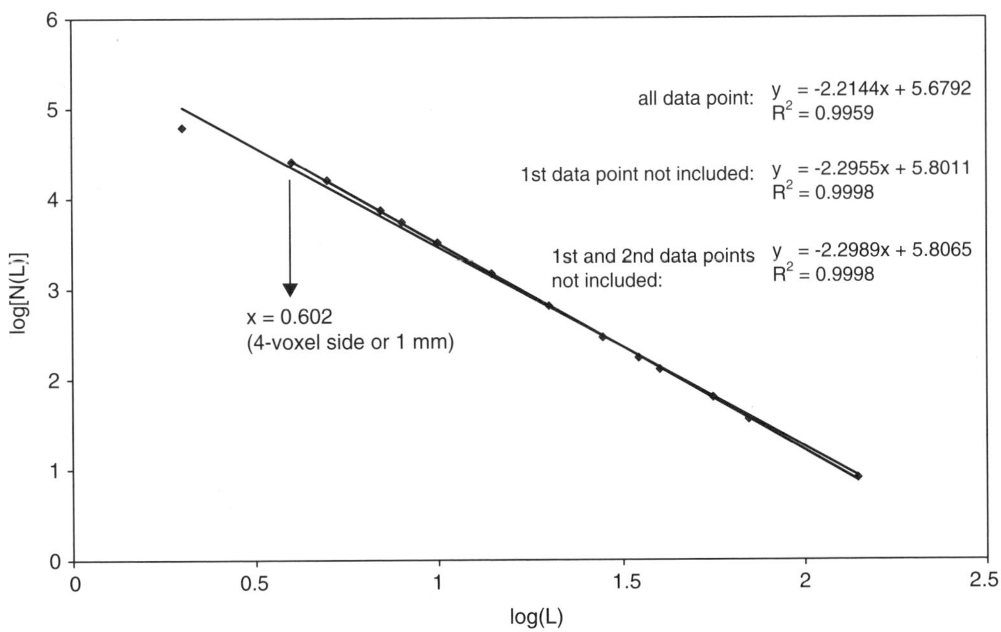

Figure 2. Fractal dimension analysis for silty shale.

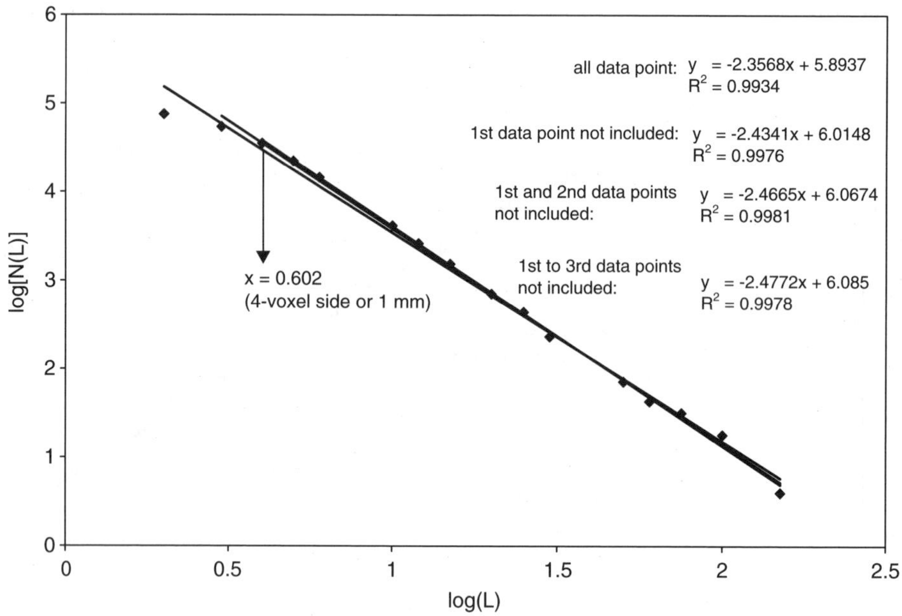

Figure 3. Fractal dimension analysis for clayey shale.

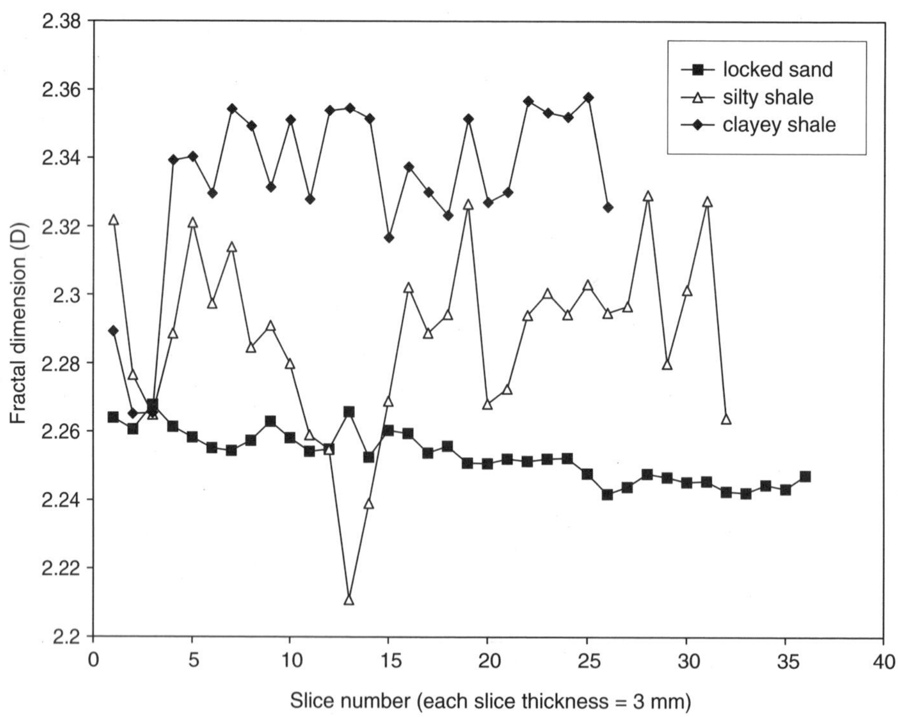

Figure 4. Fractal dimension versus sample length.

4 CONCLUSIONS

This study has demonstrated how the computer tomography (CT) data could be used to evaluate the uniformity of geomaterials from fractal dimension analysis. In addition, fractal dimension analysis can be served as a tool to determine the representative element volume (REV) of material.

ACKNOWLEDGEMENT

This study was funded by the Natural Sciences and Engineering Research Council (NSERC). Shale and locked sand specimens were supplied by Imperial Oil Canada. Alex Cheung conducted part of fractal dimension analysis.

REFERENCES

Anderson, S.H., Gartzer, C.J., Boone, J.M., & Tully, R.J. 1988. Rapid nondestructive bulk density and soil-water content determination by X-ray computed tomography. American Journal of Soil Science Society, 52: 35–40.

Anderson, S.H., Peyton, R.L., & Gartzer, C.J. 1990. Evaluation of constructed and natural soil macropores using X-ray computed tomography. Transport of water and solutes in macropores. Geoderma, 46: 13–29.

Bartoli, F., Philippy, R., Doririsse, M., Niquet, S., & Dubuit, M. 1991. Structure and self-similarity in silty and sandy soils: The fractal approach. Journal of Soil Science, 42: 167–185.

Bear, J. 1972. Dynamics of fluids in porous media. Elsevier, New York.

Brakensiek, D.L., Rawls, W.J., Logsdon, S.D., & Edwards, W.M. 1992. Fractal description of macroporosity., American Journal of Soil Science Society, 56: 157–172.

Crawford, J.W., Sleeman, B.D.S., & Young, I.M. 1993. On the relation between number-size distributions and the fractal dimension of aggregates. Journal of Soil Science, 44: 555–565.

Mandelbrot, B.B. 1983. The fractal geometry of nature. Freeman and Company, New York.

Peyton, R.L., Gartzer, C.J., Anderson, S.H., Haeffner, B.A., & Pfeifer, P. 1994. Fractal dimension to describe soil macropore structure using X-ray computed tomography. Water Research, 30: 691–700.

Turcotte, D.L. 1997. Fractals and chaos in Geology and Geophysics. Cambridge University Press, 398 pages.

Wong, R.C.K. 1999. Shear deformation of locked sand in triaxial compression. Journal of Geotechnical Testing, 23(2): 158–170.

Wong, R.C.K. & Wibowo, R. 2000. Tomographic evaluation of air and fluid flow patterns in soil columns. Geotechnical Testing Journal, 23(4): 413–422.

Zeng, Y., Gartzer, C.J., Peyton, R.L., & Anderson, S.H. 1996. Fractal dimension and lacunarity of bulk density determined with X-ray computed tomography. American Journal of Soil Science Society, 52: 35–40.

Rocks

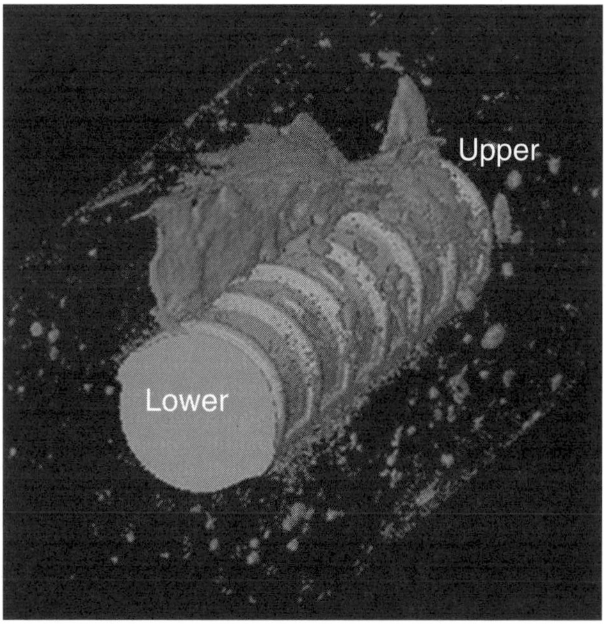

X-ray CT for Geomaterials; Soils, Concrete, Rocks – Otani & Obara (eds.)

Crack opening analysis by the X-ray CT image subtraction method

A. Sato
Faculty of Engineering, Kumamoyo University, Kumamoto Japan

D. Fukahori & K. Sugawara
Graduate School of Science and Technology, Kumamoyo University, Kumamoto Japan

ABSTRACT: A new method for the crack opening measurements of rocks by subtraction of X-ray CT images was proposed together with necessary noise reduction method, using the 3-dimensional data given by X-ray CT. This is a promising method to measure the crack opening from the difference of X-ray CT images. The characteristic point of the method is that the reduction and the elimination of fatal noise related to X-ray CT images are possible and that the accurate image processing is expected. The fundamental formulae for the crack opening measurement was firstly described as well as the necessary noise reduction technique and the data processing for the crack opening measurement. In this study, artificial cracks were simulated by a couple of semilunar shaped rock samples. In order to verify the applicability of the method to the heterogeneous materials, the rock samples were made by granite. The subtraction method was applied to the rock samples and the accuracy of the method was discussed. It was found that the influence of noises was clearly eliminated and that the crack opening distribution was accurately evaluated. It is also proved that the subtraction method is effective to the analysis of heterogeneous materials.

1 INTRODUCTION

X-ray computed tomography (CT) is well known as nondestructive medical imaging technique, which makes it possible to evaluate the attenuation of X-ray at each point within a body, by digitizing shadow pictures taken from various directions and subsequent image reconstruction. This technique has been applied for the measurements of geomaterial properties, such as soils and rock (Arthur, 1971; Verhelst et al., 1995). The migration of fluid fronts in rock has been studied by Cromwell et al. (1984), and the subtraction of CT images has been utilized to identify the water saturation process by Coles et al. (1991), Sugawara et al. (1999) and Sato et al. (2002). This technique has been also applied for evaluation of geometry of geomaterials. Sugawara et al. (1998) introduced crack projection method to evaluate crack opening and indicated that accurate evaluation of crack opening distribution is possible in the case that rock sample is relatively homogeneous. Through these studies, it has been revealed that X-ray CT is an effective tool for visualization and analysis geomaterial properties.

In this study, as a new method the X-ray CT image subtraction method for the crack opening measurements of rocks is proposed. Here, two images are constructed in the different conditions by X-ray CT. One is the condition that the inside of crack is filled with air and the other is the one filled with water. By subtracting two images, heterogeneity of rock mass can be eliminated and the information of crack can be clearly withdrawn. In the following, the fundamental formulae of the subtraction method for the crack opening measurement is firstly described as well as the necessary noise reduction technique and the data processing for the crack opening measurement, and subsequently the crack model experiments using a couple of semilunar shaped rock samples are performed in order to examine the accuracy of the method. Here granite is used as rock sample, and the accuracy and the applicability of the method to the heterogeneous materials, such as granite, are discussed.

2 X-RAY COMPUTED TOMOGRAPHY

2.1 *Principle*

The basis of formation of an X-ray CT image is the attenuation of X-rays transmitted through an object.

For one-dimensional case as shown in Figure 1, the attenuation of an X-ray beam is expressed by

$$i = i_0 \exp\left(-\int f ds\right) \tag{1}$$

where i is the intensity of the X-ray after passing through the object, i_0 is the intensity of the X-ray at source, s is the distance from the source, and f is the linear attenuation coefficient. This coefficient f is proportional to the density of the object in case that X-ray is monotonous.

By taking logarithms of Equation (1), a projection p is defined as

$$p = \ln\left(\frac{i_0}{i}\right) = \int f\, ds \tag{2}$$

From projections taken various angles of X-ray beam incidence, the filtered back projection method can be used to complete the linear attenuation coefficient at points within the object.

2.2 *X-ray CT scanner employed*

X-ray CT scanner (TOSCANER-23200) manufactured by the Toshiba Corporation is utilized in this study and major components of the scanner are schematically shown in Figure 2. An X-ray bulb operating at 300 kV/2 mA provides the radiation source from which an X-ray beam is emitted. One hundred and seventy six detectors are aligned with the X-ray source in the horizontal plane record attenuation data. The object for scanning is positioned on a traversing turntable and the X-ray beam is projected through one plane of the object as it rotates and traverses. The beam thickness can be determined with the collimators and the thickness is set to be 2 mm in this study. The X-ray source and detectors can be moved vertically with a specified interval and a three-dimensional radiographic density image is obtained if required. In the standard configuration, the pixel is a square of 0.293 mm × 0.293 mm, and the volume of a boxel is 0.1717 mm^3. Necessary time for photographing of one image is approximately five minutes. Sugawara et al.(1998, 2003) and Sato et al. (2002) have been conducted studies by same X-ray CT scanner and please refer the details of specifications and principles.

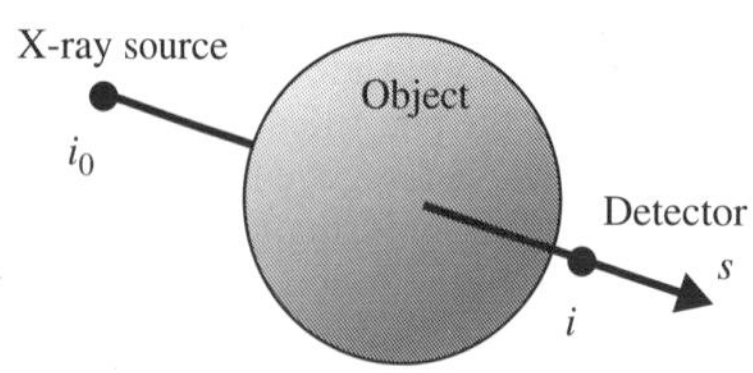

Figure 1. One-dimensional attenuation of X-ray beam.

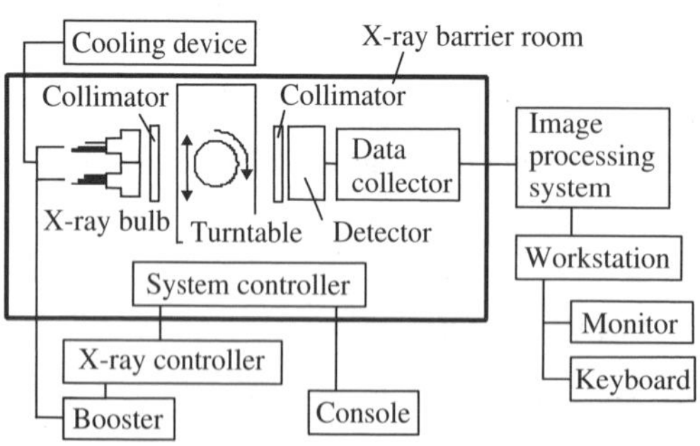

Figure 2. Composition of X-ray scanner employed.

3 THE X-RAY CT IMAGE SUBTRACTION METHOD

3.1 *Theory*

The X-ray CT image subtraction method is the method to evaluate crack opening distribution by subtracting several CT images. In this method, at least two images in different conditions are necessary, that is, the images that inside of crack is filled with different materials. Since the X-ray CT is the tool to visualize the density distributions, cracks should be filled with materials which have different density such as air and water. The information related to the crack opening can be withdrawn by subtracting these images, since the matrix of rock sample does not changed between two images.

Let us introduced the coordinate system as shown in Figure 3. A single crack exists in a material of which linear attenuation coefficient is $f_m(x)$. The origin of the coordinate system is located in the middle between crack surfaces. The x-axis is taken to be in the direction perpendicular to crack surfaces. Crack opening

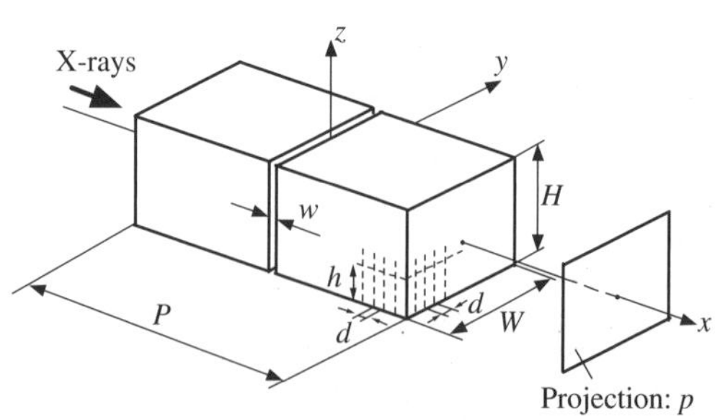

Figure 3. Analytical region including crack and coordinate system.

along x-axis is denoted by w and the position of both crack surfaces are $x = \pm w/2$. Here, it is assumed that the crack is filled with material α of which linear attenuation coefficient is $f_c^{(\alpha)}$. From equation (2), the projection along x-axis is given by

$$p^{(\alpha)} = f_m(x)\{P - w\} + f_c^{(\alpha)} w \tag{3}$$

where $p^{(\alpha)}$ is the projection in the case that inside of crack is filled with material α, and P is the length of the matrix in the x-axis direction. Here-in-after the superscript (α) represent the quantity when the inside of crack is filled with material α. Same as equation (3), the projection $p^{(\beta)}$ in the case that the crack is filled with material β of which linear attenuation coefficient is $f_c^{(\beta)}$ is also given by

$$p^{(\beta)} = f_m(x)\{P - w\} + f_c^{(\beta)} w \tag{4}$$

The subtraction method of X-ray CT images represents to take the subtraction between equation (3) and (4), and crack opening w is obtained by

$$w = \frac{p^{(\alpha)} - p^{(\beta)}}{f_c^{(\alpha)} - f_c^{(\beta)}} \tag{5}$$

As this equation (5) shows, the coefficient of attenuation of the matrix, $f_m(x)$, is not included in the equation and the crack opening is represented by the projections and coefficients of attenuation in the crack. That is, heterogeneity of the material can be eliminated by the subtraction method.

Generally X-ray CT image is given by so called CT value and equation (5) can be also expressed by CT values. The mean CT values of the material α and β are denoted by $C_c^{(\alpha)}$ and $C_c^{(\beta)}$, equation (5) is rewritten by

$$w = \frac{p^{(\alpha)} - p^{(\beta)}}{C_c^{(\alpha)} - C_c^{(\beta)}} \tag{6}$$

The projection $p^{(\alpha)}$ and $p^{(\beta)}$ are also expressed by CT values. Here the pixel numbers in the analytical region (Figure 3) in the x-, y- and z-axis directions are denoted by $\bar{P}$, $\bar{W}$ and $\bar{H}$, respectively. The number of pixels in the projection area is also denoted by $\bar{S}$ and given by

$$\bar{P} = \frac{P}{d},\ \bar{W} = \frac{W}{d},\ \bar{H} = \frac{H}{h},\ \bar{S} = \overline{WH} \tag{7}$$

where d is the length of the pixel side and h is the thickness of X-ray beam. Here pixel numbers $i = 1, 2, \ldots, \bar{P}$, $j = 1, 2, \ldots, \bar{W}$, $k = 1, 2, \ldots, \bar{H}$ are defined in the x-, y- and z-axis direction, respectively. The CT value at address (i, j, k) is denoted by $C^{(\alpha)}(i, j, k)$, the mean CT value at i, $g(i)$, is given by

$$g^{(\alpha)}(i) = \frac{\sum_j \sum_k C^{(\alpha)}(i,j,k)}{\bar{S}} \tag{8}$$

Same as equation (8), the mean CT value at i when the crack is filled with material β is given by

$$g^{(\beta)}(i) = \frac{\sum_j \sum_k C^{(\beta)}(i,j,k)}{\bar{S}} \tag{9}$$

The values $C^{(\alpha)}(i, j, k)$ and $C^{(\beta)}(i, j, k)$ take same value in the matrix of rock sample. From equations (8) and (9), the projection $p^{(\alpha)}$ and $p^{(\beta)}$ in equation (6) are given by

$$p^{(\alpha)} = \sum_i g^{(\alpha)}(i) d, \quad p^{(\beta)} = \sum_i g^{(\beta)}(i) d \tag{10}$$

3.2 *Correction of CT values in the crack*

As shown in equation (6), precise evaluation of absolute CT values in the crack is also necessary for estimation of crack opening. In the case the material α and β stated above are water and air, the difference of CT values between $C_c^{(\alpha)}$ and $C_c^{(\beta)}$ is defined as 1000. However, it is known that the measured CT values is influenced by density, size and shape of samples. Conditions of photographing, such as temperature, are also the factors which give influence to measured CT values. Therefore, appropriate correction of CT values is necessary. Here, corrected crack opening w_m is given by

$$w_m = \eta w \tag{11}$$

where η is correction coefficient. The evaluation of η is discussed in the following section.

4 NOISE ELIMINATION BY STACKING

X-ray CT is the method to visualize the distribution of density. However, X-ray CT images inevitably contain a lot of noises and the elimination of noises is indispensable for the analysis by X-ray CT images. Various kinds of image analysis methods to eliminate noises have been introduced (for example William (1978)), suitable procedure to construct X-ray CT images used for evaluation of crack opening is discussed in the following before applying the subtraction method.

The technique of stacking is commonly used as noise reduction method and the procedure of application to

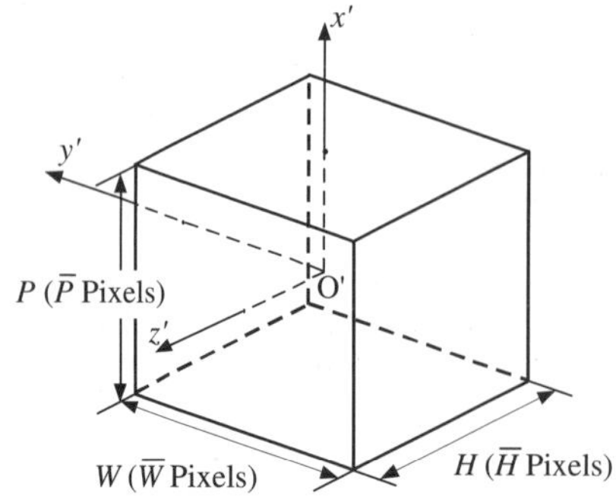

Figure 4. Cubic region for stacking.

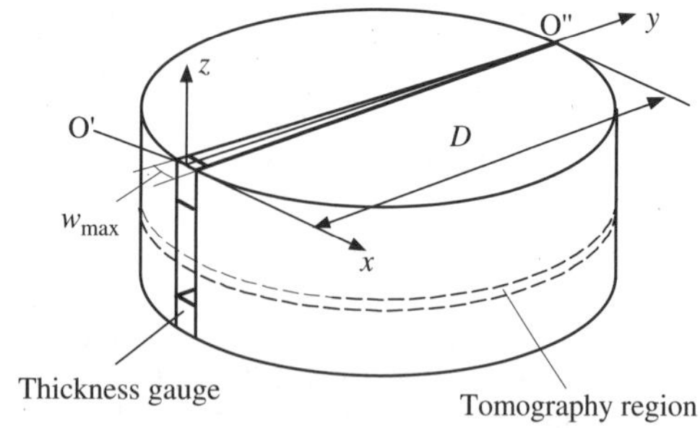

Figure 5. Geometry of rock sample.

X-ray CT images is discussed. As Figure 4 shows, cubic region is assumed and x'-, y'- and z'-axis are taken to be parallel to the each surface. The lengths in the x'-, y'- and z'-axis are denoted by P, W and H respectively, the numbers of the pixel along each axis $\bar{P}$, $\bar{W}$ and $\bar{H}$ are given by same relation as equation (7). Here also the addresses $i = 1, 2,\ldots, \bar{P}$, $j = 1, 2,\ldots, \bar{W}$, $k = 1,2,\ldots, \bar{H}$ are given to each pixel in the cubic region and each CT value at (i, j, k) is denoted by $C(i, j, k)$.

In the case that tomography is conducted n times at cross section k, it can be assumed that the measured CT value at l-th time $C_l(i, j, k)$ is divided into two components: the true CT value $C^0(i, j, k)$ and noise component $\Delta C_l(i, j, k)$, and given by

$$C_l(i,j,k) = C^0(i,j,k) + \Delta C_l(i,j,k) \tag{12}$$

By stacking n images, the mean CT value at (i, j, k), $C^*(i, j, k)$, is given by

$$C^*(i,j,k) = C^0(i,j,k) + \frac{1}{n}\sum_l^n \Delta C_l(i,j,k) \tag{13}$$

When the noise included in the CT images can be assumed to be random noise, the following relation is obtained.

$$\sum_l^n \Delta C_l(i,j,k) \approx 0 \qquad (n \to \infty) \tag{14}$$

Therefore, the noise component can be reduced by stacking plural images taken at same position in the same condition.

5 CRACK MODEL

In order to verify the accuracy of the subtraction method stated above, the crack opening measurement is conducted using semilunar shaped rock sample as show in Figure 5. The faces along the direction of diameter is assumed to be artificial crack surfaces. The thickness gauge is inserted into one end of artificial crack and linear crack opening distribution can be simulated. As Figure 5 shows, the origin of coordinate system (x, y, z) is taken at one end of the sample. The x-axis is taken in the direction perpendicular to the crack surfaces and y-axis is taken along the direction of crack surface. In this figure, w_{max} is the maximum opening of this crack and crack opening distribution is given by $w_s = w_{max}(1 - y/D)$. In this study, granite is used for rock sample as a heterogeneous material. The diameter of semilunar shaped rock sample is $D = 60$ mm and the maximum opening w_{max} is set to be 0.51 mm and 1.13 mm.

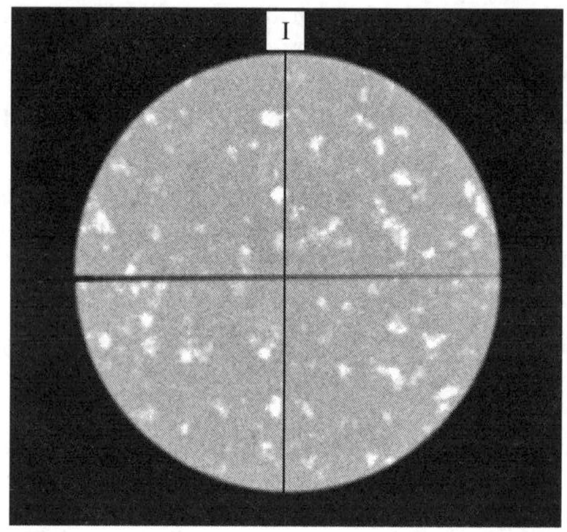

Figure 6. Single scan image of semilunar shaped sample.

6 NOISE REDUCTION

Figure 6 shows single scan image of rock sample. Here, inside of crack is filled with air. In this figure,

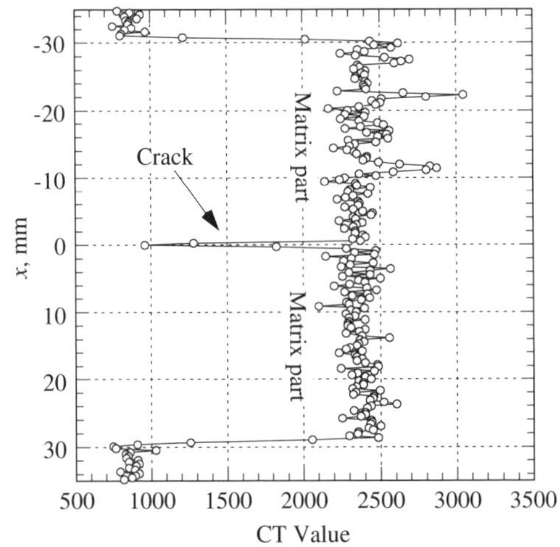

Figure 7. Distribution of CT values along line I (single scan image).

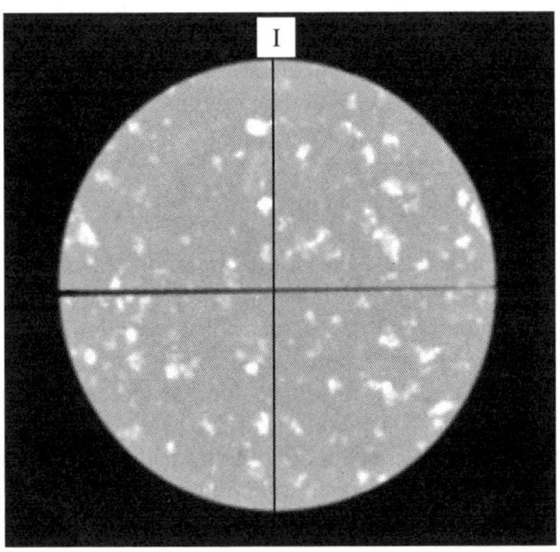

Figure 8. Reconstructed image by stacking.

relatively white parts represent the regions which have high density. Since the density of air is lower than rock, the existence of artificial crack can be easily visualized as dark region at the center of sample. Moreover, heterogeneity of granite is also confirmed. The distribution of CT value along line I is shown Figure 7. As this figure shows, the distribution of CT value is not continuous but scattered and it is confirmed that the CT image contains strong noise.

In this study, tomography was conducted 5 times at same cross section in the same condition. By applying stacking method stated above, a new image is reconstructed. The result is shown in Figure 8. It is found that the reconstructed image by stacking (Figure 8) is clearer than the single scan image (Figure 6). The

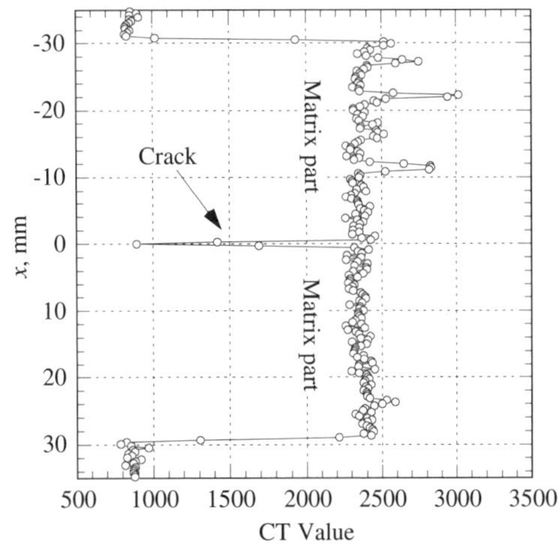

Figure 9. Distribution of CT value along line I (stacked image).

distribution of CT value along line I is also shown in Figure 9 and it is confirmed noise component is reduced by stacking. Therefore, stacking of images is useful method to reduce the noise component in the case that plural photographing by X-ray CT is possible. As for the crack opening measurements, state of crack is stable and this technique can be applied. However, more consideration is necessary when this stacking technique is applied to the visualization of transitional phenomena such as permeation process, since the nominal distribution of density is changing during photographing. As for the data analysis of transitional phenomena, please refer Sugawara et al. (1999) and Sato et al. (2002).

7 EVALUATION OF CRACK OPENING DISTRIBUTION

Two images are constructed in order to apply subtraction method. One is the case that inside of crack is filled with air (Figure 6) and another is the case that inside of crack is filled with water. An example of CT value distribution after image subtraction (along line I in Figure 8) is shown in Figure 10 and this procedure corresponds to the numerator in equation (6). As this figure shows, the value of $p^{(\alpha)} - p^{(\beta)}$ takes almost zero in the part of matrix and it is found that the heterogeneity of granite is almost canceled by the subtraction. The center of this figure represents information of crack opening and crack opening w_m is evaluated by allying this procedure along crack surfaces.

The crack opening distributions by subtraction method are shown in Figure 11, and the crack opening distributions obtained by crack projection method

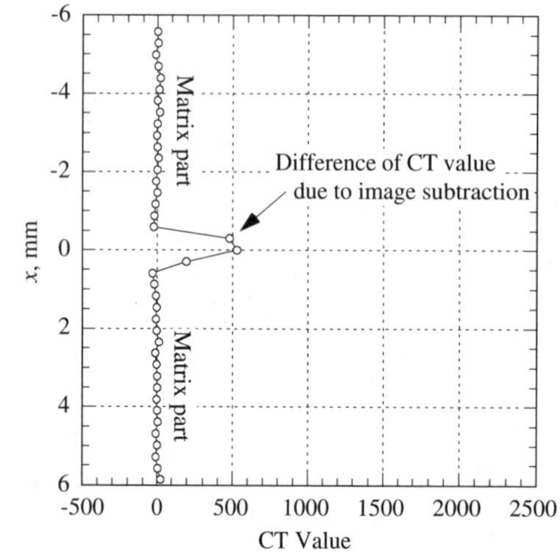

Figure 10. Distribution of CT value along line I after image subtraction.

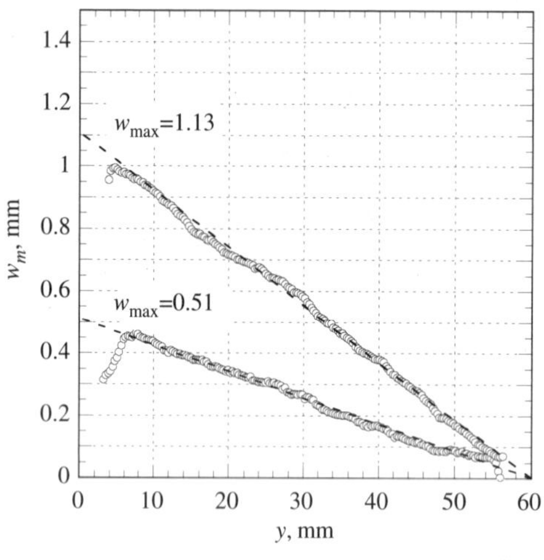

Figure 11. Result of rack opening distribution by X-ray CT image subtraction method.

are also plotted in Figure 12. As Figure 11 shows, obviously linear distribution can be obtained by the subtraction method and it is proved that subtraction between images is appropriate method to eliminate heterogeneity of the sample such as granite. The dotted line in Figure 11 represents the assumed crack opening distribution $w_s = w_{max}(1 - y/D)$. The correction coefficient η in equation (11) is evaluated in order to minimize the deviation σ_δ of measurement error $\delta = w_s - w_m$. The evaluated coefficient is $\eta = 0.86$ in the case of $w_{max} = 0.51$ mm, and this value is also apply to obtained the crack opening of $w_{max} = 1.13$ mm. Even though the resolution of X-ray CT is limited,

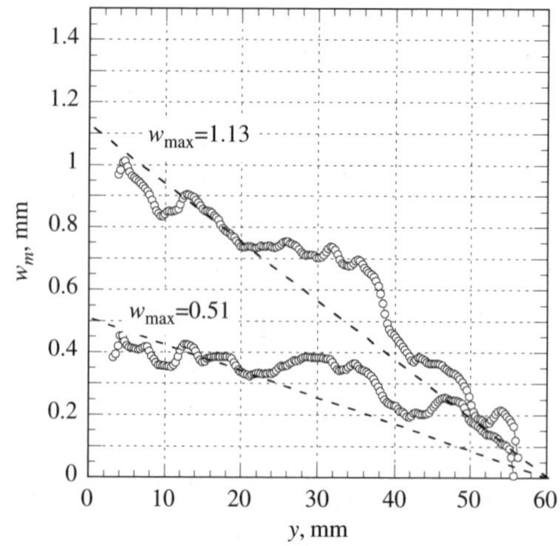

Figure 12. Result of rack opening distribution by crack projection method.

more accurate measurement of crack opening is possible by the suggested method. This result also indicates that the same correction coefficient η can be applied to the different crack opening distribution.

8 CONCLUSIONS

A new method for the crack opening measurements of rocks by subtraction of X-ray CT images was proposed together with necessary noise reduction method, using the 3-dimensional data given by X-ray CT. The fundamental formulae for the crack opening measurement was firstly described as well as the necessary noise reduction technique and the data processing for the crack opening measurement. The artificial cracks were simulated by a couple of semilunar shaped rock samples and the measurements of crack opening distribution were performed. By applying stacking method, it was found that influence of fatal noises included in reconstructed CT images was obviously reduced. The image subtraction method was applied to the reconstructed images and that the crack opening distribution was accurately evaluated. The evaluated crack distribution shows good agreement with the assumed crack opening, and it is proved that the subtraction method is effective to the crack opening measurements of heterogeneous materials.

REFERENCES

Arthur, J.R.E., 1971. New techniques to measure new parameters, *Proc. of Eoscoe Material Symp. on Stress-Strain Behavior of soils, Cambridge*, 340–346.

Coles, M.E., Muegge, E.L. and Sprunt, E.S. 1991. Application of CAT scanning for oil and gas production research, *IEEE Trans. Nucl. Sci.*, 38:510–515.

Cromwell, V., Kortum, D.J. and Bradley, D.J. 1984. The use of a medical computer tomography (CT) system to observe multi phase flow in porous media, *Soc. of Petroleum Eng., 13098, Soc. Petroleum Eng., Richardson, TX.*

Sato, A., Kubota, S., Kawaguchi, T., Ezoe, K., and Sugawara, K., 2002. Evaluation of permeability in rock by means of X-ray CT, *Proc. of ISRM Regional Symposium –3rd Korea-Japan Joint Symposium-, Korea,* 327–334.

Sato, A., Kubota, S., Kawaguchi, T., Ezoe, K., and Sugawara, K., 2002. Analysis of permeation process in rock by means of X-ray, Proc. of ISRM Int. Symp. Rock Engng. for mountainous regions, Portugal, 675–682.

Sugawara, K., Sato, A., Obara, Y. and Yanagisako, M. 1999. Measurement of permeability of rock by means of X-ray CT, *MMIJ*, 115, 11:803–808 (in Japanese).

Sugawara, K., Obara, Y. and Sato, A. 1999. Visualization of water saturation process in rock by X-rays CT, *'99 Japan-Korea Joint Symposium on Rock Engng. Fukuoka, Japan*, 503–508.

Verhelst, F., Vervoort, A., de Bosscher PH. and Marchal, G. 1995. X-ray computerized tomography, Determination of heterogeneities in rock sample, *Proc. of 8th ISRM Cong. Tokyo*, 1:105–108.

William K. Pratt, 1978. Digital image processing, Jon and Wiley & Sons, Inc. Chapter 12.

X-ray CT for Geomaterials; Soils, Concrete, Rocks – Otani & Obara (eds.)
© 2004 Swets & Zeitlinger. Lisse, ISBN 90 5809 666 1

An examination of aperture estimation in fractured rock

N. Yoshino
Maeda Co., Ltd., Japan

A. Sawada
Japan Nuclear Cycle Development Institute, Japan

H. Sato
Inspection Development Co., Ltd., Japan

ABSTRACT: Quantitative measurement of the spatial distribution of aperture is one of key factors for estimating representative values of fluid flow and transport properties in fractured rock masses. The representative values of these properties are used as input data for numerical modeling, such as a parallel plate fluid flow model. However, there are many difficulties for obtaining the spatial distribution of aperture for this purpose, due to an extremely large aspect ratio, which is the ratio of spatial extent of fracture to aperture. It has been accepted that aperture can be estimated by measuring topography of each side of the fracture surface after opening a fracture. However, this method is difficult to reproduce the initial aperture distribution since fracture aperture distribution might be changed significantly by differences of a few conditions to match two fracture surface data. Therefore, we tried to apply the conventional X-ray Computed Tomography (X-ray CT) to an artificial fracture in 10 cm granite rock block in order to check its applicability to measure actual aperture distribution. In addition, the topography of the fracture surfaces in the artificial fracture was evaluated by using three dimensional measuring apparatus which has a contact sensor (3-D sensor) and representative hydraulic properties were evaluated by the permeability tests. By comparing the aperture data by conventional X-ray CT method with those estimated from topographic data and hydraulic test data, we sorted out two major issues which should be solved, as follows; (1) Noise of CT data, which might be caused mainly by a heterogeneous distribution of rock minerals, and (2) minimal resolution of CT data.

1 INTRODUCTION

The hydrological, mechanical and geometrical properties of rock fractures are strongly affected by the aperture distribution. Various methods to estimate the fracture aperture have been reported (ex, Hakami 1995, Esaki et al. 2000). One of the most popular methods is measuring the topography of each side fracture surface after opening single fracture. However, it is difficult to reproduce initial aperture distribution since fracture aperture distribution might be changed significantly by differences of a few conditions to match upper and lower fracture surface data. The other method is direct measurement of fracture aperture at cross sections by slicing the rock samples. This method has advantage of measuring the exact aperture at each sliced surface, however this has disadvantage that it is difficult to measure all spatial data of the rock samples due to the minimum spacing of the slice.

Non-destructive inspection method such as the X-ray Computed Tomography (X-ray CT), Magnetic Resonance Imaging (MRI) and so on, is one of potential methods for measuring aperture, judging from various advantages, continuous measurement in space and measurement under the non-disturbed conditions. X-ray CT developed in the medical field is the inverse analysis method to visualize inside human body. Recently, this method is used not only in the medical field but also in the civil engineering and geological field (Sugawara et al. 1997, 1998). Authors tried to measure the aperture distribution of single fracture in the granite rock sample by using the conventional X-ray CT method to check its applicability and sort out the significant issues of application. Fracture surface topography of the rock sample were evaluated by using three dimensional measuring apparatus which has contact sensor (3-D sensor), and hydraulic properties of the fracture was also evaluated by steady state hydraulic tests, before measuring granite aperture distribution by the X-ray CT. In this paper, these data are used as the reference data for characterizing fracture surface geometry and hydraulic properties to compare with data obtained from the X-ray CT method.

As a result, we identified two main technical issues to be solved in estimation of the fracture aperture using X-ray CT.

2 SPECIFICATION OF X-RAY CT USED IN THIS STUDY

Conventional medical X-ray CT (Asteion: Toshinba Medical Co., Ltd.) was applied to scan the fracture aperture in this study. Table 1 shows the specification of this X-ray CT.

3 DETAILS OF THE TEST

3.1 *Basic properties of specimen*

A 10 cm cubic granite rock block was used as specimen in this study. It has a single artificial fracture at the middle of its height. (See Figure 1) The fracture was artificially applying compression with the edge of specimen. A 10 cm block size was chosen based on 1) almost the minimum size to study the effect of heterogeneous aperture distribution on hydraulic and tracer test and 2) almost maximum size to measure the aperture distribution using the conventional medical X-ray CT. The gouge, small fragments of rock mass caused by generating artificial single fracture, in the fracture was swept out to keep the aperture steady magnitude during a series of the examination. In this paper, the X, Y and Z axis are defined as shown in Figure 1.

Table 1. Specification of X-ray CT used in this study.

Scan time	0.5, 0.75, 1.0, 2.0, 3. 0 sec.
Reconstruction time	Min. 1 sec.
Helical scan	
Scan time	0.75, 1.0, 1. 5 sec./rotation
Continues scan time	Max. 100 sec.
Run length	Max. 139 cm.
Real time reconstruction	12 frames/sec.
X-ray tube	
Heating capacity	4.0 MHU
Cooling rate	Max.864 kHU/min.
Voltage	80, 100, 120, 135 kV
Current	30 to 300 mA
X-ray detector	Solid state, 896 channels × 22 rows
Data acquisition	896 channels × 2 slices
Slice thickness	0.5, 1, 2, 3, 4, 5, 8, 10 mm
Field of view	180, 240, 320, 400, 500 mm
Magnetic disk	
Raw data	4,000 rotations
Image data	8,000 slices
Magneto-optical disk(2.6 GB)	Raw data 1,200 rotations or image data 9,600 slices
Gantry aperture	720 mm diameter
Gantry tilt	±30 degree
Constant study control	Sure Start
On console color 3D	Standard

3.2 *Three-dimensional measuring apparatus*

Fracture surface topography was measured by the three dimensional measurement apparatus (BRIGHT710: MITSUTOYO Co., Ltd.) which has contact sensor using 1 mm diameter ruby ball at the tip of the sensor (see Figure 2). The accuracy of the three dimensional measurement apparatus ranges between 3 and 6 μm along the Z axis. The sampling interval in X–Y space parallel to the fracture surface is 1 mm in orthogonal lattice. The aperture was defined by the following procedure. Each height described in Figure 2, C1: the height of upper piece, C2: height of lower piece and A: height of the rock sample were measured, independently. The aperture, $B_{3D}(x,y)$, is calculated by:

$$B_{3D}(x,y)=A(x,y)-\{C1(x,y)+C2(x,y)\} \quad (1)$$

In this procedure, we put simple assumptions as:

- no mismatch in X–Y space of rock,
- no inclination of specimen (specimen was exact cubic block),

in facing upper piece and lower piece, because there are no objectively satisfied method to confirm these effects.

3.3 *Constant head hydraulic test*

Constant head hydraulic test was conducted to evaluate the representative hydraulic properties of the fracture. Figure 3 shows the system of hydraulic test. The fracture edge of specimen was sealed by the plastic plate glued by silicon material to avoid water leak

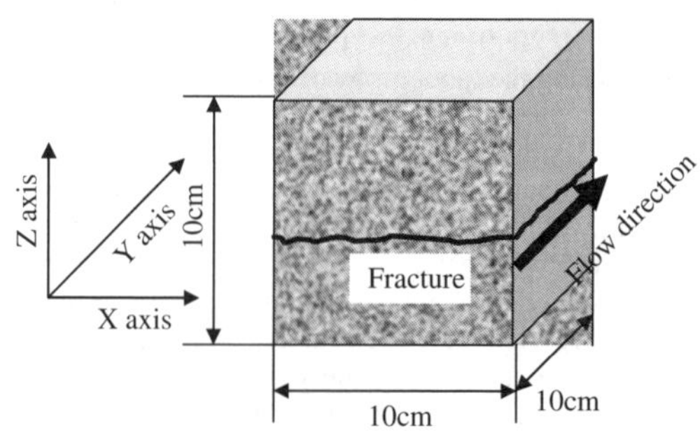

Figure 1. The specimen used in this study.

from the specimen during hydraulic test. Head value was measured by manometer at injection and withdrawal points. Flow rate at withdrawal point was automatically measured by the electrical balance meter.

3.4 *Estimation of fracture aperture using X-ray CT*

Epoxy resin (Sikadua52 normal type: SIKA Co.,Ltd.) was injected into the fracture in order to fix the aperture distribution before X-ray CT scanning. The properties used in the X-ray CT is called CT value which defined by Equation 2.

$$CTvalue = (\mu_t - \mu_w) \times K / \mu_w \tag{2}$$

where μ_t is the sample-representative linear attenuation coefficient, μ_w is the water representative linear attenuation coefficient, K is the proportional coefficient. We substitute 1000 to K in this study. Generally, CT value is proportional to the sample density. The density of granite rock and resin were approximately 2. 7 g/cm^3 and 1 g/cm^3, respectively. CT values obtained from each scanning are consisted with 512 × 512 pixel values (see Figure 4). If x and z axis length of the target area are 15 cm, the resolution of 1 pixel becomes 0.293 cm. The pitch of scanning point along y axis was set to 1 mm because the result was able to be compared with that from 3-D sensor. The variability of the CT value was affected by the scanning configurations. Generally, the larger the electrical voltage and electrical current become, the smaller the variability will be. Then 135 kV as electrical voltage and 220 mA as electrical current, which are close to the upper limitation of applied medical X-ray CT machine, were adapted in order to minimize the CT value noise. The scanning time was set to 3 second, which is also maximum configuration.

Figure 5 shows an example of CT values obtained in this examination along Z direction. An average CT value of the granite matrix is about 2000 and this value varies between 1000 and 3000. CT value at the fracture filled by lower density material compared with rock matrix became smaller than the other area. From Figure 5, it could be identified where fracture is. Additionally, it might be possible to estimate fracture

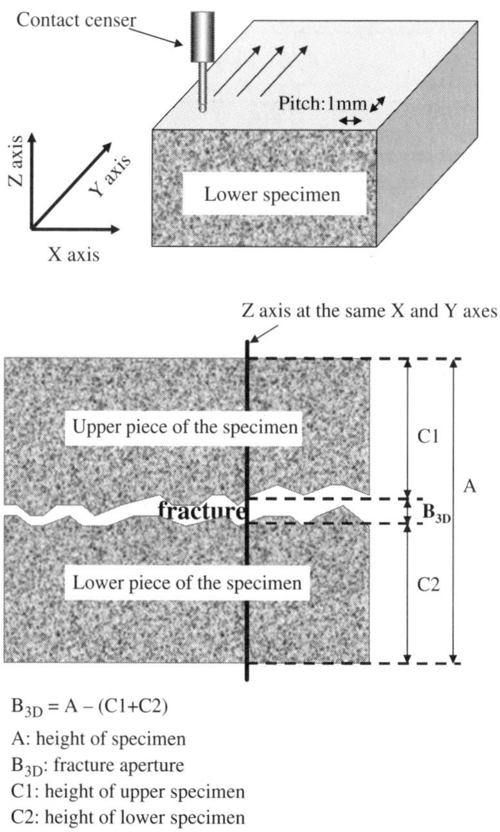

Figure 2. The procedure to define the aperture using three dimensional measurement apparatus.

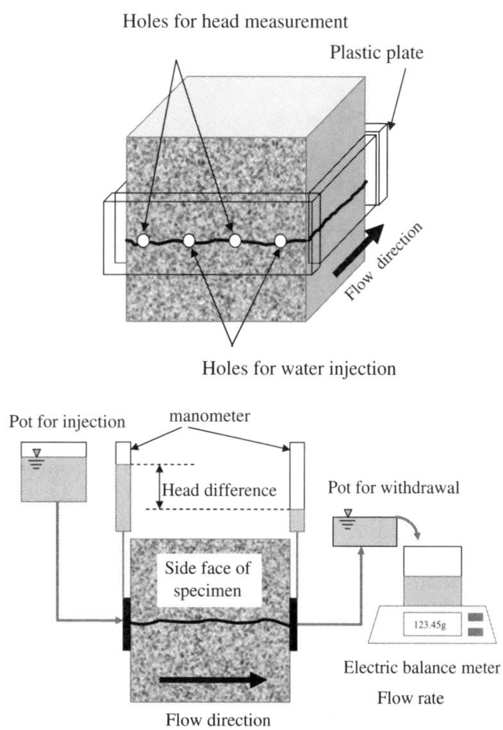

Figure 3. The hydraulic test system.

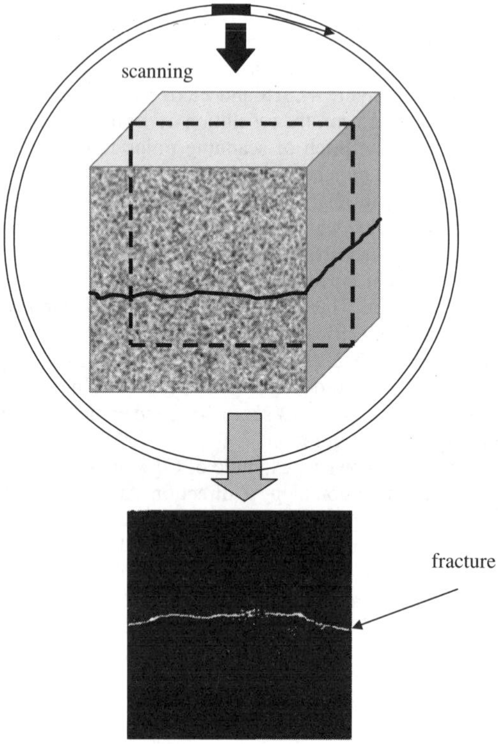

Figure 4. An example of scanning granite rock by X-ray CT.

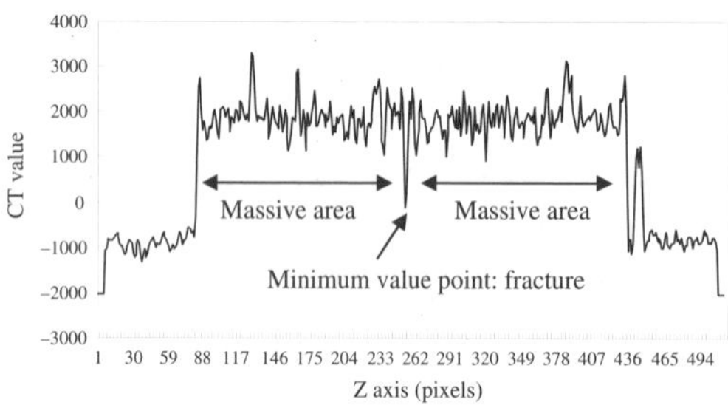

Figure 5. An example of CT value along Z axis.

aperture from this data. However, there are some difficulties to identify the interface between rock matrix and fracture, due to noise of CT value. To simplify the procedure, in this paper, we put a assumption that the boundary between rock matrix and fracture is 1000 CT value by considering difference of average CT value between rock matrix and fracture filling resin estimated from average density of each. Figure 6 shows schematic illustration to identify the boundary between the rock matrix and fracture, and to estimate the fracture aperture, B_{CT}.

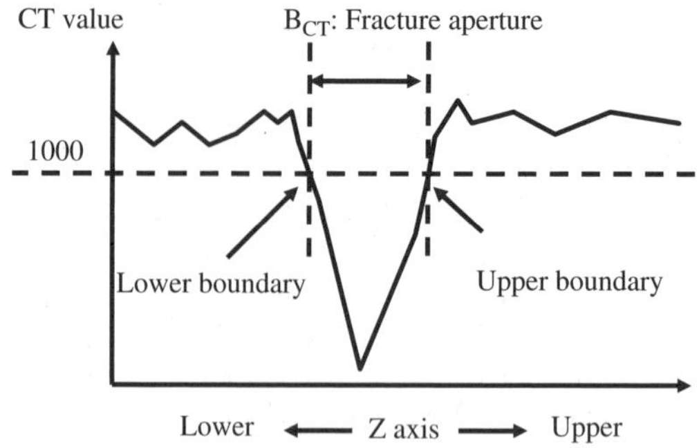

Figure 6. Boundary definition between the rock matrix and fracture in this paper.

Table 2. The result of hydraulic test.

Hydraulic gradient	1.1	1.8	2.7
Flow rate (m^3/sec)	4.32e−7	6.88e−7	9.12e−7
Transmissivity (m^2/sec)	3.93e−5	3.82e−5	3.38e−5
Hydraulic aperture (mm)	0.364	0.360	0.346

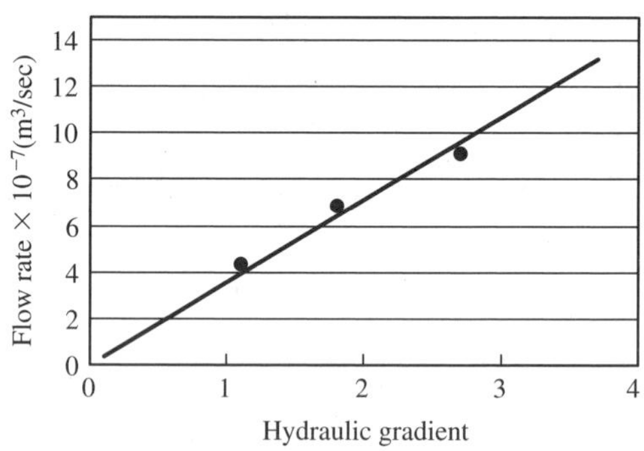

Figure 7. The relationship between hydraulic gradient and the flow rate.

4 RESULTS AND DISCUSSION

4.1 *Hydraulic test result*

Table 2 shows the result of the hydraulic tests. And Figure 7 shows the relationship between hydraulic gradient and the flow rate. There was linear relationship between them. Then the hydraulic property in the target fracture could be assumed to obey the cubic law (Snow 1965, Bianchi 1968). The representative transmissivity is about 3.5×10^{-5} (m^2/sec) and representative hydraulic aperture defined by Equation 3 is about 0.36 mm.

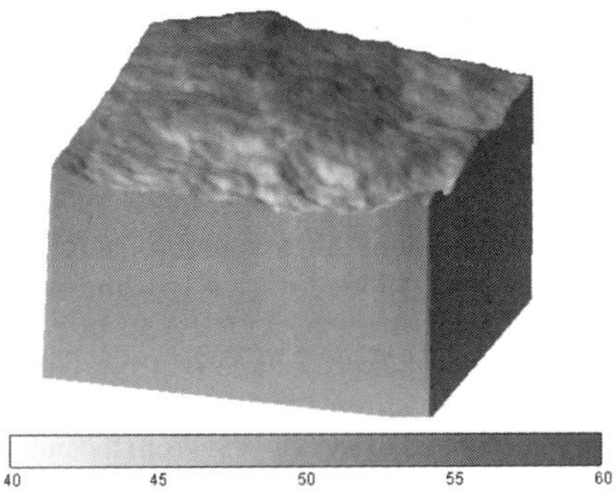

Figure 8. Fracture topography of upper piece derived from the result of 3-D sensor.

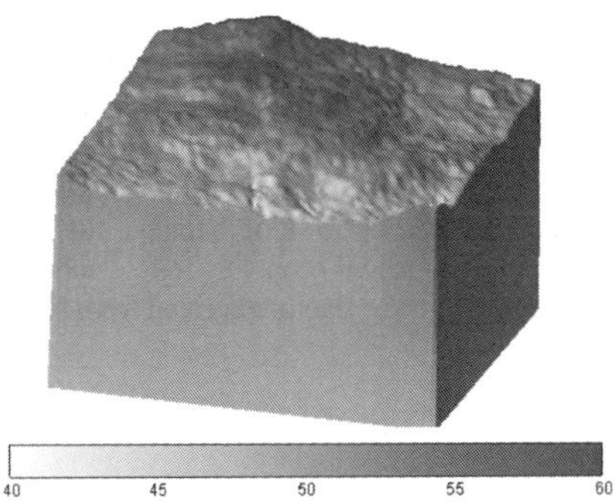

Figure 9. Fracture topography of upper piece derived from the result of X-ray CT.

$$B_H = \left(\frac{12\mu}{\rho g} \frac{L}{W} \frac{Q}{\Delta h} \right)^{\frac{1}{3}} \quad (3)$$

where μ is coefficient of viscosity, ρ is water density, g is gravity acceleration, L is the length of water flow, W is the width of fracture, Q is the flow rate, Δh is the hydraulic head difference.

4.2 *Comparison of fracture topography*

From Figure 8 to Figure 11 show the results of the fracture topography measured by 3-D sensor and X-ray CT. These results seem to be almost same shape between the topographies derived from 3-D sensor and X-ray CT. However, the result of X-ray CT seems to be more serrate shape comparing with smooth shape of one of 3-D sensor. Granite consists of several minerals which have different density (see Table 3). Then this result might be due to the noisy data of CT values which might be caused mainly by heterogeneous distribution of rock minerals. On the other hand, minimum resolution of CT data (the scale limitation of one pixel) might express this result.

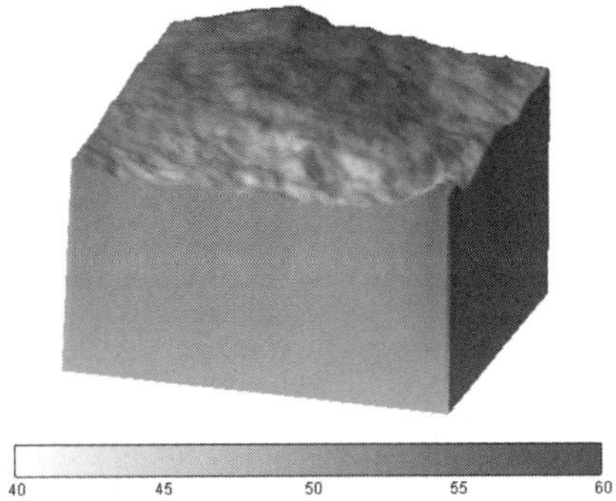

Figure 10. Fracture topography of lower piece derived from the result of 3-D sensor.

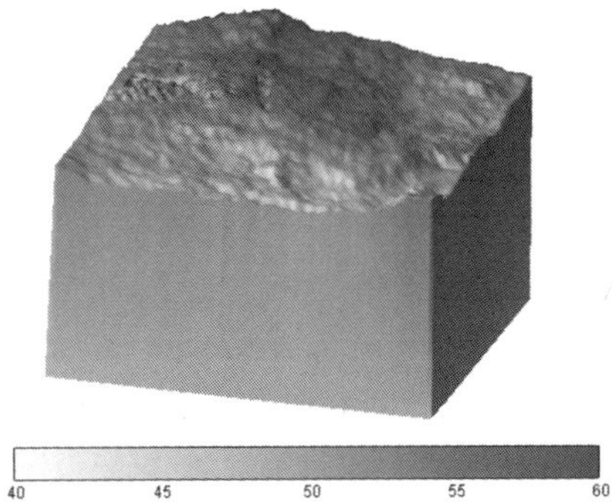

Figure 11. Fracture topography of lower piece derived from the result of X-ray CT.

Table 3. The density of granite minerals.

Mineral	Density (g/cm^3)	Average structure ratio (%)
Quartz	2.65	30
Orthoclase	2.55	30
Plagioclase	2.6–2.8	20
Biotite	2.8–3.4	10
Amphibole	2.9–3.6	10

4.3 *Comparison of the fracture aperture*

Figure 12 and Figure 13 show the estimated results of the fracture aperture. B_{CT} has larger variability than the B_{3D}. This can be identified by scattered white spots in Figure 13. Figure 14 shows the histogram of B_{3D} and B_{CT} distribution. Generally, fracture aperture distribution is described by log normal. The distribution of B_{3D} seems to obey the log normal distribution. However, the distribution of B_{CT} is truncated under $10^0 = 1.0$ mm. In addition, there are more contact areas in B_{CT} than B_{3D}. This is mainly caused by that the

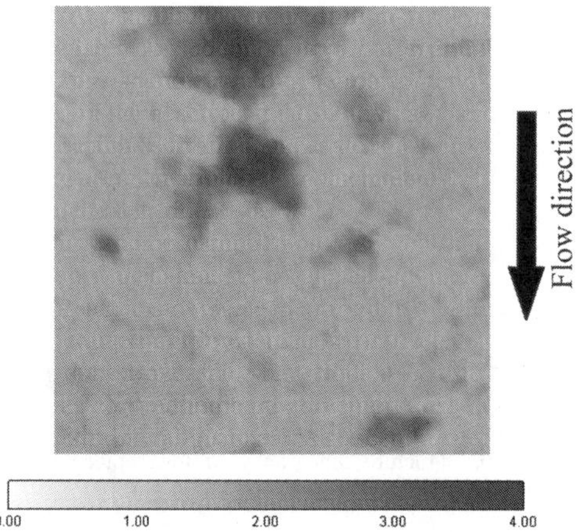

Figure 12. The fracture aperture (B_{3D}) derived from 3-D sensor.

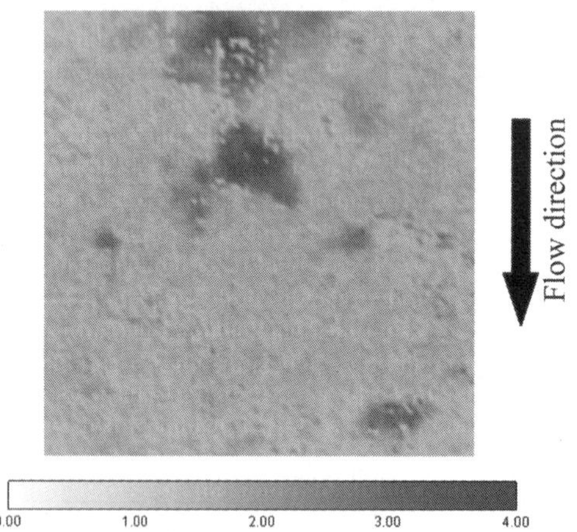

Figure 13. The fracture aperture (B_{CT}) derived from the result of X-ray CT.

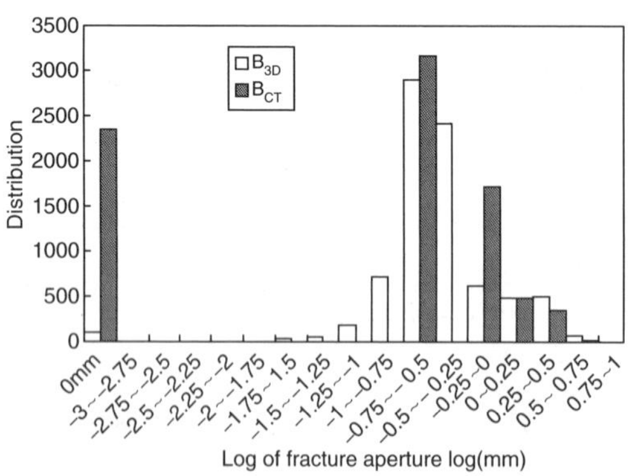

Figure 14. The histogram of B_{3D} and B_{CT}.

minimum resolution of CT data is coarser than one of 3-D sensor.

4.4 *The hydraulic property*

With assuming cubic law aperture and Darcy's law, numerical calculations have done by using MAFIC code (Miller et al. 1988) for each B_{3D} and B_{CT} data, respectively. Local trasmissivity T(x,y) at each 1 m scale finite element were estimated from cubic law. Same boundary conditions as the hydraulic tests were applied, as described in section 3.3. From the numerical calculations, representative hydraulic transmissivity was evaluated to compare with hydraulic test results.

The representative transmissivity by the numerical simulations using B_{3D} data is about $4.0 \times 10^{-5} m^2/sec$ which is similar to the value obtained from hydraulic test results. This means that the aperture distribution derived from the 3-D sensor could represent the hydraulic properties from the point of fracture aperture distribution view. On the other hand, the representative transmissivity by the numerical simulations using B_{CT} data is close to zero value because the data has much contact areas and it seems to be few connectivity for the water flow in the fracture derived from X-ray CT.

5 CONCLUSION

In this study, we examined an applicability of the conventional medical X-ray CT for estimating the fracture aperture in crystalline granite rock quantitatively, with comparing aperture distribution estimated from the topographic measurement at each fracture surface by 3-D sensor, and with comparing representative hydraulic transmissivity value between one from hydraulic tests and numerical simulation by using estimated aperture value in space from X-ray CT and 3-D sensor, respectively.

The aperture data estimated from the result of 3-D sensor was able to reproduce hydraulic tests results. But, aperture data estimated from X-ray CT data was not. Following two key issues for applying conventional X-ray CT method to measuring fracture aperture for evaluating hydraulic properties were provided and identified by the examination of obtained data.

1. Noise of CT data, which might be caused mainly by heterogeneous distribution of rock minerals
2. Minimum resolution of CT data.

In the next step, we will try to improve above these issues.

ACKNOWLEDGEMENTS

This research was conducted at Japan Nuclear Cycle Development Institute (JNC) by using X-ray CT.

Authors gratefully acknowledge to the suggestion and support by staffs of System Analysis Group in Waste Isolation Research Division in Tokai Works in JNC, especially to Masahiro Uchida and Koichiro Hatanaka. Authors also express special thanks to Kenji Tanai and Kazuhiro Matsumoto for the support of X-ray CT scanning.

REFERENCES

Bianchi, L. Snow, D. 1968. Permeability of crystalline rock interpreted from measured orientations and apertures of fractures, *Annu. Arid Zone*, 8(2), 231–245.

Esaki, T., Jinno, K., Mitani, Y., Jiang, Y., Uchida, U., Yoshino, N. 2000. Experimental and analytical Research on Shear-Flow Coupling Mechanism in Rock Joints Heisei13 progress report for the precedence-foundation engineering field-, *JNC Technical Report*, JNC TY8400 2001-005.

Hakami, E. 1995. Aperture Measurement and Flow Experiments on a Single Natural Fracture, Aperture Distribution of Rock Fractures *(Doctoral Thesis), Division of Engineering Geology Department of Civil and Engineering Royal Institute of Technology Stockholm*, Sweden.

Miller, I. Lee, G., Dershowitz, W. 1988. Mafic matrix/fracture interaction code with heat and solute transport user documentation version 1.6, *user documentation*, Golder associates Inc, Seatle WA.

Snow, D. 1965. A parallel plate model of fractured permeable media, *University of California, Berkely, Ph.D*, pp 329–331, (1965).

Sugawara, K., Kojima, R.K., Obara, Y., Satou, A., Shimada, H. 1998. Crack Opening Analysis by means of the X-rays CT. *Shigen-to-Sozai*. Vol. 114881–887.

Sugawara, K., Obara, Y., Kaneko, K., Koike, K., Ohmi, M, Aoi, T. 1997. Visualization of three-dimensional structure of rocks using X-ray CT method, *Environmental and Safety Concerns in Under ground Construction*, Lee, Yang & Chung (eds), pp769–774.

X-ray CT for Geomaterials; Soils, Concrete, Rocks – Otani & Obara (eds.)
© 2004 Swets & Zeitlinger. Lisse, ISBN 90 5809 666 1

Insight into pillar failure in experimental samples using CT visualization

E.J. Sellers
CSIR Division of Mining Technology, South Africa

A. Vervoort
K.U. Leuven, Leuven, Belgium

M.L. Drummond
Geovision CC., South Africa

ABSTRACT: A series of experiments were conducted in the laboratory on cubic samples of quartzite in order to be able to study the development of foundation failure and the effect of different pillar shapes. Three-dimensional medical CT scans of the tested samples have provided unique insight into rock fracture patterns and particularly into pillar foundation failure, and have provided a novel means of comparison to the AE locations and numerical modelling results. A method to remove beam-hardening artifacts to improve the fracture pattern reconstructions near the sample surfaces is described.

1 INTRODUCTION

Pillar failure is a significant cause of seismicity in deep level gold mines (Durrheim *et al.*, 1998). The damage caused by the seismic events causes loss of life and productivity. It is therefore very important to be able to identify the failure mechanisms and to determine the onset of pillar failure. The pillars in deep level gold mines are different to those in shallow room and pillar mines, in that they usually have much higher width to height ratios. In conventional pillar design, the pillars are expected to have width to height ratios ranging from one to eight. In deep level mines, the width to height ratios can exceed 40. Thus, these pillars exhibit only limited crushing of the edges. The main mechanism of failure is found to be shear fracturing within the foundation rocks.

The failure of pillar foundations in deep level mines has been described using numerical models (York, 1998) and the failure processes can be deduced using studies of seismic locations (Legge and Spottiswoode, 1987, Hagan, 1990, Ozbay *et al.*, 1993). However, it is very difficult to determine how failure proceeds and the final state of the fracture surfaces created by the foundation failure. It is very important to be able to properly determine these surfaces, as subsequent rock mass behaviour is controlled by sliding on the newly created surfaces leading to stress transfer mechanisms that impact on the future rock mass response.

A series of experiments were conducted in the laboratory on cubic samples of quartzite in order to be able to study the development of foundation failure, and the effect of different pillar shapes. The aim was to provide basic situations that could be used to prove newly developed three-dimensional numerical models. Good comparisons between the observed and modelled failure planes would lead to confidence in the application of the models to underground situations.

The models were monitored using acoustic emission to determine the failure processes during loading. However, it was important to be able to visualise the failure planes within the samples. To have these planes in a digital format was the most useful to be able to compare with the modelling results and AE locations and hence to assist with the study of the relationship between the failure mechanism and the pillar shape. Thus, the samples were subjected after being loaded to medical CT scanning to provide a representation of the internal structure of the fractures.

2 EXPERIMENTAL CONFIGURATION

The experiments were conducted on cubes of rock with a side length of 79.5 mm. Two types of rock were

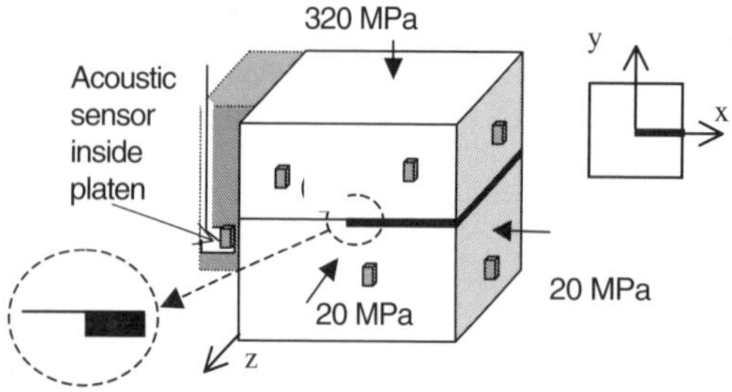

Figure 1. Experimental configuration of cubic sample with pillar (at left) and mine opening (at right). Voxel co-ordinate system xy is shown for a section and z is the slice number.

used. The first was Elsburg quartzite, a fine to medium (0.24 mm–1.52 mm) grained metamorphosed quartzwacke, with an unconfined compression strength ranging from 120 MPa to 180 MPa and a Young's modulus between 55 GPa and 65 GPa. The measured density is 2660 ± 39 kg/m^3. The second rock type was Marble Bar quartzite, a fine grained (0.072 mm–0.56 mm) metamorphosed quartz-arenite with a quartz content of 95%. The rock has a Young's modulus of 85 GPa and the unconfined compression strength is about 350 MPa. The measured density is 2670 ± 33 kg/m^3.

Figure 1 shows the sample configuration in a schematic way. Slots (at right in Figure 1) were machined into the sample to produce the pillars (at left in Figure 1). To create very high width to height pillars, and pillars with specific shapes in plan, it was necessary to cut the sample in half and machine the excavation into the top surface of the lower half. The sample was surrounded by steel platens. These contained slots that permitted placement of piezoelectric sensors around the sides of the sample to monitor the acoustic emissions associated with fracture formation. A confinement of 20 MPa was applied to the sides of the sample to represent the horizontal in-situ stresses occurring in deep mines. The load on the top surface was increased to simulate the loading of a pillar that takes place as the mined out regions increase in extent.

3 CT SCANNING PROCEDURE

X-ray computerised tomography uses the attenuation of the X-ray beam to reconstruct a section through the specimen (e.g. Verhelst *et al.*, 1995, Keller, 1998, Van Geet, 2001, Ketchem and Carlson, 2001). The basic principles of X-ray tomography are not repeated here. A multi-slice medical CT scanner (model: Siemens VolumeZoom) was used for this study. The scan spiral parameters were selected to have a radiation dose determined by 140 KeV and 180 mAs, a slice width of 0.5 mm, a colimation of 0.5 mm and a rotation time of 1 s. A standard medical reconstruction

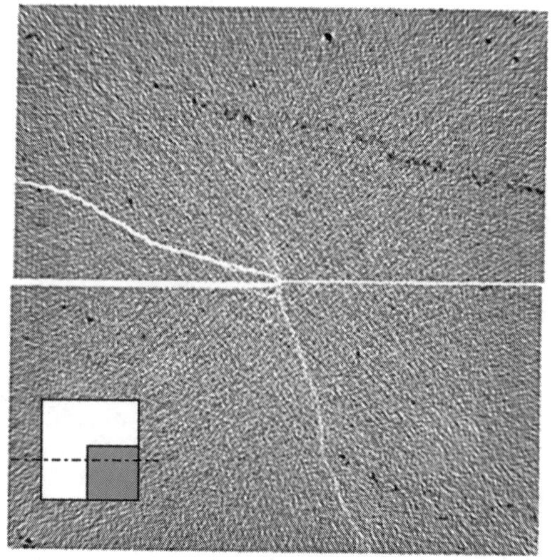

Figure 2. Ultra sharp image through pillar sample. White lines indicate low density i.e. cracks. The black line is a dense pyrite stringer. (inset shows plan view of pillar shape and line of section).

algorithm designed for the human inner ear was used. The reconstructed slice width was 0.5 mm with an increment of 0.2 mm. Two Siemens reconstruction kernel settings were used – the ultra sharp u90u and the medium smooth u30u. The same slice of one of the samples, containing 512 × 512 voxels, is shown in the ultra sharp form in Figure 2 and the medium smooth form in Figure 3.

By taking 420 slices across the sample, a three-dimensional grid of voxels of density was obtained in digital form. The VTK visualization package (Schroeder *et al.*, 1997) is an open source software library that was used to produce a three-dimensional visualization of the sample density grid. To identify the fractures (i.e. the low density regions), a "marching cubes" algorithm was used to obtain an isosurface contour of densities below a selected threshold value of CT number from the voxel grid. To save on memory, this operation was undertaken using 11 slices at a time, with one slice being common to the previous subset. Each isosurface was decimated to reduce the number of surfaces. The final isosurface is a combination of the 42 subsets that is decimated again. The isosurface contour can then be viewed to visualize the fracture shape. The program allows the superimpostion of other types of data such as acoustic emission event locations, numerical modelling results and the measured boundaries of the experimental sample. The acoustic emission can provide information on the sequence of the fracture formation and thus assist in pinpointing the onset of the pillar failure.

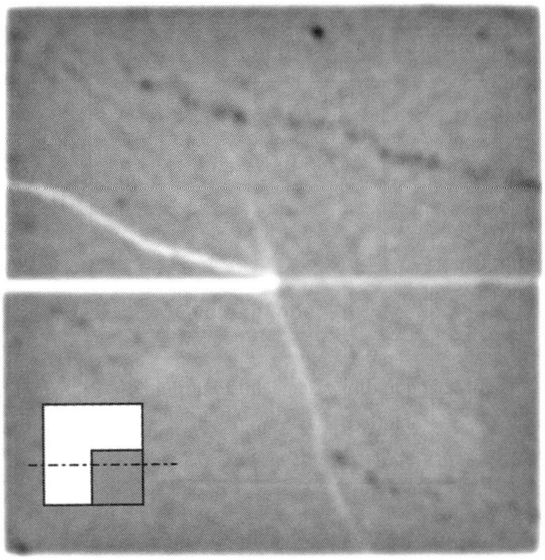

Figure 3. Medium smooth image through quarter (see previous remark) pillar sample. (inset shows plan view of pillar shape and line of section).

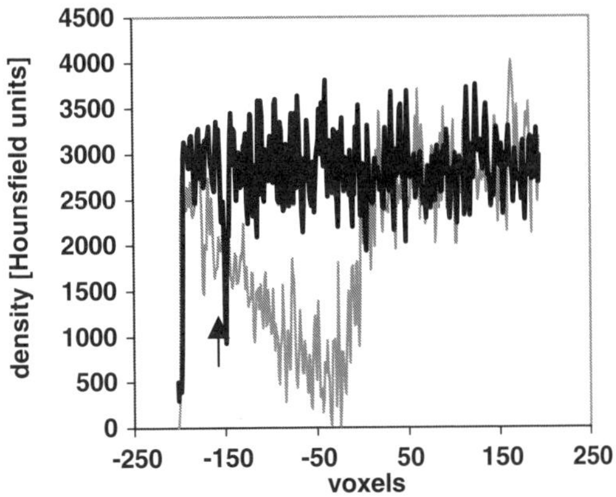

Figure 4. Two density profiles for the ultra sharp image of the quarter pillar. The lighter line is taken through the slot and the dark line at quarter of the sample height. The arrow indicates a crack.

A very beneficial advantage of having the fractures in digital format is that their positions and shapes can be directly compared with numerical model outputs. This prevents having to take numerous thin sections through the sample and to match these with sections of the model output.

4 REMOVAL OF BEAM HARDENING EFFECTS

The use of a medical scanner for CT scans of rock sample introduces beam-hardening effects (Verhelst *et al.*, 1995; Baruchel *et al.*, 2000). These effects are due to the differential attenuation of the high and low energy components within a polychromatic beam. Even though the lower energy components are attenuated more than the high-energy rays, the exiting beam has a higher energy than the incident beam (Ketchem and Carlson, 2001). The result of the beam hardening is that the outer regions of the sample are reported as being denser than the inner core. The use of a single value of the density as a contour threshold to identify the low density (i.e. fractured) regions becomes problematic as a value that is suitable in the center of the samples is not large enough to contour the fractures towards the sample edges. Increasing the threshold to capture the fractures at the edges causes the production of spurious contours within the central region.

Ketchem and Carlson (2001) highlight a number of remedies for beam hardening. The simplest is to increase the incident energy, which is not possible with a given medical CT scanner. An alternative is to use attenuating filters, however this can increase the noise in the image. The alternative that remains is the most difficult, and that is to correct the data at the image processing stage.

The following studies highlight how the images can be improved by using the data processing capabilities of the VTK software package. The first problem was to select the correct image sharpness for the scan. A series of density profiles were taken through the samples. The results of the density profiles for the ultrasharp image of Figure 2 are shown in Figure 4. Even though the image gives a very good picture of the fractures, there is considerable noise in the density profile of at least 1000 Hounsfield units. The medium smooth image of Figure 3 that looks less in focus actually produces a much less noisy image (Figure 5) that is more suitable for automatic processing.

By plotting any of the sections against the distance in voxels, it can be seen that there is a quadratic dependence of the density on the distance from the centre. This is shown in Figure 6. The beam hardening causes the cracks, which have a lower density, to be attenuated at a different rate to the solid material. The density reported for the cracks increases more rapidly than the density of the solid, and as shown in Figure 5, the cracks become less pronounced towards the sample edges. This density profile is also quadratic, as shown in Figure 6.

Thus, the image processing must seek to decrease the density at the edges and increase the amplitude of the low density spikes that indicate the cracks. This is illustrated schematically in Figure 7, where a point some distance from the center of the image has a density value $\mathbf{D}_H$ that is a fraction a/b of the distance between the curve of the low density and the curve of

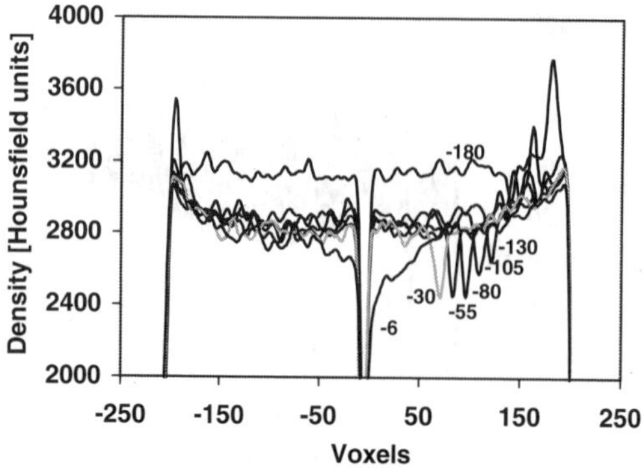

Figure 5. Density profiles for sections of the medium smooth image of Figure 3. Numbers indicate the y value of the sections.

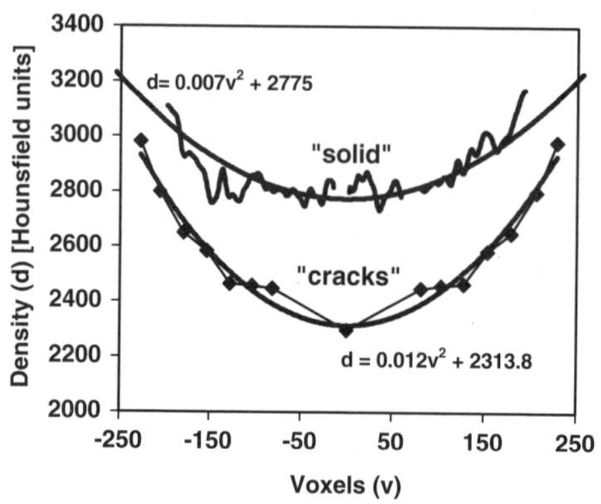

Figure 6. Quadratic functions fitted to density profiles for solid material and cracks as a function of distance in voxels (where each voxel has a side length of 0.5 mm).

the solid material. This must be transformed to a corrected density $\mathbf{D}_c$ that is equivalent to the density value it would have if situated at the centerline i.e.

$$(c/d) = (a/b) \tag{1}$$

The increase in density due to beam hardening occurs is all directions from the center of the sample and can thus be approximated by a *quadric* function. As each slice is a separate scan, there is negligible variation in the quadric surface between slices and the quadric function does not depend on the slice number z. Considering a single slice, quadric surface for the solid material is given by

$$\mathbf{D}_s(x,y,z) = d_{uo} + c_1(x^2+y^2) \tag{2}$$

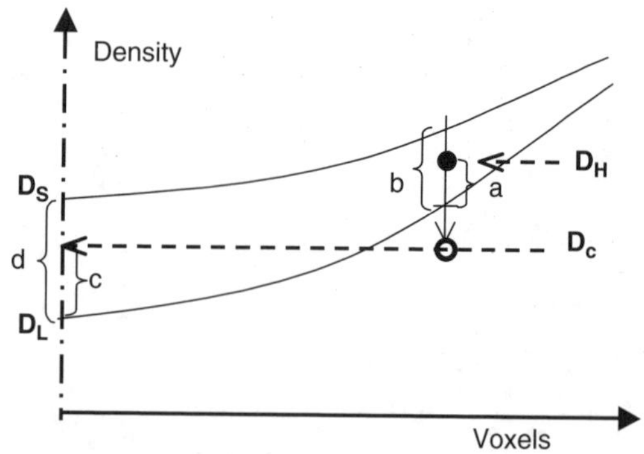

Figure 7. Schematic approach of voxel density scaling for removal of beam hardening artifacts.

and the quadric surface for the cracks is given by

$$\mathbf{D}_L(x,y,z) = d_{Lo} + c_2(x^2+y^2), \tag{3}$$

where d_{so}, c_1, d_{Lo} and c_2 are fitted constants, that are also independent of z. The corrected density surface can be expressed as

$$\mathbf{D}_c(x,y,z) = d_{L'} + (\mathbf{D}_H - \mathbf{D}_L)/(\mathbf{D}_u - \mathbf{D}_L) \tag{4}$$

where $\mathbf{D}_H$ is the original density function and the bold type denotes a function of (x, y, z) and $d_{L'} \leq d_{Lo}$. By choosing a value of $d_{L'} < d_{Lo}$, the spikes can be expanded, increasing the density contrast and improving the chances of identifying fractures near the edges of the sample.

This technique has worked successfully and it is possible in most cases to obtain 3-D pictures of the fracture surfaces that extend all the way to the sample edges. A further VTK routine was developed to separate the sample edges and the outer box so that it is possible to view the internal fractures and not be obscured by the outer surface. The final reconstruction of the image set corresponding to the slice shown in Figure 3 is given in Figure 12. Other examples are discussed in the next section.

5 PILLAR FAILURE IN DEEP LEVEL MINES

South African gold mines extract the gold bearing reefs of the Witwatersrand basin (Johnson and Schweitzer, 1996). The basin consists of a sequence of quartzite and shale layers, overlain by up to 2 km of lava. The gold bearing rocks are thin layers of about 1 m to 2 m in thickness and are distributed over many tens of km^2. Hagan (1990) demonstrated that the most damaging seismic events were located on the edges of

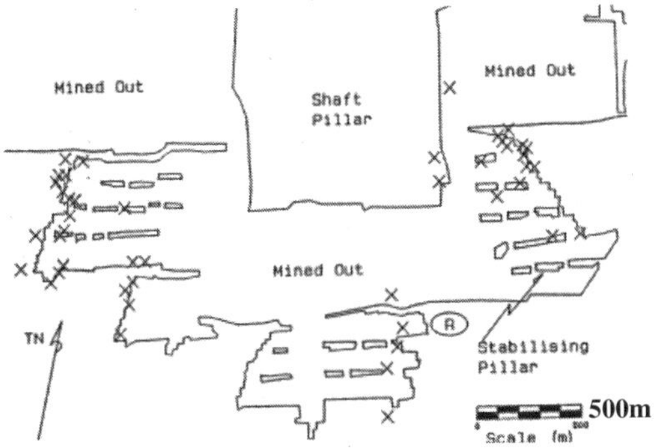

Figure 8. Plan view of a tabular gold mine with seismic events (denoted by x) delineating the failure of the pillar foundations (Hagan, 1990).

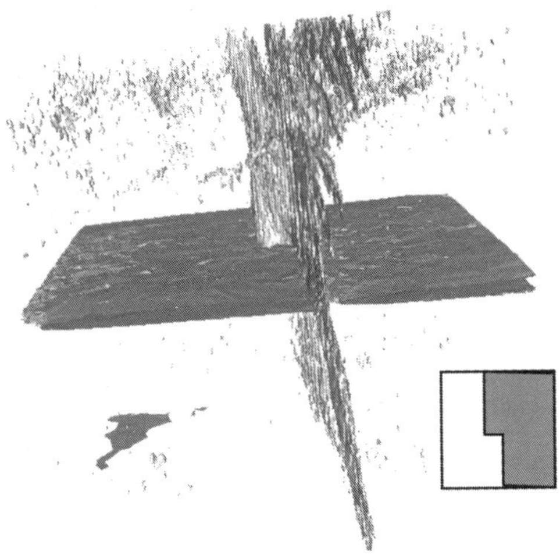

Figure 9. Fracture surface caused by lead-lag layout (lag of 10 mm) in an Elsburg quartzite block. Inset shows plan view of layout with pillar shaded.

the excavated region and along the pillars, as shown in Figure 8.

An experimental representation of the mine layout was tested and the results are shown in Figure 9. The fracture follows the stope face, arching over the excavated region where the one panel has been mined ahead of the other, as shown in the inset of Figure 9. If the stope width is sufficiently low, the excavated region tends to be closed at some distance from the face. Then as in Figure 9, the fractures dip slightly ahead of the stope face. If the excavation remains open, as for the stiffer Timeball hill quartzite sample in Figure 10, the fractures dip over the excavated region. In the experiments, an additional tensile crack forms from the edges of the sample, as defined by the lighter grey surface in Figure 10.

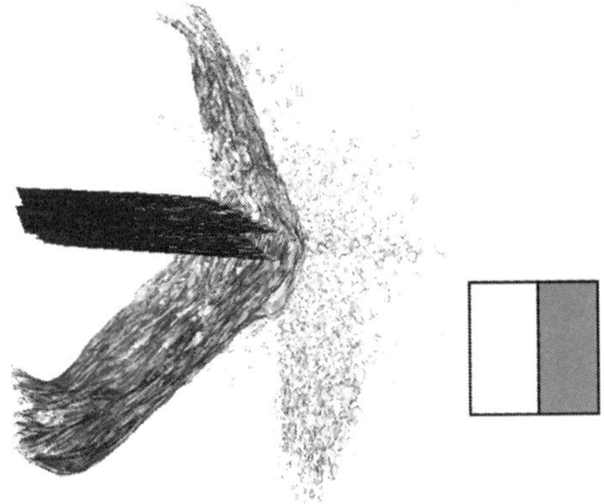

Figure 10. Fracture surface caused by pillar (without lead-lag) in a Timeball hill quartzite block. Inset shows plan view of layout with pillar shaded.

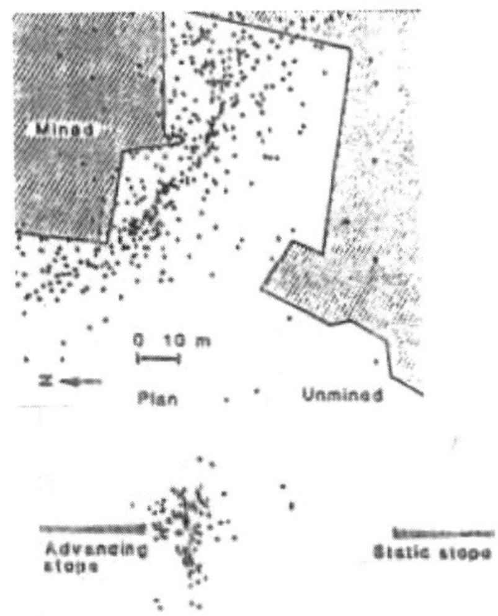

a)

b)

Figure 11. Seismic events denoting a failure plane under a pillar remaining in a gold mine in plan (a) and vertical (b) section.

6 REMNANT PILLAR

Legge and Spottiswoode (1987) reported on the mining of a rectangular shaped pillar that had been left as a peninsula within a mined out region. The subsequent mining of the pillar was monitored with a microseismic system. The seismicity was located in planes ahead of the mining face, as shown in Figure 11a. It indicated that failure occurred on a plane that followed the overall shape of the mining faces. A similar situation was tested in the experiment shown in Figure 12. In this case, one quarter of the surface was left to form a square pillar.

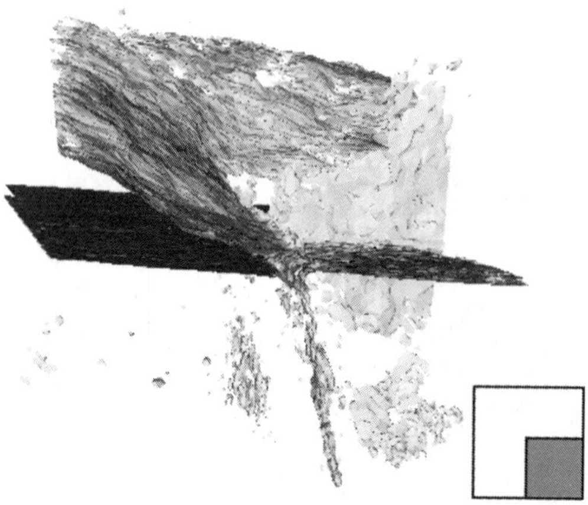

Figure 12. Fracture surface reconstructed for a quarter pillar in an Elsburg quartzite block. Inset shows plan view of layout with pillar shaded.

The isosurface contours of low-density regions in Figure 12 show how the fracture planes extend below the pillar. This is similar to the planes defined by the seismic locations in the mining situation in Figure 11b. Figure 12 also shows that the fractures on the upper side curve a considerable distance into the solid rock. As shown in Figure 1, the pillar has a discontinuity between the pillar and the upper block, but whereas the lower corner is ground into the sample. The solid, lower, corner causes the steep dipping fracture and the upper corner, with the discontinuity causes the curved fracture. A successful numerical model should be able to model the different fracture directions correctly.

7 FOUNDATION FAILURE

The underground microseismic studies by Hagan (1990) also indicated how the foundation failure occurs under a pillar between two mined out regions. These microseismic observations were correlated with observations of the induced shear zone in a tunnel below the pillar, as shown in Figure 13. One of the 2-D sections of the CT scan (Figure 14) of an experiment on a square pillar in Timeball Hill quartzite shows how the fracture plane may have looked for the case study of Figure 13. This also shows that 2-D sections are just as important as the 3-D reconstructions as they provide insight into detailed structures that may be obscured by cracks that are orthogonal to the viewing direction.

8 CONCLUSIONS

Experiments were conducted to apply a triaxial stress state to cubic samples of quartzite containing slots cut to represent various mine layout configurations applied in South African deep gold mines. Three-dimensional medical CT scans were performed on the tested samples. Visualisation software was written to reconstruct the fracture planes as isosurfaces contours of the low-density regions. Additional image processing that was required to remove beam-hardening artifacts is described. The resulting images have provided some unique insight into rock fracture patterns and particularly into pillar foundation failure. Being in digital form, they will provide a novel and easy means of comparison with the AE locations and numerical modelling results.

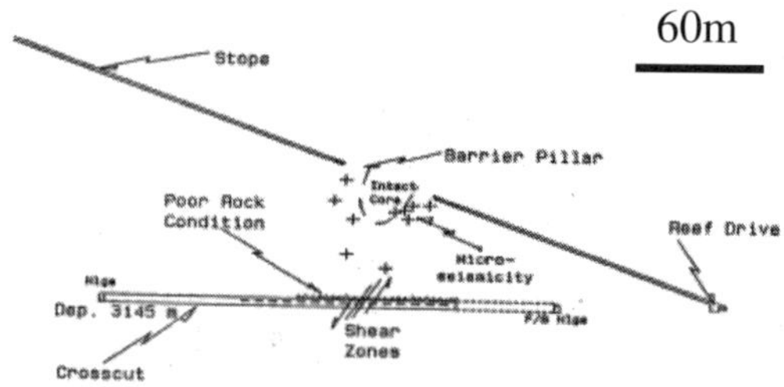

Figure 13. Foundation failure beneath a pillar defined by seismic event locations.

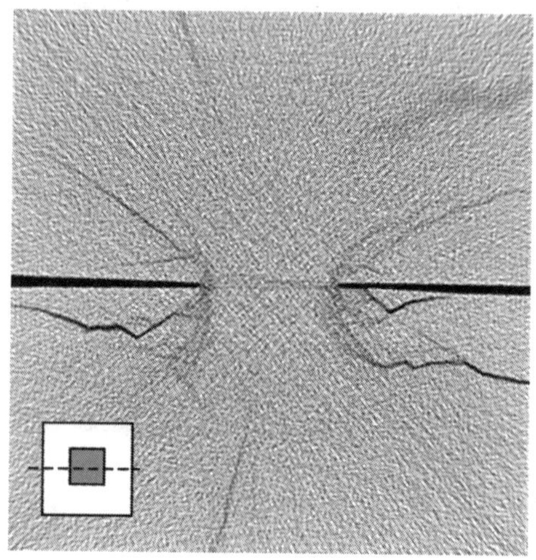

Figure 14. 2-D sections of failure underneath a square pillar in a Timeball hill quartzite block. Inset shows plan view of layout with pillar shaded.

ACKNOWLEDGEMENTS

Funding for this project was provided by the Safety in Mines Research Advisory Committee, as part of project GAP 601, and is gratefully acknowledged. The authors thank Prof. G. Marchal, Dr J. Van Cleynenbreugel and their team for the assistance during the scanning of the rock samples at the Gasthuisberg University Hospital in Leuven, Belgium.

REFERENCES

Baruchel, J., Buffière, J.-Y., Maire, E., Merle, P. and Peix, G. 2000. X-ray tomography in Material Science, General Principles, Hermes Science Publications, Paris 2000, ISBN 2-7462-0115-1, 15–21.

Durrheim, R., Haile, A., Roberts, M.C.K., Schweitzer, J.K., Spottiswoode, S.M. and Klokow, J.W. 1998.Violent failure of a remnant in a deep South African gold mine. Tectonophysics. 289, 105–116.

Hagan, T. 1990. Pillar foundations studies on a deep level South African gold mine. Rockbursts and seismicity in mines. Fairhurst (ed.) Balkema, 65–70.

Hagan, T., Durrheim, R., Roberts, M. and Haile, A. 1999. Rockburst investigation in South African mines. 9th Congr. Rock Mech. (eds Vouille & Berest) Balkema, 1089–1094.

Handley, M., Selfe, D., Viera, F., Maccelari, M. and Dede, T. 1997. Current position of strike stabilizing pillars and bracket pillars – guidelines for deep tabular orebodies. J. South Afr. Inst. Min. Metal, 103–116.

Jaeger, A.J. and Ryder, J. 1999. A handbook on rock engineering practice for tabular hard rock mines. The Safety in Mines Research Advisory Committee (SIMRAC) Johannesburg.

Johnson, R.A. and Schweitzer, J.K. 1996. Mining at depth: evaluation of alternatives. 2nd North Amer. Rock Mech. Symp. Montreal., June. Balkema, Rotterdam.

Keller, A. 1998. High Resolution, non-destructive measurement and characterization of fracture apertures. Int. J. Rock Mech. Min Sci. 35:8, 1037–1050.

Ketcham, R.A. and Carlson, W.D. 2001. Acquisition, optimization and interpretation of X-ray computed tompgraphic imagery: application to the geosciences. Computers and Geosciences, 381–400.

Legge, N. and Spottiswoode, S. 1987. Fracturing and microseismicity ahead of a deep level stope in the pre-remnant and remnant stages of mining. 6th Int. Congr. Rock Eng. Montreal, 1071–1077.

Ozbay, M. and Ryder, J. 1989. Investigations into foundation failure mechanisms of hard rock squat pillars. Int. Symp. Rock mechanics and rock physics at great depth. Pau.

Ozbay, M. Spottiswoode, S. and Ryder, J. 1993. A quantitative analysis of pillar-associated large seismic events in deep mines. 3rd Int Conf. Rockbursts and Seismicity in Mines. Kingston, 107–110.

Schroeder, W., Martin, K. and Lorensen, B. 1997. The Visualization Toolkit. An object-oriented approach to 3D graphics. Prentice Hall.

Sellers, E.J., Berlenbach, J. and Schweitzer, J. 1998. Fracturing around deep level stopes: Comparison of numerical simulation with underground observations. MJFR3, Rossmanith (ed), Balkema, Rotterdam.

Van Geet, M. 2001. Optimisation of microfocus X-ray computer tomography for geological research with special emphasis on coal components (macerals) and fractures (cleats) characterisation. PhD thesis. Katholieke Universiteit Leuven, Belgium.

Verhelst, F., Vervoort, A., De Bosscher, Ph. and Marchal, G. 1995. X-Ray computerized tomography: determination of heterogeneities in rock samples. Proc. Intl. Congr. Rock Mech. (Fujii, T. ed.), 105–108.

York, G. 1998. Numerical Modelling of the yielding of stabilizing pillar/foundation systems. J SAIMM, 281–298.

X-ray CT for Geomaterials; Soils, Concrete, Rocks – Otani & Obara (eds.)
© 2004 Swets & Zeitlinger. Lisse, ISBN 90 5809 666 1

CT real-time analysis of damage evolution of coal under compression

G. Dai
The Key Laboratory of the Exploitation of Southwest Resources & the Environmental Hazards Control Engineering, Ministry of Education, Chongqing University, Chongqing, China
Department of Geotechnical Engineering, Tongji University, Shanghai, China

G. Yin & W. Pi
College of Resource and Environmental Sciences, Chongqing University, Chongqing, China

H. Zhu & C. Xia
Department of Geotechnical Engineering, Tongji University, Shanghai, China

ABSTRACT: Using the specified loading equipment and the CT machine, the real-time computerized tomography testing of coal under the uniaxial compression was completed. Through CT scanning, the clear CT images which included the step from the micro-crack closure to the micro-crack growth, bifurcation, development, failure and the post-failure step were obtained. According to the CT values, the meso-damage evolution of coal under uniaxial compression was analyzed. Based on the results which tallies with micro-facture, cavity growth, and section forming obtained from CT scanning of coal, the study on the damage propagation of coal was carried out. It is demonstrated that in the process of unloading failure of coal is paroxysmal. At the same time, the meso-mechanism of dilatancy in coal under the condition of uniaxial compression is experimentally studied. Based on the change of the CT value and CT images obtained from scanning test, the propagation law of the meso-damage in coal is deduced. The change law of crack width and length related to creeping time has been quantitatively analyzed. In the light of the law and CT image, which are of referential for the building of damage constitutive model and damage evolution function of coal, the macro-damage process of coal under uniaxial compression in Baijiao Mine has been divided into 5 steps, the damage-weakening step, the linear step, the damage starts to evolve and damage develops steadily, the damage development speeding upand the weakening step after reaching peak. In the end, the comparison of damage variable between CT scanning and Bellonoi equation, Lemaitre equation in the process of uniaxial damage spread was obtained which resolves successfully damage discriminating "scale" problem, and the obtained results is more reasonable than Bellonoi equation and Lemaitre equation.

1 INTRODUCTION

The research of damage mechanics in rock is a basic subject, which has became more and more attractive in rock mechanics. Using CT scanning technology, Chen zheng-han, Wu zhi-wang, Yang geng-she and so on conducted a microscale-based research concerned with the configuration, distribution, evolution characteristic of various damage, and got lots of achievements, but little work on coal damage mechanics feature with adoption of CT scanning can be found in available literatures. In this paper, CT real-time scanning experiment is carried out for the spread of coal meso-damage under uniaxial compression, and the damage mechanism in coal is investigated. Finally, damage evolution equation and the corresponding constitutive are developed.

2 CT REAL-TIME TEST

2.1 *Mathematics principle of CT examining*

Through image rebuilt, the material information with different density to be shown via digital image with high resolving power. Professor Hounsfield defined the conception of CT data; CT data of certain material is,

$$H_{rm} = 1000 \times \frac{\mu_{rm} - \mu_{H_2o}}{\mu_{H_2o}} \quad (1)$$

CT data gives reflection of material density, which the higher CT data means the higher density. X-ray failing coefficient relates to material density, so the energy of X-ray can affect CT value to some extent. X-ray material absorbing coefficient (μ_{rm}) is a function of X-ray spread distance L in the material, the relationship between intensity I_2 and incident intensity I_1 is,

$$I_2 = I_1 \exp(-\int \mu_{rm} dL) \tag{2}$$

where, I_1 – incident intensity of X-ray ($ev/m^2 \cdot s$),
I_2 – intensity after passing material ($ev/m^2 \cdot s$),
L – Spread distance of X-ray (m),
μ_{rm} – Failing coefficient (m^{-1})

However,

$$\mu_{rm} = \mu_r \rho \tag{3}$$

μ_m – Failing coefficient of unit (m^2/kN), only relates to X-ray wavelength,
ρ – Density of examined material (kN/m^3).

The X-ray spiral CT machine is SIEMENMS SOMATOM plus, owed by State Key Laboratory of Frozen Soil Engineering Chinese Academy of Sciences, the space resolution is 0.35 mm × 0.35 mm, the minimum volume that can be recognized is 0.12 mm^3, the ratio of density resolution is 0.3%.

Experiment system consists of hydraulic loading sub-system, special experiment storehouse, circulatory sub-system and data sub-system. Figure 1 shows special experiment storehouse, which outside specification is 50 × 100 mm, the inner diameter is 142 mm, the axial working stoke is 40 mm, the range of strain sensor is 0–50 mm, the precision is 0.31%. Experiment storehouse locates in the CT scanning region. In order to reduce the influence of experiment storehouse material on CT scanning, experiment storehouse was machined with high quality light metal material $LY12$.

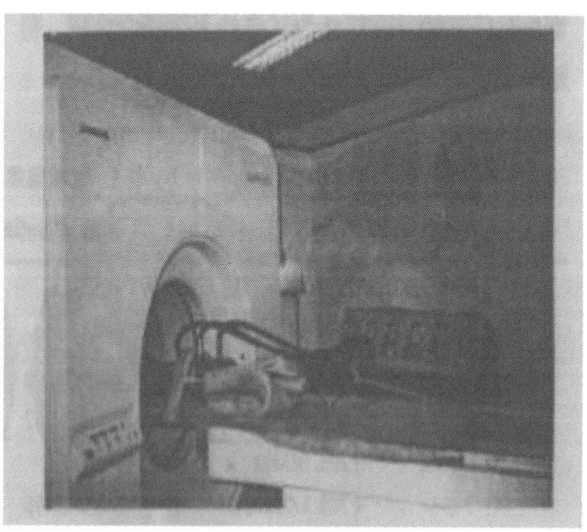

Figure 1. Device for computerized tomography.

2.2 *Experiment method*

Coal is in compression in underground engineer; therefore, the study of damage destroying mechanism under compression has significant meaning. In this test, the sample was extracted from Baijiao Mine. (The digging depth is about 500 m, unit weight is 14.928 kN/m^3, specific gravity is 1.579, contained water ratio is 2.814%, absorbed water ratio is 4.190%, and contained fracture ratio is 6.916%). First, the uniaxial compression test of coal was carried out on the MTS rigid experiment machine, the stress–strain full curve under uniaxial compression, elastic modulus, peak value and Poisson's ratio are obtained. Then the CT real-time test of meso-damage evolution of coal under uniaxial compression was carried out. During test, experiment storehouse was placed in bed horizontally, and coal sample was put in the CT scanning level. The sample is divided into four layers. During loading, scanning was carried out in different layers at the corresponding step. The image of micro-crack growth, bifurcation, development and failure were observed.

3 CT TEST RESULTS AND DAMAGE EVOLUTION IN COAL

The scanning parameters of coal sample are shown in Table 1. The numbers 1, 2, 3, 4 in Figure 2 correspond to four scanning lays from top to down separately, the thickness is 3 mm, there are 7 times scanning in process. Figures 3 to 6 show the corresponding CT image from top to down separately.

(1) Before loading, the results of scanning show that not only CT values but also CT images in every layers are not the same, even more, CT values of every zone in the same layer are different. This shows that coal in Baijiao Mine is a reprehensively initial damage medium with large quantities of micro-cavities and micro-cracks, and the initial damage is non-uniform.

(2) When σ reaches 8.591 MPa, CT data of scans (table 2) and CT data of sample have risen to some

Table 1. Parameters of CT scanning.

Voltage (KV)	120
Current (mA)	165
Time (s)	2
Mark	OM
Thick (mm)	3
Magnification factor	7.0
X/Y	10/3
Separation (mm)	20

extent, which gives indication of the initial microcavity closure, a part CT images becoming black, and coal being compressed to denser (Fig. 4).

(3) During the process of σ rising from 8.591 Mpa to 13.880 Mpa, both CT data and image of scans and coal sample have not remarkable variances. It is believed that there aren't significant changes for meso-damage of coal during this step, the curve of stress–strain is in linear step.

(4) When σ = 13.880 MPa, the increase of CT data of 2nd, 3rd scans goes on, while CT data of 1st, 4th scans continues dropping (micro-crack opening occurring), and slight dilatancy was observed in this region (table 3). According to Fig. 5, because of interaction among micro-cracks, micro-crack extension, bifurcation and connection phenomena, cracks have appeared in 1st, 4th scans, and there are macro-cracks observed in 2nd, 3rd scans, but they have not linked up. This shows that, in the same sample, damage spread characteristics differs in every lays under the same stress, that is, damage evolution is a non-uniform process. Another reason for above phenomena is the influence of end effect, which enhanced the non-uniform of damage evolution. From the continual decrease of CT data in 1st, 4th scans and the continual increase in 2nd, 3rd scans before sample failure, it can be seen that the end effect play an important role on test.

(5) When σ = 13.880 MPa, CT data of the center region of 4th scan starts to decrease, from 488.9 to 463.0, the decrease level is 5.3%, indicating meso-damage begins to evolution. At this moment,

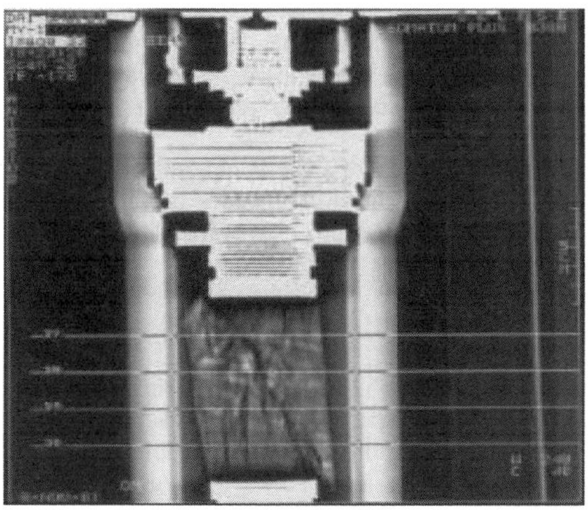

Figure 2. CT scanning and orientation line.

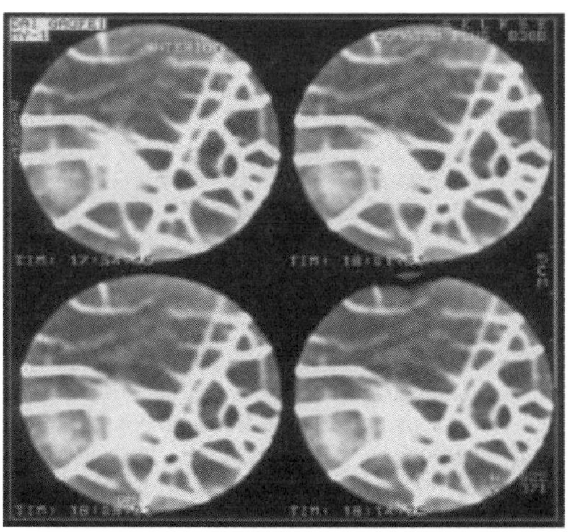

Figure 3. CT image of 1st scan.

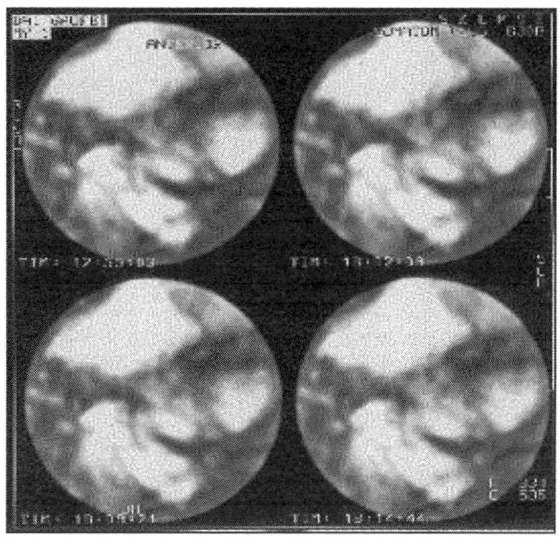

Figure 4. CT image of 2nd scan.

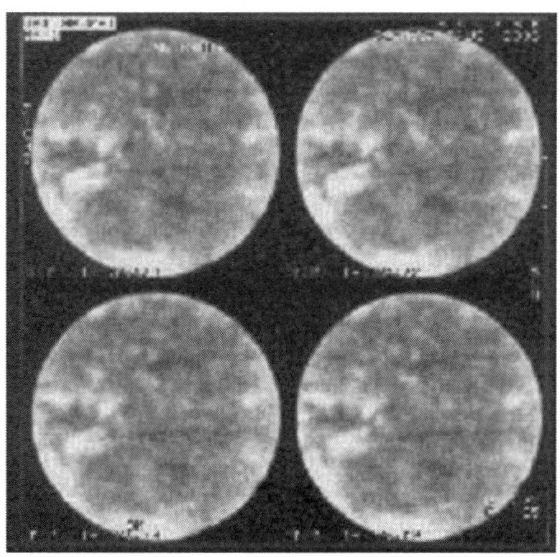

Figure 5. CT image of 3rd scan.

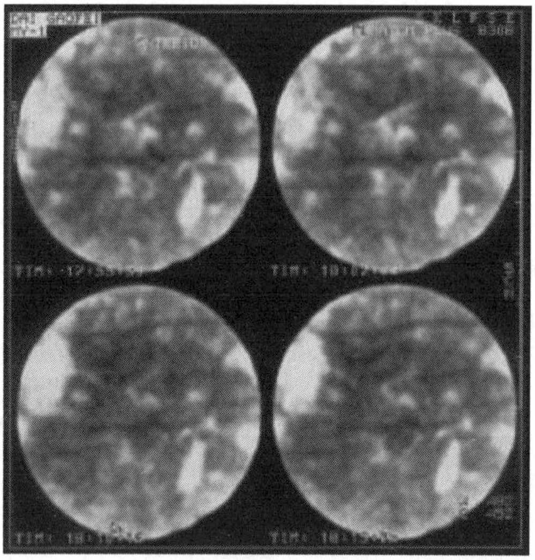

Figure 6. CT image of 4th scan.

Table 2. Stress and strain value of each scanning.

Scanning	1	2	3	4	5	6	7
σ/MPa	0	5.3	8.6	13.9	16.8	18.4	0.3
ε/‰	0	3.8	6.1	9.2	11.1	12.0	97.1

Table 3. Data in testing results of each scan.

1st scan		2nd scan		3rd scan		4th scan	
ME	SD	ME	SD	ME	SD	ME	SD
546.1	172.8	787.1	201.4	527.9	56.5	519.1	67.8
548.4	173.7	789.0	201.1	527.5	58.1	519.2	66.2
548.2	174.1	792.6	200.7	527.6	59.5	519.5	64.0
547.8	174.7	794.2	201.0	529.3	54.7	519.6	72.7
545.7	175.4	795.0	201.2	529.3	55.9	518.4	72.3
540.5	176.1	792.5	202.6	528.4	57.7	515.8	71.5
303.3	279.7	219.0	565.4	263.8	367.2	318.9	319.1

$\sigma = 75.3\% \sigma_c$ (σ_c is peak value), which can be thought as a threshold value of sample damage tentatively. This value corresponds to submit value of the stress–strain full curve under uniaxial compression, and tallies with the test result obtained by other scientists.

(6) When $\sigma = 16.802$ MPa, CT data of both corresponding regions in scans and sample starts to decrease, and quadratic difference start to increase, there are slight dilatancy occurring concerning coal sample. Because of micro-cracks interaction, micro-crack extension, bifurcation and connection, some main cracks were observed in 1st, 4th scans, and bifurcation cracks were observed in left-downward direction vertical to main crack. During the step of σ increasing from 13.880 MPa to 16.802 MPa, damage begins to evolve and stabilize.

(7) When σ come to 18.438 MPa, the decrease of CT data of corresponding regions in scans speeds up, variance component increase rapidly. According to Figures 3 and 6, the cracks that have linked up continue opening, at the same time, there are small quantities of micro-cracks sprouting. This step is a failure forewarning one, that is, this is step with higher damage evolution speed. Soon after σ come to 18.438 MPa, loading reaches peak value, the stress decreases so fast that scanning can not be completed.

(8) During the process of σ dropping to 0.284 MPa, CT data of corresponding region in scans and coal sample drop sharply, variance component increase rapidly, and the main cracks linked up broaden rapidly. Bifurcation cracks in 2nd, 3rd scans become linked up completely, forming cruciform main cracks, while many new cracks come forth, and sample destroy. The main rupture surface is not a plane, but a flex surface.

(9) In the light of experiment, under the same stress condition, the different lays of same sample show the different spread characteristics, that is, damage evolution is a non-uniform process. So the damage evolutions show the localized conditions phenomenon.

(10) As Figure 4, with the increase of stress, dilatancy phenomenon of coal sample is becoming more and more significant. The essence of is micro-cracks widen and extension, or intensification of damage evolution.

As is shown in Tables 2 and 3 that the variance of CT data and variance component is not obvious, and the ratio between the average CT data and variance component is lesser during experiment, which shows that the initial damage of coal sample has some comparability in space. This reason is that the closure between virgin fracture and flabby surface is tight, and width is very little, resulting in experiment data giving a main reflection of growth level of micro-fractures, micro-cracks, and cavities within sections, however the initial damage caused by detects of coal sample just account for damage non-uniform. There are marked differences of CT data and variance component between 2nd scan and 1st, 3rd, 4th scans, and the ratio between the average CT data and variance component of them is high, which 2nd scan and 1st, 3rd, 4th scans are differ greatly in lay structure. In fact, there is also a certain difference existing in lay structure among 1st, 3rd, 4th scans. Because of the resolving power of CT machine is 0.35 mm * 0.35 mm, CT machine is insensitive to the long and thin detects (width is less than 0.3 mm) of sample. These detects are shown as isolated cavities with chain distribution

Table 4. Testing results of coal sample.

ME	ΔME	ΔME/ME (%)	SD	ΔSD	ΔSD/SD (%)
595.0			124.6		
596.0	0.98	0.16	124.7	0.08	0.06
596.9	1.93	0.32	124.5	−0.04	−0.03
597.7	2.68	0.45	125.7	1.14	0.9
597.1	2.05	0.34	126.1	1.56	1.23
594.3	−0.75	−0.13	127.0	2.4	1.89
301.3	−293.7	−97.5	382.8	258.22	67.45

in CT image. With the increase of external force, the fracture of coal sample and every scans grow gradually, the maximum differences of CT data and variance component are 97.5% and 67.45% separately, which gives well indication of the space non-uniform of damage evolution of coal sample.

During the whole experiment process, CT data of coal sample and every scans are keeping decrease, and variance component are keeping increase, which indicate the density of coal sample and every scans is stepping down, and the difference of density distribution is stepping up. This result tallies with micro-facture, cavity growth, and section forming.

The absolute value of ΔME/ME and ΔSD/SD are becoming more and more large during experiment, which indicate that there are remarkable damages in experiment.

From the law of CT data and CT image of coal during the whole damage process under uniaxial compression, it is can be seen that there is some correspondence relation existing between the law and the stress–strain full curve of coal in Baijiao Mine. In the light of the law and CT image, the macro-damage process of coal under uniaxial compression in Baijiao Mine can be divided into 5 steps.

The first step is a damage-weakening step, during this step, CT data rises slightly relative to initial damage step, variance component decrease, density of coal increases, and the intensity enhances.

The second step is a linear step, there isn't obvious variance concerning CT data and variance component, coal is in elastic-deformation step.

During the third step, damage starts to evolve, and damage develops steadily, CT data begins to decrease, variance component rise slightly, and micro-cracks start to sprout and spread steadily.

The fourth step is a step with damage development speeding up. During this step, the decrease velocity of CT data, and the increase of variance component quicken, micro-cracks converge and link up, macro-cracks occurring, coal intensity reaches peak value quickly.

The fifth step is a weakening step after reaching peak. CT data dropped with the fastest rate, variance component rise rapidly until reached its residual intensity.

In the experiment, the maximum load is 38.02 kN, the maximum deformation is 1.253 mm, the load-deformation curve is similar to the common uniaxial experiment. CT scanning is conducted when sample deformation comes to 0, 30, 48, 73, 88, 96 percent of peak value, and structure variances in four scans are observed. In the light of load-deformation data, the load-deformation curve is completed. In order to adapt scanning orientation, the position with 3 kN load is defined as the initial position. As is evidenced in experiment, the initial density of coal sample goes up slightly with increase of load. After reaching 60 percent of peak load, the fractures in joint cementation face in coal start to expand, and the load-deformation curve fluctuates. Before coming to peak load, the regions craze suddenly and lose carrying capacity. During the first scanning, coal is in a micro-compression initial step, following close behind this step. When sample is compressed to denser a bit, the second scanning is conducted, then micro-joint gets relatively steady in coal, the third scanning is completed. With the increase of compression gradually, the inner micro-joint of coal begins to spread, at this time, the fourth scanning goes on, the inner status of coal is recorded while micro-cracks come into being, along with the further increase of compression, the inner joint spread rapidly with the local cracks occurring, then the fifth scanning is carried out, the sixth scanning is followed, which there is obvious spread of crack in coal under the compression, giving rise to coal crazing. Finally, the increase of compression causes micro-cracks link up each other, coal sample shearing destroys, and the last scanning is completed. It can be seen from Figure 2 to Figure 7, the data in the middle of the first scanning layer drops smoothly comparatively, excepting this, the data drops sharply in other parts of sample during cracking, the level is lowest in peculiar regions, variance component is the most remarkable, the compression level in initial step is 0.13%, before failure, which has dropped 0.38%, the local dropping is 1.2%, variance component changes between +1.8% and −1.8%. The average data in the second step is biggest, variance component remains steady until the sharply change of image data caused by the cracking in other scans. The change in every regions of 3rd scan is comparatively uniform, there is almost no decrease before failure. The center region of 4th scan has strong plasticity, where there is significant fluctuation concerning the average data. Although the other regions have different density, the difference of change is not obvious.

The image and CT data in 4 scans behaves differently, which results from the different lay structure. Among which, the first scan is a netted cementation of the coal and sandstone, CT data and variance component undulate slightly. The second scan is large lump

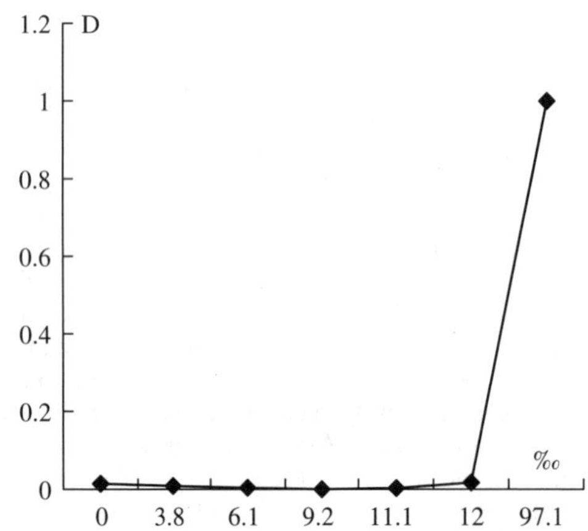

Figure 7. Relationship curve between D and ε.

crystalloid sandstone with high carrying capability in some regions, and there is the biggest increment at the edge of crystal (the obvious dislocation slippage). The 3rd, 4th scans are distributed cementation, the inner structure change showing almost no difference in every regions, ending up with forming circular cracks. It can be seen from plane slice, the sample shows typical uniaxial shearing damaging shape.

4 DAMAGE CONSTITUTIVE MODEL AND DAMAGE EVOLUTION EQUATION

4.1 *Introduction*

The CT data distribution of coal sample is quite complex and with dispersing randomicity, which do not follow general distribution law. The distribution difference of CT data in 4 scanning sections is remarkable in the same sample from top to down, which tallies with the damage phenomena given by CT scanning image, and indicates the complexity of damage characteristics in coal sample. The damage types in coal are not simple, including damages caused by fracture, joint, and cavity among mineral grains. Although coal is dominated by a certain type of damage, the other types can not be ignored.

In 1980, Grand and Kipp presented that when they were studying micro-crack spread and distribution law, the total micro-cracks sum N in unit volume and strain ε_1 in coal meets follow relationship,

$$N(\varepsilon) = k\varepsilon^m \tag{4}$$

where, k and m are material constants.

Because the damage development in coal is closely connected with micro-cracks spread and distribution,

Table 5. Damage variables of coal and its scan.

Order	1	2	3	4	Sample
1	0.0122	0.0359	0.0073	0.0024	0.0139
2	0	0.0269	0.0098	0.0024	0.0090
3	0.0008	0.0106	0.0090	0.0008	0.0041
4	0.0033	0.0033	0	0	0
5	0.0139	0	0	0.0065	0.0033
6	0.0416	0.0114	0.0049	0.0204	0.0171
7	0.9970	0.9992	0.9983	0.9951	0.9987

Table 6. Damage variables and stress, strain.

Order	σ/MPa	ε/‰	D
1	0	0	0.0139
2	5.334	3.8	0.0090
3	8.591	6.1	0.0041
4	13.880	9.2	0
5	16.802	11.1	0.0033
6	18.438	12.0	0.0171
7	0.284	97.1	0.9987

based on the microcosmic and macroscopic experiment result, when building damage model of brittle coal, it can be supposed,

(1) Coal damage is the coupling of elasticity and damage,
(2) The main body of coal damage is along stress principle axial direction, the damage tensor matrix can be selected as main diagonal matrix,
(3) Damage evolution is certain power function relationship of stress or strain.

Assuming the damage variable D of coal under uniaxial compression is,

$$D = m\varepsilon^n \tag{5}$$

where m, n are material constants, ε is axial compression strain.

Based on conception of effect stress, effect stress is,

$$\tilde{\sigma} = \frac{\sigma}{1 - D} \tag{6}$$

According to strain equivalence theory given by Lemaitre, the strain caused by effect stress on damaged material is identical to the strain caused by effective stress effect on primitive material. That is,

$$\varepsilon = \frac{\sigma}{\tilde{E}} = \frac{\tilde{\sigma}}{E} = \frac{\sigma}{(1-D)E} \tag{7}$$

$$\tilde{E} = E(1 - D) \tag{8}$$

Equation (8) is elastic modulus for damaged material, called the effective elastic modulus.

$$\sigma = E(1-D)\varepsilon \tag{9}$$

Constitutive relationship for damaged material is selected as

$$\sigma = E(1-m\varepsilon^n)\varepsilon \tag{10}$$

If

$$\varepsilon_s = \frac{1}{\sqrt[n]{m}} \tag{11}$$

Then

$$m\varepsilon^n = (\frac{\varepsilon}{\varepsilon_s})^n \tag{12}$$

Here damage variable D can be selected as,

$$D = \left(\frac{\varepsilon}{\varepsilon_s}\right)^n \tag{13}$$

So the damage constitutive relationship for coal under uniaxial stress is,

$$\sigma = E\left[1-\left(\frac{\varepsilon}{\varepsilon_s}\right)^n\right]\varepsilon \tag{14}$$

The evolution equation for damaged variable is,

$$\dot{D} = \frac{dD}{d\varepsilon} = \frac{n}{\varepsilon_s}\left(\frac{\varepsilon}{\varepsilon_s}\right)^{n-1} \tag{15}$$

where ε_s and n are material parameters for coal.

Starting from the physical mechanism through experiment, classifying its damage mechanism, then presenting damage evolution equation with a certain precision and referential meaning for engineering and its constitutive model is a feasible way for damage mechanic research. The damage evolution of coal is a non-linear process. It is difficult to describe the damage mechanism of the whole process for cracks evolution with united continuous function, therefore employing segmentation function is a practicable method.

4.2 *Constitutive model and damage evolution function in quasi-linear step*

Constitutive model in quasi-linear step is selected as line-elastic, constitutive model of coal in Baijiao Mine in quasi-linear step can be selected as,

$$\sigma = 0.45\varepsilon + 13.28\,(13.880MPa<\sigma<16.802MPa) \tag{16}$$

Damage evolution equation is,

$$D = 0 \tag{17}$$

4.3 *Constitutive model and damage evolution function in beginning damage evolution and developing steadily step*

In the light of strain equivalent theory, constitutive model is,

$$\sigma = E(1-D)\varepsilon \tag{18}$$

As can be seen in Figure 7, relationship between D and ε is similar to a section of power exponent curve, that is,

$$D = A\varepsilon\exp(B) \tag{19}$$

Taking the measured ε and σ into constitutive model, getting a few values of α_e. It is found that via comparing, when $\alpha_e = 1.10$, the error between the theory curve and the measured curve is less. Selecting $\alpha_e = 1.10$, calculating D in different stress, getting relationship between D and ε, that is evolution equation,

$$D = 0.107\varepsilon\exp(4.8099) \tag{20}$$

Taking (20) into (18), getting constitutive model and damage evolution function in beginning damage evolution and developing steadily step,

$$\sigma = E(1-0.107\varepsilon\exp(4.8099))\varepsilon \quad (16.802\text{MPa}<\sigma<18.438\text{MPa}) \tag{21}$$

4.4 *Constitutive model and damage evolution function in accelerated damage development step*

As a result of brittle characteristic of coal in Baijiao Mine, the obtained data in this step is limited. As is shown in images, there are not linear relationship existing between D and ε, after in term of power function and exponent function, founding that the exponent function result is better, therefore, the result through exponent function is selected as damage evolution equation in this step,

$$D = 0.1467\exp(2.8134\varepsilon) \tag{22}$$

Substituting equation (22) into equation (18), getting constitutive model in damage accelerated development step,

$$\sigma = E(1-0.1467\exp(2.8134\varepsilon))\varepsilon \tag{23}$$

Summing up, equation (18), (20), (22) constitute segmentation damage evolution equation of coal in Baijiao Mine before coming to peak value, and equation (19), (21), (23) constitute segmentation damage constitutive model of coal in Baijiao Mine before coming to peak value. Since scanning times are less in damage accelerated development step, the error of constitutive model is comparative large, there is a certain deviation between theory value and measured value.

Bellonoi has purposed that damage can be described with the density variety ratio $\Delta\rho/\rho_0$ in creep damage, and improved Kachanov damage variable can be shown as follow equation with adoption of conservation of mass,

$$D = 1 - \psi = -\Delta\rho / \rho_0 \tag{24}$$

Davis has defined damage variable with damage density. Lemaitre has also presented the method of measuring damage with the change of density,

$$D = (\Delta\rho / \rho_0)^{2/3} \tag{25}$$

Table 7 gives a comparison of damage variable through equation (24) and equation (25) in the process of uniaxial damage spread. From the table, it can be seen that the damage variable obtained by CT data is larger than that obtained by Bellonoi equation, and smaller than that obtained by Lemaitre equation. This is because Lemaitre supposed material damage as simple cavity damage in deducing damage variable calculation formula, which is suitable for metal and soil material. As for coal, which containing not only cavity damage but also damage caused by micro-fracture, is complicated damage. The CT data can give full expression to this characteristic, which has a general application. Calculation damage variable via CT data resolves damage discriminating "scale" problem, which mainly embodied in resolving coefficient m_0 of CT machine. At the same time, CT reorganization can be applied into different damage, and the obtained result t is more reasonable than Bellonoi equation and Lemaitre equation.

5 CONCLUSIONS

Using the specified loading equipment and the CT machine, the real-time computerized tomography testing of coal under uniaxial compression was completed. Through CT scanning, the clear CT images which included the step from the micro-crack closure to the micro-crack growth, bifurcation, development, failure and the post-failure step were obtained. According to the CT values, the meso-damage evolution of coal under uniaxial compression was analyzed. Based on the results which tallies with micro-facture, cavity growth, and section forming obtained from CT scanning of coal, the study on the damage propagation of coal was carried out. It is demonstrated that in the process of unloading failure of coal is paroxysmal. At the same time, the meso-mechanism of dilatancy in coal under the condition of uniaxial compression is experimentally studied. Based on the change of the CT value and CT images obtained from scanning test, the propagation law of the meso-damage in coal is deduced. The change law of crack width and length related to creeping time has been quantitatively analyzed. In the light of the law and CT image, which are of referential for the building of damage constitutive model and damage evolution function of coal, the macro-damage process of coal under uniaxial compression in Baijiao Mine has been divided into 5 steps, the damage-weakening step, the linear step, the damage starts to evolve and damage develops steadily, the damage development speeding up and the weakening step after reaching peak. In the end, the comparison of damage variable between CT scanning and Bellonoi equation, Lemaitre equation in the process of uniaxial damage spread was obtained which resolves successfully damage discriminating "scale" problem, and the obtained results is more reasonable than Bellonoi equation and Lemaitre equation.

Table 7. Comparison of *D* from Bellonoi, Lemaitre formula.

	1 $/10^{-2}$	2 $/10^{-2}$	3 $/10^{-2}$	4 $/10^{-2}$	5 $/10^{-2}$	6 $/10^{-2}$	7 $/10^{-2}$
Scans	1.39	0.90	0.41	0.45	0.33	1.71	0.9987
Bellonoi	0.00	0.16	0.32	0.45	0.34	0.13	0.4937
Lemaitre	0.00	1.37	2.15	2.68	2.24	1.14	0.6232

ACKNOWLEDGEMENT

This project was supported by China Postdoctoral Science Foundation and the financial supported by Visiting Scholar Foundation of Key Lab in University.

REFERENCES

Cook N. G. W. The Failure of Rock [J]. Int. J. Rock Mech. Min. Sci., 1965, 2, 389–403.

Cook N. G. W. A Note on Rock bursts Considered as A Problem of Stability [J]. J. South Afr. Inst. Min. and Metallurgy., 1965, 65 , 437–446.

Hallbauer D. K., Wagner H. and Cook N. G. W. Some observations concerning the Microscopic and Mechanical Behavior of Quartzite Specimens in Stiff, triaxial Compression Tests [J]. Int. J. Rock Mech. Min. Sci. & Geomech. Abstr., 1973, 10, 713–726.

Kawakata H., Cho A., Yanagidani T., and Shimada M. The observations of faulting in westerly granite under triaxial compression by X-ray CT scan [J]. Int. J. Rock Mech. & Min. Sci.1997, 34 (3~4), 151–162.

Lippmann H. Mechanics of "Bumps" in Coal Mines. A Discussion of Violent Deformations in the Sides of Roadways in Coal Seams [J]. Appl. Mech. Rev., 1987, 40 (8), 1033–1043.

Salamon M. D. G. and Wagner H. Role of Stabilizing Pillars in the Alleviation of Rock burst Hazard in Deep Mines [J]. Proc. 4th Int. Congr. Rock Mech., Montreal, 1979, 2, 561–566.

Sprunt E. S. and Brace W. F. Direct Observation of Micro cavities in Crystalline Rocks [J]. Int. J. Rock Mech. Min. Sci. & Geomech. Abstr., 1974, 11, 139–150.

Tapponnier P. and Brace W. F. Development of Stress~Induced Micro cracks in Westerly Granite[J]. Int. J. Rock Mech. Min. Sci. & Geomech. Abstr., 1976, 13, 103–112.

Verhelst F., Vervoort A. Debosscher P. H. and Leuven K.U. X-ray computerized topography, Determination of heterogeneities in rock samples [J]. In, S. Sakuraied. Proceedings of the 8th International Congress on Rock Mechanics. Rotterdam, A.A. Balkema, 1995, 105–108.

Zhao Y., Huang J. and Wang R. Real~Time SEM Observations of the Micro fracturing Process in Rock During a Compression Test [J]. Int. J. Rock Mech. Min. Sci. & Geomech. Abstr., 1993, 30(6), 643–652.

Zhang Wohua and Valliappan S. Analysis of Random Anisotropy Damage Mechanics Problems of Rock Mass [J]. Part I-Probability Simulation, Part II-Statistical Estimation. Rock Mech. Rock Engng., 1990, 23, 241–259.

Zubelewicz O. C. and Mroz Z. Numerical Simulation of Rock Burst Processes Treated as Problems of Dynamic Instability [J]. Rock Mech. Rock Eng., 1983, 16, 253–274.

X-ray CT for Geomaterials; Soils, Concrete, Rocks – Otani & Obara (eds.)
© 2004 Swets & Zeitlinger. Lisse, ISBN 90 5809 666 1

Lateral displacement and failure of Akiyoshi marble in the post-failure condition observed by X-ray CT

S. Murata & T. Saito
Kyoto University, Kyoto, Japan

M. Imamura
Chuo Kaihatsu Corporation, Chiba, Japan

ABSTRACT: For the specimen of Akiyoshi marble, post-failure lateral displacement was measured by twelve radial displacement transducers mounted around the rock specimen in every 30-degree. Moreover, the lateral displacement and the failure condition was inspected by X-ray CT. The specimens used for this inspection were prepared by unloading at several interesting points appeared in a triaxial compression test. From this study, followings were concluded. First, the isotropic lateral displacement is caused by the development of small failures uniformly occurring in the specimen. Second, the anisotropic lateral displacement is caused by the development of localization of the small failure in the specimen, and the anisotropic displacement increases in the direction that the localization occurs. Third, the lateral displacement clearly increases with the increase in slide along a generated fracture if it has been generated. Thus, the progress of lateral displacement was successfully related to the failure of the specimen.

1 INTRODUCTION

To estimate the stability of rock caverns is one of the most important problems on mining and civil engineering. For the caverns, the stability is usually estimated from rock wall displacement such as convergence during the excavation, but it is not always estimated correctly on the stage of design. Because the deformation behavior of rock in the loosed region around the caverns is not sufficiently clear. In the loosed region, rock would be failed and deform plastically or slide along the fractures. Therefore, it is necessary to understand the deformation behavior of rock in failed condition for the correct stability estimation of caverns.

Near the wall of caverns, the stress condition is equal to that of the specimen under a triaxial compression test, and the rock wall displacement corresponds to the lateral displacement of the specimen. We have investigated the lateral displacement of rock specimen especially in the post-failure condition under the triaxial compression test. From the investigation, it was clarified that the isotropic deformation governs the lateral displacement before an apparent fracture is generated, and the slide along the fracture governs the lateral displacement after the fracture is generated (Saito et al. 1997, 1998(a), 1998(b)).

In this study, for the specimen of Akiyoshi marble, the post-failure lateral displacement is measured by twelve radial displacement transducers mounted around the specimen in every 30-degree. Moreover, the failure condition is inspected by using an X-ray CT scanner in order to discuss the relation between them clearly.

2 EXPERIMENTAL PROCEDURE

2.1 *Specimen and triaxial compression test*

Cylindrical Akiyoshi marbles whose size is 30 mm in diameter and 60 mm in length was used for a specimen. This is because marbles are more plastic than the other kinds of rock under the triaxial compression test even with low confining pressure and it is easy for us to control the progress of failure. Both end surfaces of the specimen were polished to be enough smooth and parallel. The specimens had no apparent heterogeneity. This was confirmed by X-ray CT. Typical uniaxial compressive strength, Young's modulus and Poisson's ratio of the specimens are shown in Table 1.

It is impossible for us to observe the specimen by X-ray CT under the triaxial compression test. Therefore, specimens were unloaded at interesting points on the differential stress vs. axial strain curves (stress–strain

Table 1. Mechanical properties of Akiyoshi marble determined by the uniaxial compression test.

Uniaxial compression strength	74 MPa
Young's Modulus	38 GPa
Poisson's ratio	0.38

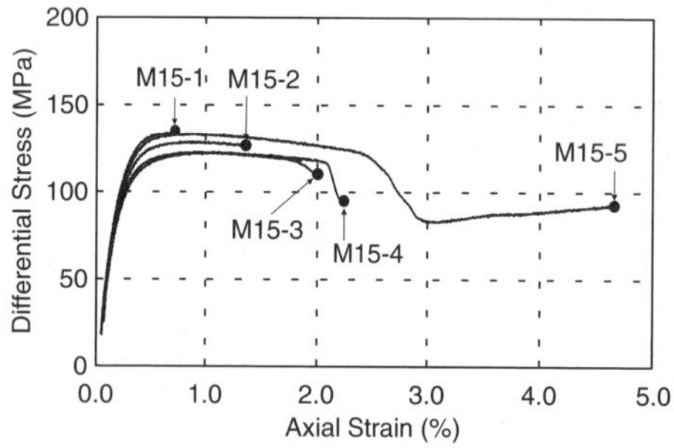

(a) Small confining pressure (15MPa)

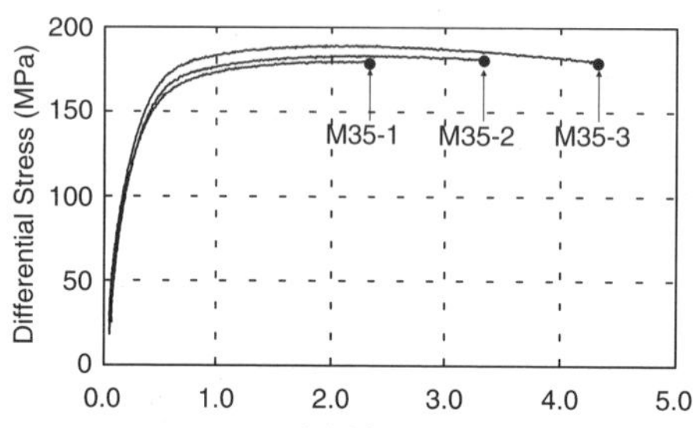

(b) Large confining pressure (35MPa)

Figure 1. Stress–strain curves obtained from the triaxial compression tests for the specimens of the X-ray CT.

curves) shown in Figure 1-(a) and Figure 1-(b) and inspected the failure condition by X-ray CT. The unloading points are the strength failure point (M15-1), just before the large stress-drop (M15-2), during the large stress-drop (M15-3), just after the large stress-drop (M15-4) and the axial displacement of 3 mm, that is, the end of the test (M15-5) for the small confining pressure of 15 MPa. They are the strength failure point (M35-1), during the strain softening (M35-2) and the axial displacement of 3 mm (M35-5) for the large confining pressure of 35 MPa. From Figure 1, we can know that the unloading points were well set at the characteristic point of failure condition, although the stress–strain curves are little different each other. Thus, the specimen of different failure condition for the X-ray CT observation was obtained.

The triaxial compression test were performed under the constant axial displacement rate of 0.0375 mm/minute until the stress–strain curve reached the unloading point with keeping the confining pressure constant. In this study, as shown in Figure 1, the confining pressure was set to 15 MPa and 35 MPa in order to investigate the influence of confining pressure on the failure condition in the specimen.

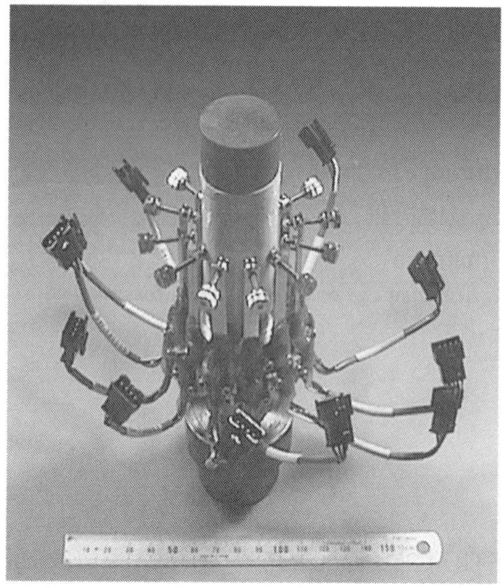

Figure 2. The lateral displacement transducers mounted around the cylindrical specimen.

2.2 *Measurement of lateral displacement*

Under the triaxial compression test, radial displacement was measured in the center cross section by 12 displacement transducers of cantilever type. Their sensitivity is 1750×10^{-6}/mm and their capacity is 3 mm. They were mounted around the specimen in every 30-degree by fixing them around the iron pedestal as shown in Figure 2.

The specimen was glued on the pedestal in order to reduce the relative displacement between the specimen and the displacement transducers. The heat shrinkage tube used for a jacket to protect the specimen from the invasion of hydraulic oil was enough hard. Therefore, the deformation of it is ignorable. Moreover, thin Teflon film was attached in order to reduce the friction acting at the measuring points. Thus, the 12 radial displacements were measured with the axial load and axial displacement.

2.3 *X-ray CT observation*

The X-ray CT scanner possessed by Japan National Oil Corporation was used for this study. The specification of the CT scanner is shown in Table 2.

In the X-ray CT observation, a cross sectional image of the specimen is obtained as the distribution of CT number determined by the next equation.

Table 2. The specification of the X-ray CT scanner.

Generation	Second generation (traverse/rotation)
X-ray tube voltage (maximum)	320 Kev
Scan field (maximum)	250 mm (diameter) × 600 mm (length)
Resolution (minimum pixel size)	0.15 mm × 0.15 mm
Slice width	1.0, 2.0, 4.0 (mm) (selectable)
Inspection time	3.5 minute/slice
Display	512 × 512 matrix

$$\text{CT number} = K\frac{\mu - \mu_w}{\mu_w} \qquad (1)$$

where μ is X-ray absorption coefficient of a specimen; μ_w is that of water, and K is a conversion coefficient. Since the CT number of air is −1000 and that of water is zero, the value of K is usually set to 1000. Generally, soft materials have small CT number and hard materials have large CT number.

The X-ray of long wavelength, soft X-ray, is easily absorbed and has small penetration ability, but the X-ray of short wavelength, hard X-ray, is not absorbed so easily and has large penetration ability. As a result, the hard X-ray remains as X-ray penetrates the specimen. Therefore, in the CT image, the center part of the specimen shows small CT number because the specimen becomes relatively soft at that part. This phenomenon is called beam hardening. It should be removed in order to estimate the failed region correctly from the CT image.

For each specimen, twenty cross sections of 2 mm thick were observed to the center region of 40 mm long. The cross sectional image was taken before and after the triaxial compression test at the same position, and then, the difference between them in CT number was calculated in order to remove the beam hardening effect supposing it should be unchangeable.

3 EXPERIMENTAL RESULTS

3.1 *Results of lateral displacement measurement*

For each specimen, radial displacement measured in the 12 directions is shown in Figure 3. The numbers beside each axis show the displacement number.

From this figure, followings are recognized for the case of small confining pressure (15 MPa), in which the apparent fracture was generated. First, the radial displacement is isotropic before the large stress-drop, because the shape of radar chart for the specimen M15-1 and M15-2 is almost circle. Moreover, parallel movement of the specimen has been occurred, because the center of the radar chart for these specimens moves

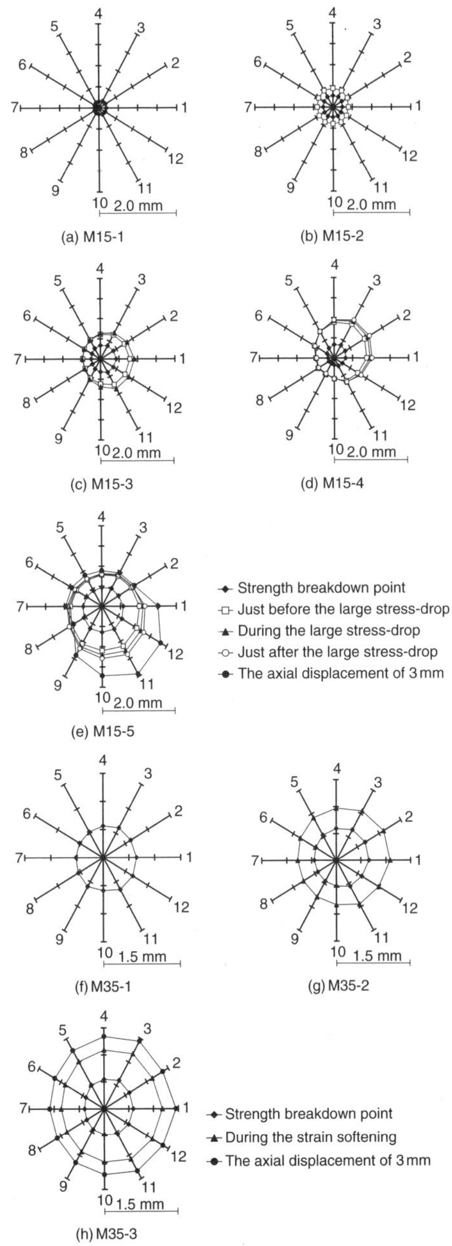

Figure 3. Distribution of the lateral displacement measured in the triaxial compression test for each specimen.

from the origin. Second, radial displacement increases in some directions, but it almost stops increasing in the other directions after the large stress-drop shown in the radar chart of the specimens M15-4 and M15-5. This anisotropic displacement is probably caused by the slide along the generated fracture.

On the other hand, it is recognized that the radial displacement increases isotropically for the case of large confining pressure (35 MPa), in which the apparent fracture was not generated.

3.2 *Result of the X-ray CT*

CT images of each specimen are shown in Figure 4. The upper images are the volume-rendering image generated from the twenty cross sectional images and the lower images are the cross sectional image obtained at the center of the specimen. They show the change of CT number between before and after the triaxial compression test. The reduction of CT number becomes large as the failure progresses. The direction of the CT images corresponds to that of the radar chart shown in Figure 3, that is, the right direction of the CT images is the direction of the displacement transducer No. 1.

For the case of small confining pressure (15 MPa), it is recognized that the small failures occur uniformly in the specimen and does not clearly localize before the large stress-drop. In the CT image during the large stress-drop, however, it is recognized that the small failures localize along a line to be a fracture in the volume-rendering image. This localization is also recognized in the cross sectional image slightly. Furthermore, it is recognized that the fracture is generated in the CT image of just after the large stress-drop and the shape and aperture of the fracture become much clear in the CT image of axial displacement of 3 mm. The aperture would be yielded by the slide along the generated fracture surface.

For the case of large confining pressure (35 MPa), it is recognized that the small failure occurs uniformly in all specimens without generating a fracture, and the uniformly occurring small failure increases gradually.

4 DISCUSSION

4.1 *Change of lateral displacement behavior*

As authors have published, the lateral displacement of the specimen is mainly composed from next four components shown in Figure 5 (Saito et al. 1997, 1998(a), 1998(b)). They were (a) isotropic deformation, (b) anisotropic deformation, (c) parallel movement and (d) slide along the generated fracture. The component (c) must be caused by the testing condition such as the parallelism between the end surfaces of a specimen and it would not relate to the failure of the specimen

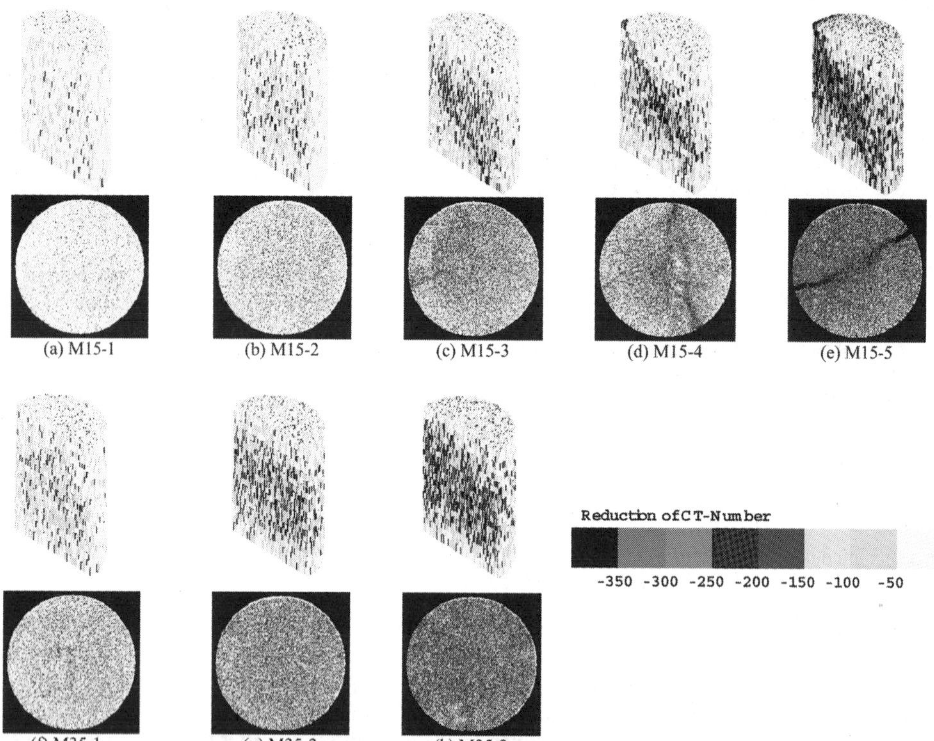

Figure 4. Volume-rendering image generated from the twenty cross sectional images and the cross sectional image obtained at the center of the specimen for each specimen.

directly. In addition, the component (d) should appear after an apparent fracture has been generated.

These components can be described as a function of the radial direction, θ, as follows.

(a) Isotropic deformation:

$$u_{r1}(\theta) = C_1 \tag{2}$$

where C_1 is the magnitude of isotropic deformation.

(b) Anisotropic deformation:

$$u_{r2}(\theta) = C_2 \cos^2 \theta \tag{3}$$

where C_2 is the length of major axis of the anisotropic displacement ellipse.

(c) Parallel movement:

$$u_{r3}(\theta) = C_3 \cos\theta \tag{4}$$

where C_3 is the movement of the center of specimen.

(d) Slide along a generated fracture:

$$u_{r4}(\theta) = \begin{cases} C_4 \cos\theta & (|\theta| \le \alpha) \\ -C_4 \cos\theta & (\alpha < |\theta| \le \pi) \end{cases} \tag{5}$$

where C_4 is the horizontal displacement yield by the slide and α is determined by the position of generated fracture as shown in Figure 5. Representing Equation (5) by fourth-order Fourier series, following equation is obtained.

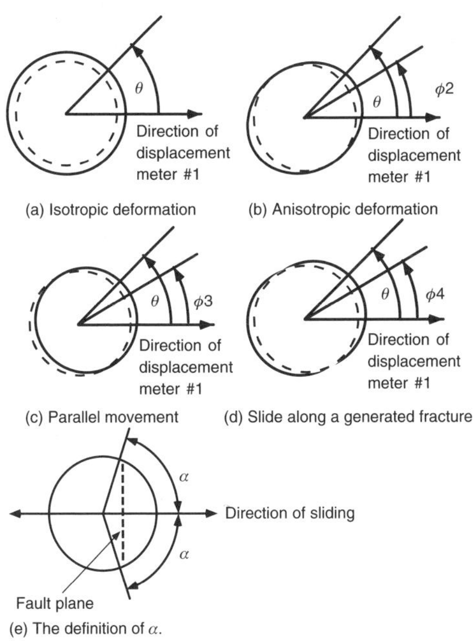

Figure 5. The four components of lateral deformation.

$$u_{r4}(\theta) = C_4 f(\theta) \tag{6}$$

$$\begin{aligned} f(\theta) = {} & \frac{2\sin\alpha}{\pi} + 2\left(\alpha - \frac{\pi}{2} + \frac{\sin 2\alpha}{2}\right)\cos\theta \\ & + 2\left(\sin\alpha + \frac{\sin 3\alpha}{3}\right)\cos 2\theta \\ & + 2\left(\frac{\sin 2\alpha}{2} + \frac{\sin 4\alpha}{4}\right)\cos 3\theta \\ & + 2\left(\frac{\sin 3\alpha}{3} + \frac{\sin 5\alpha}{5}\right)\cos 4\theta \end{aligned}$$

Thus, the lateral displacement is represented by the summation of these four components as

$$\begin{aligned} u_r(\theta) = {} & C_1 + C_2\cos^2(\theta - \phi_2) \\ & + C_3\cos(\theta - \phi_3) + C_4 f(\theta - \phi_4) \end{aligned} \tag{7}$$

where ϕ_2, ϕ_3, and ϕ_4 are the phase angle of each component measured from the direction of the displacement transducer No. 1, and the coefficients, C_1, C_2, C_3 and C_4, represent the magnitude of each component in the lateral displacement. Therefore, if these coefficients and phase angles are determined from the result of radial displacement measurement, the behavior of lateral displacement can be estimated quantitatively.

In this study, $u_r(\theta)$ was first determined from the measured data, and then, the coefficients were determined from the coefficient of fourth-order Fourier series of $u_r(\theta)$. Among the parameters, ϕ_4 and α were directly determined from the specimen after the test. Moreover, the coefficient C_4 was ignored for the analysis to the case of large confining pressure in which the apparent fracture was not observed.

The analytical results for the specimens, M15-5 and M35-3, which were loaded until the axial displacement reaches 3 mm, are shown in Figure 6-(a) and Figure 6-(b) respectively. In these figures, stress–strain curve is also drawn to indicate the variation of stress for each confining pressure.

For the case of small confining pressure (15 MPa), following are recognized from Figure 6-(a). The component C_1 starts increasing from the start of loading and it starts rapidly increasing when the specimen can be thought to be yielding. This increase of the component C_1 continues until a little after the start of the large stress-drop. The component C_3, in contrast to the component C_1, increases with almost constant rate even after the yielding point. However, since the component C_3 would not relate to the failure of the specimen directly, the component C_1 governs the lateral displacement of the specimen from the start of loading to a little after the start of the large stress-drop. After that, the component C_1 stops increasing. Alternatively, the component C_4 appears and starts rapidly increasing, and it governs the lateral displacement.

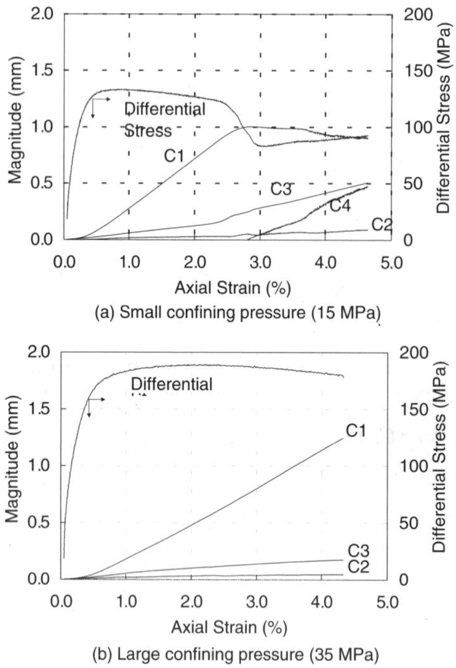

Figure 6. The variations of each component of lateral deformation under the triaxial compression test.

Although the component C_2 is recognized after the strength failure point and it becomes large during the large stress-drop, it is small through the test.

On the other hand, for the case of large confining pressure (35 MPa), following are recognized from Figure 6-(a). The component C_1 starts increasing from the start of loading and it starts rapidly increasing when the specimen can be thought to be yielding. Although the component C_3 and C_2 appear from the start of loading and increases with almost constant rate, they are much smaller than the component C_1 through the test. Therefore, the component C_1 governs the lateral displacement of the specimen through the test. In this case, the large stress-drop does not appear, and the component C_4 does not appear as a result.

4.2 *Lateral displacement and failure in the specimen*

The behavior of lateral displacement must closely relate to the progress of failure in the specimen. In this section, therefore, we will discuss the relation between them comparing Figure 6 and Figure 4.

As mentioned above, in the case of small confining pressure, the isotropic displacement governs the lateral displacement until a little after the start of the large stress-drop. Moreover, in the case of large confining pressure, the isotropic displacement governs the lateral displacement through the test. Looking at the corresponding CT images to these stages of failure condition, small failures occur uniformly in the specimen. Therefore, the isotropic displacement must be caused by the uniformly occurring small failures.

Next, during the large stress-drop, the component of anisotropic deformation becomes a little large and the component of slide along a generated fracture appears. Looking at the corresponding CT images to this stage of failure condition, the small failure localized along the line to be a fracture, and then, the localization of them progresses and a fracture is generated at the end of the large stress-drop. In addition, the anisotropic displacement increases in the direction that the localization occurs. Therefore, it can be though that the lateral displacement changes from isotropic to anisotropic as the failure in the specimen changes from uniform failure to localized failure in this stage.

Finally, lateral displacement clearly increases by the slide along the generated fracture if it has been generated. This is confirmed by the cross sectional CT image of axial displacement of 3 mm that shows the aperture of the generated fracture becomes large compared to that observed in the CT image of just the end of large stress-drop.

5 CONCLUSION

In this study, we clarified the development process of lateral displacement of Akiyoshi marble under a triaxial compression test in relation to the failure in the specimen by using X-ray CT. The followings are concluded for the isotropic Akiyoshi marble as a result.

1. The isotropic lateral displacement is caused by the development of small failures uniformly occurring in the specimen.
2. The anisotropic lateral displacement is caused by the development of localization of the small failure in the specimen, and the anisotropic displacement increases in the direction that the localization occurs.
3. The lateral displacement clearly increases with the increase in slide along the generated fracture if it has been generated.

REFERENCES

Saito, T., Murata, S. and Takehara, H. 1997. Postfailure lateral displacement of rock specimen under the triaxial compression test, *Proc. of the 1st ARMS*, Seoul/Korea: 439–444.

Saito, T., Takehara, H. and Murata, S. 1998. The deformation analysis of circular tunnel based on the results of post-failure lateral displacement under the triaxial compression test, *Proc. of the 10th Japan Symp. on Rock Mech.*: 563–568 (in Japanese).

Saito, T., Murata, S., Imamura, M. and Sasao, H. 1998. The radial deformation of rock specimen in the post-failure region under the triaxial compression test, *Shigen-to-Sozai*, 114: 901–908 (in Japanese).

X-ray CT for Geomaterials; Soils, Concrete, Rocks – Otani & Obara (eds.)
© 2004 Swets & Zeitlinger. Lisse, ISBN 90 5809 666 1

X-ray CT observations of strain localization and failure in two porous sandstones

P. Bésuelle
Laboratoire Sols, Solides, Structures, CNRS-UJF-INPG, Grenoble, France

ABSTRACT: The localized failure of two porous sandstones in triaxial compression is presented in the transition between the brittle and ductile regimes. X-ray computed tomography (CT) is used to characterize the deformation bands in post-mortem specimens. Such a tool is useful to study the volumetric strain inside the bands and to describe the band patterning. It is found that deformation bands are dilative when the specimens are loaded at low confining pressure and are compactive at high confining pressure. The patterns of shear banding depend also on the confining pressure, with either a single band or a complex pattern of several bands. This evolution of strain localization is associated to a change of rock behavior before localization. These observations highlight the brittle-ductile transition where failure in the brittle regime is associated to strain localization and failure in the ductile regime is associated to a cataclastic flow.

1 INTRODUCTION

The advantages in using X-ray CT scan to study the strain localization phenomenon in geomaterials, and more specifically in rocks, are well known (*e.g.*, Raynaud *et al.* 1989; Vinegar *et al.* 1991; Kawakata *et al.* 1999). The two major advantages are that the method is nondestructive and can be used for a same specimen at several steps of loading, and that the method gives 3D information on the mass density field evolution in a whole specimen.

The aim of this study is to analyze the transition between brittle and ductile regime of failure in porous rocks. Brittle failure is generally associated to strain localization or faulting, whereas the ductile regime is generally associated to a diffuse shear-enhanced compaction (*e.g.,* Wong *et al.* 1997). This paper summarizes and compares for the first time two recent studies (Bésuelle *et al.* 2000, 2003) which deal with this aspect. The two works have been performed with two different sandstones, two different load cells, two different X-ray CT systems, and two different microscope techniques. We concentrate here on what we can and what we cannot see with X-ray CT apparatuses.

The first part of the paper describes the test conditions, the second part describes the mechanical behavior of the two sandstones, and the third part shows the results obtained by tomography on post-mortem specimens. A discussion finally compares the X-ray CT observations with microscope characterizations.

2 TESTED MATERIALS AND EXPERIMENTAL DEVICES

2.1 *Materials*

The two tested rocks are natural pink sandstones coming from the Vosges mountains in eastern France, at Woustviller and Rothbach quarries. They are quite similar, the studied Woustviller sandstone has a porosity of 22%, a mean grain size of about 0.3 mm and is composed of quartz (93%) with a few percent of feldspar and white mica. The Rothbach sandstone specimens come from the same block studied by David *et al.* (1994), the rock has a porosity of about 20.3% (average of the connected porosity measured on each studied samples), a mean grain size of about 0.23 mm and is composed by quartz (68%), feldspar (16%), clay (~12%) and oxides and mica (3%). Specimens axis were perpendicular to the bedding.

2.2 *Experimental conditions*

The two sandstones were tested with two different triaxial (axisymmetric) compression cells. Woustviller sandstone was tested in Grenoble (Bésuelle *et al.* 2000) with a cell which can sustain a confining pressure of 60 MPa while Rothbach sandstone was tested in Stony Brook, USA (Bésuelle *et al.* 2003) with a confining pressure lower than 140 MPa. The experimental conditions are quite similar. A first step of the test is to apply an isotropic stress in the specimen by increasing the confining pressure, the specimen being separated from the confining fluid by a thin membrane. The second step of the test is the deviatoric loading, which is obtained by increasing the axial stress via an axial piston while keeping the confining pressure constant. The axial loading is controlled in displacement, with a strain rate of about $10^{-5}\,s^{-1}$.

The Woustviller sandstone specimens had a diameter and a height of 40 mm and 80 mm, respectively. They were tested dry after exposing them to a temperature of 100°C for a few days. Deformation of the specimens was measured with seven internal transducers, three in the axial direction and four in the lateral directions (Bésuelle & Desrues 2001). Such a device allows to detect the emergence of strain localization in the specimen. Specimen ends were in contact with smooth enlarged platens and were lubricated with a mixture of vaseline and stearic acid to minimize friction. Specimens were unloaded after failure and two of them were afterwards analyzed by X-ray CT and then by electronic microscope (on thin sections).

The Rothbach sandstone specimens had a diameter and a height of 18.1 mm and 38.1 mm, respectively. They were saturated with distilled water. Axial strain was computed from the displacement of the cell piston measured by an external transducer. Adjustment of a pressure generator kept the pore pressure constant to 10 MPa during the deviatoric loading step, and the pore volume change was recorded. An *effective stress* is defined here as the global stress minus the pore pressure. The ends of the specimens were also lubricated with the same mixture as for Woustviller sandstone, but the platens contained several shallow grooves to insure pore fluid drainage, which is less favorable for a frictionless interface. Specimens at different stages of deformation were unloaded and retrieved from the pressure vessel for subsequent X-ray CT imaging. Some of the specimens were analyzed by optical microscope to measure crack density field on thin sections.

2.3 *X-ray CT apparatuses*

The two sandstones have been analyzed in two different X-ray CT apparatuses which are both medical scanners. Imaging of the Woustviller sandstones specimens were conducted at the Laboratoire de Mécanique et Acoustique in Marseille, France. The beam energy was 73 keV, the X-ray tube voltage was 120 kV, the detector had 31 channels and each pixel represented a $0.7 \times 0.7\,mm^2$ surface projected onto the medium plane of the slice, which had a thickness of 2 mm. Imaging of the Rothbach sandstones specimens were conducted at the Institut Français du Pétrole in Rueil-Malmaison, France. The X-ray tube voltage was 130 kV, the detector contained 1024 channels and the pixel size was $0.2 \times 0.2\,mm^2$ for a slice thickness of 1.5 mm.

For these two apparatuses, a set of 1D projections of the attenuation profile through a slice of the specimen (perpendicular to the specimen axis) was measured for different angular positions around the specimen. The 2D slice was reconstructed by a mathematical algorithm and a 3D reconstruction was computed from several adjacent slices. Then, reconstruction of slices parallel to the specimen axis could be obtained. For the Rothbach sandstone specimens, imaging of slices parallel to the specimen axis had also been directly performed.

3 MECHANICAL BEHAVIOR

The mechanical responses obtained are shown in Figure 1 (numbers in front of each curves correspond to the effective lateral stress). Compressive stresses and strains are taken positive. The deviatoric stress is defined as the axial stress minus the lateral stress (confining pressure). The deviatoric stress *vs.* axial strain curves for Woustviller sandstone (Fig. 1a) and for Rothbach sandstone (Fig. 1b) are quite similar for effective lateral stresses smaller than 60 MPa. The peak axial strain for Rothbach sandstone is higher, however this might be due to the fact that the axial displacement is measured outside the cell, and therefore takes into account the cell compliance, while internal transducers were used for Woustviller sandstone. In this range of confining pressures, the deviatoric stress increases during loading up to a peak and then decreases toward a residual stress. The peak stress and residual stress increase with the lateral stress value, however, for Woustviller sandstone, the peak stress at 60 MPa confining pressure is lightly smaller than for 50 MPa. With Rothbach sandstone, for 90 MPa and 130 MPa effective lateral stress, a peak stress is not clearly visible, and residual stress still increases with confining pressure. However, at 90 MPa, in the deviatoric stress *vs.* axial strain curve, a deviation from the initial linear part of the curve, followed by a peak and a short strain softening occurs at a smaller value than for the test at 55 MPa effective lateral stress.

As far as volumetric behavior is concerned (Figs. 1c, d), contractancy occurs at the beginning of the loading and, depending on the lateral stress, one gets either dilatancy (stronger at low effective lateral stresses) or contractancy at high lateral stresses (shear-enhanced compaction). However, it should be noted that axial strain and volumetric strain after strain localization (close to the stress peak) are only representative of a structural behavior of specimens and should be considered with caution.

The failure envelope (stress peaks locus) in the deviatoric stress *vs.* effective mean stress plane for

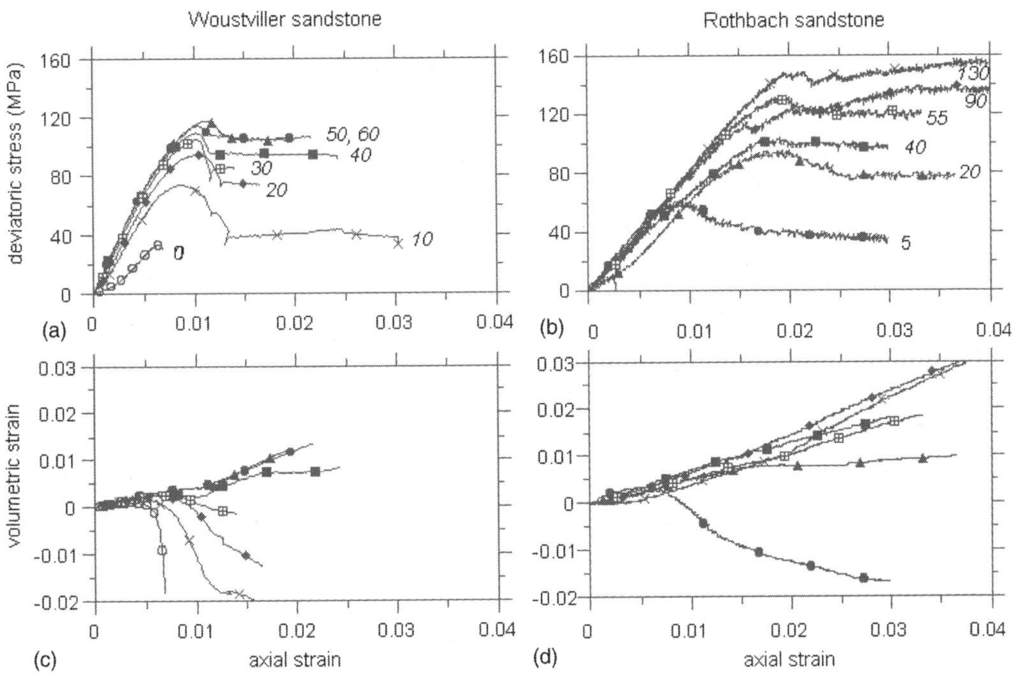

Figure 1. Deviatoric stress *vs.* axial strain and volumetric strain *vs.* axial strain for Woustviller sandstone and Rothbach sandstone tested in triaxial compression at several confining pressures.

Woustviller sandstone shows a positive slope between 0 and 50 MPa lateral stress and a negative slope between 50 and 60 MPa. For Rothbach sandstone, the curve has a positive slope up to 130 MPa, except if one considers for the test at 90 MPa the first stress peak discussed previously. In that case, there is a negative slope between 55 and 90 MPa. Other tests would be necessary to clarify this aspect.

4 STRAIN LOCALIZATION OBSERVATIONS BY X-RAY CT IMAGING

The Woustviller sandstone specimens were obtained from a block which had a slight heterogeneity, not visible by simple observation, corresponding probably to the bedding. The upper portion was less dense than the lower portion of the specimen, the mass densities measured by water impregnation being 1.955 and 1.982 g/cm^3, respectively. This heterogeneity can be observed by X-ray CT imaging of the specimens where the upper part is slightly darker then the lower part.

Also, the Rothbach sandstone specimens had a heterogeneity, which is well visible on the X-ray images. Thin bands, a few millimeters thick, are less dark than outside and are sub-perpendicular to the specimens axis. These heterogeneities correspond to the initial bedding and the X-ray absorption difference can be explained, either by mass density difference or by mineralogy composition difference, or both. However, optical microscopic observations suggest that these bands are associated with a change of grain size and porosity.

4.1 *Woustviller sandstone*

Two specimens tested at 30 MPa and 50 MPa lateral stress (up to an axial strain of 0.019 and 0.015, respectively) have been X-ray CT imaged. Visual inspection of the specimens after testing allows to see that the specimen at 30 MPa had externally one to two parallel white bands. Figure 2 shows the CT images of several adjacent slices in the part of the specimen where strain localization occurred. The band is darker than in the rest of the specimen, which means that this band has a porosity greater than the mean porosity of the specimen. The position of the band in the slices depends on the slice elevation, because the band is inclined with respect to the specimen axis. The band is not perfectly plane, and the porosity inside the band is not uniform. At intermediate elevations, the porosity in the band near the surface of the specimen is higher than the porosity in the band far from the surface. The reconstruction of the specimen in a plane

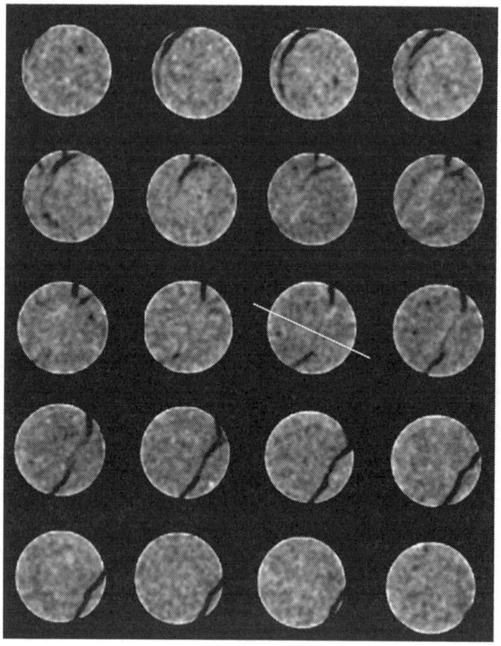

Figure 2. X-ray CT imaging of several slices at different elevations of a Woustviller sandstone specimen tested at 30 MPa lateral stress. The white line gives the direction of reconstruction.

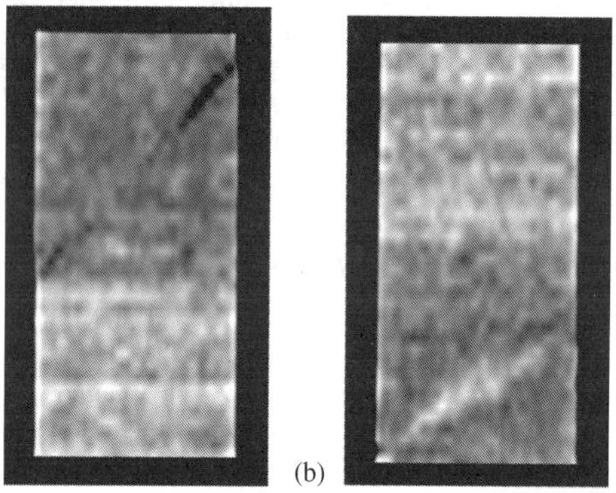

(a) (b)

Figure 3. Reconstructions of the Woustviller sandstone specimens tested at 30 MPa (a) and 50 MPa (b) lateral stress. Planes of reconstruction correspond to the directions of white lines in Figures 2 and 4, respectively.

parallel to the specimen axis (indicated by the white line in Fig. 2) is shown in Figure 3a. The initial heterogeneity of the specimen can easily be observed, the deformation band occurred in the more porous part of the specimen. The band is well observable in the reconstruction.

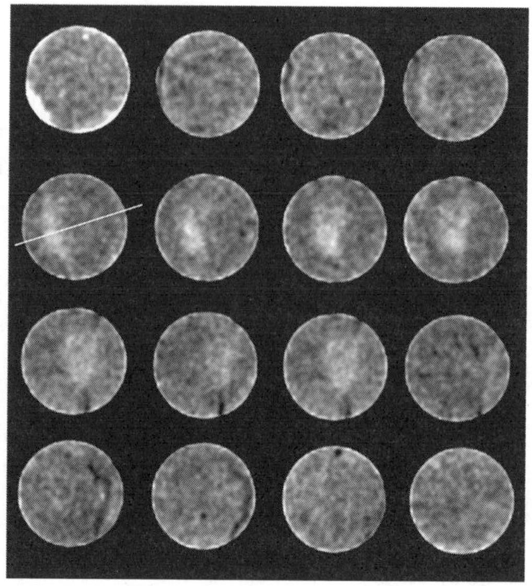

Figure 4. X-ray CT imaging of several slices at different elevations of a Woustviller sandstone specimen tested at 50 MPa lateral stress. The white line gives the direction of reconstruction.

Figure 4 shows different slices of the specimen tested at 50 MPa confining pressure. For this specimen, visual observation of the specimen revealed several conjugated bands. However, the reconstruction of the specimen in a plane parallel to its axis (Fig. 3b), shows only a single band. The band is larger than the band in the previous specimen and not so well defined. In the band and near the surface of the specimen, the porosity is higher than the mean porosity of the specimen. In the core of the specimen, the porosity in the band is smaller than the mean porosity of the specimen. Note that the predominance of one shear band over the others was also detected with internal lateral transducers.

4.2 *Rothbach sandstone*

X-ray CT images of twelve specimens tested at 5, 20, 40, 55, 90 and 130 MPa effective lateral stress were performed. Two samples tested at 5 MPa up to an axial strain of 0.029 (corresponding to the residual stress plateau) and 0.017 (after the peak and just before to attain the residual stres) show the same strain localization patterning (Figs 5–6a). In each slice, several dark zones were observed to radiate from an approximately circular zone. Both the diameter of the concentric zone and the spacing between the radial zones vary with the elevation of the slice. Such a pattern is composed of a cone centered on the specimen axis and a set of shear bands associated with V-shape pairs.

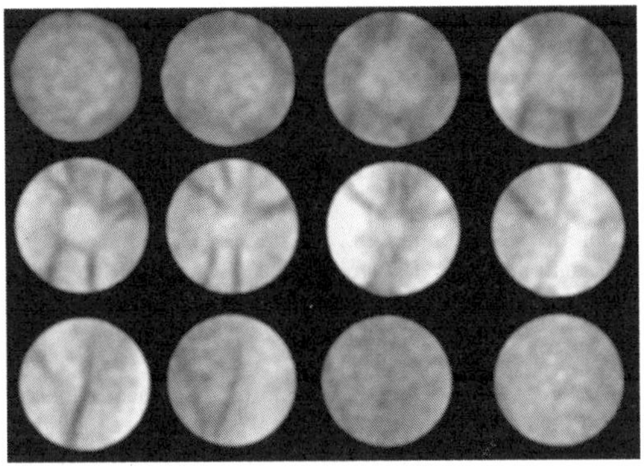

Figure 5. X-ray CT imaging of several adjacent slices of a Rothbach sandstone specimen tested at 5 MPa of effective lateral stress.

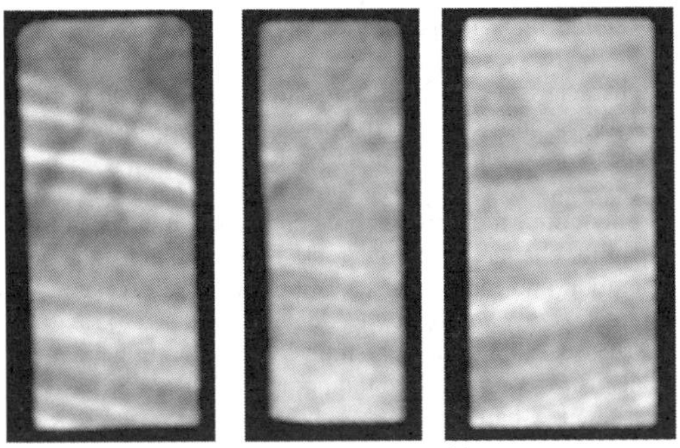

(a) (b) (c)

Figure 6. X-ray CT imaging of slices parallel to the specimen axis of Rothbach sandstone specimens tested at 5 MPa (a), 20 MPa (b) and 55 MPa (c) of effective lateral stress. Sub-horizontal bright bands correspond to the initial bedding.

Two samples have been tested at 20 MPa effective lateral stress, up to an axial strain of 0.034 (on the residual stress plateau) and 0.021 (before to attain the residual stress). A simple dark band can be seen on the first specimen (Fig. 6b), similarly to Woustviller sandstone at 30 MPa (Fig. 3a), and nothing is visible on the second specimen, probably due to the smaller maximum loading axial strain.

For the specimens tested at 40 MPa effective lateral stress, nothing can be observed on the X-ray images. At 55 MPa, a cone of slightly higher mass density seems to have developed on a specimen (Fig. 6c), near the upper end. Given the low resolution, it is difficult to unambiguously evaluate to what extent these represent strain localization features. At 90 MPa and 130 MPa effective lateral strain, nothing can be observed on the images, which could be clearly attributed to strain localization and not to the initial bedding.

5 DISCUSSION

The observations on Woustviller sandstone indicate the existence of dilating shear band in the specimen tested at low effective lateral stress and of compactive shear band at higher lateral stress. The X-ray images have been compared with a measurement of the surfacic porosity on thin section by electronic microscope. Where one observes a dark band by X-ray CT, one also observes a band of damaged grains. The external part of the band is characterized by grain cracking and a higher porosity than outside the band while the central part of the band is characterized by a cataclastic deformation (grain crushing) and a very high porosity. For the specimen where one observes a white band on the X-ray image (decrease of the porosity), one also observes (with the microscope) a band, the external part of which is characterized by a grain cracking and a lower surfacic porosity than outside the band, whereas the central part of the band is characterized by a cataclastic deformation and a very high porosity. These measurements are consistent with X-ray CT images but with more details in the spatial composition of the band. Due to the resolution of the X-ray apparatus, only a compacting band appears, resulting from the averaging of the thin dilating central part of the band and the larger contracting external part of the band.

The experimental results have also been compared with theoretical prediction. A bifurcation analysis corresponding to the possible occurrence of a shear band was presented by Bésuelle (2001). The theoretical model predicts that shear bands are dilative at low confining pressure and compactive at higher confining pressure, with a continuous evolution from one behavior to the other.

For Rothbach sandstone, the observations of strain localization are more delicate. At 5 MPa effective lateral stress, a complex pattern of localization, including a central cone and some external radial and inclined bands appeared. Such a pattern was already observed in sand specimens (Desrues *et al.* 1996; Alshibli *et al.* 2000; Desrues 2003). Apparently, no such pattern was observed in Woustviller sandstone. It is possible that the grooves in the loading platens of the experimental apparatus used for Rothbach sandstone had an influence on that. Indeed, such a pattern respects more the axisymmetric condition of the test than a single band pattern. At 20 MPa, only a single band seems to exist.

At higher lateral stress, no structure of localization is clearly visible on X-ray CT images. However, the measurements of the crack density field by optical microscope show that the specimens were damaged (Bésuelle *et al.* 2003). At 40 MPa and 55 MPa effective lateral stress, a substantial damage by grain cracking is apparent near one or both the ends of the sample. High-angle conjugate zones initiated from the sample corner. At 55 MPa, locations of high-angle conjugate zones in the thin section roughly correspond to those where an axisymmetric compacting cone was vaguely resolved by CT (Fig. 6c). At 90 MPa lateral stress, microscopic observation shows a damage zone at the ends of specimen on a portion which represents approximately the half of the specimen. At 130 MPa, intense cracking (grain crushing) was observed on about 2/3 of the specimen, and several localized and elongated clusters (like bands) were identified in the central part of the sample. The orientation of these clusters is mainly sub-horizontal. Such structures could be interpreted as compaction band in which essentially compactive strain without shear is concentrated.

From a theoretical point of view, the model predicts that, if localization occurs during the tests in an intermediate range corresponding to around 40 and 55 MPa and even more, there is essentially a shear mechanism, without volume changes (Bésuelle *et al.* 2003). This result could explain why the damage zone observed by microscope cannot be observed by X-ray CT imaging. For the test at 130 MPa, the sub-horizontal bands, which are expected to be compaction bands, could not be observed by X-ray CT because they can be mistaken with the initial bedding of Rothbach sandstone. A differential measurement, before and after the test, would be needed to identify the existence of strain localization by X-ray CT.

It can be concluded that the transition between the brittle regime and the ductile regime (generally associated to a diffuse damage and a shear-enhanced compaction) is characterized by a continuous evolution of strain localization, from dilative shear band to compactive shear band and finally to compaction band.

As a conclusion, X-ray CT imaging is a very powerful tool to study the strain localization in terms of porosity evolution and band patterning. However, it appears that this tool cannot detect the damage when no volume change is implicated as it can occur in porous rocks in the brittle-ductile transition. Of course, this conclusion would not apply if the CT apparatus resolution is sufficient to observe cracks in grains.

ACKNOWLEDGEMENTS

The author thanks Frédéric Mazerolle who performed the X-ray CT measurements at the Laboratoire de Mécanique et Acoustique and Camille Schlitter who performed the CT measurements at the Institut Français du Pétrole.

REFERENCES

Alshibli, K.A., Sture, S., Costes, N.C., Frank, M.L., Lankton, M.R., Batiste, S.N. & Swanson R.A. 2000. Assessment of localized deformations in sand using X-ray computed tomography. *Geotechnical Testing Journal* 23: 274–298.

Bésuelle, P. 2001. Compacting and dilating shear bands in porous rock: Theoretical and experimental conditions. *Journal of Geophysical Research* 106(B7): 13435–13442.

Bésuelle, P., Baud, P. & Wong, T.-F. 2003. Failure mode and spatial distribution of damage in Rothbach sandstone in the brittle-ductile transition. *Pure and Applied Geophysics* 160: 851–868.

Bésuelle, P., & Desrues, J. 2001. An internal instrumentation for axial and radial strain measurements in triaxial tests. *Geotechnical Testing Journal* 24: 193–199.

Bésuelle, P., Desrues, J. & Raynaud, S. 2000. Experimental characterisation of the localisation phenomenon inside a Vosges sandstone in a triaxial cell. *Int. J. of Rock Mechanics and Mining Sciences* 37: 1223–1237.

David, C., Wong, T.-F., Zhu, W. & Zhang, J. 1994. Laboratory measurement of compaction-induced permeability changes in porous rock: implications for the generation and maintenance of pore pressure excess in the crust. *Pure and Applied Geophysics* 143: 425–456.

Desrues, J. 2003. Tracking strain localization in geomaterials using computerized tomography. This issue.

Desrues, J., Chambon, R., Mokni, M. & Mazerolle F. 1996. Void ratio evolution inside shear bands in triaxial sand specimens studied by computed tomography. *Géotechnique* 46: 529–546.

Kawakata, H., Cho, A., Kiyama, T., Yanagidani, T., Kusunose K. & Shimada, M. 1999. Three-dimensional observations of faulting process in Westerly granite under uniaxial and triaxial conditions by X-ray CT scan, *Tectonophysics* 313: 293–305.

Raynaud, S., Fabre, D., Mazerolle, F., Géraud, Y. & Latière, H.J. 1989. Analysis of the internal structure of rocks and characterization of mechanical deformation by a non-destructive method: X-ray tomodensitometry. *Tectonophysics* 159: 149–159.

Vinegar H.J., De Waal, J.A. & Wellington, S.L. 1991. CT studies of brittle failure in Castlegate sandstone. *Int. J. of Rock Mechanics and Mining Sciences* 28: 441–448.

Wong, T.-F., David, C. & Zhu, W. 1997. The transition from brittle faulting to cataclastic flow in porous sandstones: mechanical deformation. *Journal of Geophysical Research* 102: 3009–3025.

X-ray CT for Geomaterials; Soils, Concrete, Rocks – Otani & Obara (eds.)
© 2004 Swets & Zeitlinger. Lisse, ISBN 90 5809 666 1

X-ray tomography characterization of microfissuration on rocks generated by freeze-thaw cycles

A. Rodríguez-Rey, V.G. Ruiz de Argandoña, L. Calleja & L.M. Suárez del Río
Departamento de Geología, Universidad de Oviedo, Oviedo, España

C. Celorio
Servicio de Radiología, Hospital Alvarez-Buylla (SESPA), Mieres, España

ABSTRACT: The X-ray computed tomography (CT) technique has been applied to the study of samples of the "Laspra Stone", a dolomitic rock used in historical buildings of Oviedo (N of Spain), subjected to freeze-thaw cycling test to evaluate the internal damage and its evolution. This Non-Destructive Technique allows the damage to be observed and followed after each cycle without the need of destroying the sample. The specimens, 50 mm cubes, were imaged under a fourth generation X-ray medical equipment using a working conditions of 120 kV and 100 mA. The X-ray CT images of the untested rock show a distinct anisotropy due to a sedimentary layering with bands of different porosity. We present a method for the quantification of the internal damage due to the ageing tests based on the evolution of the CT numbers associated to the cracks in the successive images of sections obtained by CT. The relationship between the damage and the petrographic characteristics of the rock has been established. Cracks begin at the sample surface and grow both in depth and thickness in successive cycles.

1 INTRODUCTION

Ageing tests are fundamental in the study of the durability of monumental stones since the evolution of damage and its relation to the petrographic characteristics of rocks provides interesting information. The quantification of damage can be done by indirect measures (mass loss, some physical properties variation, etc.); the evaluation of damage was based on the superficial observation (ASTM, 2002) and, if the observation of its progression from inside were needed, it would be necessary to destroy the sample and in this case, it is no longer available for successive cycles. The X-ray computed tomography (X-ray CT) is a non-destructive technique (NDT) that has been applied increasingly in the study of rocks properties and fluid flow in porous media, as in many cases keeping the material during and after the study is necessary. A review of about the general applications of this technique can be found in Duliu (1999) and more precisely in Van Geet et al. (2000) and Ketcham and Carlson (2001).

The X-ray CT allows the quantification of the damage produced, especially if we are talking about microcracks; the apparition of new microcracks and the increasing width of the existing ones can be followed along the successive studying cycles. The apparition and morphology of microcracks are features that can be used for the quantification of the damage produced in the accelerated ageing tests. Besides that, fracture width is an important parameter in determining the flow and characteristics of fractured media. Specific X-ray CT studies of different kinds of microfisuration on rocks can be found in Johns et al. (1993), Vinegar et al. (1991), Verhelst et al. (1995), Montemagno & Pyrak-Nolte (1995 and 1999), Keller (1997, 1998) and Gouze et al. 2003.

A procedure that provides some changes in the method by Keller (opus cit.) for the quantification by CT number of the internal damage produced in freeze-thaw cycles is presented, from the study of the crack width on a dolomotic rock used in the construction of historic buildings in Oviedo (N of Spain). Former studies by means of this technique about the effects produced inside the rock samples subjected to alteration cycles can be seen in Ruiz de Argandoña et al. (1999).

2 STUDIED MATERIAL AND EXPERIMENTAL PROCEDURE

The "Laspra Stone" is a Paleogen dolomitic rock of microcrystalline texture mainly composed of dolomite

(90%), quartz (5%) and clay minerals (5%), with a sedimentary layering characterised by different porosity. Dolomite crystals are of micrite size; quartz grains, between 20 and 100 μm, are uniformly distributed in the rock (Fig. 1). The four specimens used were cubes 50 mm edge and the studies have been done in conventional X-ray CT equipment of fourth generation used routinely in medical practice (General Electric SYTEC 3000); the working conditions have been 120 kV and 100 mA.

Each specimen was sliced under X-ray CT into 50 virtual sections, 1 mm thick, spaced 1 mm apart, thus X-ray CT information of the whole cube was obtained (Fig. 2); the images are 512 × 512 pixels in size with a spatial resolution of 450 μm which, allowed us to determine microcracks until 30 μm, addjusting the reconstruction field.

After the initial characterisation by X-ray CT, the samples were subjected to freeze-thaw ageing tests between −15° and +10°C. The specimens were

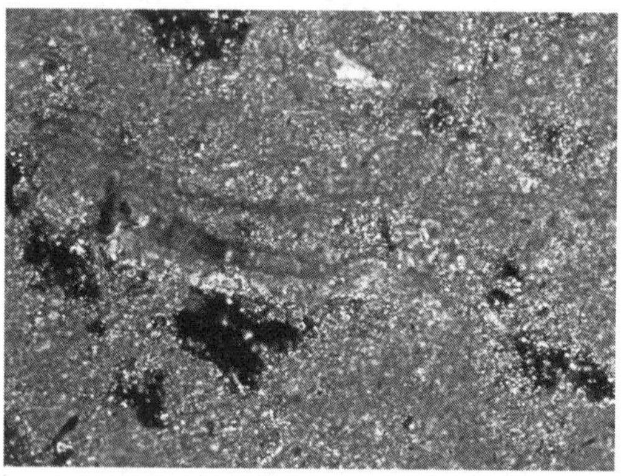

Figure 1. Appearance of the texture under a petrographic microscope (polarized light, crossed polars, width 0.250 mm).

saturated in water (at 20°C) under vacuum for 24 hours; afterwards the samples are frozen until −15°C in 30 minutes, keeping the temperature during 2.5 hours, finally it is increased until +10°C in 30 minutes and kept at this value for another 2.5 hours. The duration of each cycle was 6 hours. After each cycle the specimens were dried at 60°C and studied under X-ray CT.

3 METHOD FOR THE DAMAGE QUANTIFICATION

A cylindrical pattern of the rock material itself, about 22 mm of diameter and 35 mm of length, that has been cut longitudinally has been built, polishing the different faces with carborandum of grain 1000 and later, with diamond paste of 9 μm with the aim of removing the roughness originated on the faces during the cutting process and of decreasing the generated artefacts. Later on, a series of metal plates (1 mm to 50 μm thick, with intervals of 50 μm), have been introduced between the two parts of the cylinder, and images of this "built crack" have been obtained under X-ray CT (Fig. 3). The two halves were firmly held together with a clamp during scanning and the lower polished surface was levelled, to produce a horizontal fracture plane. In the perpendicular direction to each crack, the variation of the CT number values have been studied, establishing not only its minimum value but also the "integrated area" (surface limited between the average value of CT number in a given line and the distribution of the CT number values along the crack width, Fig. 4).

When the minimum values of the CT number in each artificial "crack" are represented opposite to its width (Fig. 5), the existing lineal relation between both values is observed.

When relating the widths of the artificial cracks to their "integrated areas", the linear relationship obtained

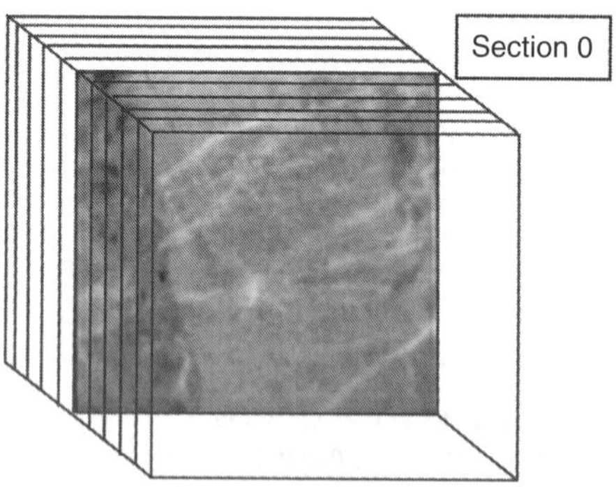

Figure 2. Sketch showing the arrangement of the virtual sections imaged by X-ray CT.

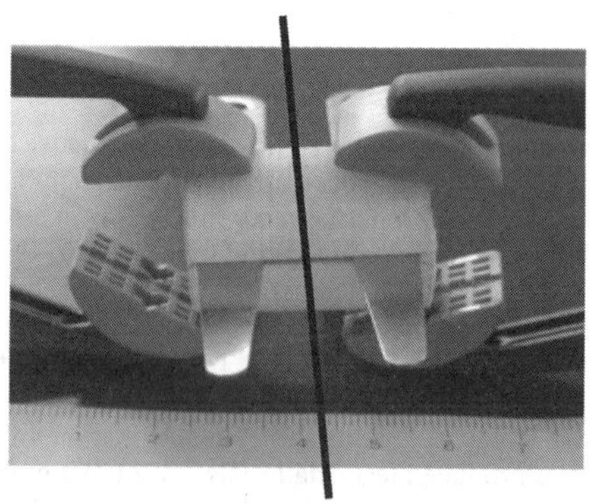

Figure 3. Device built for the simulation of artificial cracks, with indication of the plan studied by means of X-ray CT.

is still better (Fig. 6), for this reason and from the equation of the defined straight line, once the "integrated area" of each crack in this rock material is known, its width can be determined with rather accuracy.

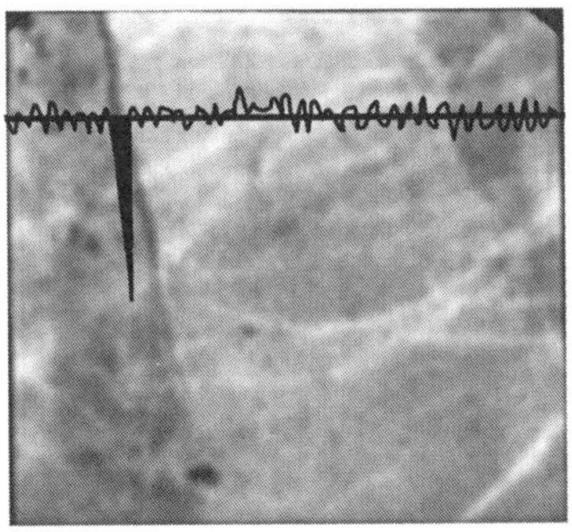

Figure 4. Variation of CT number (HU) through a perpendicular section to the crack. The black area is the one considered in our studies.

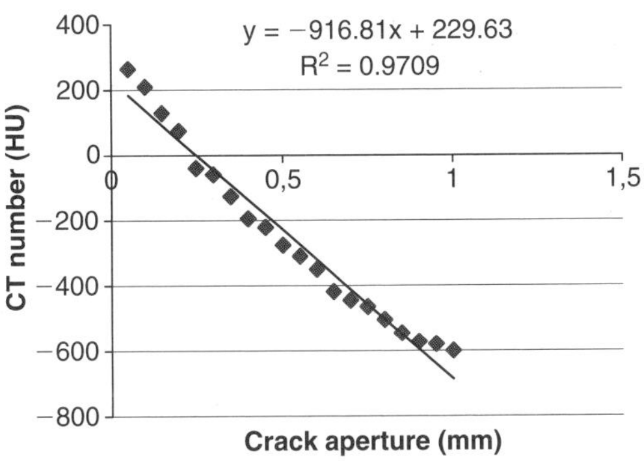

Figure 5. Relation between the minimum values of the CT numbers (HU) and the openings of the cracks (mm).

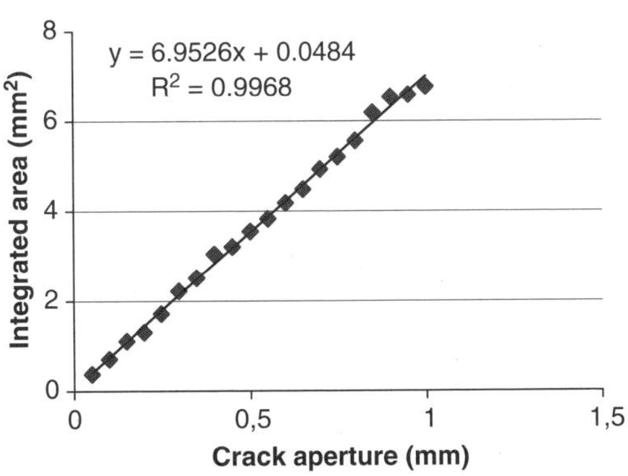

Figure 6. Relationship between the integrated areas (mm^2) and the widths of the cracks (mm).

4 RESULTS

4.1 *Petrophysic information*

Before subjecting the samples to the freeze-thaw cycles, the X-ray CT has been used to estimate some physical properties of the rock.

Once the instrumental equipment has been calibrated at a value of CT number of −1000 Houndsfield Units (HU) for the air and 0 for water, in pre-cycling samples an average radiological density has been determined for the dried sample of 1350 HU with a standard deviation of 27. As it is an almost mono-mineral rock and, due to its small size of grain, the observed variability in the rock is due mainly to differences in porosity.

According to several authors (Raynaud et al., 1989; Geraud et al., 1993, 1998a and b; Orsi et al., 1994, Boespflug et al., 1995; Amos et al., 1996 and Tsuchiyama et al., 2000) there is a direct relationship between the radiological densities, the mineralogical compositions and the porosities. Applying this to the studied rock, some values of total porosity about 21.7 % and of density in the dried rock about 2046 kg/m^3 have been obtained, values close to the meassured ones by means of classical techniques (porosity 27.6 % and bulk density 1970 kg/m^3, Ruiz de Argandoña et al., 1999), which indicates the validity of the technique to make a close estimation of the properties without using destructive tests.

Layers of different porosity have been observed (Fig. 7). In the X-ray CT image the medium grey areas correspond to the normal microcrystalline

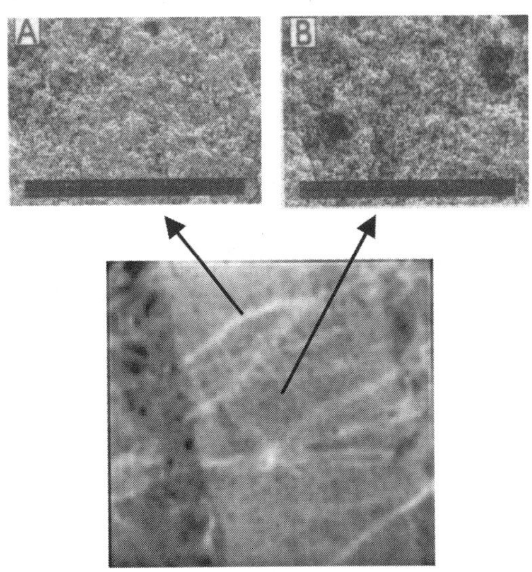

Figure 7. Appearance under X-ray CT (A) and SEM (B) of the areas with different porosity (SEM images width 140 μm).

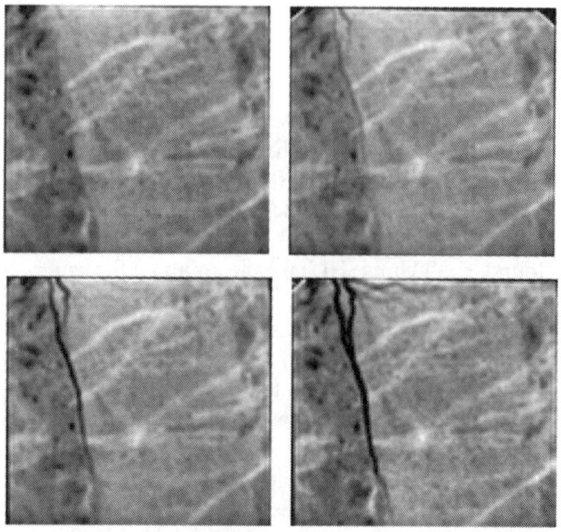

Figure 8. Images of the studied section after 4 (upper, left), 5 (upper, right), 6 (lower, left) and 7 (lower, right) cycles.

texture of the rock, while the brighter areas belong to zones of lower microporosity and the darker areas are zones with higher microporosity; these differences in porosity have been cheked using a Scanning Electron Microscope (SEM).

4.2 *Quantification of the damage produced and petrophysic interpretation*

To make the study easy, from all the tested samples, one, where an only crack was developed, has been chosen, making the study itself on the central area of the cube (Section 0) (Fig. 2).

The studies referring not only to the evolution in the width of the crack, but also to the depth it reached have been made at different depths (each 5 mm) with regard to the superior surface of the sample. In some cases, these studies were made every mm, to obtain more precision.

For the measurement of the "integrated area", some authors always use the same average reference value of the rock, independent of the area of the study. In this case and although the rock was rather homogeneous in relation to the mineralogy, given the existence of an oscillation due to its associated microporosity and with an irregular line, it has been preferred to work with specific values of each area and not with the average value of the rock; so, for each studied area, first the average value at each depth was determined in the non-tested sample, being this the one which was used together with the former ones in the same areas and depth after each cycle.

An example of the images which the crack studies were used with for 4th, 5th, 6th and 7th cycles can be seen in Figure 8; where we observe how the crack grows,

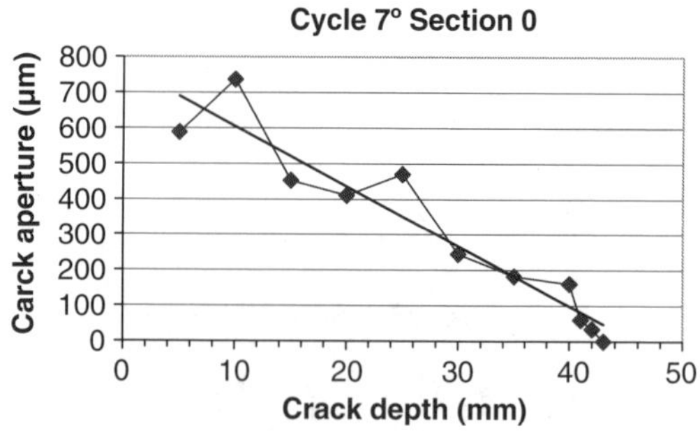

Figure 9. Evolution of the crack width in cycle 7th section 0.

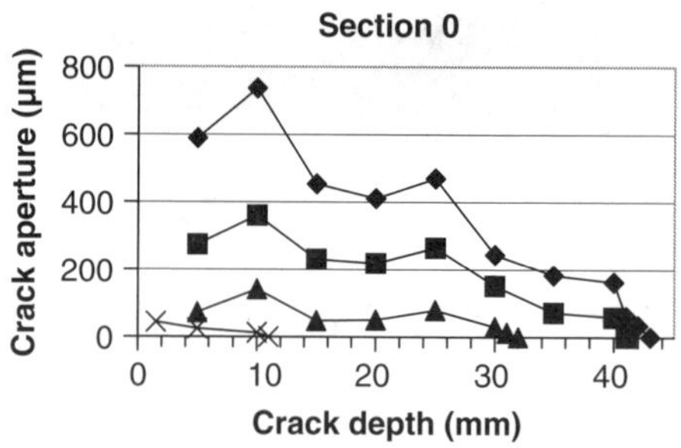

Figure 10. Crack widths opposite depth and number of cycles 7th (upper), 6th , 5th and 4th (lower).

both in width and in depth, together with the number of cycles.

When comparing the evolution of the crack width to its depth after cycle 7 (Fig. 9) it is observed that the crack width decreases from the surface to inside, getting to disappear approximately at 43 mm from the surface.

It has been stated that there are three depths where the crack width increases more than the average trend (10, 25 and 40 mm). This behaviour is taken as due to the fact that the porosity is greater in this area, which allows the absorption of a greater amount of water that, with the stress originated by the increase in volume during the freezing process, produces a greater wideness of the crack. At 5 and 15 mm of depth, the crack width is less than the average, due to the fact that, at these depths, the porosity is less and, therefore, also the stress originated during the freezing (Fig. 7).

In Figure 10, the evolution of the width together with the number of cycles at different depths is represented. It can be observed that cracking starts in the 4th cycle and the evolution trend of the width together with the depth is similar every cycle.

It can be seen that, except for cycle 4th, the crack width is greater than the average at 10, 25 and 40 mm depth; this variation is greater every time with the

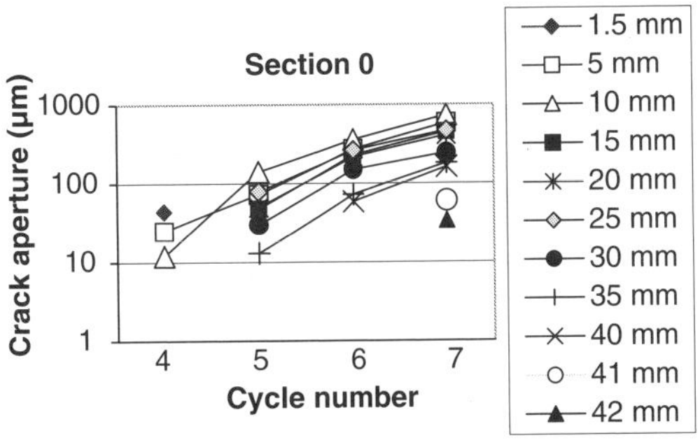

Figure 11. Evolution of the crack width opposite the studied number of cycles and depth.

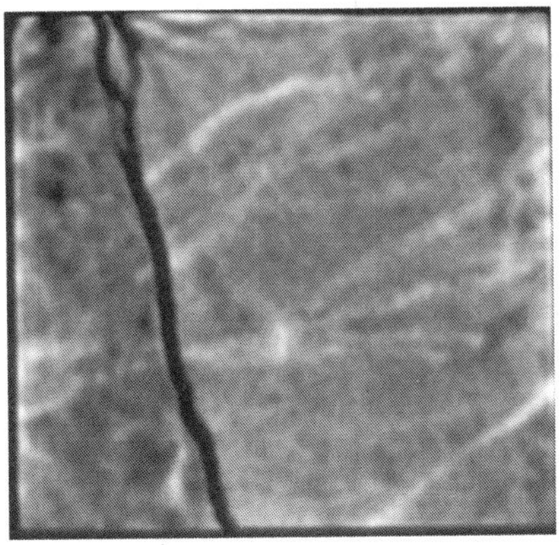

Figure 12. Appearance of the studied plane after 8th cycle.

number of cycles due to the progressive increase of porosity. There is an opposite tendency in the areas of less porosity (at 5 and 15 mm).

In Figure 11, the evolution of the crack width and the number of cycles for each studied depth have been represented. Once the cracking starts, there is a good semilogarithmic relationship increasing the crack width along the number of cycles at every depth; reaching the other side of the sample and breaking it at cycle 8th (Fig. 12).

5 CONCLUSIONS

Under X-ray CT technique, the total porosity and the density of the dried rock have been determined with an acceptable accuracy; on the other hand, the existence of a textural anisotropy has been stated, due to the presence of an irregular distribution of porosity.

Before the microcracking study of a rock under X-ray computerised axial tomography, it is necessary to establish a pattern of the same rock type, so the relation between the widths of the cracks and the integrated area is defined.

For "Laspra Stone" subjected to freeze-thaw cycles, once the cracks start on surface, their width and depth increase as well.

The influence of porosity on the width of the cracks has been defined, so, in those areas where cracking is bigger, the crack width is also bigger than the average trend.

ACKNOWLEDGEMENTS

This research was financially supported by the "Consejeria de Cultura", Principado de Asturias, Spain. Projects: PB-ESE-99-09C, PC-CIS01-56, PB-EJS01-24 and Ministerio de Ciencia y Tecnología, Acción integrada España-Francia: MCT-02-ACC-HF2001-0083.

REFERENCES

Amos, C.L., Sutherland, T.F., Radzijewski, B., & Doucett, M. 1996. A rapid technique to determine bulk density of fine-grained sediments by X-ray computed tomography, *Journal of Sedimentary Research,* 66 (5): 1023–1024.

ASTM. 2002. Standard test method for evaluation of durability of rock for erosion control under freezing and thawing conditions (D 5312–97), *Annual Book of ASTM Standards*, Vol. 04.08.

Boespflug, X., Long, B.F.N. & Occhietti, S. 1995. CAT-scan in marine stratigraphy: a quantitative approach, *Marine Geology*, 122: 281–301.

Duliu, O.G. 1999. Computer axial tomography in geosciences: an overview, *Earth-Science Reviews*, 48: 265–281.

Géraud, Y., Mazerolle, F. & Raynaud, S. 1993. Essai de quantification de la porosité d´un granite altéré utilisation du scanner médical (tomodensitomètre X), *Bull. Soc. Géol. France,* 164 (2): 243–253.

Géraud, Y., Mazerolle, F. Cardon, H. Vidal, G. & Caron, J.M. 1998. Anisotropie de connectivité du réseau poreux d´une bande de cisaillement ductile, *Bull. Soc. Géol. France*, 169 (5): 645–654.

Géraud, Y., Mazerolle, F. Raynaud, S. & Lebon, P. 1998. Crack location in granitic samples submitted to heating, low confining pressure and axial loading, *Geophys. J. Int.*, 133: 553–567.

Gouze, P., Noiriel, C., Bruderer, C., Loggia, D. & Leprovost, R. 2003. X-ray tomography characterization of fracture surfaces during dissolution, *Geophysical Research Letters*, 30 (5): 1267.

Johns, R.A., Steude, J.D., Castanier, L.M. & Roberts, P.V. 1993. Nondestructive measurementts of fracture aperture in crystalline rocks cores using X ray computed tomography, *Journal of Geophysical Research*, 98 (B2): 1889–1900.

Keller, A. 1997. High resolution CAT imaging of fractures in consolidated materials, *Int. J. Rock Mech. Min. Sci.* 34 (3–4): paper no. 155.

Keller, A. 1998. High resolution, non-destructive measurement and characterization of fracture apertures. *Int. J. Rock Mech. Min. Sci.*, 35 (8): 1037–1050.

Ketcham, R.A., & Carlson, W.D. 2001. Acquisition, optimisation and interpretation of X-ray computed tomographic imagery: applications to the geosciences, *Computers & Geosciences*, 27 (4): 381–400.

Montemagno, C.D., & Pyrak-Nolte, L. 1995. Porosity of natural fracture networks, *Geophysical Research Letters*, 22 (11): 1397–1400.

Montemagno, C.D., & Pyrak-Nolte, L. 1999. Fracture network versus single fractures: Measurement of fracture geometry with X-ray tomography, *Phys. Chem. Earth* (A), 24 (7): 575–579.

Orsi, T.H., Edwards, C.M. & Anderson, A.L. 1994. X-ray computed tomography: a non-destructive method for quantitative analysis of sediment cores, *Journal of Sedimentary Research* (A), 64: 690–693.

Raynaud, S., Fabre, D., Mazerolle, F., Géraud, Y. & Latière, H.J. 1989. Analysis of the internal structure of rocks and characterization of mechanical deformation by a non-destructive method: X-ray tomodensitometry, *Tectonophysics*, 159: 149–159.

Ruiz de Argandoña, V.G., Rodríguez-Rey, A., Celorio, C., Suárez del Río, L.M., Calleja, L. & Llavona, J. 1999. Characterization by computed X-ray tomography of the evolution of the pore structure of a dolomite rock during freeze-thaw cyclic test, *Phys. Chem. Earth* (A), 24 (7): 633–637.

Tsuchiyama, A., Hanamoto, T., Nakashima, Y, & Nakano, T. 2000. Quantitative evaluation of attenuation contrast of minerals by using a medical X-ray scanner, *Journal of Mineralogical and Petrological Sciences*, 95: 125–137.

Van Geet, M., Swennen, R. & Wevers, M. 2000. Quantitative analysis of reservoir rocks by microfocus X-Ray computerised tomography, *Sedimentary Geology*, 132: 25–36.

Verhelst F., Vervoort, A., De Bosscher, Ph. & Marchal, G. 1995. X-ray computerized tomography: determination of heterogeneities in rock samples In *8th International Congress on Rock Mechanics (ISRM), Tokyo*.

Vinegar, H.J., De Waal, J.A. & Wellington, S.L. 1991. CT Studies of brittle failure in Castlegate sandstone. *Int. J. Rock Mech. Sci. & Geomech. Abstr.*, 28 (5): 441–448.

X-ray CT for Geomaterials; Soils, Concrete, Rocks – Otani & Obara (eds.)
© 2004 Swets & Zeitlinger. Lisse, ISBN 90 5809 666 1

Microstructure observation in deformed geomaterials using microfocus X-ray computed tomography

T. Takemura & M. Oda
Saitama University, Saitama, Japan

M. Takahashi
National Institute of Advanced Industrial Science and Technology, Tsukuba, Japan

ABSTRACT: The three-dimensional microstructure of a shear band in sand and a shear plane in rock was observed by means of microfocus X-ray computed tomography (CT). In a shear band of Toyoura sand, the column-like structure reported by Oda & Kazama (1998) can also be observed in microfocus X-ray CT images. Outside a shear band, columns grow parallel to the compression direction. Inside the shear band, on the other hand, columns are bent along with the accumulation of shear strain, and extremely large voids grow between the inclined columns. In Inada granite deformed beyond a peak point (failure), microcracks grow along a shear plane in particular. Using X-ray CT, we measured apertures of microcracks in the rock with success. Furthermore, change in the aperture with increasing confining pressure was observed using a newly designed confining pressure vessel equipped with microfocus X-ray CT. It was found that the microfocus X-ray CT, along with the newly designed confining pressure vessel, provides a powerful tool for constructing clear images of individual particles, voids and cracks in non-destructive manner.

1 INTRODUCTION

Under a microscope, geomaterials (e.g., soil and rock) are characterized by three-dimensional (3D) structure formed by constituent elements such as pores, voids and cracks, and their mechanical and hydrological properties are deeply related to the microstructural aspects. In order to discuss the mechanics of such geomaterials on a microstructure-basis, accordingly, details on the 3D microstructure are needed. A stereology-based analysis provides one of the methods to estimate 3D microstructure. Using the method, in fact, we can qualitatively estimate the geometrical properties such as orientation, density and size distribution (e.g. Dehoff, 1968; Kanatani, 1984; Oda, 1984; Kuo et al., 1998). Recently, Takemura & Oda (2002) have shown that the results of stereology-based method are in agreement with microscopic observations using an optical microscope equipped with a universal-stage. Although the stereology-based method is very useful for the purpose, time-consuming and tedious work is needed to do so. More importantly, a sample must be cut along several planes to analyze the structure.

In the past decade, based on computer technology, X-ray computed tomography (CT) was developed so efficiently that we can now use it to investigate 3D microstructure of geomaterials (Fredrich et al., 1995; Ohtani et al., 2001). A problem is that a conventional type of X-ray CT did not give spatial resolution accurate enough to separate individual particles and voids in granular sand and to recognize each microcrack in rock. Recently, however, microfocus X-ray CT was developed to solve the difficulty. Using this technology, we can easily identify microcracks even if they are just a few microns in thickness (Hirono et al., 2002; Takahashi et al., 2002; Oda et al., 2003).

Oda & Kazama (1998) analyzed microstructure of Toyoura sand developed in a shear band using an optical microscope and thin sections. They concluded that microstructure of granular sand changes dramatically while inelastic deformation is accumulating. That is, column-like structure grows first inside the shear band in the direction parallel to the compression axis, and then the columns are bent along with the accumulation of shear strain. In this paper, we will show that the similar observation can easily be done using microfocus X-ray CT. An important point is that this can be done in 3D as well as in a non-destructive manner.

Using Inada granite deformed beyond a peak stress in a triaxial test, we also show that microcracks can directly be observed using the present system. The 3D fabric of microcracks in deformed Inada granite has already been analyzed by means of the crack tensor and stereology method (Oda et al., 2002a; Takemura & Oda, 2002; Takemura & Oda, 2003). In these studies, however, we did not succeed in detecting the details of 3D geometrical properties such as shape, aperture and connectivity.

Finally, a new triaxial vessel equipped with microfocus X-ray CT is designed to observe directly the change in the crack aperture with increasing confining pressure.

2 MICROFOCUS X-RAY COMPUTED TOMOGRAPHY

X-ray CT is a method to construct a 3D image by means of detecting 3D-distribution of attenuation coefficients through a material. This is non-destructively done, and as a result, the X-ray CT provides a very powerful tool for observing microstructure of geomaterials (e.g. Orsi et al., 1994; Van Geet et al., 2000; Hirono et al., 2003).

In this study, we used an X-ray CT system, SHX225, assembled by the TESCO Corporation (Figure 1). In this system, the maximum voltage is 225 kV, and focal spot size is 5 μm. The so-called third generation CT system, which makes it possible to record X-ray attenuation at many angles by rotating an object on a computer-controlled rotation manipulator stage, is used in this instrument (Figure 2(a)). X-ray attenuation data is detected by a 12 bit CCD (charge-coupled device) camera, and the recorded attenuation data are analyzed to reconstruct two-dimensionally an internal attenuation image of an object by means of a numerical technique known as filtered back projection. The resolution of 2D images is 1024 × 1024 pixels in this system. To obtain a clear boundary image between substances having different attenuation coefficients, X-ray source must be small enough to minimize scattering zones on an X-ray detector, image intensifier (Figure 2(b), (c)).

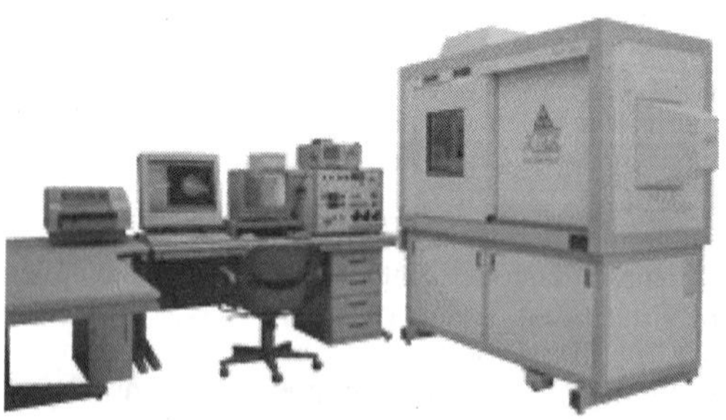

Figure 1. Microfocus X-ray system assembled by TESCO corporation and the CT system (BIR ACTIS+3) used.

3 MICROSTRUCTURE OF SHEAR BAND IN TOYOURA SAND

3.1 *Sample*

A sample was first selected from the ones reported by Oda and Kazama (1998) to observe its microstructure using the X-ray CT system.

A uniform sand (called Toyoura sand) with a mean grain size of 0.206 mm was selected for testing. A rectangular parallelopiped sample 180 mm high, 160 mm wide and 80 mm thick was formed such that the void ratio was about 0.65. The sample was sheared using plane strain apparatus under a constant minor principal stress of $\sigma_3 = 49$ kPa until a major shear band was generated. The sample was then fixed in place using polyester resin mixed with a solvent (see Oda & Kazama (1998) for more detail). Then, for X-ray CT analyses, a cylindrical sample 24 mm in diameter and 38 mm high was cored in the central part of the sample in the direction normal to the major shear band. In this study, we observed the cylindrical sample with special interest in 3D structure of particles and associated with voids in the shear band.

Oda & Kazama (1998) have already reported the microstructure in and out of the shear band by means of a microscope and thin section method. The main

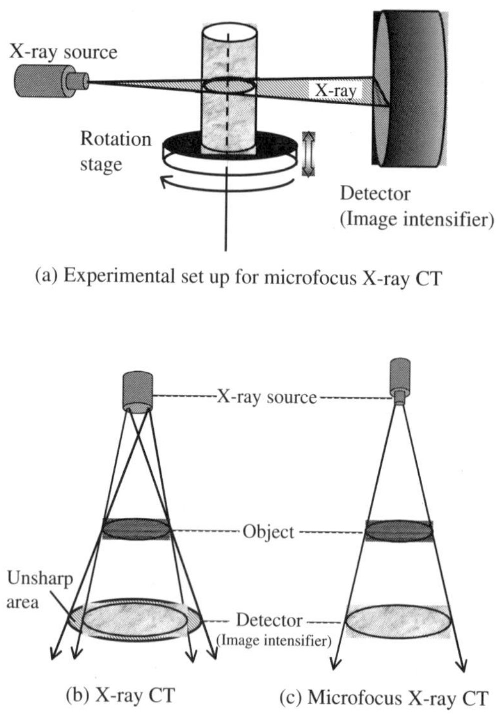

Figure 2. Illustration of the microfocus X-ray CT system.

objective is therefore to compare their results to the images obtained from the microfocus X-ray CT.

3.2 *Microstructure by microfocus X-ray CT*

Two-dimensional images reconstructed from the central part of a 3D image are shown in Figure 3 where x_1 stands for the maximum compression axis and x_3 the minor principal axis. Extremely large voids are clearly seen within a narrow band (called shear band). We can also see such large void using a thin section-optical microscope method (e.g., Oda & Kazama (1998)). Someone may suggest, however, that such large voids can be artificially formed in the preparation process of thin sections. In fact, the particles may sometimes drop out of the sample during the preparation of thin sections. However, since this microfocus X-ray CT is a non-distractive method, we can say that these large voids are no doubt generated along with shear banding, reflecting the micro-mechanism leading to the formation of the shear band.

4 MICROCRACK IN DEFORMED INADA GRANITE

4.1 *Sample and procedure*

A granitic rock, called Inada granite, was next examined. It consists of quartz (37% by volume), alkali feldspar (24%), plagioclase (33%), biotite and other minerals (6%). The mean grain size is about 2.0 mm. We can detect three orthogonal planes called rift, grain and hardway in the field. For convenience, three orthogonal directions were chosen normal to these planes as the reference axes x_i ($i = 1, 2, 3$), and a plane normal to one axis x_i is called the x_i-plane.

3D microstructural observation was carried out using a sample, which was loaded until a major shear plane was formed. The sample was loaded normal to the hardway plane under an 80 MPa confining pressure so that the cylindrical axis was parallel to x_3. A cylindrical sample 10 mm high 5 mm in diameter was cored from the damaged sample in the direction perpendicular to the shear plane using a high stiffness boring machine (Figure 4). The cylindrical sample was placed on a rotation stage, and a 3D image of 4.8 mm high and 9 mm diameter was constructed using 240 2D images, each of 20 μm thickness.

4.2 *Fault-related microcrack*

Figures 5 and 6 show 2D images taken from the 3D image, called a tomography image. Figure 5 shows a tomography image taken parallel to the shear plane. In these X-ray CT images, the color contrast reflects difference in the density of mineral (or element); that is, the white portions indicate the places where high density minerals exist. On the other hand, open microcracks appear as dark lines in these images.

We can distinguish two types of microcracks. One type is the microcracks developed along mineral grains, and is called the grain boundary cracks. The orientation is variable. For example, some grain boundary cracks are oriented normal to the axial stress direction (called the load normal grain boundary cracks). The grain boundary crack is not sharp, but is rather undulated

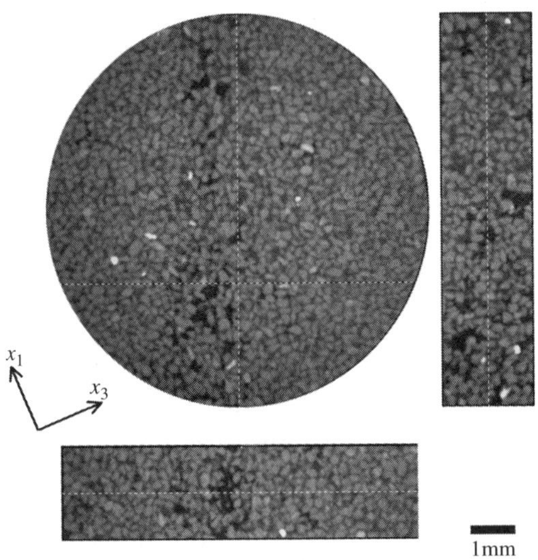

Figure 3. Two-dimensional X-ray attenuation image around a shear band reconstructed from 3D image (source voltage and current are 130 kV and 150 μA).

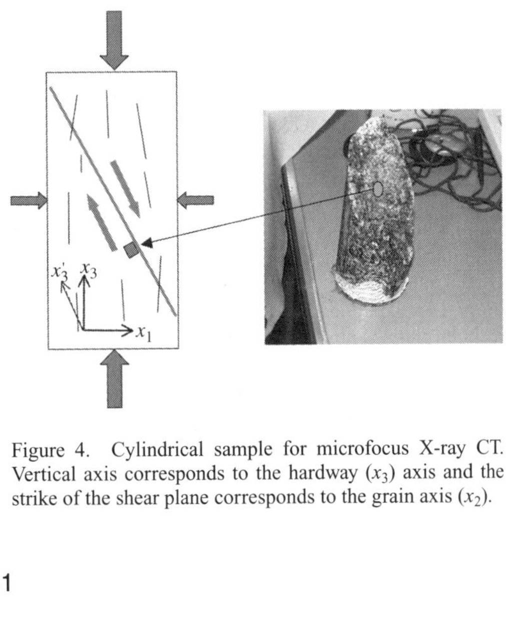

Figure 4. Cylindrical sample for microfocus X-ray CT. Vertical axis corresponds to the hardway (x_3) axis and the strike of the shear plane corresponds to the grain axis (x_2).

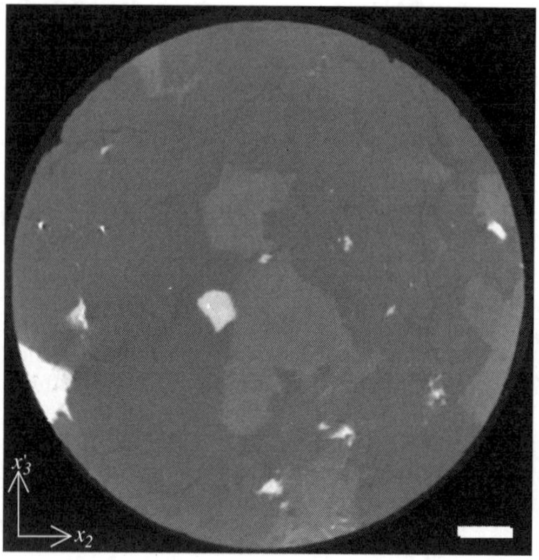

Figure 5. Two-dimensional X-ray attenuation image around a shear plane reconstructed from 3D image (source voltage and current are 90 kV and 110 μA). This image was taken at a depth of 1.1 mm from the shear plane. The horizontal axis corresponds to the grain axis (x_2); and the vertical axis is in the direction inclined at about 30 degrees to the hardway axis (x'_3). Scale bar is 1 mm.

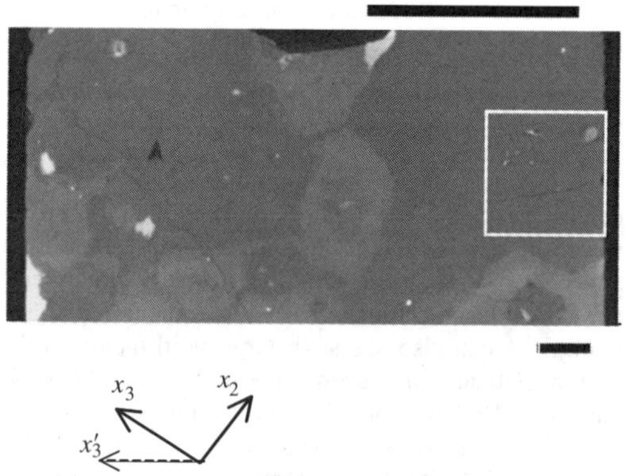

(a)

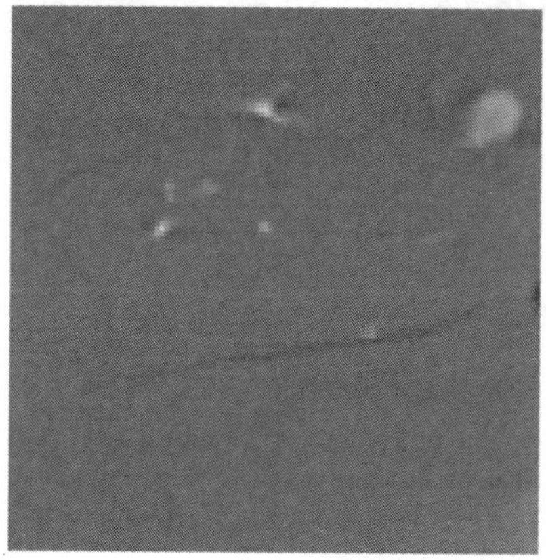

(b)

Figure 6. (a) Two-dimensional X-ray attenuation image around a shear plane reconstructed from 3D image (source voltage and current are 90 kV and 110 μA). This image is perpendicular to the shear plane, the upper surface corresponds with the shear plane, and x_3 is the loading axis. Scale bar is 1 mm. (b) The image expanded from the white frame of image (a). Scale bar is 1 mm.

along the mineral grain boundary. We can sometimes see a small open pore at which a few grain boundary cracks are intersected. Another type is composed of very sharp microcracks, as shown in Figure 7(a), whose orientation is preferentially parallel to the axial stress direction. This type of microcracks is mainly developed in quartz grains, and cuts through two or more quartz grains.

Oda et al. (2002a) proposed a failure mechanism. That is, failure starts when cracks grow so densely that a rock actually turns out to be an assembly of disintegrated blocks, and shear bands develop as a result of the sliding and/or rolling of the disintegrated blocks. Takemura & Oda (2002, 2003) also proposed a microstructural model leading to development of a shear plane. Rolling and sliding of disintegrated blocks in the post failure region are caused by combined action between the load-normal generated grain boundary cracks and the high crack density in quartz. If this is the case, we should observe many load-normal grain boundary cracks of large apertures around a shear plane. The X-ray CT image seems to support the proposed model. It should also be noted that the grain boundary cracks surely cause dilatancy in the post failure region.

It is well known that microcrack growth is closely related to generation of a network of water flow through damaged granite. If this is the case, their apertures are important when assessing their contribution to permeability. We measured, with success, apertures by mean of the image analysis. The maximum aperture was found to be 15–30 μm (Figure 6(b)).

4.3 *Microcrack squeeze by confining pressure*

The aperture of 15–30 μm was measured under an air pressure. It should be noted, however, that microcracks may be closed when subjected to a confining pressure. In fact, for example, permeability of damaged Inada granite sample, which was loaded until failure occurred, is about $9.0 \times 10^{-17}\,m^2$ under a 2 MPa effective confining pressure. (Note that the permeability of

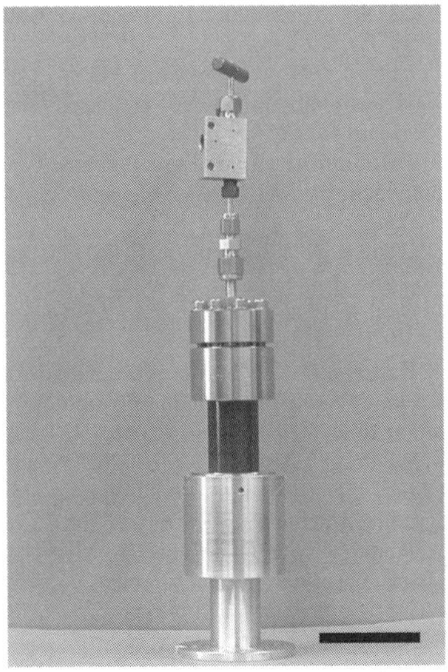

Figure 7. Confining pressure vessel. Central black portion is made from carbon fiber. The upper part is connected to a pressure pump to increase confining pressure by water. Scale bar is 5 cm.

intact Inada granite is about $2.0 \times 10^{-19}\,m^2$ (Oda et al., 2002b)). However, the permeability decreases down to $6.0 \times 10^{-18}\,m^2$ when the effective confining pressure increases up to 25 MPa, which corresponds to the pressure at about 1000 m in depth. Closure of microcracks no doubt causes the decrease of permeability. Inada granite shows a nonlinearity relation between confining pressure and volumetric strain, at least up to 140 MPa confining pressure (Oda et al., 2002b). This result also suggests that the crack aperture changes as a function of the confining pressure.

In order to observe the change of microcrack aperture under confining pressure by means of microfocus X-ray CT, we developed a new confining pressure vessel (Figure 7). The cell should be made of material having low X-ray attenuation, and, at the same time, should have high strength to sustain a cell pressure as high as 140 MPa. We selected carbon fiber for it since carbon fiver has high tensile strength as well as low specific gravity. The inside space of the vessel is 40 mm high and 10 mm in diameter.

Using the vessel, we observed the change of microcrack aperture in the same damaged Inada granite when subjected to confining pressure. To set the sample under the confining pressure, it was sealed by acrylic resins. Figure 8(a) shows a two-dimensional X-ray attenuation image taken parallel to the shear plane; and the microcrack, which might be a grain boundary crack, is open (see in the white circle in the figure). However, we cannot detect an open microcrack in the same area under 25 MPa confining pressure (Figure 8(b)), although some microcracks, for example the upper left side of the image, still show dark lines corresponding to aperture. This result suggests that the stiffness may be different from microcrack to microcrack. That is, some microcracks are easily closed under the pressure of 25 MPa, and others are not.

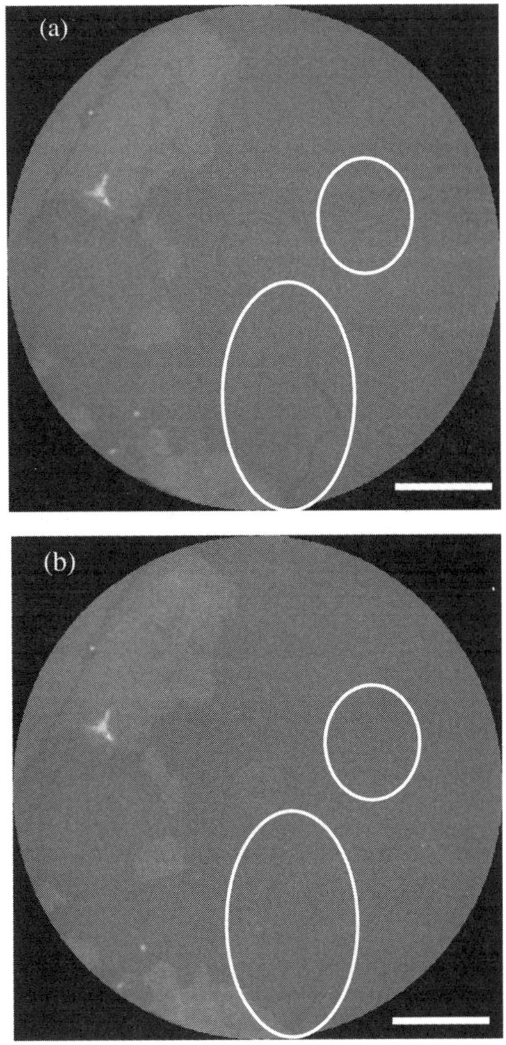

Figure 8. Two-dimensional X-ray attenuation image under (a) air pressure and (b) 25 MPa confining pressure (source voltage and current are 90 kV and 110 μA). Scale bar is 1 mm.

It can now be said that the newly designed cell can be used to observe directly the microcrack growth and the aperture change. Such observation will provide us useful information in the study of rock permeability.

5 CONCLUDING REMARKS

We observed the fault-related microstructure of granular sand and damaged rock three-dimensionally using microfocus X-ray CT. We also succeeded in measuring microcrack aperture and its change under confining pressure using a newly designed triaxial vessel. We can confidently say that microstructural-based study on geomaterial will greatly advance if microfocus X-ray CT is used concurrently with data-analysis methods.

In near future, a triaxial compression cell equipped with microfocus X-ray CT will be developed, which makes it possible to observe the evolution of microcracks during brittle failure. Since microfocus X-ray CT can distinguish water from air, we will be able to trace movement of fluid associated with failure.

ACKNOWLEDGMENT

The authors would like to thank Mr. A. Murakoshi, Mr. H. Hirai and Mr. T. Hishinuma of TESCO Corporation for their assistance in using the microfocus X-ray CT.

REFERENCES

DeHoff, R. T. & Rhines, F. N., 1968, *Quantitative microscopy*, McGraw-Hill, New York.

Fredrich, J. T., Menendez, B. & Wong, T. F., 1995, Imaging the pore structure of geomaterials, *Science*, 268, 276–279.

Hirono, T., Yokoyama, T., Takahashi, M., Nakashima, S., Yamamoto, Y. & Lin, W., 2002, Nondestructive observation of internal structure in sediments and rocks using microfocus X-ray CT system, *Jour. Geol. Soc. Japan*, 108, 606–609. (*in Japanese with English abstract)*

Hirono, T., Takahashi, M. and Nakashima, S., 2003, In-situ visualization of fluid flow image within deformed rock by X-ray CT. *Engineering Geology*, 70, 37–46.

Kanatani, K., 1984, Distribution of directional data and fabric tensors. *Int. J. Engrg. Sci.* 22, 149–164.

Kuo, C-, Y., Frost, J. D. & Chameau, J. -L. A., 1998, Image analysis determination of stereology based fabric tensor, *Géotechnique*, 48, 515–525.

Oda, M., 1984, Similarity rule of crack geometry in statistically homogeneous rock masses, *Mechanics of Materials*, 3, 119–129.

Oda, M., Katsube, T. & Takemura, T., 2002a, Microcrack evolution and brittle failure of Inada granite in triaxial compression tests at 140 MPa, *Jour. of Geophys. Res.*, 107, ECV9-1-17.

Oda, M. & Kazama, H., 1998, Micro-structure of shear band and its relation to the mechanism of dilatancy and failure of granular soils, *Géotechniqu.* 48, 465–481.

Oda, M., Takemura,T. & Aoki, K., 2002b, Damage growth and permeability change in triaxial compression tests of Inada granite, *Mechanics of Materials,* 34, 313–331

Oda, M., Takemura, T. & Takahashi, M.; Microstructure in shear band observed by microfocus X-ray computed tomography, *Géotechniqu.* (*In press*)

Ohtani, T., Nakano, T., Nakashima, Y. & Muraoka, H., 2001, Three-dimensional shape analysis of miarolitic cavities and enclaves in the Kakkonda granite by X-ray computed tomography, *Jour. Struct. Geol.*, 23, 1741–1751.

Orsi, T.H., C.M. Edwards, and A.L. Anderson, 1994, X-Ray Computed Tomography: A Non-Destructive Method for Quantitative Analysis of Sediment Cores, *Jour. of Sedimentary Res.*, 64, 690–693.

Takahashi, M., Lin, W., Hirono, T. & Yamamoto, Y., 2002, On visualization of inner microstructure in rocks by microfocus X-ray CT, *Jour. Japan Soc. Eng. Geol.,* 43, 235–238. (*in Japanese with English abstract*)

Takemura, T. & Oda, M., 2002, Three-dimensional fabric analysis of microcracks associated with brittle failure of granitic rocks. *Jour. Geol. Soc. Japan*, 108, 453–464. (*in Japanese with English abstract*)

Takemura, T. & Oda, M., Stereology-based fabric analysis of microcracks in damaged granite, *Tectonophysics. (submitted)*

Van Geet, M., Swennen, R. & Wevers, M., 2000, Quantitative analysis of reservoir rocks by microfocus X-ray computerized tomography, *Sedimentary Geol.*, 132, 25–36.

X-ray CT for Geomaterials; Soils, Concrete, Rocks – Otani & Obara (eds.)
© 2004 Swets & Zeitlinger. Lisse, ISBN 90 5809 666 1

Visualization of bond failure in a pull-out test of rock bolts and cable bolts using X-ray CT

F. Ito & T. Aoki
Taisei Corporation, Tokyo, Japan

Y. Obara
Kumamoto University, Kumamoto, Japan

ABSTRACT: The patterns of the failure in a pull-out test are visualized by X-ray CT scanner to supply the basic data for the detail discussion of the bond failure of rock bolt and cable bolt in this paper. In the pull-out test, a comparison was made between two types of cable bolts and rock bolts. From the results, it is shown that the microscopic failure mechanism is evaluated as the different failure mode. Then the support effect of rock bolts and cable bolts are discussed.

1 INTRODUCTION

Rock bolts have been used as a primary support member of underground openings in the last two decades. However, a clear explanation for the support effect of rock bolts has not been made sufficiently. In order to clarify the support effect of rock bolts, the failure mechanism in a pull-out test of them has been discussed. Then a main support effect was explained by bond strength of rock bolts. For a design of fully grouted bolts using convergence in underground opening, the analytical solution based on elasto-plasticity in the axisymmertic problem was suggested (Indraratna et al. 1990). A finite difference method using equations based on the convergence-confinement curves of a bolted tunnel was proposed and then the effects of the distance from the bolted section from tunnel face, bolt spacing and end plate were discussed (Oreste et al. 1996). Furthermore, the behavior of rock bolt under dynamic loading was discussed (Tannant et al. 1995).

Recently, cable bolts have also been applied to underground openings as a new support member. The support effect of cable bolt has been discussed by many researchers (Yazici et al. 1992, Kaiser et al. 1992, Hyett et al. 1992). In Japan, the challenging effort to produce the rational support system using both rock bolt and cable bolt has been conducted in The Second TOMEI highway tunnel with a large section of about 200 m (Oreste et al. 1996, Tanaka 2000). Furthermore, in this trial, the cost of the support system is focused on. To minimize the cost, first of all, the effect of the support members must be examined much more quantitatively than before.

On the other hand, numerical models of fully grouted bolt and cable bolt are used for the design of tunnel. In a numerical analysis, the bond failure is assumed to occur between the bolt and cement grout, and then the mechanical behavior of them is modeled by shear spring and slider (Brady 1988). The constants of the model are determined by the result of pull test in a field. Furthermore, the constitutive law for the bond failure cable bolt was proposed (Hyett et al. 1995). This low is derived in consideration with the failure of bolt–grout interface and grout annulus, and the interaction between them. In this research, the failure within grout is observed by a scanning electron microscope (SEM). Thus the visible area is so narrow. Therefore it is necessary to visualize wider area globally and to discuss the failure mechanism of bolt–grout interface, grout and rock mass.

In this paper, patterns of the failure in a pull-out test are visualized by X-ray CT scanner to supply the basic data for the detail discussion on the bond failure of rock bolt and cable bolt. In the pull-out tests, a comparison was made between two types of cable bolts and rock bolts. From the results, it is shown that the microscopic failure mechanism is evaluated as the different failure mode. Then the support effect of rock bolts and cable bolts is discussed (Ito et al. 2001, Obara et al. 2002).

2 PULL-OUT TEST

The pull-out tests were conducted on four types of bolt grouted into an artificial rock with cement paste in laboratory. The artificial rock made by concrete. The dimension of it is 100 cm in height with a base of 50 cm by 50 cm. After 14 days cure of the artificial rock, a hole having a diameter of 65 mm for installation of a bolt is drilled with a depth of 40 cm. The bolts (rock bolts and cable bolts) are grouted with cement paste. The cement used in the grout is portland cement. The water – cement ratio is 0.35. The embedment length of the bolt is 35 cm in all cases of the test. The pull-out test is performed after 17 days when the bolts were grouted. The mechanical properties of the artificial rock and grout are summarized in Table 1.

The bolts used in this test are shown in Figure 1. The geometry and yielded force are summarized in Table 2. Two types of rock bolt are used: a deformed bolt with a diameter of 25 mm in Case 1 and a twist bolt with a diameter of 24 mm in Case 2, respectively. Two types of cable bolt are used: a plane strand cable bolt in Case 3 and a bulb strand cable bolt (so called Garford bulb cable bolt) in Case 4. The diameter of both cable bolts is 15.2 mm. These cable bolts are often used at mines in Canada and Australia.

The pull-out test setup is illustrated in Figure 2. The bolts are pulled by a hollow ram jack linked an electric oil pump, which is installed on a bearing plate. The pulling force is measured by a pressure cell of the oil pump. The end plate and nut are equipped at end of bolt. The anti-rotation device is adopted in a pulling head coupler. The bolt displacement is estimated as the mean value calculated by values measured by two

Table 1. Mechanical properties of artificial rock and cement.

	ρ [kg/m^3]	UCS [MPa]	UTS [MPa]	E [GPa]	ν
Artificial rock (concrete)	2410	82.3	4.83	35.1	0.22
Grout (cement paste)	2060	89.7	3.59	21.2	0.25

ρ: Density; UCS: Uniaxial compressive strength, 21 days cure in concrete and 17 days cure in grout; UTS: Tensile strength by disk test; E: Young's modulus; ν: Poisson's ratio.

Table 2. Mechanical properties of bolts.

	Bolt shank (Threaded portion)		
	Cross sectional area [mm^2]	Ultimate strength [kN]	Yield strength [kN]
Case 1: Deformed bolt	506.7 (353)	247.9 (172)	173.5 (121)
Case 2: Twist bolt	445.9 (353)	308 (244)	227 (180)
Case 3: Plain strand cable bolt	138.7	261	222
Case 4: Bulb strand cable bolt	138.7	261	222

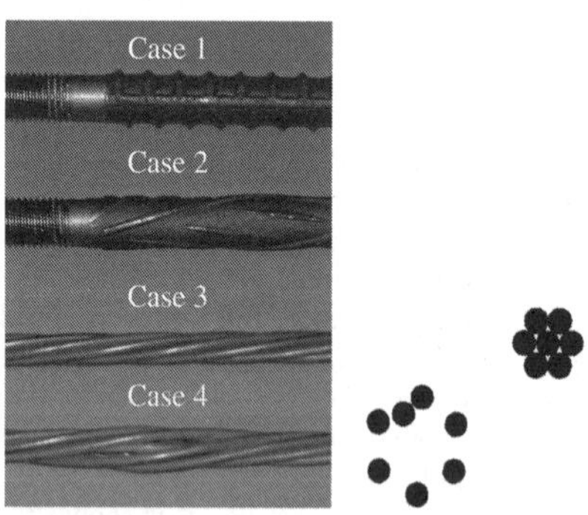

Figure 1. The rock bolts and cable bolts used in the pull-out test; deformed bolt in Case 1, twist bolt in Case 2, plane strand cable bolt in Case 3, bulb strand cable bolt in Case 4 in order from top.

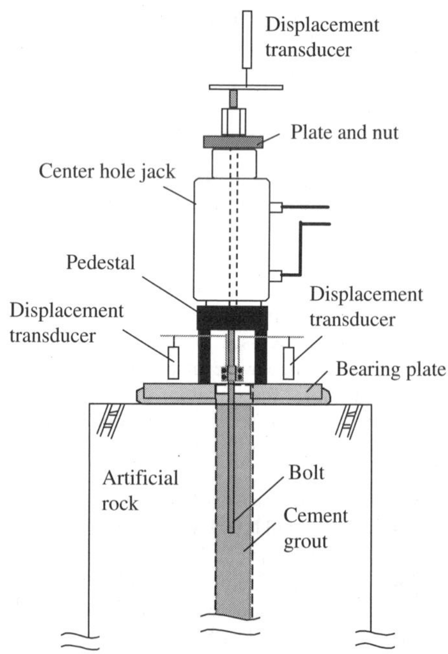

Figure 2. Schematic set-up of the pull-out test.

displacement transducers. In addition, a pulling rate of the test is 0.05 kN/min. The force and displacement are recorded by a personal computer at every 0.5 kN.

3 RESULTS OF PULL-OUT TEST

Figure 3 shows the load–displacement curves for each case. The results show the strong influence of bolt type on the deformational behavior. In both Case 1 and Case 2 using the rock bolts, the rock bolts cannot be pulled out up to end of this test, and then the part of screw for holding the bolt with a nut is yielded. In the load–displacement curves, the point that the bolt begins to slide away from elastic behavior is defined as the yield point. The yield forces of the load – displacement curves in Case 1 and 2 are 170 kN and 215 kN, respectively, and then these values are greater than those in Case 3 and 4. The initial stiffness of them is greater than that in Case 3 and 4, and the displacement at the yield point is smaller. If the rock bolt is not yielded, the maximum force of the rock bolt is considered to be greater. However, the displacement of rock bolt is seemed to be smaller than that in Case 3 and 4 as ever.

The load–displacement curves in Case 3 and 4 show ductile behavior. In Case 3, that is approximated by the bi-linear curves. On the other hand, that in Case 4 is linear up to the yield point, and then is approximately hyperbolic curves. The load–displacement curve is dependent on the radial confining pressure, and the curve in Case 4 is similar to that for higher confinement in the pull test performed by Hyett et al. (1992). Therefore, the bulb strand cable bolt in Case 4 has the great effect of the radial confining pressure. It is considered that the bulb of the cable bolt plays a role like an asperity of joint plane and that the radial confining pressure, namely the stress perpendicular to the grout-bolt interface is induced due to the movement of the cable bolt along the borehole axis. On the other hand, the plane strand cable bolt is also considered to have the effect of the radial confining pressure. However, the effect in Case 3 is smaller than that in Case 4, and then the plane strand cable bolt is pulled out after the yield point, maintaining a constant lower load.

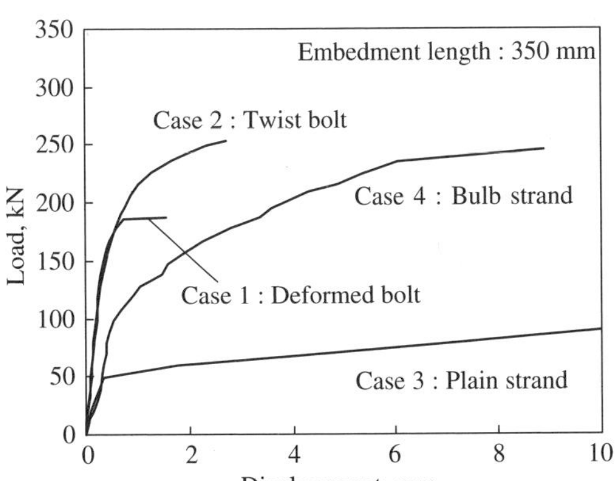

Figure 3. Load–displacement curves of four cases in the pull-out test.

The difference of the load–displacement curve in each case is seemed to be caused by the mechanism of the bond failure. To clarify this failure mechanism, it is indispensable to observe invisible area. From this point of view, an X-ray CT is adopted to examine what happens along the axis of fully grouted bolts as the bond failure.

4 VISUALIZATION OF FAILURE USING X-RAY CT

4.1 *X-ray CT scanner*

X-ray Computed Tomography (CT) is well known as a nondestructive medical imaging technique. A usual X-ray photograph is shadow picture to indicate the features of attenuation of an X-ray beam through a body.

The attenuation of X-ray beams through the object is firstly utilized to reconstruct a two dimensional image of the object, and subsequently a three dimensional image is built laminating the two dimensional images. When X-ray beam propagates through the one-dimensional homogeneous object in Figure 4, the intensity of the X-ray flux at the source i_0 in terms of the number of photons that enter the specimen changes to that value of i after the attenuation of X-ray flux through the object. The attenuation of X-ray beams is expressed as follows (Hagiwara et al. 1990, Kasahara et al. 1993):

$$i = i_0 \exp(\int f_m dr) \tag{1}$$

where r is a distance from the source, f_m is the beams, and then is a constant material property for the linear

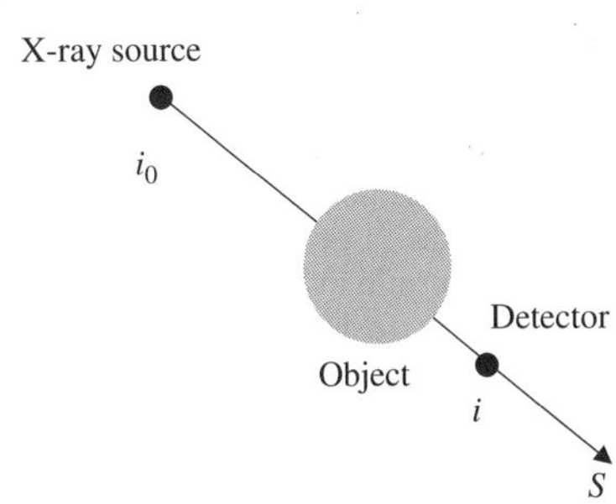

Figure 4. One-dimensional X-ray attenuation.

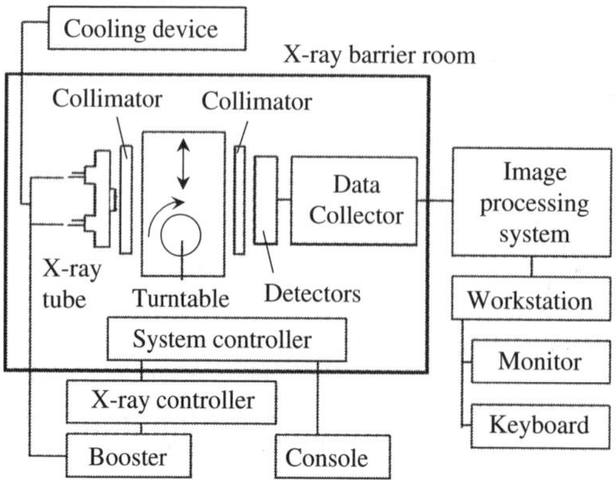

Figure 5. Composition of X-ray scanner.

absorption coefficient. The linear absorption coefficient is mainly a function of the radiometric density of materials and of the energy of X-ray beams, and then is a constant material property for the X-ray with one single energy level.

The projection p is defined by

$$p = \ln(i_0 / i) = \int f_m dr \qquad (2)$$

The projection is required to be measured for various angles of incidence, to compute the linear absorption coefficient at each point by the Filtered Back Projection Method (Kak et al. 1987).

In the image processing analysis, following so called "CT-value" is used:

$$CT - value = \frac{\mu_t - \mu_w}{\mu_w} \kappa \qquad (3)$$

where μ_t: linear absorption coefficient at scanning point; μ_w: linear absorption coefficient for water; and κ: constant for projection. Here, it is noted that this constant is fixed to a value of 1000. Thus, the CT-value of air should be -1000 because the linear absorption coefficient for air is almost zero, and then the CT-value of water is 0. The CT images are presented with shaded gray or black color for low CT-value and light gray or white color for high CT-value as all the subsequent black and white images. The total number of levels on these colors is 256, namely gray-level image.

The system of the X-ray CT scanner used here is TOSCANER-23200 min in Figure 5, developed for an industrial use by the Toshiba Corporation (Sugawara et al. 1887, 1999, Otani et al. 2000, 2001). In this apparatus, the collimated X-ray is penetrated from all around the circumference of a specimen by rotating and traversing the turntable. The detected data are assembled and the cross sectional images are reconstructed using

Table 3. Specification of X-ray CT scanner (TOSCANER-23200 min, TOSHIBA Cop.).

Scan type	Traverse/rotation
Power of X-ray	300 kV/200 kV
Maximum size of specimen	400 mm in diameter, 600 mm in height
Thickness of X-ray beam	0.5 mm, 1 mm, 2 mm
Spatial solution	0.2 mm (diameter of hole) for steel bar of 20 mm diameter

image data processing device by means of the filtered back projection method. Then, the image is displayed on the monitor of engineering workstation. By using all these cross sectional images around the circumference of the specimen, the three dimensional images can be reconstructed. The contents of the specification on the X-ray CT scanner are shown in Table 3. The medical CT scanners are most commonly equipped with a 140 kV X-ray tube while the industrial ones used here is equipped with a 300 kV X-ray tube. Thus, it is easily realized that the capacity of scanning for the industrial use is much higher than that of medical one.

The CT-value map is obtained as a discrete set of numbers, supposed to represent the average value over small pixel. In the standard configuration, the size of each pixel is 0.293 mm by 0.293 mm by X-ray beam thickness.

4.2 *Failure of cement grout*

After the pull-out test, the coring from the artificial rock is conducted to obtain the cross sectional image of the specimen by the X-ray CT as shown in Figure 6. The diameter of the specimen is 100 mm. The location of scanning perpendicular to the core axis is from 10 mm to 110 mm below the upper surface of the artificial rock with every 1 mm. Therefore the total number of sections is 100 in each case. The location of the cross sectional images at every 10 mm is also shown in the figure.

An example of cross-sectional gray-level image which consists of 256 colors is shown in Figure 7. The dark region in the image shows low density area while the region of relatively light color shows that of high density. The black area around specimen and the white area at the center of specimen represent the air and the bolt, respectively.

Figure 8 shows the cross sectional gray-level images at every 10 mm from 10 mm to the bottom of specimen below the upper surface of the artificial rock in each case. The number of cross sections in the figure is corresponding to the location number in Figure 6. In Case 1, a deformed bolt is shown. Thin fractures are produced radially in the first two images, then the primary fracture is spirally induced anti-clockwise in the upper part of the specimen.

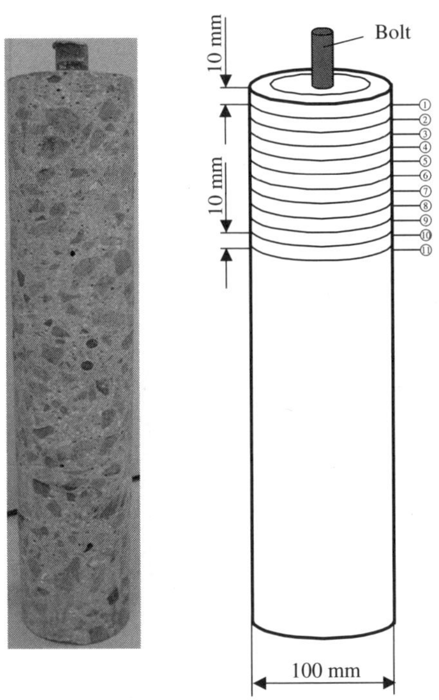

Figure 6. Drilled specimen and scanning locations indicated in Figure 8.

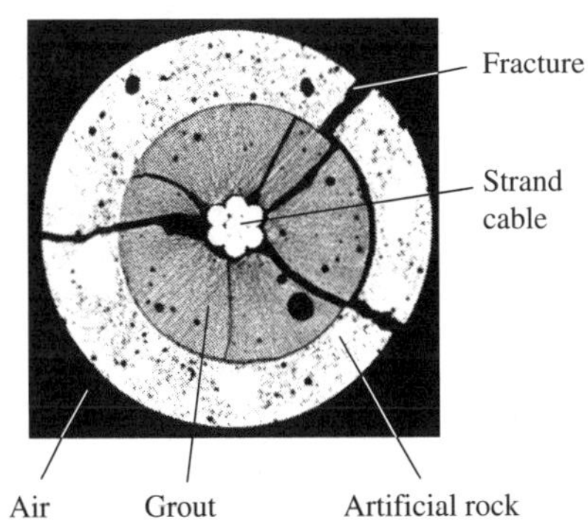

Figure 7. Gray-level image of scanning (256 colors).

However, in the lower part, it is induced almost. The fracture reaches the boundary between the artificial rock and the cement grout, then propagates along the boundary.

As the rock bolt used in Case 2 is a twist bolt, the anti-clockwise spiral fracture in the cement grout is predominant. It is noted that the surface of twist bolt has spiral lugs. No. 6 and 7 images show the typical pattern of the bond failure. Namely, the fracture initiates from the bolt–grout interface and propagates spirally to the boundary between the artificial rock and the cement grout. Then the fracture propagates along the boundary as the artificial rock and the cement grout are separated each other. It is considered that the degree of the twist in Case 2 is larger than that in Case 1.

In Case 3, the plane strand cable bolt is used. The radial splitting is observed within the cement grout in all sections. The number of the radial fractures is four or five. These fractures are rotated along the spiral lugs of the cable bolt. It is clear that the propagation of fractures is little affected by pores, nevertheless there are many pores within the cement grout.

In Case 4, the bulb strand cable bolt is used. The bulb is located at 150 mm depth from the ground surface of the artificial rock. Therefore, the sectional images are in the upper region of the bulb. Three thick fractures are observed. These fractures penetrate through not only the cement grout but also the artificial rock. The rotation of the fractures observed in Case 3 is difficult to confirm in Case 4.

4.3 *Discussion of failure mechanism*

Two failure modes in pull-out test on the deformed bar from grout have been summarized by Hyett et al. (1992) One is radial splitting of a surrounding grout, the other is shearing of the reinforcement against the surrounding grout. The radial splitting mechanism is induced by the wedging action between the lugs of the bar and the grout. This exerts an outward pressure on the inside of the grout annulus that is balanced by the induced circumstantial tensile stress within the annulus.

According to the results in this research, it is clear that the failure mechanism is dependent on the type of used bolts, that is the shape of the lugs of the bolt. In Case 2, the lugs of the twist bolt is spiral. Therefore, the failure mode within the grout is spiral with the twist too. In this case, the state of stress within the grout annulus may be calculated by the theory of twist.

On the other hand, the failure mode in Case 3 and 4 that the strand cable bolt is used shows the radial splitting mechanism. This mode is induced by the wedging effect which the grout is yielded by the movement of the bar, and then the inner pressure on the inside of the grout annulus can be exerted due to the dilation of the yielded grout near the bolt–grout interface (Kaiser et al. 1992, Hyett et al. 1995). The failure mode in Case 4 is very similar to that of the result shown in Figure 9. This failure is observed in the experiment that a hollow cylinder made by cement mortal is submitted to almost uniform inner pressure of the center hole by expansive cement, without outer pressure (Mori et al. 2000). It is concluded that the failure in Case 3 and 4 is induced by inner pressure on the bolt–grout interface. In addition, the inner pressure at the

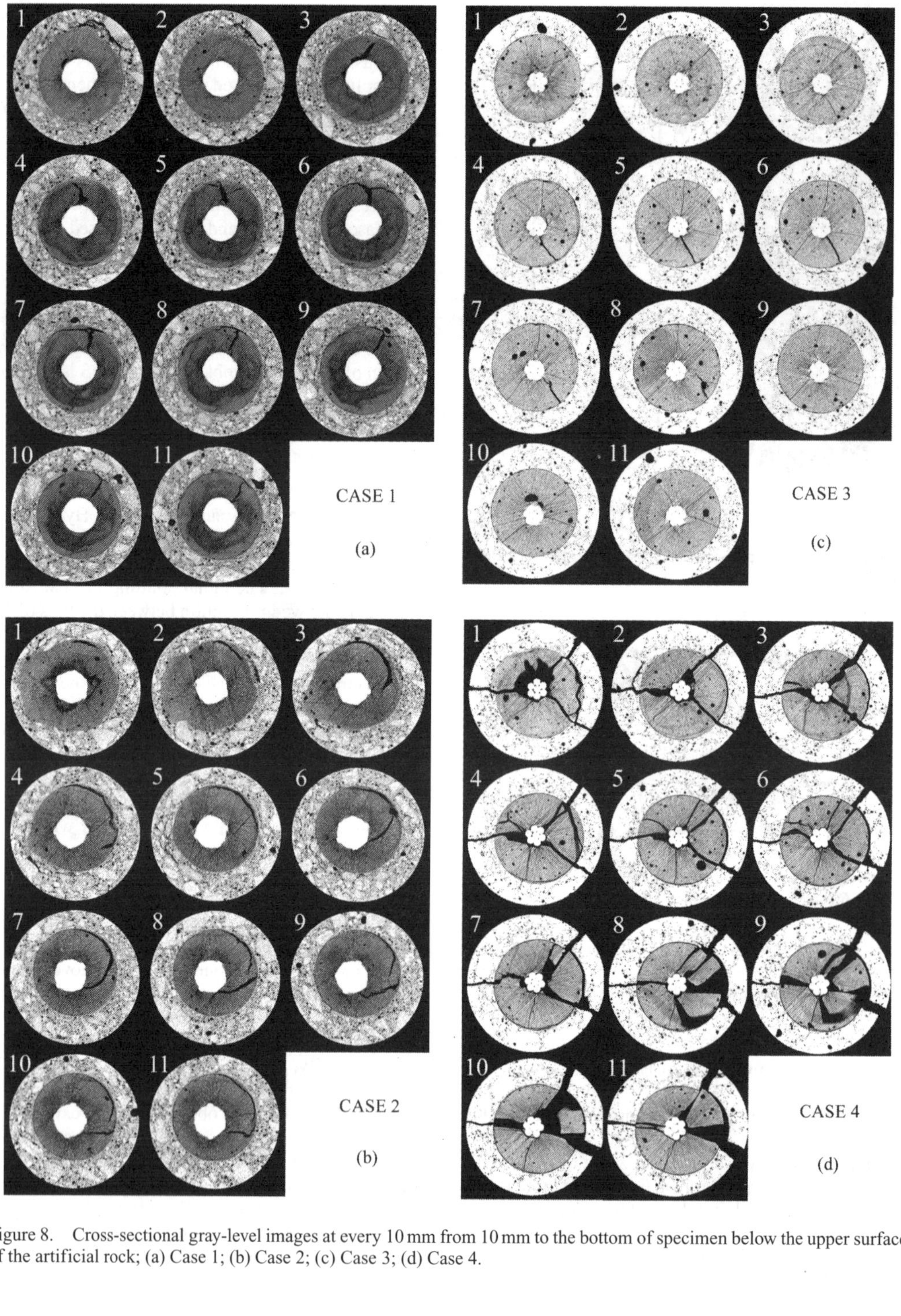

Figure 8. Cross-sectional gray-level images at every 10 mm from 10 mm to the bottom of specimen below the upper surface of the artificial rock; (a) Case 1; (b) Case 2; (c) Case 3; (d) Case 4.

failure is 3.5 times of the tensile strength of the cement mortal used in this experiment. However, the radial fractures in Case 3 are rotated along the spiral lugs of the cable bolt. This means that the effect of twist also involves slightly in failure. On the other hand, the rotation of the radial fractures is not observed in Case 4. This result may be caused by the bulb of the cable bolt.

It is very difficult to clarify when the failure in each case occurs, using these X-ray CT images. Because the specimen is drilled after the pull-out test. In Case 4, it was confirmed that the failure was occurred at the core drilling. This means that the large residual stress remains within the grout annulus after unloading in the pull-out test. Accordingly, the residual stress was relieved due to core drilling, and then the failure occurred. Comparing the degree of the failure in Case 3 with Case 4, it is concluded that the value of the residual stress in Case 4 is greater than that in Case 3. This is considered to result from the effect of the bulb equipped in the strand cable bolt. In Case 1 and 2, the fracture which aperture is large is induced within the cement grout without failure within the artificial rock. Therefore, it is considered that the failure occurs during the pull-out test.

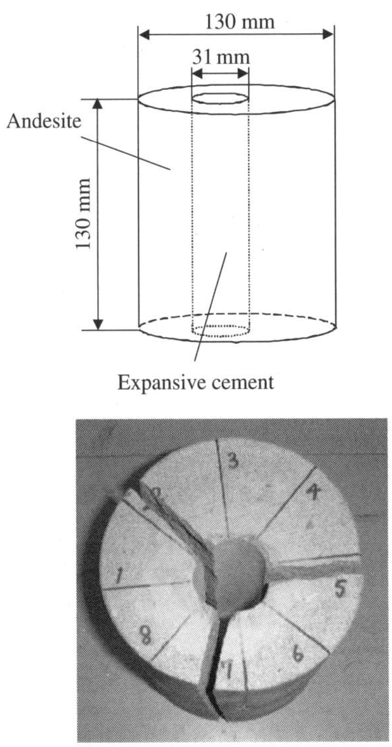

Figure 9. Fracture of hollow cylinder with inner pressure by expansive cement.

Putting together these results, it is indicated that the support effect of the rock bolt in Case 1 and 2 is primarily the twist rather than the inner pressure, and that in Case 3 and 4 is dominated by the inner pressure and the slight twist.

The failure mode reflects the support mechanism of rock bolts and cable bolts. Therefore, it is necessary to visualize the occurrence of fracture at arbitrary load/displacement stage. It is concluded that the X-ray CT can be effective tool for the visualization of the failure in the pull-out test.

Figure 10 shows the three dimensional images for Case 1 of the deformed bolt specimen, Case 2 of the twist bolt specimen and Case 3 of the plain strand specimen, based on 100 cross-sectional gray-level images. As found in cross-sectional images in Figure 8, successive failure plane can be specified clearly. In the case of rock bolts the anti-clockwise spiral fracture in cement grout is predominant due to the surface of rock bolts, spiral lugs and ribs. On the other hand, in the case of cable bolt, two types of failure are obtained. One is bond failure along the bolt–grout interface. The other one is spiral failure due to the radial tension stress caused by inner pressure on the bolt–grout interface (Obara et al. 2002, Aoki et al. 2002).

It is clear that failure patterns can not be explained by simple frictional model like slider. Therefore, much attention must be paid to twist failure for rock bolts and spiral failure for cable bolts. Three dimensional images help us to understand failure mechanism at invisible area and develop the numerical model for actual mechanical behavior.

5 CONCLUSIONS

In order to visualize the bond failure of rock bolts and cable bolts, the pull-out test was conducted and the X-ray CT is applied to the specimen drilled from the artificial rock after the pull-out test. From the visualization of the bond failure, it was clarified that the failure mode of cement grout is different in type of bolts. Namely, the failure mode within the grout is spiral with the twist in Case 1 and 2, in which a deformed bolt and twist bolt are respectively used. On the other hand, the failure mode in Case 3 and 4, which the plan strand and bulb strand cable bolt are respectively used, shows the radial splitting mechanism. The radial splitting mechanism exerts the confining pressure. It is clear that these differences are dependent on the shape and existence of lugs of the bars.

Putting together theses results, it is concluded that the support effect of the rock bolt in Case 1 and 2 is primarily the twist rather than the inner pressure, and that in Case 3 and 4 is dominated by the inner pressure and the slight twist.

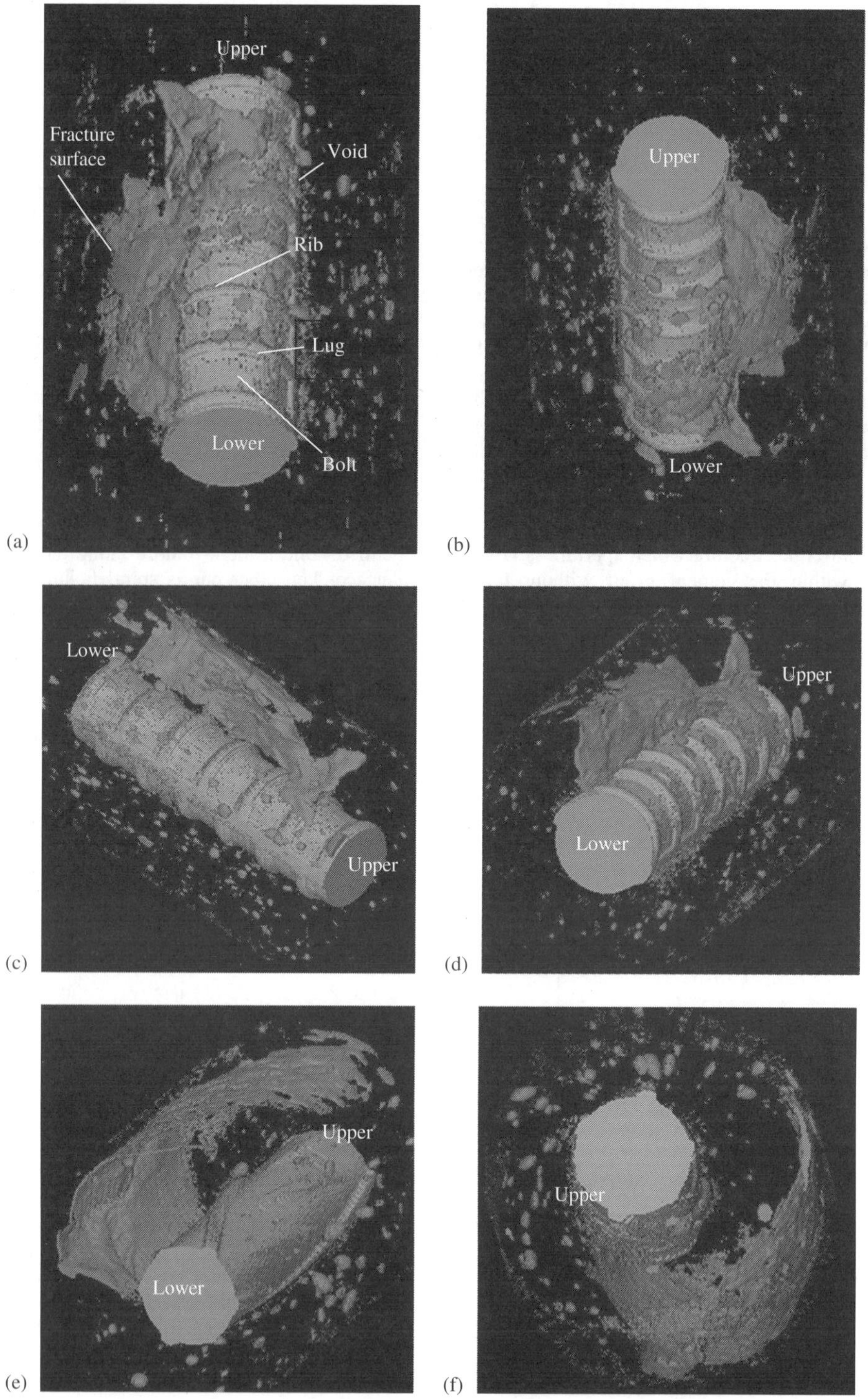

Figure 10. Three dimensional images; (a, b, c, d) Case 1 of the deformed bolt specimen; (e, f, g, h) Case 2 of the twist bolt specimen; (i, j, k, l) Case 3 of the plain strand specimen.

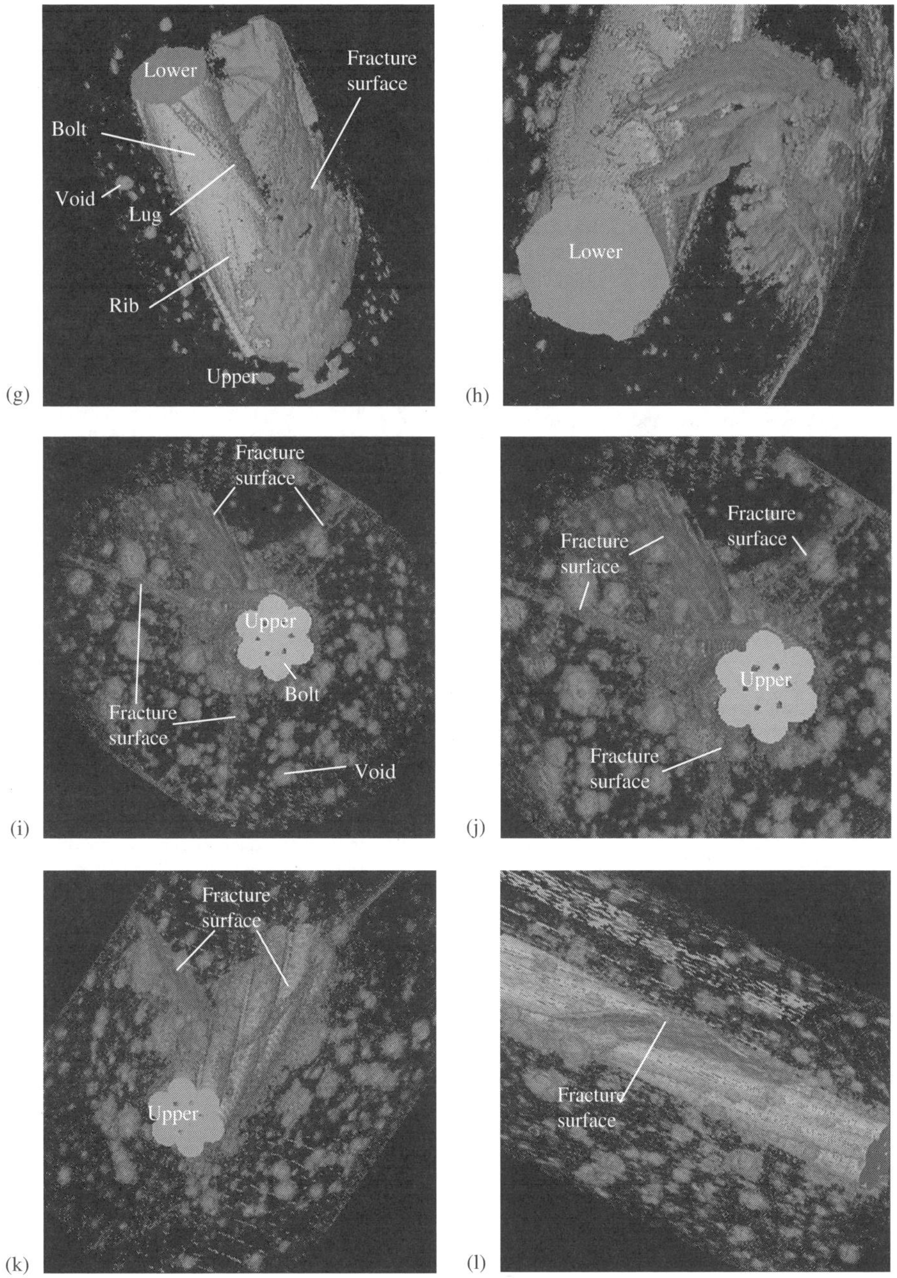

Figure 10. (Continued)

REFERENCES

Aoki, T., Y. Maeno, K. Shibata and Y. Obara, Laboratory pull-out tests of cablebolts, Proc. of EUROCK 2002 Conference, Portuguese (Funchal), 2002, pp.599–606.

Indraratna, B. and P.K. Kaiser, Design for grouted rock bolts based on the convergence control method, *Int. J. Rock Mech. Min. Sci. & Geomech. Abstr.*, 1990, Vol.27, No.4, pp.269–281.

Ito, F., F. Nakahara, R. Kawano, S.S. Kang and Y. Obara, Visualization of failure in a pull-out test of cable bolts using X-ray CT, Construction and Building Materials, 2001,Vol.15, pp.263–270.

Oreste, P.P. and D. Peila, Radial passive rockbolting in tunneling design with a new convergence-confinement model, *Int. J. Rock Mech. Min. Sci. & Geomech. Abstr.*, 1996, Vol.33, No.5, pp.443–454.

Tannant, D.D., R.K. Brummer and X. Yi, Rockbolt behaviour under dynamic loading: field tests and modeling, *Int. J. Rock Mech. Min. Sci. & Geomech. Abstr.*, 1995, Vol.32, No.6, pp.537–550.

Yazici, S. and P.P. Kaiser, Bond strength of grouted cable bolts, *Int. J. Rock Mech. Min. Sci. & Geomech. Abstr.*, 1992, Vol.29, No.3, pp.279–292.

Kaiser, P.P., S. Yazici and J. Nose, Effect of stress change on the bond strength of fully grouted cables, *Int. J. Rock Mech. Min. Sci. & Geomech. Abstr.*, 1992, Vol.29, No.3, pp.293–306.

Hyett, A.J., W.F. Bawden and R.D. Reichert, The effect of rock mass confinement on the bond strength of fully routed cable bolts, *Int. J. Rock Mech. Min. Sci. & Geomech. Abstr.*, 1992, Vol.29, No.5, pp.503–524.

Tanaka, H. and S. Aoyama, Trial construction of a tunnel having a large cross sectional area in the Second Tomei Highway, The third Shimizu tunnel, *J. Tunnels and underground*, 2000, Vol.31, No.9, pp.15–23, 25–35 (in Japanese).

Brady, B. and L. Lorig, Analysis of rock reinforcement using finite difference methods, Computer and Geotechnics, 1988, Vol.5, pp.123–149.

Hyett, A.J., W.F. Bawden, G.R. Macsporran and M. Moosavi, A constitutive law for bond failure of fully-grouted cable bolts using a modified Hoek cell, *Int. J. Rock Mech. Min. Sci. & Geomech. Abstr.*, 1995, Vol.32, No.1, pp.11–36.

Hagiwara, T. and T. Nanba, Generation of Proximity Function for Naturally Fractured Reservoir Simulator Using X-ray CT Scanner System, presented at the Eleventh Workshop for the IEA, Collaborative Project on EOR, Paris, 1990

Kasahara, J. and Y. Tomoda, An introduction to computerized geoscience, University of Tokyo Press, 1993, pp.180–185 (in Japanese).

Kak, A.C. and M. Slaney, Principles of computed tomographic imaging, IEEE PRESS, 1987, pp.49–110.

Sugawara, K., Y. Obara, K. Kaneko, K. Koike, M. Ohmi and T. Aoi, Visualization of three-dimensional structure of rocks using X-ray CT method, Proc. of 1st Asian Rock Mechanics Symp. Korea (Seoul), 1887, pp.769–774.

Sugawara, K., Y. Obara and A. Sato, Visualization of water saturation process in rock by X-rays CT, Proc. of '99 Japan-Korea Joint Symposium on Rock Engineering, Japan (Fukuoka), 1999, pp.503–508.

Obara, Y., Y. Maeno, R. Kawano, F. Ito and F. Nakahara, Bond failure of rock bolts and cable bolts in a pull-out test, *J. of JSCA*, 2002, pp.97–106 (in Japanese).

Otani, J., T. Mukunoki and Y. Obara, Application of X-ray CT method for characterization of failure in soils, Soils and Foundations, 2000, Vol.10, No.2, pp.111–118.

Otani, J., T. Mukunoki and Y. Obara, Evaluation of progressive failure in soils using industrial X-ray CT scanner, Proc. of 10th IACMAG, USA (Arizona), 2001, to be published.

Mori, T. and A. Hirata, Laboratory fracture experiment of rock using expansive cement, Proc. of Annual Meeting of MMIJ Kyushu Branch, 2000, pp.34–36 (in Japanese).

X-ray CT for Geomaterials; Soils, Concrete, Rocks – Otani & Obara (eds.)
© 2004 Swets & Zeitlinger. Lisse, ISBN 90 5809 666 1

Analysis of wetting process of rock by means of X-ray CT

K. Sugawara, D. Fukahori, T. Iwatani, T. Ikutake & S. Kubota
Graduate School of Science and Technology, Kumamoto University, Japan

ABSTRACT: Subtraction of X-ray CT images is utilized for the quantitative analysis of the unsaturated wetting process of a porous rock. A multi-stage pressurization procedure is applied to a one-dimensional water permeation experiment, and in which the migration of water through a rock specimen is precisely monitored by means of the X-ray CT. Case examples make clear that the subtraction of X-ray CT images is an effective procedure available for the evaluation of the volumetric water content at each point within a rock specimen. Analyzing the forward speed of the wetting front and the distribution of the pore-water pressure, the coefficient of permeability of rock is evaluated along with the magnitude of the matric suction, which plays an important role to determine unsaturated wetting flows.

1 INTRODUCTION

Knowledge of water flow in rock is of fundamental importance for rock engineering and oil and gas production, and in particular for the design and the construction of radioactive repositories, since the mass transfer phenomenon of radioactive nuclear matter deeply associates with water current in rock strata, which is expected to play an important role as a natural barrier (Stephansson 1997). Various techniques and methods have been developed to determine the permeability for a wide range of rock and soil (Fredlund & Rahardjo 1993), and also in order to analyze the water flow, the mass transfer process and so on (Fetter 1993).

X-ray CT is one of effective tools available for the investigation of the mass transfer phenomena in rock and soil. This is known as a nondestructive medical imaging technique (Hounsfield 1972), which makes it possible to evaluate the attenuation of X-ray at each point within a body, by digitizing shadow pictures taken from various directions and subsequent image reconstruction (Kak & Slaney 1988).

Several authors have investigated the potential use of X-ray CT for geo-materials, beginning with a pioneering paper from Arthur (1971). Tillard Ngan et al. (1992) and Desrues et al. (1996) reported on the use of X-ray CT for the measurement of sand density, and Vinegard et al. (1991) showed how heterogeneities and density change in rock could be analyzed with this technique. Cromwell et al. (1984), Coles et al. (1991), Verhelst et al. (1995), Sugawara et al. (1998a, 1999a, 1999b) and Sato et al. (2002) studied the migration of water in rock by X-ray CT, while Sugawara et al. (1997) utilized X-ray CT to examine the three-dimensional structure of rock. Otani et al. (2002) studied the strain localization with failure of soil. Sugawara et al. (1998b, 1999c) successfully utilized the images subtraction method to measure the distribution off the aperture of cracks in rock. From these pioneering studies, it has been clarified that the X-ray CT is a promising tool in the research of geo-mechanics.

This paper explains how the wetting process can be analyzed by means of the X-ray CT method and subsequent data processing. One-dimensional water permeation experiment of multi-stage pressurization is presented to make clear the wetting process of a porous rock specimen. The subtraction of X-ray CT images is proposed to evaluate the volumetric water content at each point within the specimen. It will be clarified that the images subtraction is a promising procedure available not only for the visualization, but also for the quantitative analysis of the wetting process. Moreover a new scheme is proposed to formulate the distributions of the volumetric water content, the flow rate of water and the pore-water pressure, along with the procedure to evaluate the coefficient of permeability and the matric suction simultaneously. Case examples make clear the significant role of the effective confining pressure and the matric suction in determining unsaturated wetting flows.

2 X-RAY COMPUTED TOMOGRAPHY

2.1 *Principle*

The basis of formation of an X-ray CT image is the attenuation of X-rays transmitted through an object. For a one-dimensional case illustrated in Figure 1, the attenuation of an X-ray beam is expressed by

$$i = i_o \exp(- \int f\, ds), \tag{1}$$

where i is the intensity of the X-ray after passing through the object, i_o is the intensity of the X-ray at source, s is the distance from the source, and f is the linear attenuation coefficient called the radiographic density. The radiographic density is a measure for the attenuation by traversing a unit length.

By taking logarithms of Equation (1) a projection P is defined as

$$P = \ln(i_o/i) = \int f\, ds. \tag{2}$$

From projections taken various angles of X-ray beam incidence, the filtered back projection method can be used to complete the linear attenuation coefficient at points within the object (Takagi & Shimoda 1991).

An image formed by X-ray CT is called a radiographic density map. In the present paper, the magnitude of the radiographic density f is expressed by the CT value. The CT value, represented by CT, is taken as being $CT = 0$ in air and $CT = 1000$ in water. In the equation form, it can be written as follow:

$$CT = 1000\, f / f_w \tag{3}$$

where f_w is the radiographic density of water. The CT values are integers and the radiographic density map can be displayed as a digital image.

2.2 *X-ray CT scanner employed*

This work made use of an industrial X-ray CT scanner (TOSCANER-23200) manufactured by the Toshiba Corporation. Major components of the scanner are schematically shown in Figure 2.

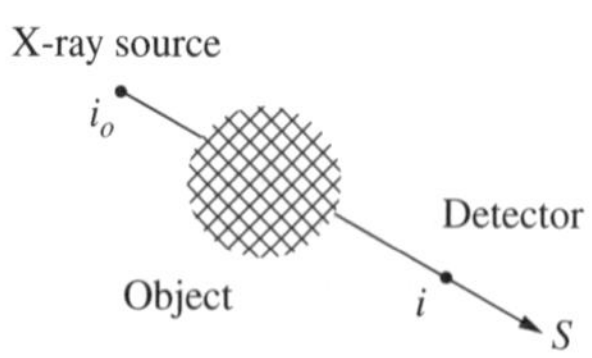

Figure 1. One-dimensional attenuation of X-ray beam.

An X-ray bulb operating at 300 kV/2mA provides the radiation source from which an X-ray beam is emitted. 176 detectors aligned with the X-ray source in the horizontal plane record attenuation data. The object for scanning is positioned on a traversing turntable and the X-ray beam is projected through one plane of the object as it rotates and traverses. The beam thickness is determined with collimators. The X-ray source and detectors can be moved vertically with a specified interval and so a three-dimensional radiographic density image of an object may be obtained if required.

A few attenuation profiles are recorded for each incidence by the 176 detectors, and a set of profiles is utilized to reconstruct a tow-dimensional CT image. The beam thickness was set in 2 mm in the following experiments, and the radiographic density of each pixel was given as an average over a 2 mm thick. In the standard configuration, the pixel is a square of 0.293 mm × 0.293 mm, and the volume of a boxel is 0.1717 mm^3. The time required for a cross-sectional image is about 5 minutes.

2.3 *X-ray beam hardening*

Linear attenuation coefficient f is proportional to the radiometric density of the object, and approximately in inverse proportion to the photon energy of X-ray beam used. Then it is noteworthy that the linear attenuation coefficient f is a constant material property for the X-ray of one single energy level (Kak & Slaney 1988). This is the basis of X-ray CT.

X-ray beams putted to practical use is, however, a mixture of X-rays of various energy levels. Thus in the process of passing through the object, an X-ray of low energy may swiftly attenuate, though an X- ray of high energy still maintains its original energy level. This phenomenon is called the X-ray beam hardening, which causes an error in the evaluation of the radiometric density. This is the limitation and disadvantages of X-ray CT presently available.

The error due to the X-ray beam hardening is generally observed as a shift of the CT value in the object and

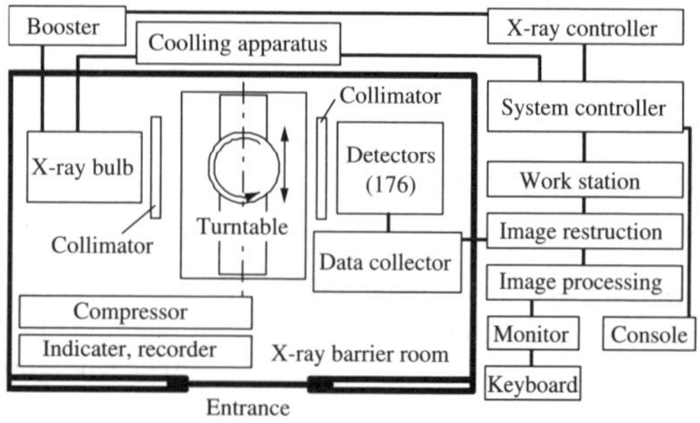

Figure 2. Composition of X-ray CT scanner employed.

background regions. For example, the CT value varies with the object dimensions, along with background materials. Simultaneously the CT value varies with the location in the object, even if the radiometric density of the object is completely uniform. In general, the CT value obtained in the outer region of the object is larger than that in the central region. This is called the cupping effect, since the distribution of the CT value describes a curved surface of concave like a cup. Additionally the CT values decrease with the increase of object dimensions. This is also associated with the X-ray beam hardening. In order to minimize the influence of the X-ray beam hardening, the higher photon energy is required for X-ray scanning, as well as the optimization of object dimensions.

2.4 *Noise problems*

The radiographic density map involves noises arisen from various causes, and the noise elimination is a significant problem to obtain a clear image. In the case that the object is placed in air, the surface of the object is a kind of noise source, since there is generally a great difference in the CT value between the object and the atmosphere. In order to reduce the difference and noises along the surface, an X-ray scanning in water can be recommended. The edge is also a noise source. For instance, in the case that the object has a cross section of square, noises are generated from four corners, and generally form conjugate noise bands. To eliminate such a noise, the covering with oiled soil can be recommended. Since an oiled soil has a nearly same CT value with geo-materials such as rock, the edge noise can be eliminated by this procedure. Additionally various data processing methods can be applied for the noise elimination, which include the simple data stacking and averaging over some area (Takagi & Shimoda 1991).

2.5 *Subtraction of CT images*

Subtraction of radiographic density maps has been proposed for the quantitative measurement of crack opening profiles (Sugawara et al. 1998b, 1999c). This technique is successfully utilized in the present study. In order to analyze the time-dependent water permeation process, the change in the volumetric water content at each point in rock is determined by the subtraction between two CT images scanned at different times. The procedure will be described in the following paragraph.

It is noteworthy that the reliability of quantitative evaluation with the images subtraction is limited by the X-ray beam hardening. The error is considered to be composed of two elements. One is an error due to the shift of the CT value, which can be concretely observed as the difference of the CT values in the background regions. The other is an error related to the degrees of the cupping effect. The CT values in the object empirically form a concaved surface, and its curvature increases with the mean CT value in the object. Thus the images subtraction provides the results deeply influenced by the cupping effect, and a correction of the CT value at each point involves great difficulties. Calibration using a set of standard specimens may present a possible solution.

Error can be estimated as follows, to assess the reliability of the images subtraction analysis. The relation between the true CT value: CT and the measured one CT_m can be expressed as follows:

$$CT = CT_m + e, \tag{4}$$

where e represents the error of the CT value, and the subtraction form is as follows:

$$\Delta CT = \Delta CT_m + \Delta e, \tag{5}$$

where Δ represents the subtraction. By assuming Equation (5), the change in the radiographic density Δf can be written from Equation (3), as follows:

$$\Delta f = f_w \, \Delta CT/1000 - f_w \, \Delta e/1000. \tag{6}$$

The second term of right side represents the error of the radiographic density due to the error of the CT value. The precise images subtraction analysis may require a correction on Δf, according to Equation (6). However it involves great difficulties, in particular in the evaluation of Δe in the object. Thus, in this paper, the measurement of Δe in the background regions is proposed to assess the degrees of the error in the object, as a way presently available.

3 TEST APPARATUS & PROCEDURE

3.1 *Experimental apparatus*

Apparatus consists of a cylindrical pressure vessel and control systems, as shown in Figure 3. To avoid from the attenuation of X-ray, the pressure vessel is made from acrylic resin. Heater and thermostat are installed in the vessel to maintain a constant water temperature of ranging from 30°C to 60°C.

By the compressor-regulator system, a hydraulic head of water of from atmospheric pressure to 500 kPa is applied to a cylindrical rock specimen set on the specimen rest. The rock specimen is placed under a specified constant head of water, and the X-ray scanning is performed on a fixed cross section perpendicular to the cylindrical axis of the pressure vessel, with specified time intervals.

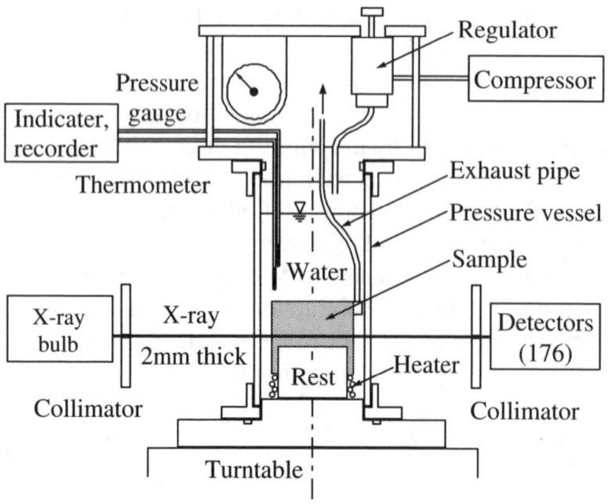

Figure 3. Apparatus for pressurization experiments.

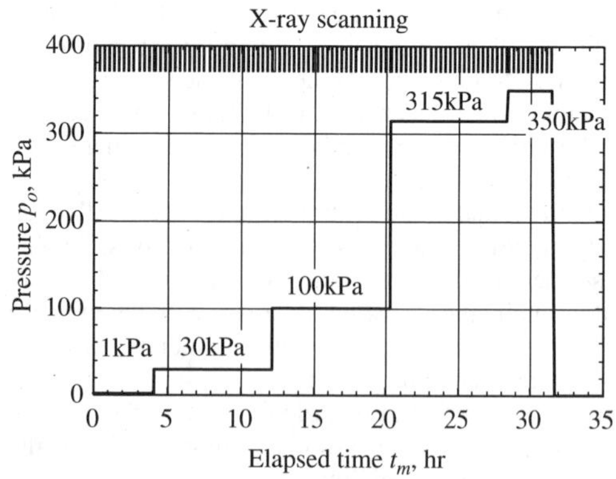

Figure 5. Pressure-time record of the water permeation test with the multi-stage pressurization.

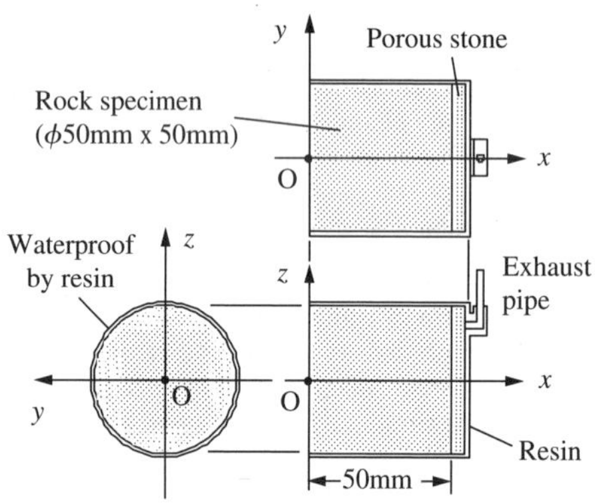

Figure 4. Cylindrical specimen and the co-ordinates.

3.2 *Specimen preparation & experimental procedure*

Kimachi sandstone was tested by two kinds of the pressurization experiment, the water permeation test and the hydrostatical compression test, using the apparatus in Figure 3, in water of 30°C with a deviation of 0.1°C. Prior to the tests, the traditional saturation method (ISRM 1979) was applied and the porosity was measured as 21% and the dry density as 2.54 g/cm^3 (Sugawara et al. 1998c).

In order to clarify the saturated wetting flow and the unsaturated wetting flow in porous rock, a water permeation test was conducted by applying a multi-stage pressurization procedure of from atmospheric pressure to 350 kPa. The hydrostatical compression test was carried out to investigate the deformation effect of rock and water in the pressure vessel.

Figure 4 shows a cylindrical specimen of ϕ50 mm × 50 mm and the co-ordinates (x, y, z). Cylindrical side surface was coated with resin to form an impermeable seal. On a flat end of the specimen, a porous stone of ϕ50 mm × 5.2 mm and an exhaust pipe were fixed, which allowed air to discharge. The circumference of them was also sealed by resin. By such a sealing of 0.6 mm~1 mm thick, water is allowed to permeate only from the unsealed flat end-surface called the inlet.

3.2.1 *Water permeation test*

At the first step the fully dry specimen was scanned by X-ray. For this purpose the specimen was dried at 105°C for 96 hours, and completely rapped with an impermeable foil. The CT image obtained at this step was utilized as the standard image for the following images subtraction analysis.

After removing the impermeable foil, the water permeation test was started, and monitored by X-ray scanning as shown in Figure 5. The pressure was increased step-by-step, and the X-ray scanning was taken place at 20 minutes intervals for each pressure stage, providing 98 CT images in total. After the water permeation test, the specimen was saturated by the traditional saturation method and tested by X-ray scanning.

In the water permeation test, the volumetric water content can be evaluated by the images subtraction scheme. It is generally defined in percent as a ratio of the volume of water to the total volume of the specimen. This definition is extended and applied to each boxel, and the volumetric water content ϕ_w has been defined as follows:

$$\phi_w = (CT - CT_d)/1000 \tag{7}$$

where CT denotes the CT value of a given boxel and CT_d is that when the rock is fully dry.

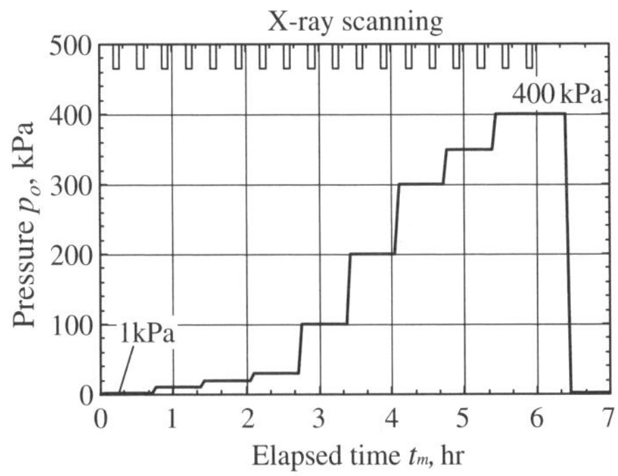

Figure 6. Pressure record of hydrostatical compression.

3.2.2 *Hydrostatical compression test*
The rock specimen processed as in Figure 4 was completely coated with resin, and provided to the hydrostatical compression test. The pressure record is shown in Figure 6.

The increment of density $\Delta\rho$ in the hydrostatical compression test can be defined from the principle of the CT images subtraction as follows:

$$\Delta\rho = (CT - CT_o)/1000, \quad (8)$$

where CT denotes the CT value at the pressure p_o and CT_o is the standard value when the specimen is at $p_o = 1$ kPa.

4 EXAMPLES OF IMAGE SUBTRACTION

4.1 *Cross-sectional CT image*

Figure 7 shows an example of cross-sectional image, obtained by the hydrostatical compression test. A rectangular in the center part corresponds to the cross section of the rock specimen and a porous stone, which are surrounding by water, and a dark gray ring is the cross section of the pressure vessel. Outer black zone surrounding the ring is air.

4.2 *Images subtraction in hydrostatic compression*

The pseudo-images in Figure 8 are cross-sectional images of rock specimen, and the mean CT value in each attached figure is calculated by stacking the CT data of neighboring five boxels into the y-axis direction, that is the mean value within a volume of 146.5 mm^3. The distribution of the mean CT value is relatively flat in both cases, excluding the data indicated by white circles immediately neighboring the end surface of specimen. The subtraction image is given in Figure 8(c), with the change in dry density $\Delta\rho$ computed by

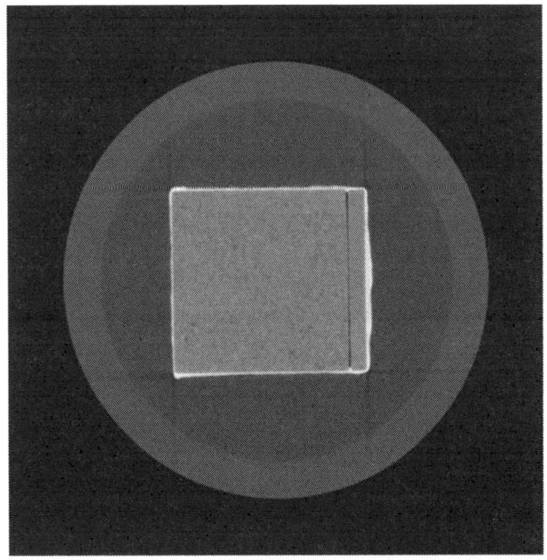

Figure 7. A cross-sectional CT pseudo-image, the hydrostatical compression test.

Equation (8). The density change evaluated is very small, and un-uniform. This may be related to heterogeneities in rock.

The relation between the density change $\Delta\rho$ and the pressure p_o is as summarized in Figure 9. White circle represents the average of $\Delta\rho$ of rock specimen, and the painted circle is that of background water measured in a middle domain of a volume of 2.4 cm^3. The theory of elasticity requires that the density change $\Delta\rho$ is in a direct proportion to the increment of the volumetric strain $\Delta\varepsilon_v$, and $\Delta\varepsilon_v$ coincides with the ratio of the increment of the pressure Δp_o to the Bulk modulus K. The equation form is as follows:

$$\Delta\rho = \rho\Delta\varepsilon_v = \rho\,\Delta p_o / K. \quad (9)$$

From Equation (9), two broken lines in Figure 9 are obtained, by assuming $\rho = 1$ g/cm^3 and $K = 0.45$ GPa for water, and $\rho = 2.5$ g/cm^3 and $K = 1$ GPa for Kimachi sandstone. The results show that the change in the CT value is very small, as forecasted by the theory of elasticity in the experimental range.

4.3 *Images subtraction in water permeation test*

A typical example is given in Figure 10, (a) the initial image of fully dry condition and (b) the case of $p_o = 30$ kPa, at the time of $t_m = 10.1$ hr from the commencement of water permeation test. The mean CT value is computed by stacking the CT data of neighboring five boxels into the y-axis direction. In Figure 10(a), the distribution of the mean CT value is slightly concaved by the cupping effect, and it increases with

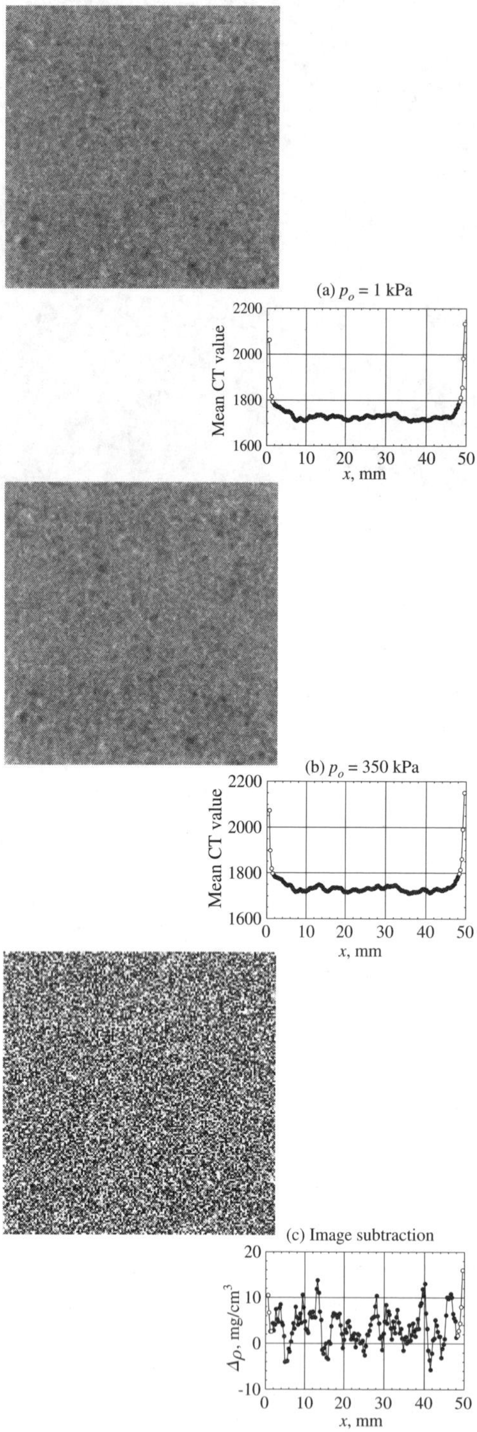

Figure 8. An example of the images subtraction, the hydrostatical compression test.

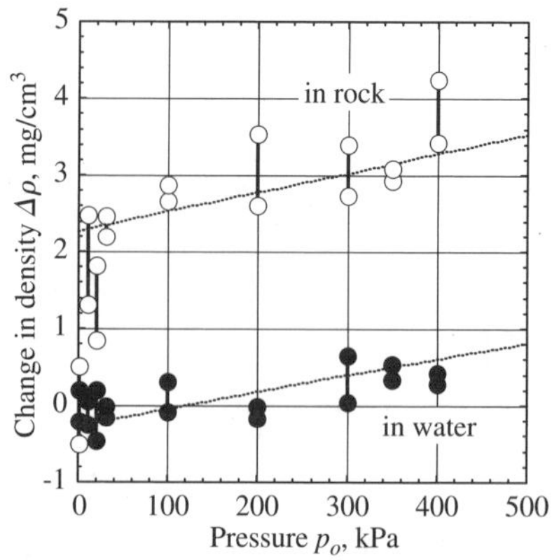

Figure 9. Change in density of rock and water in the pressure vessel, the hydrostatical compression test.

approaching to the inlet, as indicated by white circles. In Figure 10(b), the mean CT value clearly increases at the inlet side, corresponding to the water permeation from the inlet. The subtraction image in Figure 10(c) shows that the wetting front describes a plane approximately parallel to the inlet surface.

The volumetric water content ϕ_w in Figure 10(c) is obtained by substituting the mean CT values into Equation (7). The distribution of ϕ_w along the X-axis has a plateau immediately neighboring the inlet.

In front of the plateau, the value of ϕ_w decreases with the distance from the inlet, and it becomes zero at the wetting front. Between the front and the outlet $x = 50\,\text{mm}$, the value of ϕ_w is always nearly zero, as expected in a dry region. The convergence to zero in the dry region proves the high reliability of the present images subtraction.

Figure 11 shows the images of the volumetric water content obtained by the CT images subtraction. It is clearly observed that the wetting front can advance with time, approximately being parallel to the inlet surface. In the case of $t_m = 30\,\text{hr}$, the front seems to be slightly curved. This suggests the ununiformity of the porosity. The pores and cracks in rock can play a role of the reservoir, then the advance of front is deeply related to the porosity in front.

In order to confirm the reliability of the present CT images subtraction, the mean CT values in the background regions of water and air were measured, as in Figure 12. The absolute value of Δe increases with the increase of the mean CT value in rock. This suggests that the error of ϕ_w may reach to 0.01 in maximum at the final stage of the present water permeation test.

4.4 *CT image of specimen at fully saturated state*

The images subtraction between the fully saturated specimen and the dry one is expected to be available

(a) Initial image

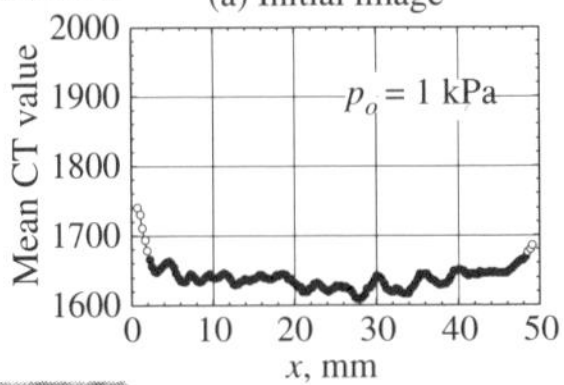

(b) Image of water permeation

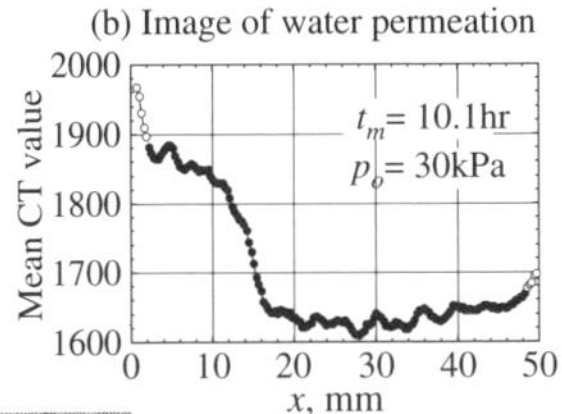

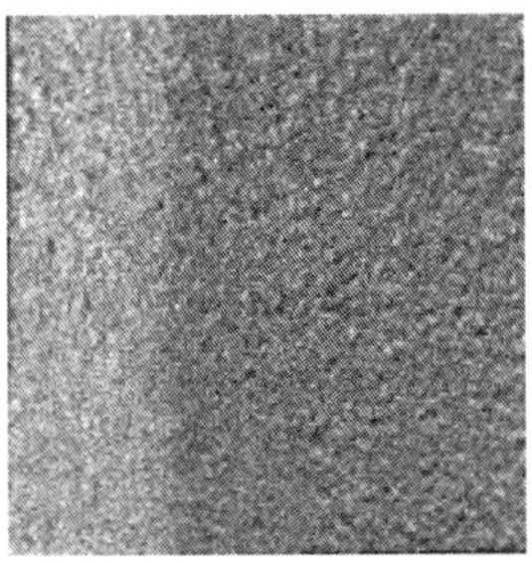

(c) Image subtraction

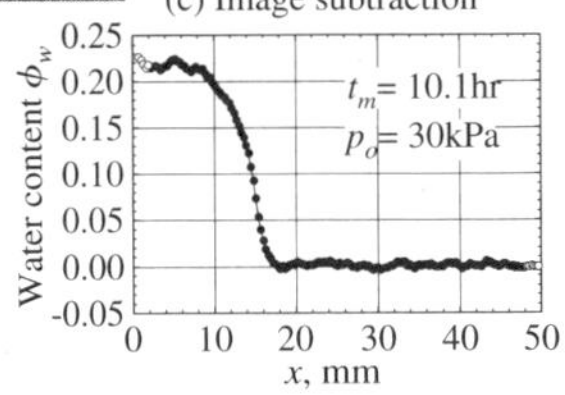

Figure 10. An example of the image subtraction, the water permeation test.

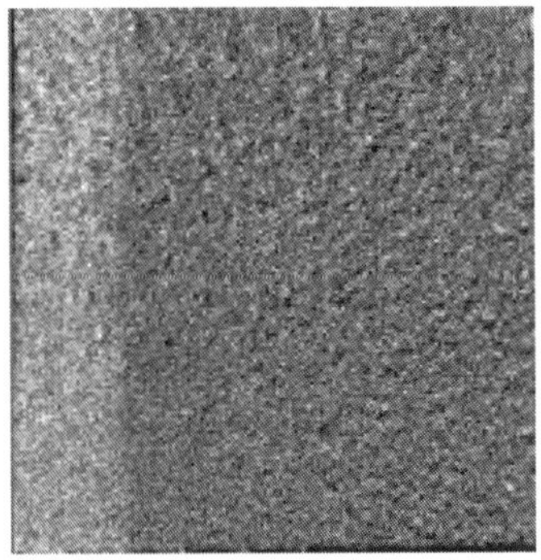

(a) Subtraction image of $t_m = 5$ hr.

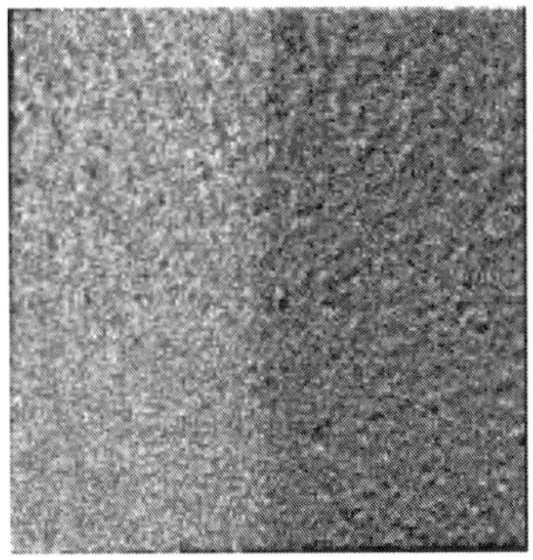

(b) Subtraction image of $t_m = 20$ hr.

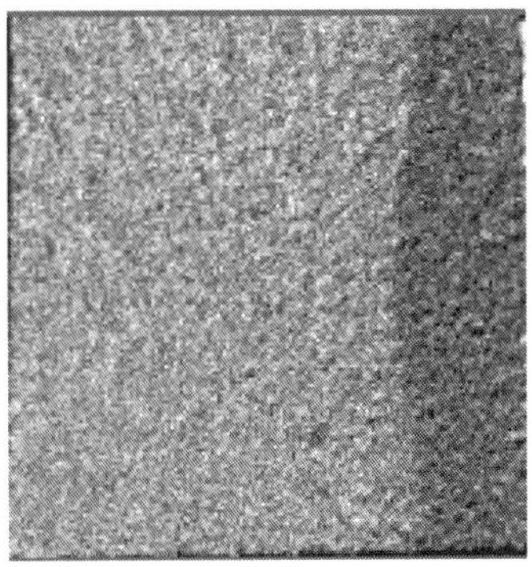

(c) Subtraction image of $t_m = 30$ hr.

Figure 11. Pseudo-images of the volumetric water content obtained by the CT images subtraction.

for the evaluation of porosity ϕ_r of rock. A case example is given in Figure 13. The distribution of the mean CT value in the fully dry case is relatively flat, but that in the fully saturated case is clearly concaved. Then it is clear that the degree of the cupping effect is greater in the later. Such a difference between (a) and (b) clearly shows that the cupping effect can increase with increasing the mean CT value in the object.

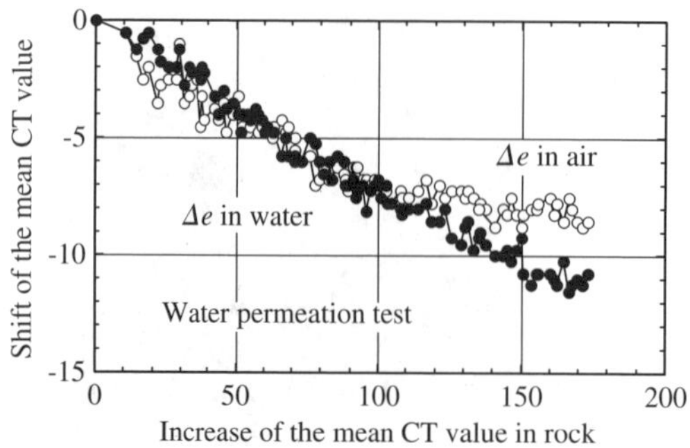

Figure 12. Change of mean CT value in the background.

The porosity is estimated to be 30%, as shown in Figure 13(c), by averaging the porosity along the x-axis. Comparing to $\phi_r = 21\%$ determined by the traditional saturation method, the discrepancy is significant. This indicates that the present estimation of porosity involves a huge error caused by the X-ray beam hardening. Then it can be concluded that the error of the present images subtraction analysis may increase with the advance of wetting front. Additionally it can be concluded that the overall evaluation of porosity using a fully saturated specimen has a great difficulty in the case that the porosity is greater than 0.21.

5 THEORETICAL CONSIDERATION ON THE ONE-DIMENSIONAL WATER PERMEATION

5.1 *Fundamentals*

One-dimensional wetting flow consists of two kinds of flow, a saturated wetting flow and an unsaturated one, as in Figure 14. The time-dependent total length L of the wetting flow region is given by

$$L = L_S + L_U, \tag{10}$$

where L_S is the length of the saturated wetting flow region and L_U is the unsaturated wetting flow region.

The saturated wetting flow is described from the law of conservation of water mass:

$$du_w / dx = -\,d\phi_w / dt, \tag{11}$$

and the Darcy law:

$$u_w = -\,k / \mu_w \cdot dp_w/dx, \tag{12}$$

where u_w is the flow rate of water, $d\phi_w/dt$ is the increase rate of the volumetric water content ϕ_w, p_w is the pore-water pressure, k is the coefficient of permeability, μ_w is the coefficient of viscosity of water (μ_w = 7.92 $\times 10^{-6}$Pas at 30°C), and dp_w/dx is the gradient

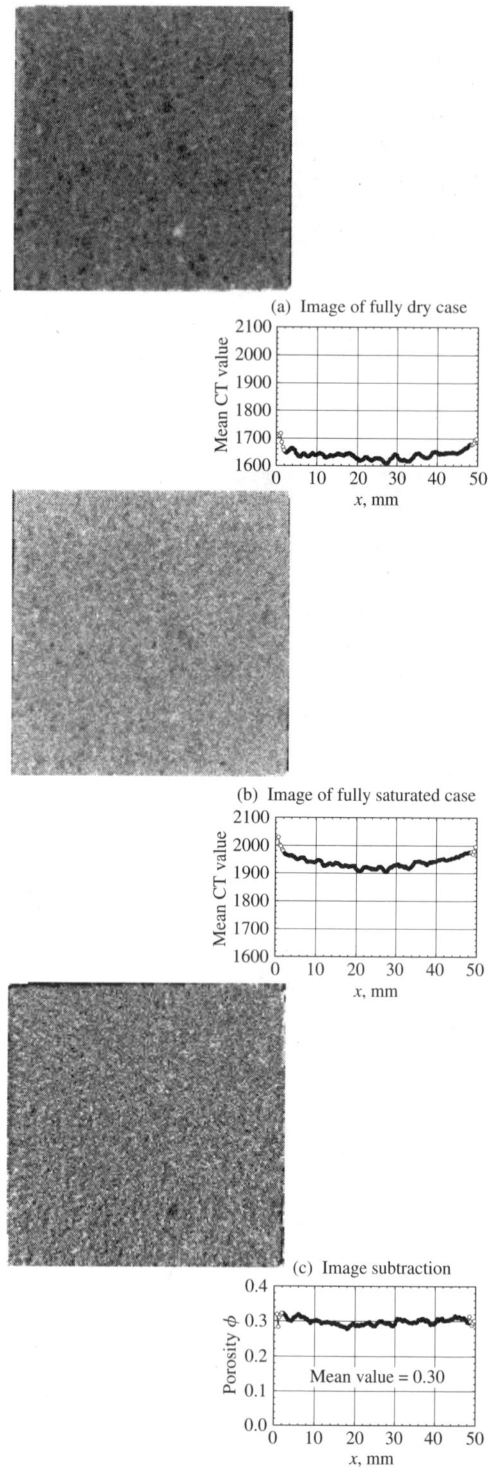

Figure 13. CT images subtraction to evaluate the porosity.

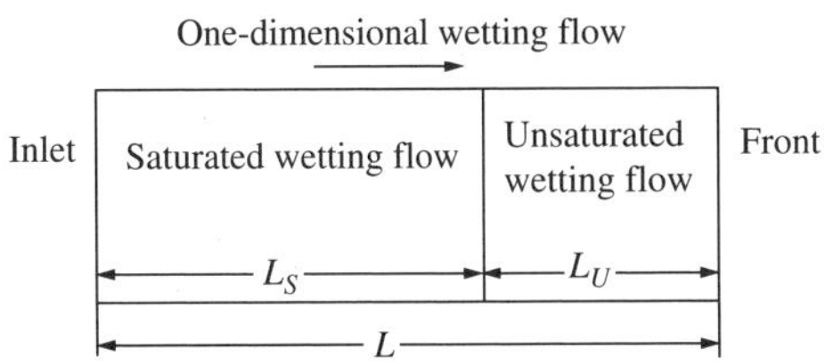

Figure 14. One-dimensional wetting flow.

of p_w referred to the horizontal co-ordinate x. In Equations (11) and (12) the flow rate of water u_w is an apparent one that is the volume of water permeated per a unit section per a unit time. The real flow rate u_{real} in pores is given by dividing u_w by the volumetric water content ϕ_w, as follows:

$$u_{real} = u_w/\phi_w. \tag{13}$$

In the unsaturated case, the flow is the two-phase flow of water-air mixture. The real flow rate of the mixture, represented by $u_{m\ real}$, is given as the sum of the real flow rate of air $u_{a\ real}$ and the real flow rate of water $u_{w\ real}$. This is written as follows:

$$u_{m\ real} = u_{a\ real} + u_{w\ real} \tag{14}$$

Considering the volumetric contents of air and water, the components are written as follows:

$$u_{a\ real} = \phi_a\ u_{m\ real}/\phi_m,\ u_{w\ real} = \phi_w\ u_{m\ real}/\phi_m, \tag{15}$$

where ϕ_a denotes the volumetric air content and ϕ_w is the volumetric water content, and ϕ_m is the sum of ϕ_a and ϕ_w. Since the later ϕ_m is equivalent of the porosity ϕ_r, we obtain

$$\phi_r = \phi_m = \phi_a + \phi_w. \tag{16}$$

In the same manner, the apparent flow rate of the mixture, represented by u_m, is defined as the sum of the apparent flow rate of air u_a and the apparent flow rate of water u_w. This is written as follows:

$$u_m = u_a + u_w. \tag{17}$$

If we use the real flow rate of $u_{m\ real}$, the components u_a and u_w are written as follows:

$$u_a = \phi_a\ u_{m\ real}, \quad u_w = \phi_w\ u_{m\ real}, \tag{18}$$

and $u_w = \phi_w\ u_{m\ real}$, (19)

then we obtain the following relations:

$$u_m/\ \phi_m = u_a/\ \phi_a = u_w/\ \phi_w = u_{m\ real}. \tag{20}$$

Equation (20) is available for the evaluation of $u_{m\ real}$ and u_a from u_w and ϕ_w. The apparent flow rate of water u_w will be obtained from the volumetric water content ϕ_w, basing upon the conservation law of water mass, as discussed in the following.

Considering the relations in Equation (20), the Darcy flow of the water-air mixture in the un-saturated wetting region is described as follows:

$$u_{m\ real} = -\ k/\mu_m \cdot dp_m/dx/\phi_m, \tag{21}$$

where μ_m is the coefficient of viscosity of water-air mixture, ϕ_m is the volumetric content of the mixture of equivalent to the porosity and dp_m/dx represents the gradient of pressure in the water-air mixture referred to the horizontal co-ordinate x.

The matric suction p_S, which is produced by the surface tension on the surface of air, is defined as the difference between the pore-air pressure and the pore-water pressure (Fredlund & Rahardjo 1993), as follows:

$$p_S = p_a - p_w, \tag{22}$$

where p_a is the pore-air pressure and p_w is the pore-water pressure. In general, the magnitude of the matric suction p_S in the unsaturated wetting flow region is considered to vary with the volumetric air content ϕ_a, since the dimensions of air changes with ϕ_a. However in order to simplify the equation, the uniformity for the matric suction is assumed in the unsaturated wetting region. By this simplification, the pressure gradient dp_m/dx in Equation (21) can be replaced with dp_w/dx.

In order to evaluate the coefficient of viscosity μ_m of water-air mixture in Equation (21), the following relation can be assumed.

$$\mu_m = (\mu_a\phi_a + \mu_w\phi_w)/\phi_m. \tag{23}$$

Thus the apparent flow rate of water u_w is expressed from Equations (20) and (21) as follows:

$$u_w = -\ k\ \phi_w/(\mu_a\phi_a + \mu_w\phi_w) \cdot dp_w/dx. \tag{24}$$

Therefore, when the contribution of air is negligibly small, Equation (24) is completely equivalent to Equation (12).

Basing upon the consideration mentioned above, Equations (11) and (12) were applied to the analysis of wetting process. The conservation of mass of water given by Equation (11) describes that the flow rate of water u_w can be determined from the volumetric water content ϕ_w obtained from the images subtraction analysis. Additionally the Darcy law given by Equation (12) describes that the pore-water pressure p_w is determined from the flow rate of water u_w. For the computation, Equations (11) and (12) will be rewritten in a time-independent form.

5.2 *Pore-water pressure in saturated flow*

Saturated wetting flow is defined by $d\phi_w/dt = 0$, and characterized by a constant flow rate, as shown in Figure 15. From the fact that the pores are fully saturated with water, the pressure at the front is equivalent to the atmospheric pressure p_{atm}. If the coefficient of permeability k is a constant, the pore-water pressure p_w is solved as follows:

$$p_w = p_o - (p_o - p_{atm}) \cdot (x/L_s), \tag{25}$$

where p_o is the inlet pressure and L_S is the length of the saturated wetting flow region.

In general, the coefficient of permeability k of porous rock can be expressed as a function of the effective confining pressure σ, as follows:

$$k = k_o \cdot (\sigma/\sigma_o)^{-m}. \tag{26}$$

where k_o represents the coefficient of permeability at $\sigma = \sigma_o$ and m is an index number. In the present water permeation test, the effective confining pressure is given by the difference between the hydrostatic pressure p_o and the pore-water pressure p_w, as $\sigma = p_o - p_w$.

In this case, the pore-water pressure p_w is given as follows:

$$p_w = p_o - (p_o - p_{atm}) \cdot (x/L_S)^{1/(1-m)}. \tag{27}$$

5.3 *Flow rate of water at the inlet*

For the saturated wetting flow, the flow rate u_w is given by

$$u_w = u_{IN} = u_{SF} = E/L_S, \tag{28}$$

where

$$E = k_o/\mu_w \cdot (\sigma_o)^m/(1-m) \cdot (p_o - p_{atm})^{(1-m)}. \tag{29}$$

It is noteworthy that the flow rate u_w is in inverse proportion to the length L_S.

Equation (29) is the basis for the evaluation of the coefficient of permeability k_o at $\sigma = \sigma_o$ and the index number m as a materials constant, as demonstrated in the following paragraph. The value of E will be concretely evaluated through the numerical analysis of the inlet flow rate u_{IN}. It will be given from the integration of the volumetric water content ϕ_w obtained by the CT-images subtraction.

5.4 *Length of wetting flow regions*

Unsaturated wetting flow having a length of L_U is produced by the matric suction p_S defined by Equation (22), as illustrated in Figure 16. This region is characterized by a negative pore-water pressure of $p_w, < p_{atm}$.

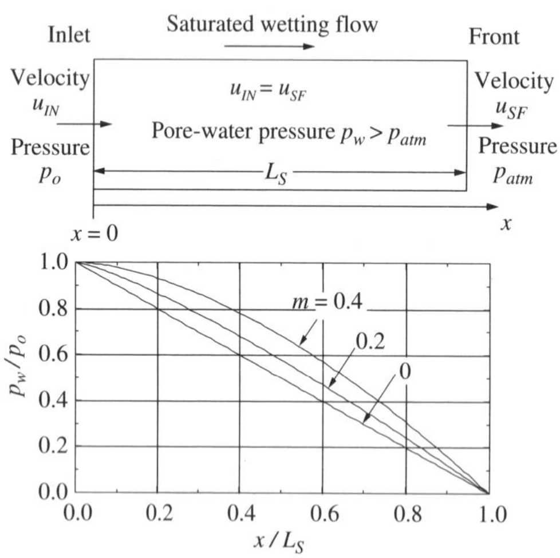

Figure 15. Positive pore-water pressure in the saturated wetting flow region.

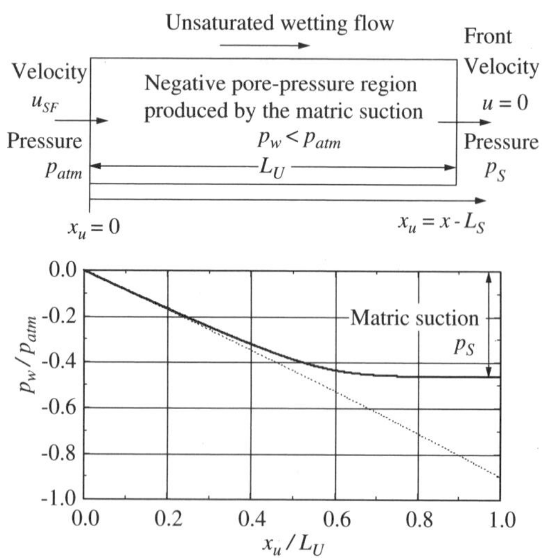

Figure 16. Negative pore-water pressure in the un-saturated wetting flow region.

In the case of $L_U = 0$, the advance of the front dL_S in an infinitesimal time of dt can be forecasted from the volume of the water permeated per a unit sectional area. In a differential equation form, it is expressed by

$$\phi_r\, dL_S = u_w\, dt \quad \text{when } L_U=0, \tag{30}$$

where ϕ_r is the porosity of rock. Substituting Equation (28) into (30), we obtain

$$L_S\, dL_S = E/\phi_r\, dt, \tag{31}$$

and the following relation by an integral.

$$L_S = C_S \cdot t^{0.5}, \tag{32}$$

where

$$C_S^2 = 2E/\phi_r \text{ when } L_U=0. \tag{33}$$

The value of the coefficient C_S can increase with the inlet pressure p_o.

By referring to Equation (32), the length of the unsaturated wetting flow region L_U is expressed by introducing the coefficient C_U, as follows:

$$L_U = C_U \cdot t^{0.5}. \tag{34}$$

Then the total length L is expressed as follows:

$$L = C \cdot t^{0.5}, \tag{35}$$

where

$$C = C_S + C_U. \tag{36}$$

5.5 *Flow rate of water at the inlet*

The volume of water permeated into rock specimen is equivalent to the product of the total length L and the mean volumetric water content of the wetting flow region. In the equation form, it is written as follows:

$$F = L\, \phi_{w\,mean}, \tag{37}$$

where F is the total volume of water permeated per a unit area and $\phi_{w\,mean}$ is the mean volumetric water content in the range of from x = 0 to $x = L$.

By differentiating F with respect to time t, the flow rate of water at the inlet $x = 0$ can be obtained as follows:

$$u_{IN} = dF/dt. \tag{38}$$

Then substituting Equation (37) into Equation (38), we obtain

$$u_{IN} = \phi_{w\,mean} \cdot C/2 \cdot t^{-0.5}. \tag{39}$$

Thus the fundamental formulation to evaluate the magnitude of the coefficient E in Equation (29) is written as follows:

$$2E = C_S\, C \cdot \phi_{w\,mean}. \tag{40}$$

5.6 *Normalization of the fundamental equations*

The fundamental equations (11) and (12) can be written in a time-independent form. For this purpose, the normalized flow rate of water U is introduced as follows:

$$U = u_w/u_{IN} \tag{41}$$

Moreover the normalized co-ordinate ξ as follows:

$$\xi = x/L. \tag{42}$$

Thus we obtain the time-independent fundamental equations as follows:

$$dU/d\xi = \xi/\phi_{w\,mean} \cdot d\phi_w/d\xi, \tag{43}$$

$$dp_w/d\xi = A \cdot (p_o - p_w)^m \cdot C/C_S \cdot U \tag{44}$$

where

$$A = (p_o - p_{atm})^{(1-m)}/(1-m). \tag{45}$$

The mean volumetric water content $\phi_{w\,mean}$ within the region L are required to compute the normalized flow rate U from the distribution of ϕ_w by Equation (43), and the index number m and the ratio of the coefficients C and C_S are required to evaluate the distribution of the pore-water pressure p_w by Equation (44). In the following paragraph, focusing on the evaluation of the coefficient of permeability k and the matric suction p_S, the necessary data processing will be discussed.

6 ANALYSIS OF THE WATER PERMEATION PROGRESS

6.1 *Characteristics of the distribution of volumetric water content*

The distributions of the volumetric water content ϕ_w along the X-axis are summarized in Figure 17, which are obtained from the CT images subtraction and stacking procedure. To make clear the characteristics of wetting process, an example is given in Figure 18. The profile of ϕ_w is composed of three regions, the plateau region of immediately neighboring the inlet,

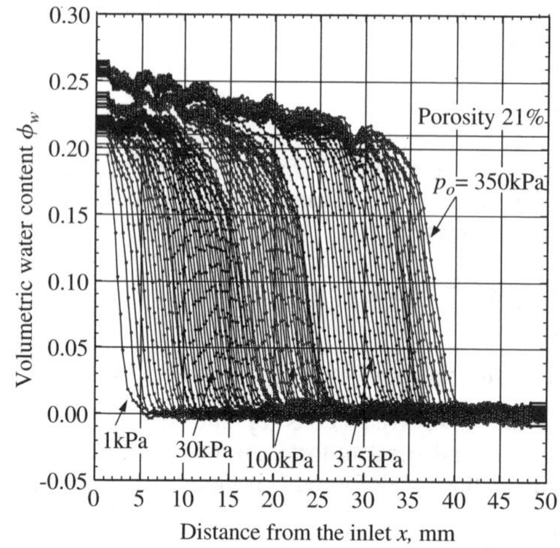

Figure 17. Time-dependent profiles of the volumetric water content.

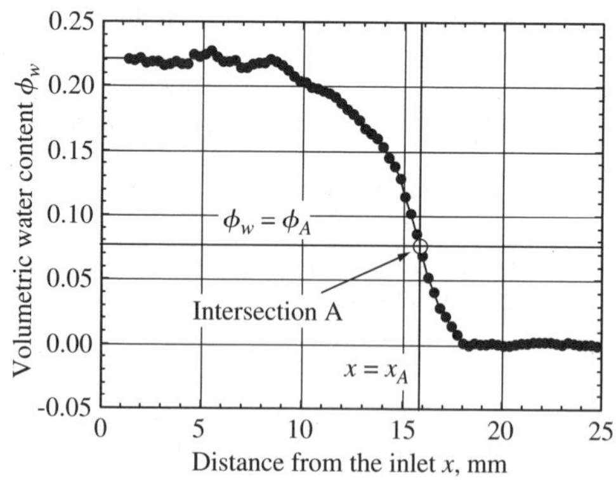

Figure 19. Definition of the intersection (x_A, ϕ_A) for the forward speed analysis.

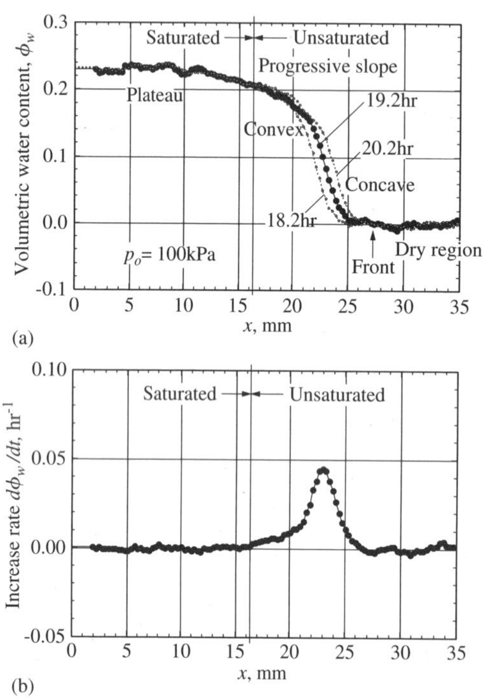

Figure 18. Characteristics of the water permeation process; (a) volumetric water content ϕ_w versus x; (b) increase rate of ϕ_w.

the progressive slope in front of the plateau region and the flat region corresponds to a dry area. The plateau corresponds to the saturated region, and the progressive slope to the unsaturated region.

At the inlet side, the volumetric water content ϕ_w increases with the inlet pressure p_o, exceeding the porosity 21%. This suggests the presence of the error. If there is no error, this means an unsaturation. In other words the compressive air remains in pores, and ϕ_w can increases with the compression of air in pores. However this interpretation is doubtful. It has to be emphasized that the data in the inlet side is very susceptible to the cupping effect.

The increase rate $d\phi_w/dt$ in the plateau region is smaller than that in the progressive slope region, as shown in Figure 18(b). This means that the water flow in the plateau region keeps approximately a constant flow rate dependent upon the inlet pressure p_o and the coefficient of permeability k.

The increase rate $d\phi_w/dt$ in the progressive slope region has a peak at a point near the center of the region. Additionally the value of ϕ_w becomes zero at the front of the region. These results state that the flow rate of water u_w decreases in the unsaturated wetting flow region with approaching to the front, and that it becomes zero at the front. Concerning to the shape of progressive slopes in Figures 17 and 18, it can be noted that the ϕ_w–x curves are similar with each other, and the rear half of each curve is of convex and the front half is concaved. This is one of significant characteristics of unsaturated wetting flows. It is not influenced very much by the inlet pressure p_o.

6.2 *Forward speed of water permeation*

In order to evaluate the time-dependent lengths of L, L_S and L_U, the forward speed of the progressive slope was examined. For this purpose, the x co-ordinate of a point of $\phi_w = \phi_A$ is investigated on the curve of $\phi_w - x$, as illustrated in Figure 19.

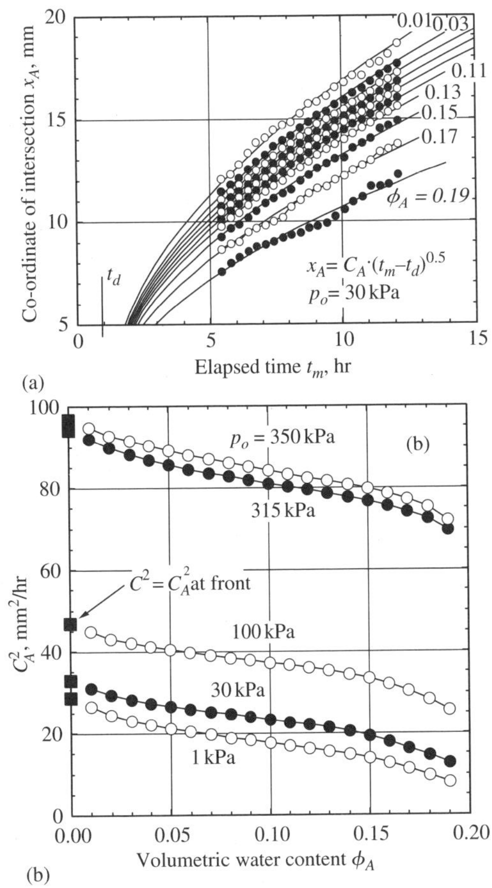

Figure 20. Analysis of the forward speed.

The intersection (x_A, ϕ_A) moves on a line of $\phi_w = \phi_A$, and the co-ordinate x_A was expressed as

$$x_A = C_A \cdot t^{0.5}, \tag{46}$$

where C_A is a coefficient of depending upon the value of ϕ_A, and t is the equivalent elapsed time. The time t can be expressed as follows:

$$t = t_m - t_d, \tag{47}$$

where t_m is the elapsed time measured from the commencement of the water permeation test, and t_d represents a time correction for each pressure stage.

As illustrated in Figure 20(a), the evaluation of C_A was carried out in a range of from $\phi_A = 0.01$ to $\phi_A = 0.19$ with an interval of 0.01, excluding the data of in an hour from the beginning of each pressure stage. Since the coefficient C_A is dependent upon the volumetric water content ϕ_A, it is plotted as a function of ϕ_A, as in Figure 20(b). The curves of C_A^2 with similar form and different levels are obtained. Therefore it is clear that C_{AI}^2 consists of two parts, and it can be expressed as follows:

$$C_A^2 = C_{AI}^2 + C_{AII}^2. \tag{48}$$

The first term C_{AI}^2 represents the unsaturated part, depending upon the value of ϕ_A. This corresponds to the unsaturated wetting flow region of negative pore-water pressure. The second term C_{AII}^2 is the saturated part of depending upon the inlet pressure p_o. This corresponds to the saturated wetting flow region of positive pore-water pressure.

The value of C in Equation (35) can be defined as the value of C_A at $\phi_A = 0$. Figure 20(b) shows an example of extrapolation to determine the value of C. However, it has to be pointed out that a precise determination of C involves great difficulties, since the fluctuation of ϕ_w makes the front to be unclear. In the following analysis, the value of L was given by Equation (35), using the value of C indicated by the black square in Figure 20(b).

The coefficient C_S in Equation (32) corresponds to the coefficient C_{AII} in Equation (48). The value of C_S becomes zero at $p_o = p_{atm}$, then the precise evaluation of C_S is difficult in the case of $p_o = 1$ kPa. Therefore by shifting the curves of $C_A^2 - \phi_A$ as shown in Figure 21(a), the value of C_{AI}^2 was firstly computed from the data of $p_o = 30$ kPa~350 kPa. The value of C_{AI} at the front was assumed to be a constant, represented by C_D. Subsequently the values of C_S^2 are determined as the subtraction of C_D^2 from C^2. The results obtained are as indicated in Figure 21(b), and the value of C_S at $p_o = 1$ kPa was computed by the extrapolation.

Based upon the theoretical considerations in 5 and the characteristics of the forward speed of the progressive slope mentioned above, the relation between the coefficients C and C_S was expressed as follows:

$$C^2 = C_S^2 + C_D^2. \tag{49}$$

Moreover the coefficient C_U in Equation (34) was computed by

$$C_U = C - C_S. \tag{50}$$

The coefficients C, C_S, C_U and C_D evaluated are summarized in Figure 22. The pressure dependency of the coefficients will be discussed through the evaluation of the coefficient of permeability of rock based on Equation (29), and from the simulation of the flow rate of water and the pore-water pressure based on Equations (43) and (44).

6.3 *Volume of water permeated*

The flow rate of water u_{IN} at the inlet $x = 0$ is obtained by differentiating the volume of water F, permeated

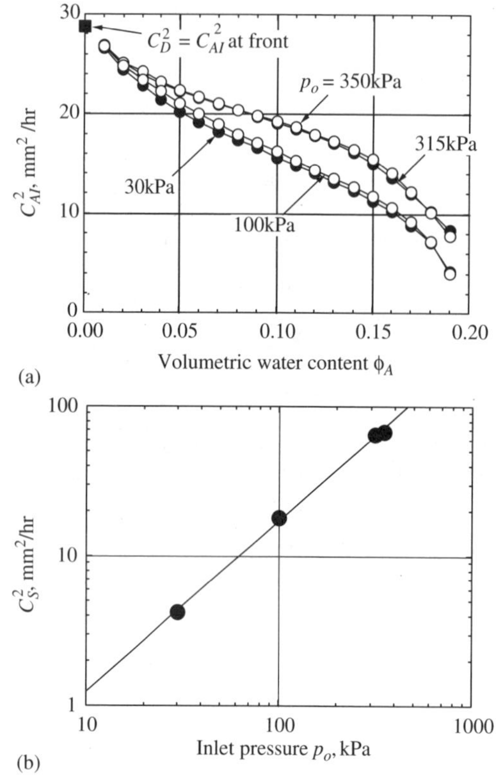

Figure 21. Evaluation of the coefficients C_D and C_S.

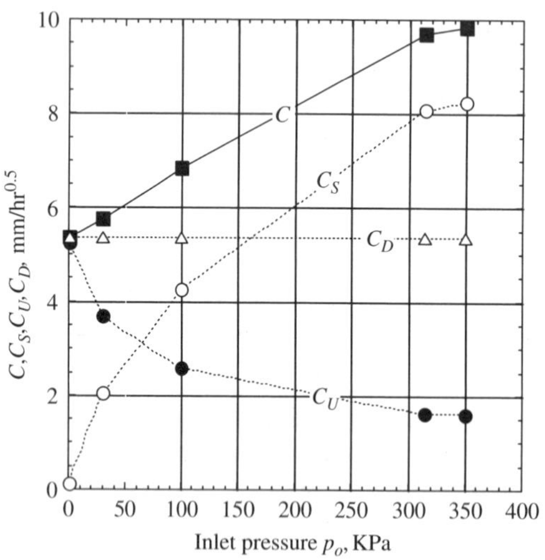

Figure 22. The coefficients C, C_S, C_U and C_D versus the inlet pressure p_o.

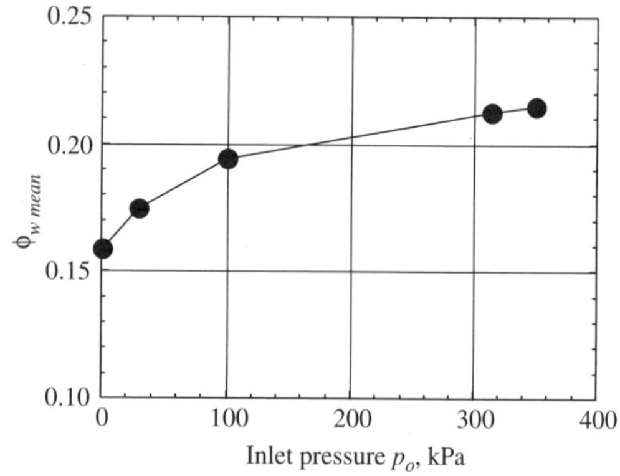

Figure 23. The mean value of the volumetric water content $\phi_{w\,mean}$ in the wetting region of length L, depending upon the inlet pressure p_o.

into the specimen through a unit section, with respect to t. Additionally the volume of water F is given as the product of the length L and the mean of the volumetric water content $\phi_{w\,mean}$ of the wetting region. Here, the mean value $\phi_{w\,mean}$ is depending upon the inlet pressure p_o as shown in Figure 23. It may converge to the porosity of rock with increasing the inlet pressure.

6.4 *Normalized profile of volumetric water content*

Normalized profiles of the volumetric water content ϕ_w are summarized in Figure 24, as a function of the dimensionless co-ordinate $\xi = x/L$. In the figure, small painted circles represent the data of after an hour from the beginning of each pressure stage, and smooth curves are the moving averages respectively. The moving average of time-independent form is available for the computation of the flow rate by Equation (43), and subsequently for the computation of the pore-pressure by Equation (44).

The white circle in the figure represents the point of $\xi = L_S/L = C_S/C$, which is computed with the values of C_S and C in Figure 22. This is the boundary between the saturated wetting flow region and the unsaturated wetting flow region. Then the pore-water pressure p_w is expected to be equivalent to the atmospheric pressure p_{atm}.

As discuss in the following paragraph, when the pore-water pressure is computed by substituting the ratio of $L_S/L = C_S/C$ into Equation (44), it can be expected that the absolute value of the pore-water pressure converges to the matric suction at the front $\xi = 1$. In order to satisfy this requirement, the value of C_S is improved step-by-step. The line near the white circle, in Figure 24, represents the improved solution of the boundary. It can be pointed out that the correction

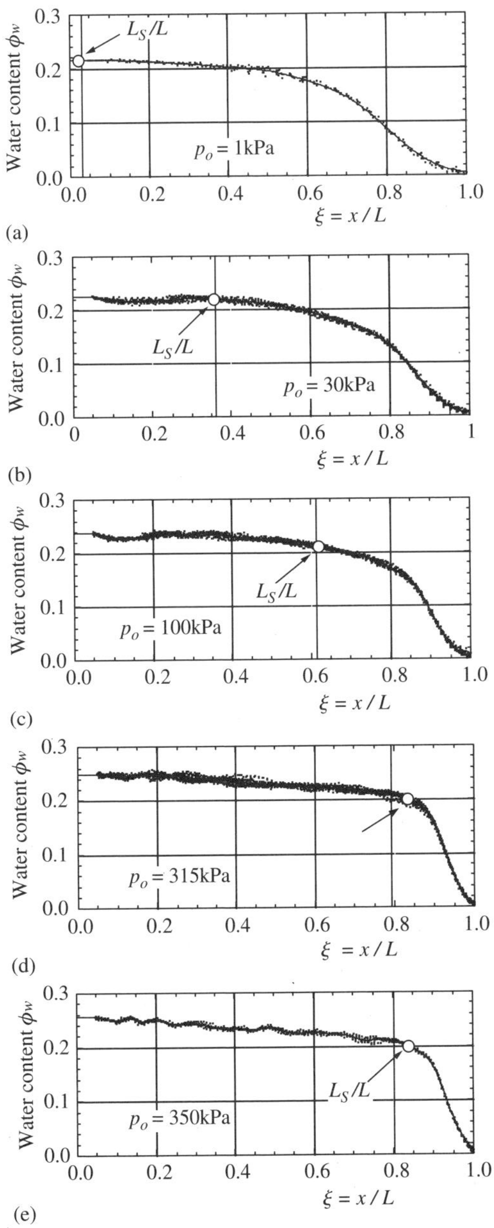

Figure 24. Time-independent expression of volumetric water content ϕ_w.

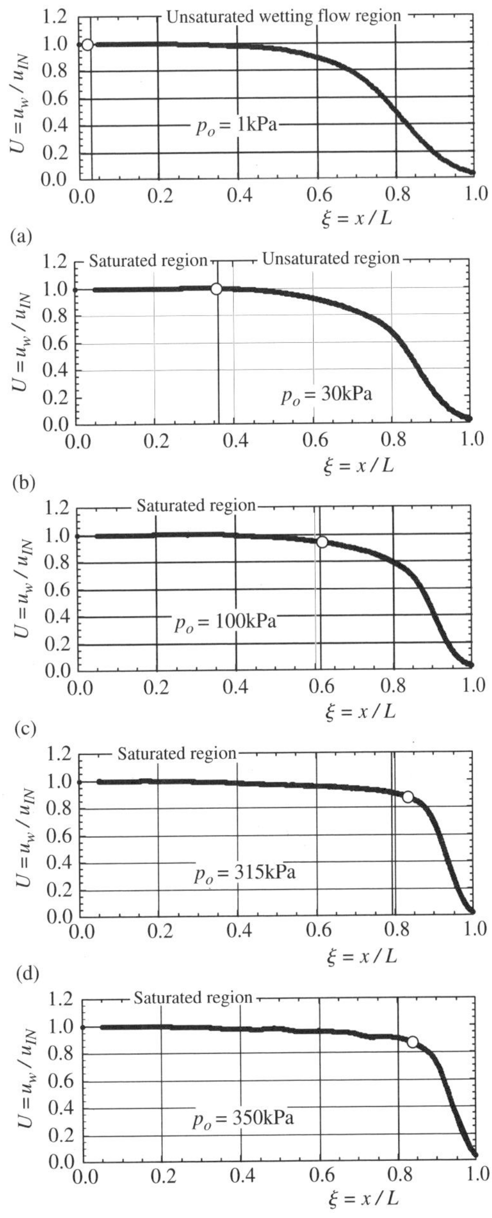

Figure 25. Normalized flow rate of water calculated by Equation (43).

is required about the values of C_S at $p_o = 315$ kPa and 350 kPa.

6.5 *Normalized flow rate of water*

The normalize flow rate U of water was numerically determined by Equation (44), and illustrated in Figure 25. The computation was conducted by assuming that the value of U is unity at $\xi = 0$. And the mean values $\phi_{w\,mean}$ in Figure 22 were used as well as the moving average of ϕ_w in Figure 23.

In the case of $p_o = 30$ kPa, the value of U is unity in the saturated wetting flow region. Additionally in the unsaturated wetting flow region, the value of

U decreases with increasing the distance from the inlet, and finally becomes nearly zero at the front $\xi = 1$. This rational result indicates the reliability of the CT images data. However in the case of $p_o = 100$ kPa, the value of U at the boundary is slightly smaller than unity. Similar decreases of U in the saturated wetting flow region are also observed in the cases of $p_o = 315$ kPa and 350 kPa. These irrationalities are associated with the error in the volumetric water content in the inlet side due to the cupping effect.

Comparing Figure 25 to Figure 24, it is clear that the distribution of U is similar to that of ϕ_w, respectively. But there is a clear difference. As discussed in 5, it is caused by the air flow in the unsaturated flow region.

Since the normalized real flow rate $U_{m\ real}$ is given by U/ϕ_w, as described in Equation (20), the analysis of the normalized flow rate of water can be followed by the analysis of the two-phase flow of water-air mixture. In particular it may provide the valuable information to investigate the flow of air in the unsaturated wetting flow region, and to analyze the matric suction mechanism. Such an advanced analysis of the two-phase flow of water-air mixture in the unsaturated wetting flow region will be reported in near future by the authors, using the data in Figures 24 and 25. In particular, it will be conducted with a reliable data in the cases of $p_o = 1$ kPa~100 kPa.

7 EVALUATION OF PERMEABILITY OF ROCK

7.1 *Observation equations*

Estimation of the permeability is upon Equations (21) and (32). By substituting Equation (40) into Equation (29), the observation equation is given in a time-independent form, as follows:

$$A \cdot (p_o - p_{atm})^{(1-m)} = E, \tag{51}$$

Where

$$A = k_o/\mu \cdot (\sigma_o)^m/(1-m), \tag{52}$$

$$E = \phi_{w\ mean} \cdot C_S C/2. \tag{53}$$

The observation equations obtained from the multi-stage pressurization experiment are solved as a simultaneous equation by the mean square method, to evaluate the coefficient of permeability k_o, and the index number m, assigning a specified value to σ_o.

For this purpose the logarithms of Equation (51) is taken, as follows:

$$\log A + (1-m) \cdot \log(p_o - p_{atm}) = \log(E). \tag{54}$$

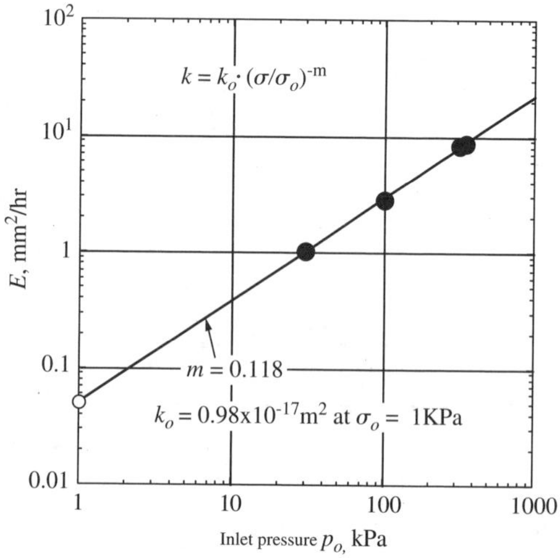

Figure 26. Preliminary estimation of the permeability of Kimachi sandstone.

Namely, by the linear relation between $\log(E)$ and $\log(p_o - p_{atm})$, the unknown parameters k_o and m are determined.

7.2 *Preliminary evaluation of permeability*

A case example of the permeability determination is presented in Figure 26. This is a preliminary one, using the data in Figures 22 and 23. Here the data at $p_o = 1$ kPa were excluded, since the precise value of C_S was unknown at this stage.

The measurement represented by painted circles well agrees with a line of Equation (52), then it can be concluded that Equation (26) is hold in porous rock. The value of E at $p_o = 1$ kPa was evaluated as $E = 0.050$ mm^2/hr by the extrapolation, then $C_S = 0.119$ mm/hr$^{0.5}$ and $C_S/C = 0.022$.

The most suitable value of the coefficient of permeability k_o was evaluated as $k_o = 0.98 \times 10^{-17}$ m^2 at $\sigma_o = 1$ kPa and the index number m as 0.118. The rationality of the results can be examined by the subsequent analysis of the pore-water pressure.

7.3 *Computation of pore-water pressure*

The computation of the pore-water pressure p_w is numerically carried out, basing on Equation (44). Equation (44) states that the distribution of the pore-water pressure p_w is only dependent upon the value of C_S/C, in the case the index number of m and the normalized flow rate U are known. Moreover it is theoretically expected that the absolute value of the pore-water pressure converges to the matric suction p_S at the front $\xi = 1$. The maric suction p_S is a kind of

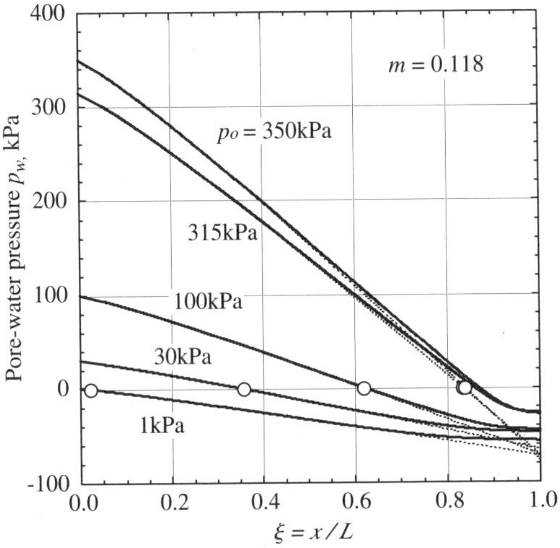

Figure 27. Preliminary computation of the pore-water pressure by Equation (44), using the normalized flow rate in Figure 25.

materials constant, being independent upon the inlet pressure p_o. Therefore the pore-water pressure p_w at $\xi = 1$, calculated by Equation (44), is considered to be available for the improvement of the ratio C_S/C.

The pore-water pressure evaluated by Equation (44) is shown in Figure 27, with solid curves. In this computation, the relation of $p_w = p_o$ was assumed at the front $\xi = 0$, and the normalized flow rate U in Figure 25 was used with the value of $m = 0.118$. White circles in the figure represent the atmospheric pressure points of $\xi = C_S$/C, which are the boundaries between the saturated wetting flow region and the unsaturated wetting flow region. Broken curves indicate the pore-water pressure obtained by Equation (27), passing through the boundary of the atmospheric pressure respectively. In Figure 27, the pore-water pressures at the front $\xi = 1$ vary in a range of from -26 kPa to -72 kPa. This result shows that the preliminary analysis is not reliable. Then some correction is required about the value of C_S/C.

However the correction of the ratio *Cs/C* results in the change of the magnitudes of E and m. Then the iterative procedure is required to obtain a more rational evaluation. The iteration consists of the permeability analysis and the computation of pore-water pressure.

7.4 *Improvement of solution*

The step-by-step improvement of the coefficient of permeability and the matric suction was taken placed, as shown in Figure 28. In the present procedure the distributions of the normalized flow rate U in Figure 25 were used along with the values of C in Figure 22.

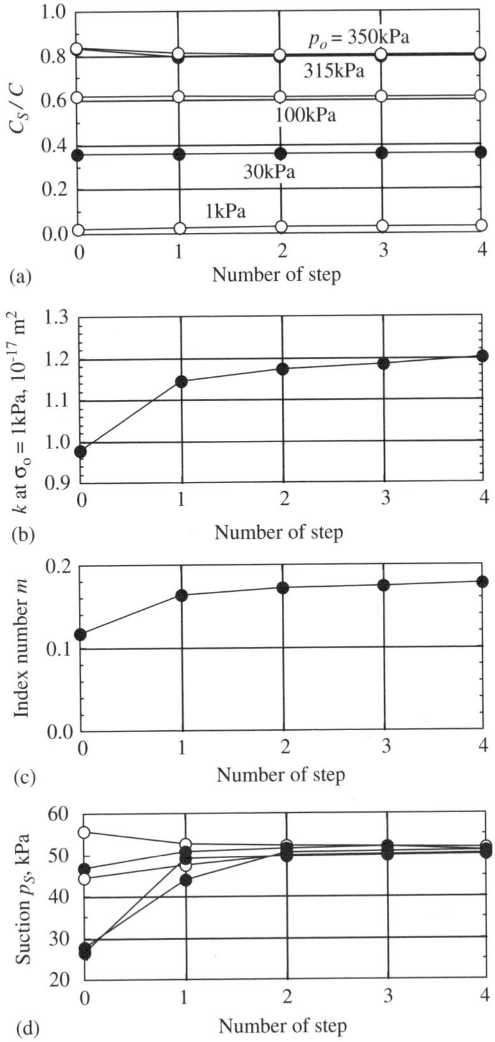

Figure 28. Iterative determination of the coefficient of permeability and the matric suction by the improvement of variables m and C_S/C.

Namely, these data were held in the iteration, and the value of m and the ratio C_S/C were assumed to be variables.

As indicated in Figure 28, the convergence was obtained by the iteration of four steps. The most suitable values of Kimachi sandstone are determined as follows: the coefficient of permeability $k = 1.20 \times 10^{-17}\,\mathrm{m}^2$ at the effective confining pressure $\sigma = 1$ kPa, the index number $m = 0.178$ and the matric suction $p_S = 51$ kPa.

Comparing the solution to the preliminary one, it can be noted that the magnitudes of k, m and p_S changes

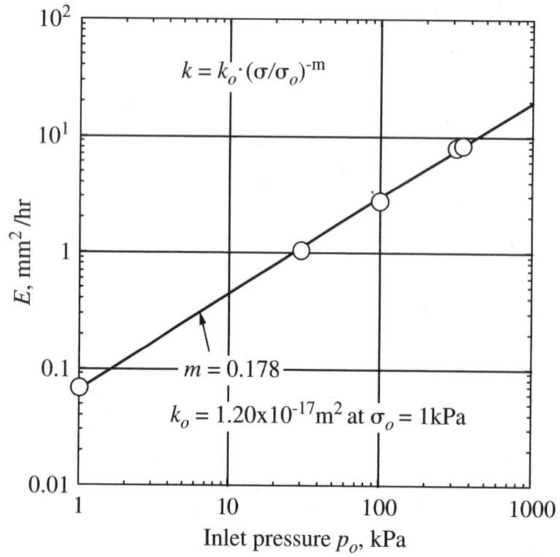

Figure 29. Solution of permeability, Kimachi sandstone.

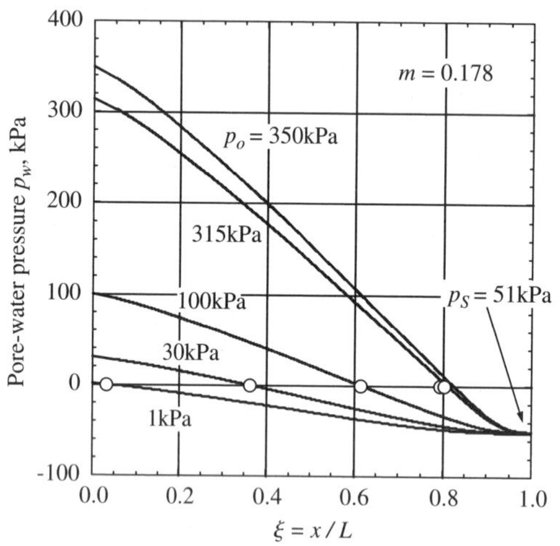

Figure 30. Solution of the pore-water pressure p_w, Kimachi sandstone.

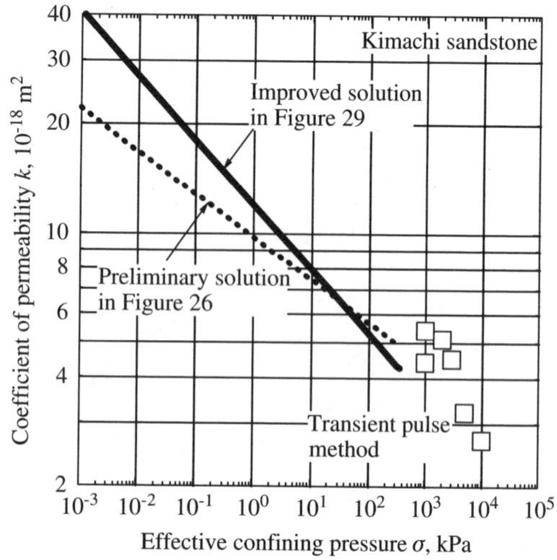

Figure 31. Effective confining dependency of the coefficient of permeability, Kimachi sandstone.

sensitively in response to the given ratio C_S/C. This suggests that the present procedure is essential for the evaluation of the coefficient of permeability and the matric suction by means of the CT images subtraction technique.

The solution of the coefficient of permeability is shown in Figure 29, and the distribution of the pore-water pressure p_w is given in Figure 30. From the curve fitting in Figure 29, it can be reconfirmed that Equation (52) well agrees with the measurement, and that Equation (26) is acceptable to describe the effective confining pressure dependency of the permeability of porous rock.

Figure 30 shows that the pore-water pressure p_w converges to the matric suction $p_S = 51$ kPa at the front $\xi = 1$. The pressure curves of $p_o = 1$ kPa~100 kPa pass through the atmospheric pressure state at the boundary between the saturated wetting flow region and the unsaturated wetting flow region indicated by white circles in the figure. However in the cases of $p_o = 315$ kPa and 350 kPa, the disagreement in the location is clearly observed. Then it was concluded that the data of $p_o = 1$ kPa~100 kPa are more reliable and rational than those of $p_o = 315$ kPa~350 kPa.

The pore-water pressure computation based on Equation (44) is considered to be essential, in particular, to evaluate the two-phase flow of water–air mixture in the unsaturated wetting flow region. It can be concluded that the subtraction of CT images and subsequent data processing can provide the fundamental information for the unsaturated wetting flow within porous rock.

7.5 *Comparison with the transient pulse method*

In order to clarify the effective confining pressure dependency of the permeability, the improved solution was compared to the measurement by the transient pulse method (Brace et al. 1968, Takahashi et al. 1998), as shown in Figure 31. The preliminary solution is given for reference.

The results obtained by the two methods are compatible with each other, though there is a clear difference in the range of the effective confining pressure σ. The transient pulse data are in a higher range of σ, and clearly indicate that the permeability k decreases with increasing the value of σ. The decreasing rate is considered to be similar, though the transient pulse data vary widely. From the comparison in Figure 31, it can be concluded that the subtraction of CT images is available for the quantitative evaluation of the permeability of porous rock. In particular it can be emphasized that the present procedure to determine the permeability and the matric suction at once is promising in a pressure range of much smaller than the traditional method, such as the transient pulse method.

8 CONCLUDING REMARKS

Wetting process of Kimachi sandstone of porosity 21% and dry density 2.54 g/cm^3 was studied by a one-dimensional water permeation experiment with the multi-stage pressurization in a range of from 1 kPa to 350 kPa. The X-ray CT was successfully applied, and the subtraction of X-ray CT images was proposed as a promising tool presently available for the visualization of the wetting process and for the quantitative evaluation of the volumetric water content at each point within rock specimen. Moreover a new scheme was proposed to formulate the distributions of the volumetric water content, the flow rate of water and the pore-water pressure, along with the iterative scheme to evaluate the coefficient of permeability and the matric suction. The proposal was supported by case examples.

Principle of the X-ray CT method has been briefly described in the present paper, along with the functions of the X-ray CT scanner employed. The requirement for a precise images subtraction was discussed to avoid from the error due to the X-ray beam hardening and the cupping effect. Additionally in order to assess the reliability of the images subtraction, the error estimation using CT values in the background regions was proposed.

Special apparatus was presented for a one-dimensional water permeation experiment with the multi-stage pressurization, to avoid from the X-ray attenuation. The apparatus was firstly applied to the hydrostatical compression test to investigate the influence of compression of rock and background water, and subsequently to the water permeation test to evaluate the influence of the effective confining pressure and the matric suction upon the wetting process.

Significant characteristics of the one-dimensional water permeation were clarified by the X-ray CT data processing. The flow rate of water at the inlet was clarified to be in inverse proportion to the square root of the elapsed time. In the same manner the forward speed of wetting front is in inverse proportion to the square root of the elapsed time, and the distance of the wetting front from the inlet increases proportionally with the square root of the elapsed time. Moreover within the wetting region, which consists of the saturated wetting flow region and the unsaturated wetting flow region in front, the pore-water pressure at the boundary between the two regions is equivalent to the atmospheric pressure, and the absolute value of the pore-water pressure at the wetting front is equivalent to the matric suction. Basing on these characteristics, the distribution of the volumetric water content was summarized as a function of the dimensionless co-ordinate.

The characteristics of water flow rate were clarified by the numerical analysis based upon the conservation law of mass, using the distribution of the volumetric water content measured by the CT images subtraction. Additionally the characteristics of the pore-water pressure were concretely evaluated, basing upon the Darcy law applicable to both of the saturated and unsaturated wetting flow regions.

Iterative scheme to evaluate the coefficient of permeability and the magnitude of the matric suction simultaneously has been presented as a practical usage of the X-ray CT. Presenting a successful case example, the significance of the effective confining pressure in determining the permeability of rock was discussed, as well as the important role of the matric suction in the unsaturated wetting flow. Moreover the coefficient of permeability of porous rock was confirmed to decrease with increasing the effective confining pressure in a wide range, by comparing the results obtained to the transient pulse data.

It can be concluded that the subtraction of CT images and subsequent data processing provide the essential data for the analysis of wetting process within porous rock. It can be announced that the data presented by this study is utilized to analyze the two-phase flow of water-air mixture in rock, near future. Additionally, it can be noted that the X-ray CT is also applicable to the investigation of a drying process of rock.

REFERENCES

Arthur, J.R.E. 1971. New techniques to measure new parameters, Proc. of Roscoe Material Symp. on stress-strain behaviour of soils, G.T. Foulis, Cambridge, pp. 340–346.

Brace, W.F., Walsh, J.B. and Frangos, W.T. 1968. Permeability of granite under high pressure, *J. Geophys.*, Res. 73, pp. 2225–2236.

Coles, M. E., Muegge, E.L. and Sprunt, E.S. 1991. Application of CAT scanning for oil and gas production research, *IEEE Trans. Nucl. Sci.*, 38: 510–515.

Cromwell, V., Kortum, D.J. and Bradley, D.J. 1984. The use of a medical computer tomography system to observe multiphase flow in porous media, Sci. of Petroleum Eng., Paper No. 13098, Richardson, Tx, USA.

Desrues, J., Chambon, R., Mokni, M. and F. Mazerolle F. 1996. Void ratio evolution inside shear bands in triaxial sand specimens studied by computed tomography, Geotechnique, 46, 3, 529–546.

Fetter C.W. 1993. Contaminant Hydrogeology, Prentice-Hall, Inc.

Fredlund, D.G. and Rahardjo, H. 1993. Soil mechanics for unsaturated soils. John Wiley & Sons, Inc., New York, pp. 64–106 and pp. 150–177.

Hounsfield, G.N. 1972. A method of and apparatus for examination of a body by radiation such as X- or Gamma-Radiation: London, British Patent No. 1283915.

International Society of Rock Mechanics. 1979. Suggested methods for determining water content, porosity, density, absorption and related properties and swelling and slake durability index properties, *Int. J. Rock Mech. & Min. Sci.*, 16, 141–156.

Kak, A.C. and Slaney, M. 1988. Principles of Computerized Tomographic Imaging, IEEE Press 1988, New York, USA.

Otani, J., Mukunoki, T. and Obara, Y. 2002. Characterization of failure in sand under triaxial compression using industrial X-ray CT scanner, *International Journal of Physical Modeling in Geotechnics.,* 2, 15–22.

Sato, A., Kubota, S., Kawaguchi, T., Ezoe, K. and Sugawara, K., 2002. Evaluation of permeability in rock by means of X-ray CT, Proc. of ISRM Regional Symposium – 3rd Korea-Japan Joint Symposium, Seoul, Korea, pp. 327–334.

Stephansson, O. The importance of rock stress measurement and its interpretation for rock disposal of hazardous waste. Rock Stress, eds by K. Sugawara & Y. Obara, A.A. Balkema, Rotterdam, pp. 3–13 1997.

Sugawara, K., Obara, Y., Kaneko, K., Koike, K., Ohmi, M. and Aoi, T. 1997. Visualization of three-dimensional structure of rocks using X-ray CT method, Proc. of 1st ARMS, Seoul, Korea, Vol. 2, pp. 769–774.

Sugawara, K., Obara, Y., Aoi, T. and Kojima, R. 1998a. Visualization of water permeation within rock using the X-ray CT. Proc. of 10th Jpn. Symp. on Rock Mech., pp. 341–346.

Sugawara, K., Kojima, R., Obara, Y. Sato, A. and Shimada, H. 1998b. Crack opening analysis by means of the X-ray CT. J. MMIJ, 114(12), 881–887. (in Japanese).

Sugawara, K., Reid, T.R., Yanagisaki, M. and Kawaguchi, T. 1998c. Measuring the coefficient of permeability of rock by X-ray computed tomography, Memorial Report 1998-5 of Rock Mechanics Laboratory, Graduate School of Science & Technology, Kumamoto University.

Sugawara, K., Sato, A., Obara, Y. and Yanagisako, M. 1999a. Measurement of permeability of rock by means of X-ray CT. J. MMIJ, 115(11), 803–808. (in Japanese).

Sugawara, K., Obara, Y. and Sato A. 1999b. Visualization of water saturation process in rock by X-rays CT, '99 Japan-Korea Joint Symposium on Rock Eng., Fukuoka, Japan, pp. 503–508.

Sugawara, K., Sato, A. and Obara, Y. 1999c. Crack opening analysis using X-rays CT data, Proc. of 9th Int. Congress on Rock Mechanics, ISRM, Paris, France, pp.1019–1022.

Takagi, M. and Shimoda, H. 1991. Handbook of Image Analysis. Tokyo University Publication.

Takahashi, M., Zhang, M., Lin W., Nishiyama, S. and Li, X. 1998. Hydraulic head, hydraulic gradient and storage coefficient within specimen during laboratory permeability tests, J. MMIJ, 114(12), 888–894. (in Japanese).

Tillard-Ngan, D., Desrues, J., Raynaud, S. and Mazerolle, F. 1992. Strain localization in the Beaucarire marl, Geotechnical engineering of hard soils-soft rocks, Balkema, pp. 1679–1686.

Verhelst, F., Vervoort, A., de Bosscher, P.H. and Marchal, G. 1995. X-ray computerized tomography, Determination of heterogeneities in rock sample, Proc. of 8th ISRM Cong., Tokyo, Japan, Vol. 1, pp. 105–108.

Vinegard, H.J., de Waal, J.A. and Wellington, SL. 1991. CT studies of brittle failure in Castlegate sandstone, *Int. J. Rock Mech. Min. Sci. & Geomech. Abstr.,* 28, 5, 441–448.

X-ray CT for Geomaterials; Soils, Concrete, Rocks – Otani & Obara (eds.)
© 2004 Swets & Zeitlinger. Lisse, ISBN 90 5809 666 1

Analysis of water flow in rock by a Tracer-aided X-ray CT

K. Sugawara, D. Fukahori, T. Iwatani & S. Kubota
Graduate School of Science and Technology, Kumamoto University, Japan

ABSTRACT: A new scheme named the Tracer Density Time-Integration Method (TDTIM) is proposed to evaluate the ununiformity of a steady water flow in rock by means of the X-ray CT. Transport diffusion phenomenon of a tracer is analyzed to determine the distribution of flow rate. Tracer mainly composed of potassium iodide is utilized, preparing the viscosity of water-tracer mixture to be equivalent to pure water in a wide range of the tracer density. The CT images subtraction technique is applied to evaluate the tracer density at points within a rock specimen. Subsequent time-integration of the tracer density provides the simultaneous linear equation for the pore-water pressure, and the flow rate of water is determined, basing upon the Darcy law. Case examples clarify that the present method is a promising tool available for evaluating the fluctuation of water flow deeply influenced by heterogeneities in rock.

1 INTRODUCTION

Mass transport phenomena in geo-materials, such as a diffusion of pollutant in soil and rock and a transport diffusion borne by water current, are of importance for the environmental geo-science and technology. In particular the evaluation of the water flow in rock strata and the transport diffusion phenomenon with water flow are significant for the design and construction of radioactive repositories in future, since the outflow of radioactive nuclear matter if it occurs deeply associates with water flow in rock, which is expected to play an important role as a natural barrier. In the present paper, focusing on the visualization of a steady water flow in saturated porous rock by means of the X-ray CT, a new scheme named the Tracer Density Time-Integration Method (TDTIM) is proposed.

X-ray CT is one of effective tools available for investigating the mass transfer phenomena in rock (Sugawara et al. 1997). This is well known as a non-destructive medical imaging technique, which makes it possible to evaluate the attenuation of X-ray at each point within a body, by digitizing shadow pictures taken from various directions and subsequent image reconstruction (Hounsfield 1972, Kak & Slaney 1988). The CT images subtraction technique (Sugawara et al. 1998a, 1999) is applied, in the present study, for the quantitative evaluation of the density of a tracer, which is injected to visualize the steady water flow.

The TDTIM is upon the analysis of the transport diffusion of a tracer with steady water flows in rock. The tracer composed of the potassium iodide (KI) is utilized, preparing the viscosity of a water-tracer mixture to be equivalent to pure water in a wide range of the tracer density. Theory and practice of the method are presented and discussed, including a necessary experimental procedure and subsequent data processing. The X-ray scanning with a specified time interval is conducted to evaluate the time-dependent tracer density at each point within the rock specimen, and the numerical integration of the tracer density with respect to time is performed to complete the simultaneous linear equation for the pore-water pressure, basing upon the conservation law of mass. Solving it the distribution of the pore-water pressure is determined, and the flow rate of water at a given point is evaluated from the differentiation of pore-water pressure, based on the Darcy law. Case study makes clear that the present method is a promising tool available for evaluating the two-dimensional field of the steady water flow deeply influenced by heterogeneities in rock.

2 THEORY OF THE TDTIM

The TDTIM is a scheme to evaluate the distribution of flow rate in a steady state within a porous rock fully saturated with a water-tracer mixture. This is upon the measurement of the variation of the tracer density with the transport diffusion. If the viscosity of the water-tracer mixture is independent upon the tracer density, both of the pore-water pressure and the flow rate of water are steady. This is the basis of the TDTIM.

The X-ray CT can provide the image of the CT value proportional to the radiographic density, and it is utilized to evaluate the tracer density at points in the rock specimen. The evaluation is based upon the direct proportion between the tracer density and the subtraction of the CT values. Then the CT images subtraction is an essential procedure of the TDTIM, along with the data processing for time integration. In this paragraph, it is described how the distribution of flow rate is determined, basing on the Darcy law and the conservation law of mass.

A boxel with dimensions of $2\Delta x$, $2\Delta y$ and Δz is considered, but the steady flow is assumed to be two-dimensional. Location of the boxel is expressed as (i, j) by the number of boxel, as shown in Figure 1, and also as (x_o, y_o) by the x-y co-ordinates of the center. Four boxels of $(i-1, j)$, $(i+1, j)$, $(i, j-1)$ and $(i, j+1)$, immediately neighboring the boxel (i, j), are taken into consideration.

The CT value of the boxel (i, j) is represented by $CT(i, j, t)$, as a function of location (i, j) and time t. The subtraction $\Delta CT(i, j, t)$ between the CT image at a given time t and the standard image of $t = 0$ can be defined as follows:

$$\Delta CT(i, j, t) = CT(i, j, t) - CT(i, j, t{=}0). \tag{1}$$

Additionally, the tracer density is expressed by $\rho_T(i, j, t)$, as a function of location (i, j) and time t. This is defined as the mass of the tracer (solute) in a unit

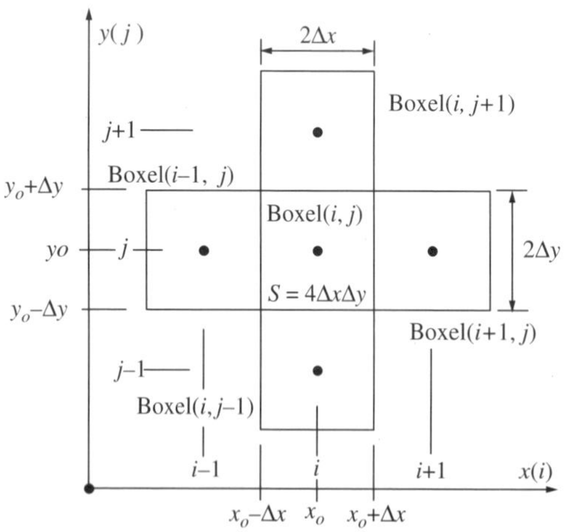

Figure 1. Boxel (i, j) and the co-ordinates (x, y).

volume of the water-tracer mixture (solution). The direct proportion between the tracer density and the subtraction is assumed as follows:

$$\rho_T(i, j, t) = \kappa \cdot \Delta CT(i, j, t) \tag{2}$$

where κ is a constant. The proportional relation in Equation (2) will be examined by experiments in the following paragraph, along with the preparation of the tracer and the practice of CT images subtraction.

To formulate the conservation law of mass, it is assumed that the tracer density at each section surrounding the boxel (i, j) is equivalent to the mean between the neighboring boxels. For example, the tracer density on the section of $x = x_o - \Delta x$, having an area of $2\Delta y\Delta z$, is given as follows:

$$\rho_T(x_o-\Delta x, y_o, t) = \{\rho_T(i-1, j, t) + \rho_T(i, j, t)\}/2. \tag{3}$$

Flow rate u is positive when water flows in the positive x-axis direction, and the flow rate v is positive for flow in the positive y-axis direction. These are independent upon time t, and given from the Darcy law as follows:

$$u = -k/\mu \cdot dp/dx, \qquad v = -k/\mu \cdot dp/dy, \tag{4}$$

where k denotes the coefficient of permeability of rock, μ is the viscosity of water-tracer mixture, and p is the pore-water pressure. In Equation (4), the isotropy of permeability is assumed in a boxel scale. If the viscosity μ is a constant in a wide range of the tracer density, the water flow is steady.

Equation (4) is able to be re-written in the form of a difference equation. For instance, the flow rate u at $x = x_o - \Delta x$ is given as follows:

$$u(x_o-\Delta x, y_o) = -k/\mu \cdot \{p(i, j) - p(i-1, j)\}/(2\Delta x), \tag{5}$$

where $p(i, j)$ is the pore-water pressure at the center of the boxel (i, j). Then the conservation law of mass for the tracer is expressed as follows:

$$\begin{aligned} &\rho_T(x_o-\Delta x, y_o, t) \cdot u(x_o-\Delta x, y_o) \cdot 2\Delta y\Delta z\Delta t \\ &- \rho_T(x_o+\Delta x, y_o, t) \cdot u(x_o+\Delta x, y_o) \cdot 2\Delta y\Delta z\Delta t \\ &+ \rho_T(x_o, y_o-\Delta y, t) \cdot v(x_o, y_o-\Delta y) \cdot 2\Delta x\Delta z\Delta t \\ &- \rho_T(x_o, y_o+\Delta y, t) \cdot v(x_o, y_o+\Delta y) \cdot 2\Delta x\Delta z\Delta t \\ &= -\Delta\rho_T(x_o, y_o, t) \cdot \phi(x_o, y_o) \cdot 4\Delta x\,\Delta y\Delta z, \end{aligned} \tag{6}$$

where $\Delta\rho_T$ denotes the increment of the density in an infinitesimal time increment Δt, and ϕ is the porosity of rock. The term of the right side represents the mass increase for the tracer within the boxel (i, j) in a time increment Δt. By substituting Equations (3) and (5) into Equation (6), in the case of $\Delta x = \Delta y$, we obtain

$$\{\rho_T(i-1,j,t)+\rho_T(i+1,j,t)+\rho_T(i,j-1,t)+\rho_T(i,j+1,t)+4\rho_T(i,j,t)\}\cdot p(i,j)$$
$$-\{\rho_T(i-1,j,t)+\rho_T(i,j,t)\}\cdot p(i-1,j)$$
$$-\{\rho_T(i+1,j,t)+\rho_T(i,j,t)\}\cdot p(i+1,j)$$
$$-\{\rho_T(i,j-1,t)+\rho_T(i,j,t)\}\cdot p(i,j-1)$$
$$-\{\rho_T(i,j+1,t)+\rho_T(i,j,t)\}\cdot p(i,j+1)$$
$$=\mu/k\cdot 2S\cdot \phi(x_o,y_o)\cdot \Delta\rho_T(i,j,t)/\Delta t. \quad (7)$$

where $S = 4\Delta x\,\Delta y$: the area of a pixel.

Time-integration of the tracer density $\rho_T(i, j, t)$ in a range of from $t = 0$ to $t = \infty$, is expressed as follows:

$$\Phi(i,j)=\int \rho_T(i,j,t)dt. \quad (8)$$

This is called the time-integrated tracer density in the present paper. Since the time-integration of the density rate $\Delta\rho_T/\Delta t$ is negligibly small, Equation (7) is re-written in a time-integrated form as follows:

$$\{\Phi(i-1,j)+\Phi(i+1,j)+\Phi(i,j-1)+\Phi(i,j+1)+4\Phi(i,j)\}\cdot p(i,j)=\{\Phi(i-1,j)+\Phi(i,j)\}\cdot p(i-1,j)$$
$$+\{\Phi(i+1,j)+\Phi(i,j)\}\cdot p(i+1,j)$$
$$+\{\Phi(i,j-1)+\Phi(i,j)\}\cdot p(i,j-1)$$
$$+\{\Phi(i,j+1)+\Phi(i,j)\}\cdot p(i,j+1) \quad (9)$$

In order to express the time-integrated tracer density using the CT value, we can define

$$C(i,j)=\int \Delta CT(i,j,t)dt. \quad (10)$$

By substituting Equations (2) and (10) into Equation (9), we obtain

$$\{C(i-1,j)+C(i+1,j)+C(i,j-1)+C(i,j+1)+4C(i,j)\}\cdot p(i,j)=\{C(i-1,j)+C(i,j)\}\cdot p(i-1,j)$$
$$+\{C(i+1,j)+C(i,j)\}\cdot p(i+1,j)$$
$$+\{C(i,j-1)+C(i,j)\}\cdot p(i,j-1)$$
$$+\{C(i,j+1)+C(i,j)\}\cdot p(i,j+1) \quad (11)$$

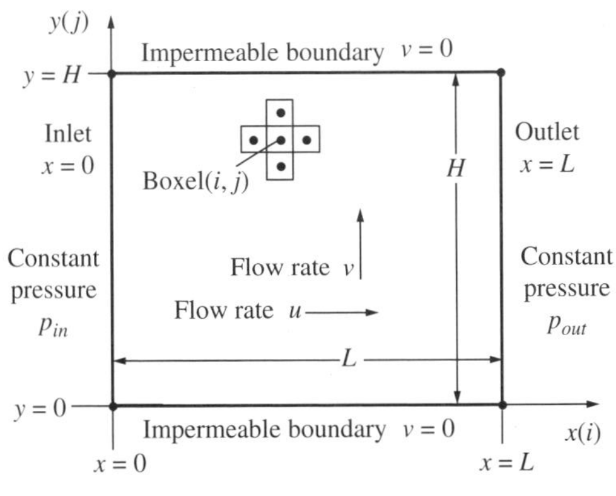

Figure 2. Rectangular region for the TDTIM analysis and the boundary conditions.

When the values of $C(i, j)$ are known, Equation (11) is a simultaneous linear equation for the pore-water pressure $p(i, j)$. In this study, $C(i, j)$ is also called the time-integrated tracer density.

Equation (11) is applied to solve the steady flow within a rectangular region of $L \times H$, as shown in Figure 2. A constant pressure p_{in} is given on the inlet $x = 0$, along with a constant outlet pressure p_{out} at $x = L$. On the impermeable boundaries of $y = 0$ and H, the flow rate v can be assumed to be zero.

Since the time-integrated tracer density $C(i, j)$ is numerically obtained from the X-ray CT image data as discussed in the following paragraph, the pore-water pressure $p(i, j)$ is obtained as the solution of Equation (11). Then the flow rate (u, v) is obtained by the differentiation of the pressure, as follows:

$$u(i,j)=-k/\mu\cdot\{p(i+1,j)-p(i-1,j)\}/(4\Delta x), \quad (12)$$

$$v(i,j)=-k/\mu\cdot\{p(i,j+1)-p(i,j-1)\}/(4\Delta y) \quad (13)$$

Equations (12) and (13) require precise values of the coefficient of permeability k and the viscosity μ of water-tracer mixture to compute the flow rate at a given point. However the determination of local permeability has great difficulties, then in this study the flow rate is computed in a normalized form by the mean flow rate u_{mean} in the x-axis direction. Additionally the time-integrated tracer density $C(i, j)$ is expressed in a normalized form with the mean value E of $C(i, j)$ in the analytical region. The details are described in the following paragraph.

3 PREPARATION OF TRACER

The tracer having a high density was prepared with the potassium iodide and a medical contrast medium being called urografin on the market. The viscosity was measured by the capillary viscometer, as summarized in Figures 3 and 4.

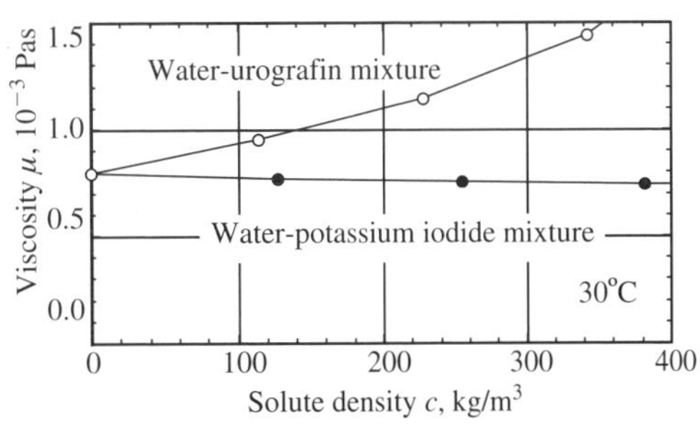

Figure 3. Viscosities of the water-urografin mixture and the water-potassium iodide mixture.

The solute density c in Figure 3 denotes the mass of solute in a unit volume of solution. The viscosity of a water-urografin solution increases with the concentration of the urografin, and conversely the viscosity of the water-potassium iodide mixture slightly decreases with increasing the density of potassium iodide at a constant temperature. Thus a suitable mixing of them is expected to provide the viscosity equivalent to pure water.

The viscosity of the water-tracer mixture used in this study is shown in Figure 4, as a function of the tracer density ρ_T defined as the mass of tracer in a unit volume of the water-tracer mixture. The tracer is a mixture of the potassium iodide and the urografin in a ratio of 1.0:0.12 in mass. The viscosity μ is almost constant in a range of from $\rho_T = 0$ to $\rho_T = 400\,\text{kg/m}^3$, which completely coincides with that of pure water. Then it is concluded that the present tracer makes no-disturbance of the steady water flow.

The density of water-tracer mixture ρ_M is the sum of the tracer density ρ_T and the water density ρ_W. The later is defined the mass of water in a unit volume of the water-tracer mixture. These are summarized in Figure 5, as a function of the mass ratio $r = M_T/M_M$, where M_T: the mass of tracer; M_M: the mass of water-tracer mixture. The mixture density ρ_M and the tracer density ρ_T increase with increasing the value of r, but the water density ρ_W decreases. The water density ρ_W becomes smaller than the density of pure water $\rho_{PW} = 1000\,\text{kg/m}^3$. This is a significant point in the quantitative evaluation of the tracer density ρ_T by means of the CT images subtraction.

The density difference $\Delta\rho$ of pure water and the water-tracer mixture can be expressed as follows:

$$\Delta\rho = \rho_M - \rho_{PW}. \tag{14}$$

The linear relation between the tracer density ρ_T and the density difference $\Delta\rho$ is held as in Figure 5(b). This is a significant point in the evaluation of the tracer density ρ_T, which is required to complete the fundamental Equation (11). Based on the direct proportional relation between ρ_T and $\Delta\rho$, the tracer density ρ_T will be evaluated, as discussed in the following paragraph, from the measurement of the density difference $\Delta\rho$ by means of the CT images subtraction.

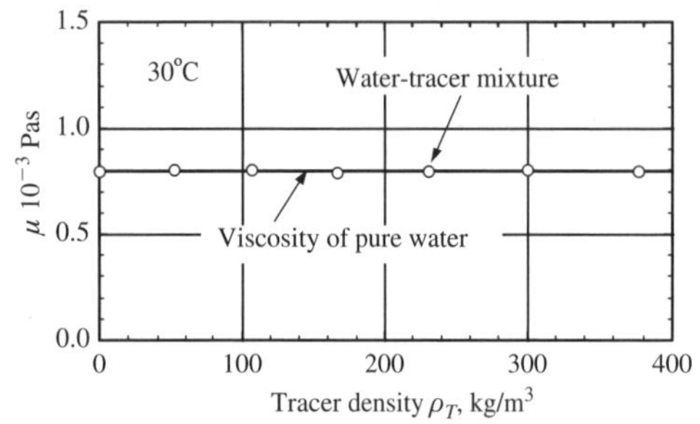

Figure 4. Viscosity of the water-tracer mixture.

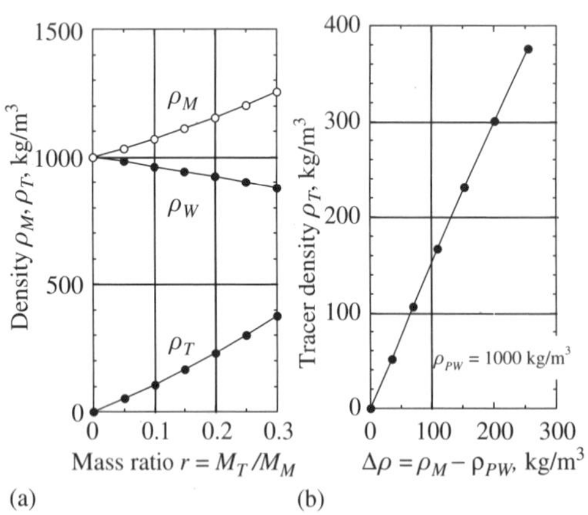

Figure 5. Relations among the density of the water-tracer mixture ρ_M, the tracer density ρ_T, the water density ρ_W and the density difference $\Delta\rho$.

4 X-RAY CT SCANNER EMPLOYED

This study made use of an industrial X-ray CT scanner (TOSCANER-23200) manufactured by the Toshiba Corporation, schematically shown in Figure 6. An X-ray bulb operating at 300 kV/2mA provides the radiation source from which an X-ray beam is emitted. 176 detectors aligned with the X-ray source in the horizontal plane record attenuation data. The rock specimen for scanning is positioned on a traversing turntable and the X-ray beam is projected tf hrough one plane of the specimen as it rotates and traverses.

A few attenuation profiles are recorded for each incidence by the 176 detectors, and a set of profiles is used to reconstruct a two-dimensional CT image. The beam thickness was set in 2 mm in the present study. The pixel is a square of 0.293 mm × 0.293 mm, and the volume of a boxel is set to be 0.1717 mm^3. The

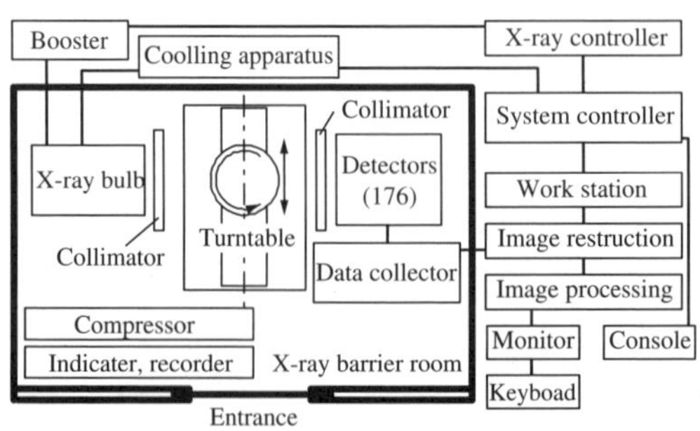

Figure 6. Composition of the X-ray CT scanner.

time required for a cross-sectional image is about 5 minutes. The magnitude of the radiographic density is expressed by the CT value. The CT value, represented by CT, is taken as being $CT = 0$ in air and $CT = 1000$ in water.

5 TEST APPARATUS AND PROCEDURE

5.1 *Experimental apparatus*

Apparatus consists of a cylindrical pressure vessel and control systems, as in Figure 7. In order to avoid from the attenuation of X-ray, the pressure vessel is made from acrylic resin. Heater and thermostat are installed in the pressure vessel to maintain a water temperature at 30°C. With the compressor-regulator system, a hydraulic head of 300 kPa is applied to a rock specimen. The X-ray scanning is performed on a fixed cross section.

5.2 *Processing the rock specimen*

Kimachi sandstone of the porosity 21% and the dry density 2.54 g/cm^3 was tested (Sugawara et al. 1998b). In order to produce the one-dimensional water flow in Kimachi sandstone, it was processed into a specimen of ϕ50 mm × 50 mm, as shown in Figure 8. Excluding a flat end surface at $x = 0$, the circumference was coated with resin to form an impermeable seal.

5.3 *Preliminary water saturation*

At the preliminary step the specimen was fully saturated by the traditional saturation method (ISRM 1979), and scanned by X-ray in the pressure vessel fulfilled with water of 30°C. For this purpose the specimen was dried at 105°C for 96 hours. The CT image at this step is used as the standard image for the CT images subtraction.

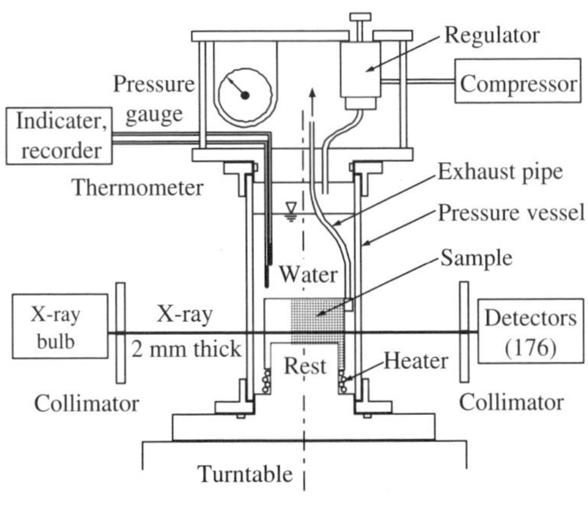

Figure 7. Experimental apparatus.

The original CT image is shown in Figure 9. As indicated in the attached figure, the cupping effect is negligibly small, but the CT value has noises of a high frequency. To eliminate the noises, a local averaging with a moving window was taken place (Takagi & Shimoda 1991). As shown in Figure 10, a square window of 13 boxels × 13 boxels was used, and the CT value of the center boxel was renewed by the mean CT value within the window.

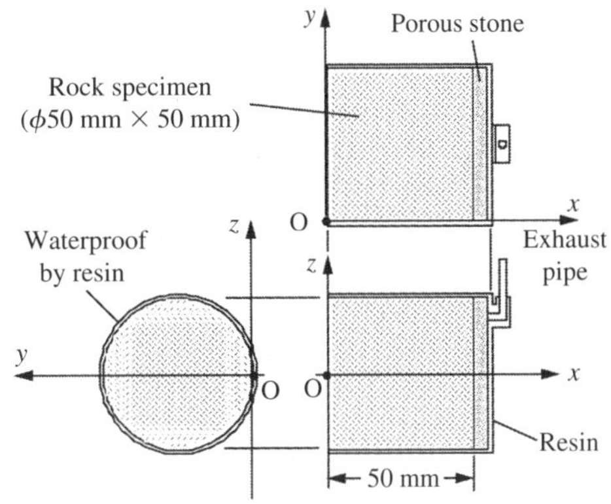

Figure 8. Cylindrical rock specimen.

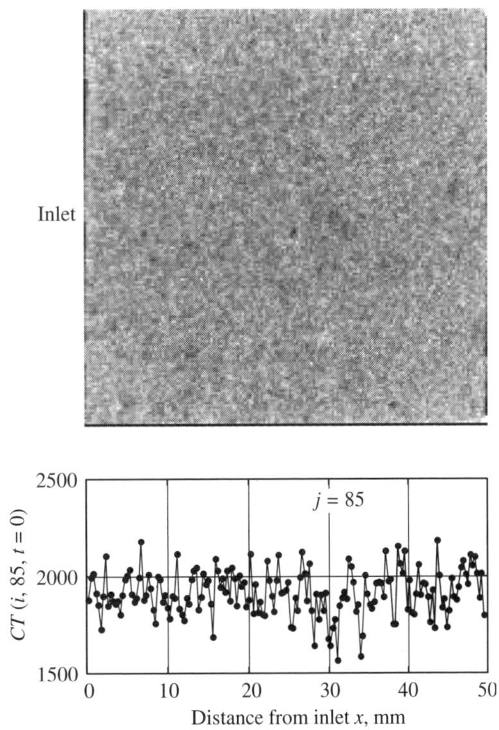

Figure 9. Original CT image of saturated specimen.

Figure 11 shows the processed CT image of the preliminary step. It can be confirmed that the local averaging provides an image of no light and dark irregularities. In the following analysis, CT images are processed by the local averaging of 13 boxels × 13 boxels, and utilized for the CT images subtraction to evaluate the tracer density.

5.4 *Injection of water-tracer mixture*

Test is started by the water-tracer mixture injection in the pressure vessel. The water-tracer mixture of

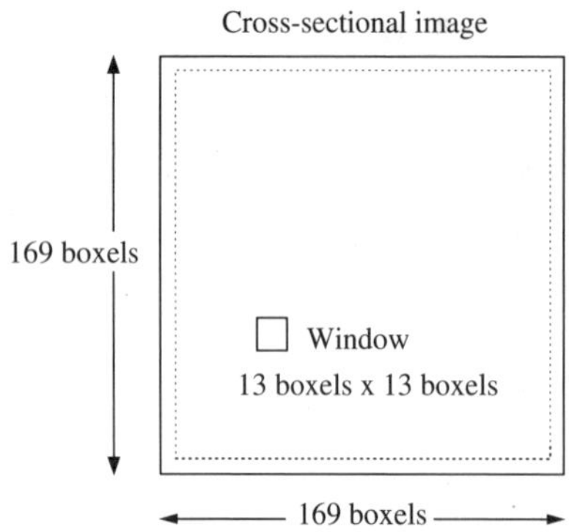

Figure 10. Local averaging procedure.

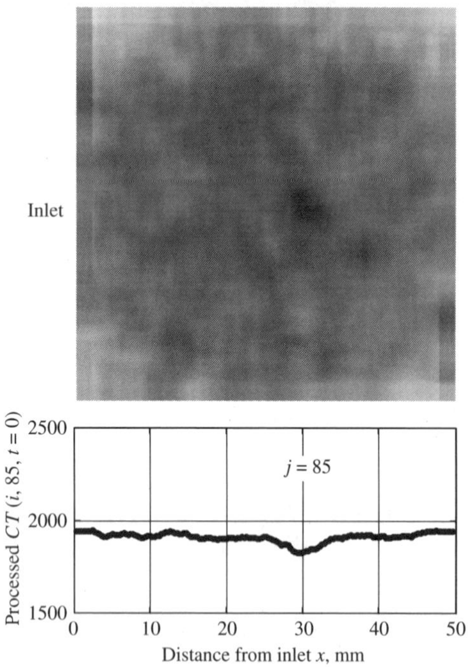

Figure 11. Processed CT image of saturated specimen.

376 kg/m^3 was injected from the inlet $x = 0$ under a pressure of 300 kPa and a temperature of 30°C. The injection process was monitored by the X-ray CT with 20 minutes intervals. After the injection of five hours, the water-tracer mixture in the vessel was completely removed and replaced with pure water. This was followed by the pure water injection.

5.5 *Subsequent injection of pure water*

Following to the water-tracer mixture injection, the pure water injection of 45 hours was conducted under a steady pressure of 300 kPa and a constant temperature of 30°C, along with the X-ray scanning of 20 minutes intervals.

6 EVALUATION OF TRACER DENSITY

6.1 *The CT images subtraction*

In the TDTIM, a time-series of the image $\Delta CT(i, j, t)$ is used instead of the tracer density image $\rho_\square(i, j, t)$ to evaluate relative values of the time-integrated tracer density, since the direct measurement of the tracer density ρ_T has great difficulties. In this section, it is described how the tracer density $\rho_\square$ can be evaluated by the CT images subtraction.

The CT value of the water-tracer mixture varies with the mass ratio r as shown in Figure 12. The CT data in the figure are obtained by the X-ray scanning for the solution in a glass container having an inner diameter of 12 mm. The X-ray scanning was taken place five times, and the CT values on a central line of the container were evaluated by the stacking procedure. Figure 12(b) shows that the mean CT value of the solution is proportional to the mass ratio r. In Figure 12(a), the cupping effect is clearly found out from a curved distribution in the case of $r = 0.15$.

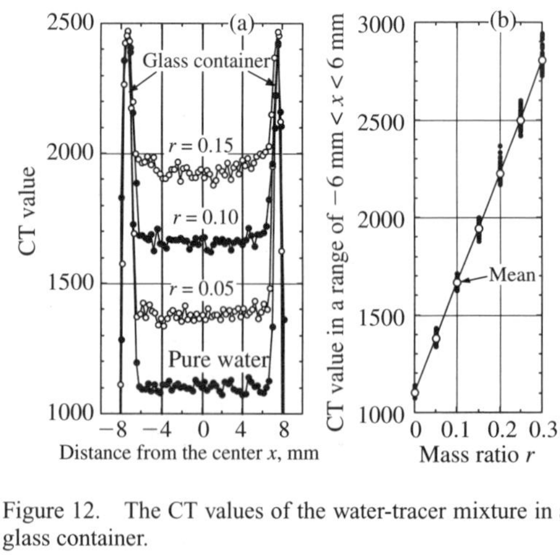

Figure 12. The CT values of the water-tracer mixture in a glass container.

From the principle of the X-ray CT, the CT data is related to the solution density ρ_M. Then the CT images subtraction ΔCT between the solution and the pure water provides an image of the density difference $\Delta\rho = \rho_M - \rho_{PW}$. It cannot give the image of ρ_T, in a direct manner. Then the direct proportional relation between the images subtraction ΔCT and the density difference $\Delta\rho$ is required to evaluate the tracer density ρ_T, along with the direct proportional relation between the density difference $\Delta\rho$ and the tracer density ρ_T. The later relation is satisfied as shown in Figure 5. The former relation is given in Figure 13.

Figure 13 shows that the subtraction ΔCT of the CT values increases with the density difference $\Delta\rho$. However the direct proportion is held in a limited range of $\Delta CT < 560$. Then it can be noted that the CT images subtraction has a clear limitation to evaluate the tracer density ρ_T within the glass container.

When the CT images subtraction is applied to the injection tests, the effect of porosity ϕ is considered to be of importance, since the subtraction $\Delta CT(i, j, t)$ between the CT image at a given time t and the standard image of $t = 0$ is related to the change in mass in pores. If the tracer density in pores is constant, the value of $\Delta CT(i, j, t)$ is reduced with decreasing the porosity. Then, it can be noted that the allowable range for the tracer density may become wider in the injection tests. Within the allowable limit, the CT images subtraction can provide an image equivalent to the tracer density image. It can be noted that the allowable limit may be expressed by the CT value, and it can be given as $\Delta CT < 560$ from the experiment in Figure 12.

Conclusively the relative value of tracer density is obtained by the CT images subtraction. In other words, the tracer density can be expressed in values relative to a standard. Thus the flow rate and the time-integrated tracer density are presented in a normalized form.

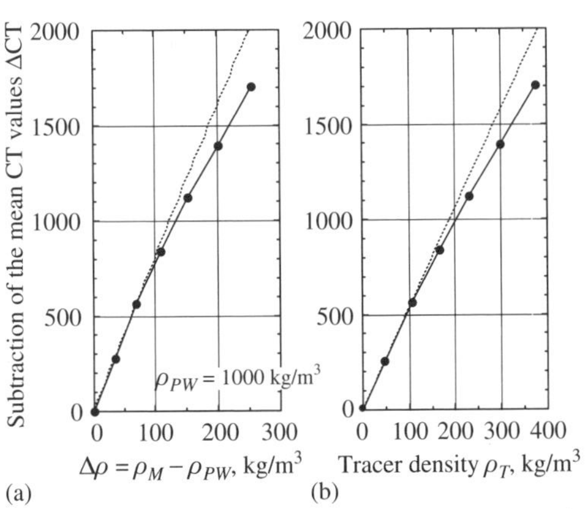

Figure 13. Subtraction of the mean CT values versus the density difference $\Delta\rho = \rho_M - \rho_{PW}$, and the tracer density ρ_T.

6.2 *Tracer density images obtained*

Figure 14 shows the image of the tracer density obtained by the CT images subtraction after the local averaging procedure. The increase of the tracer density is represented with white. Then the images describe

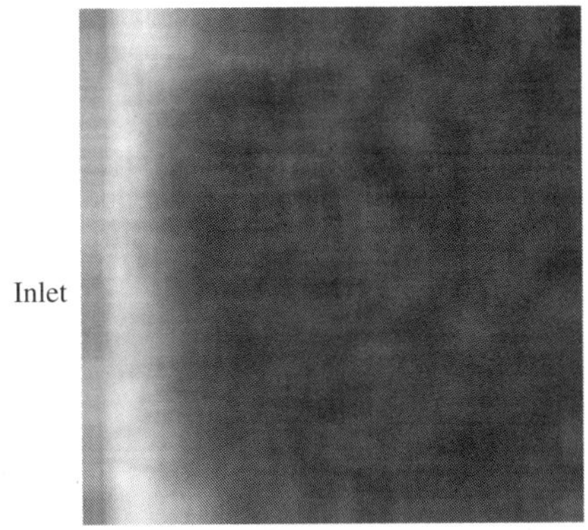

(a) Tracer density image at t = 6 hr.

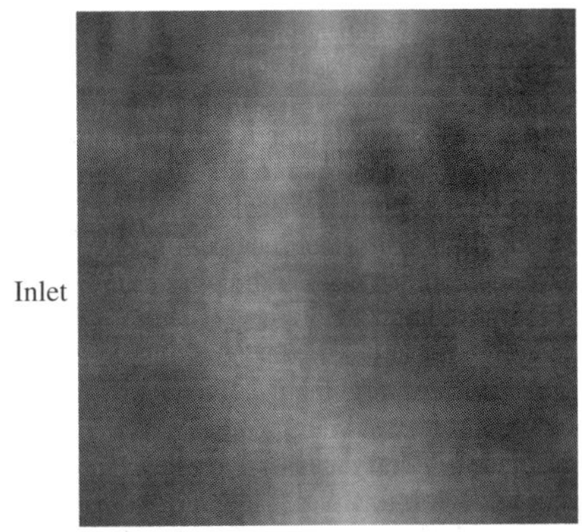

(b) Tracer density image at t = 18 hr.

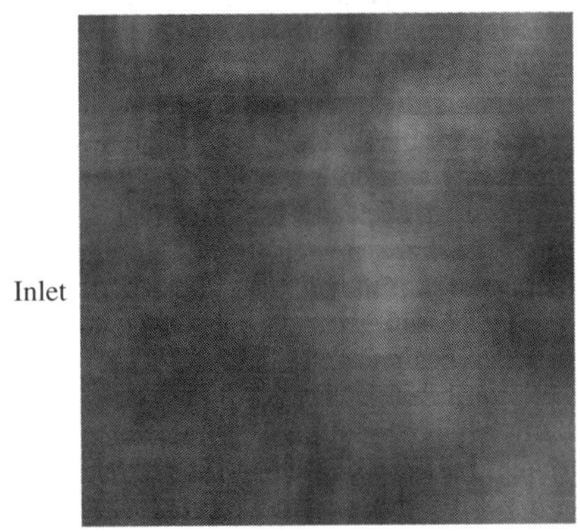

(c) Tracer density image at t = 30 hr.

Figure 14. Examples of tracer density image obtained by the CT images subtraction.

that the tracer injected from the left hand moves to the right hand in the figure, with water flow. At the stage of $t = 6$ hr, the tracer advance is limited in a narrow region near the inlet, and a remarkable advance is observed near impermeable boundaries. This suggests that the flow rate is relatively high near the boundaries. At the stage of $t = 18$ hr, the high-density zone forms a curved band in the center of the specimen. This is also associated with the ununiformity of the flow. As observed clearly in the image of $t = 30$ hr, the distribution of the tracer density becomes flatter in the downstream area, step by step with time. This is a significant characteristic of the transport diffusion phenomenon.

7 WATER FLOW ANALYSIS BY THE TDTIM

7.1 *Time integrated tracer density*

The time-integrated tracer density $C(i, j)$ defined by Equation (10) was calculated with a time-series of $\Delta CT(i, j, t)$. An example is shown in Figure 15. In the figure, the subtraction is expressed by $\Delta CT_m(i, j, t)$, and the time-integrated tracer density by $C_m(i, j)$. The subscript m represents the measurement.

The precise evaluation of $C(i, j)$ needs the X-ray scanning of a short time interval as continuously as possible, and it is hoped to measure over a fairly long period. In this case example, the tracer density: $\Delta CT(i, j, t)$ was measured with 20 minutes intervals, and the time-integrated tracer density: $C(i, j)$ was computed as $C_m(i, j) = 1467$ hr.

In order to complete the simultaneous linear equation (11) for the pore-water pressure $p(i, j)$, the time integration must be performed for all of boxels within the analytical region of $L = H = 50$ mm, from the start of the injection of water-tracer mixture until the time required for the tracer density to be completely

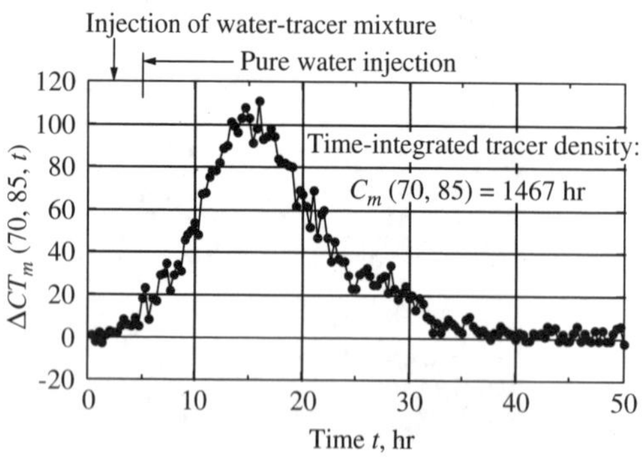

Figure 15. Example of the subtraction $\Delta CT_m(i, j, t)$ of the CT values equivalent to the tracer density as a function of time t, and the time-integrated tracer density $C_m(i, j)$.

reduced in the region. However the execution has great difficulties, since the precise measurement of a long period is needed in particular for the evaluation in the downstream area. Thus, a data processing based on the conservation law of mass was adopted to improve the time-integrated tracer density: $C(i, j)$. Namely, the measured value $C_m(i, j)$ was processed for the mass of the tracer passing through a plane perpendicular to the x-axis to be uniform along the x-axis.

For this purpose, the mean flow rate u_{mean} in the analytical region was utilized as the approximate value of flow rate $u(x, y)$. And, the mean $D_m(x)$ of $C_m(x, y) = C_m(i, j)$ in the y-axis direction was defined, along with the mean E_m of $D_m(x)$ in the x-axis direction. In the equation form, these are written as follows:

$$D_m(x) = \int C_m(x, y)dy/H, \quad E_m = \int D_m(x)dx/L. \tag{15}$$

The distribution of $D_m(x)$ is illustrated in Figure 16. $D_m(x)$ varies along the x-axis, but a fluctuation is relatively small in the region A. However, in the downstream region B, the value of $D_m(x)$ decreases monotonously with approaching the outlet $x = 50$ mm.

The two kinds of data processing scheme can be recommended, as follows:

$$C(x, y) = C_m(x, y) \cdot E_m / D_m(x), \tag{16}$$

$$C(x, y) = C_m(x, y) + E_m - D_m(x), \tag{17}$$

where $C(x, y)$ denotes the processed value of the time-integrated tracer density of the boxel (i, j). The combination of Equations (16) and (17) is also considered to be acceptable.

Equation (16) is pertinent in the region A in Figure 16. But Equation (17) is considered to be more suitable in the region B, since it can provide rational results of positive, even if $C_m(x, y)$ is negative. In the

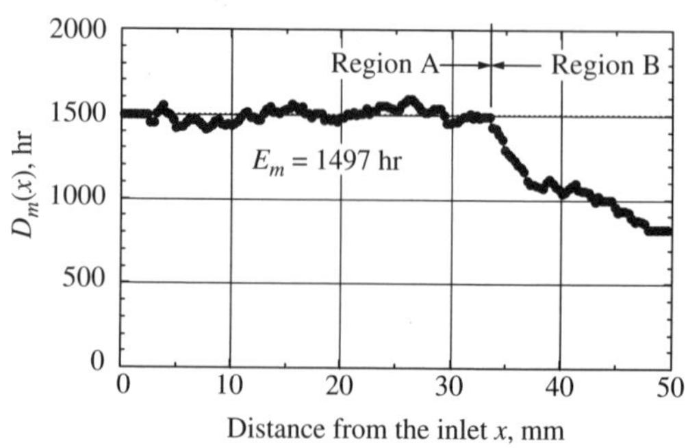

Figure 16. Example of the distribution of $D_m(x)$.

following, Equation (16) was applied for the region A, and Equation (17) was for the region B. The mean E_m was calculated in the region A, as $E_m = 1497$ hr. The results obtained are shown in Figure 17.

The pseudo-images of the time-integrated tracer density $C(i, j)$ is given in Figure 18. In the figure $C(i, j)$ is expressed in a form normalized by the mean value E_m. White region represents a high value area of $C(i, j)$, and it corresponds to a region of relatively low flow rate. Conversely a black region is a low value area of $C(i, j)$, and of relatively high flow rate.

7.2 *Pore-water pressure analysis*

The pore-water pressure $p(i, j)$ is given by solving the simultaneous linear equation (11). Figure 19 shows a bird's-eye view of the pore-water pressure. The pressure gradient in the y-axis direction is very small, comparing to that in the x-axis direction.

7.3 *Flow rate analysis*

The flow rate u in the x-axis direction is shown in Figure 20, and the flow rate v in the y-axis direction is given in Figure 21. These are normalized by the mean velocity u_{mean} in the x-axis direction.

It can be noted from Figures 20 and 21 that the steady water flow measured is not uniform. It is deeply associated with the fluctuation of the pore dimensions and the heterogeneity of rock. The flow rate u in the center part of the inlet, represented by b in the figure, has a relatively small value, though being higher in the regions denoted by a and c in the figure. This is compatible with the ununiform tracer advance mentioned in 6 previously. Additionally it can be pointed out that the ridges and valleys in Figure 20 have continuities in the y-axis direction. This may be caused by the anisotropy of a sedimentary

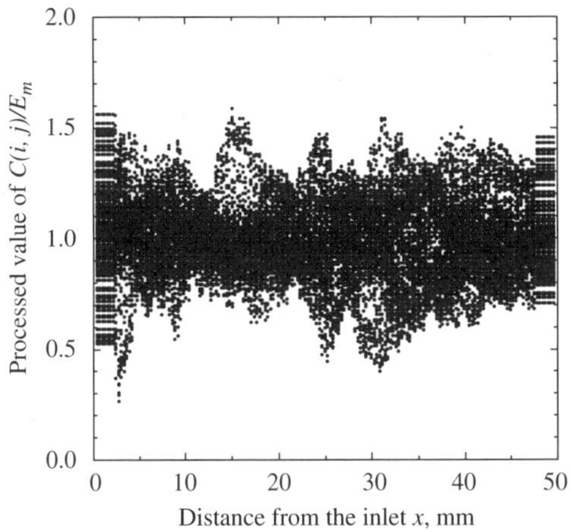

Figure 17. Distribution of $C(i, j)/E_m$.

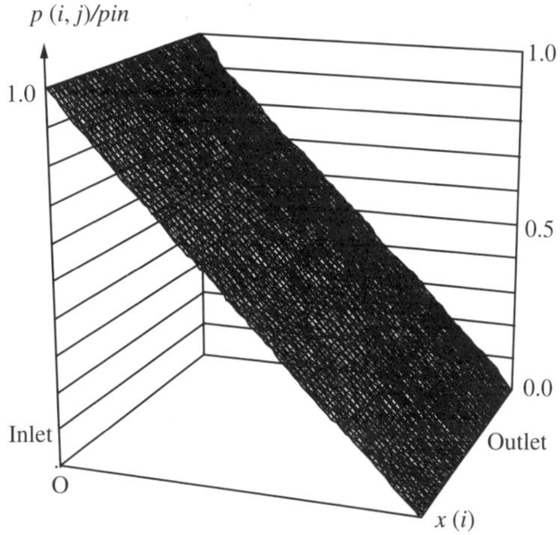

Figure 19. Pore-water pressure solved.

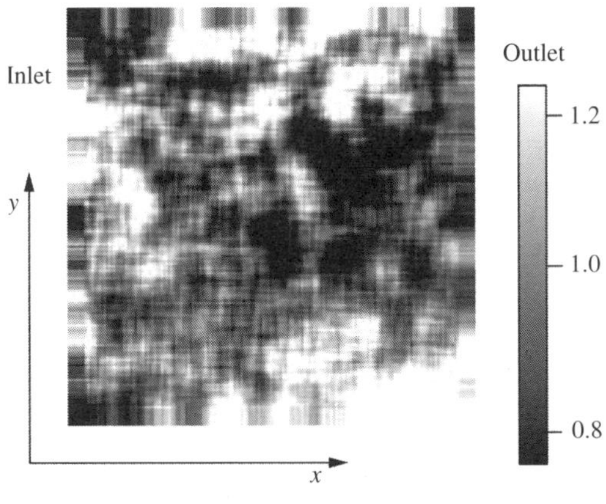

Figure 18. Pseudo-image of $C(i, j)/E_m$.

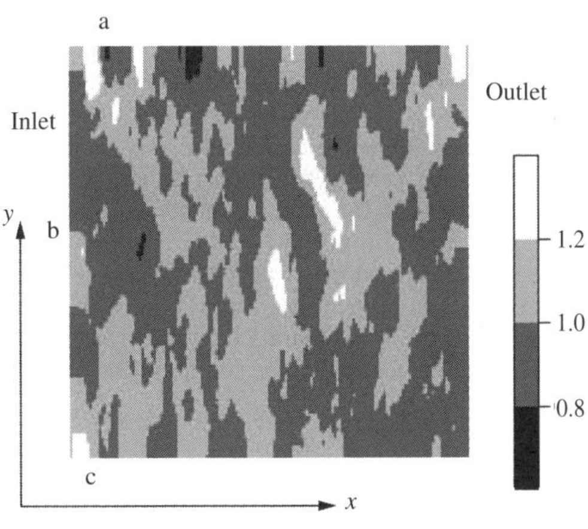

Figure 20. Distribution of u/u_{mean}.

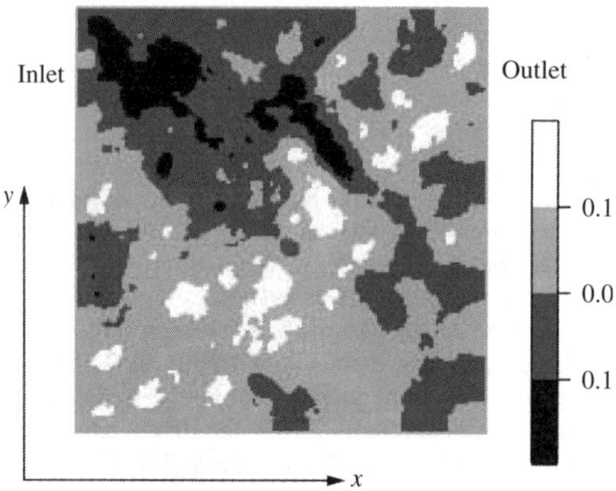

Figure 21. Distribution of v/u_{mean}.

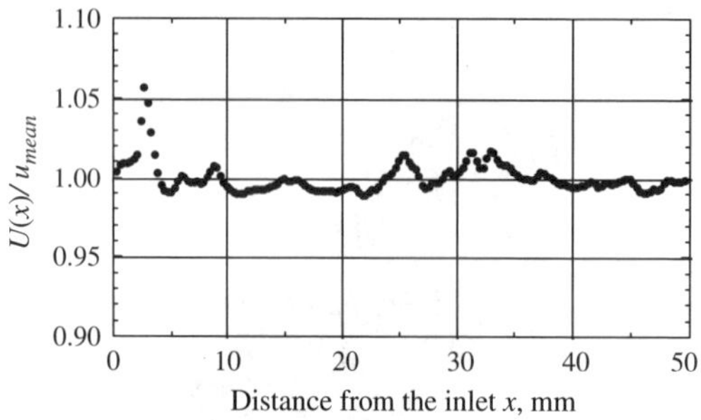

Figure 22. Distribution of the mean flow rate $U(x)$.

rock. In Figure 21, the distribution of v is approximately symmetry with respect to the center axis of the specimen. But the value varies with the location, associating with the changes in the flow rate u.

In order to prove the reliability of the present analysis, the uniformity of flow rate in the x-axis direction was investigated, by introducing the mean flow rate $U(x)$:

$$U(x)= \int u(x, y)dy/H. \tag{18}$$

Figure 22 shows the distribution of $U(x)$. Excluding a few fluctuations, a fairly uniform distribution has been obtained. Thus the assumption for the present data processing can be concluded to be acceptable in this example. If $U(x)$ cannot satisfy the specified allowance of uniformity, the iterative improvement procedure is required. To evaluate the limits allowed, the investigation of the distribution of $u(i, j)$ is indispensable, as given in Figure 23. A significant peak near the inlet indicates that the solution near the inlet is not reliable.

7.4 *Statistical characteristics of flow rate*

The statistical distribution of the flow rate is shown in Figure 24. This is the normal distribution paper, and

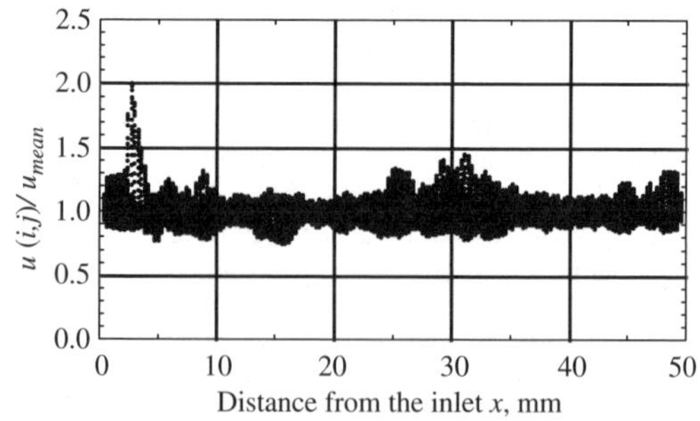

Figure 23. Distribution of the flow rate $u(i, j)$.

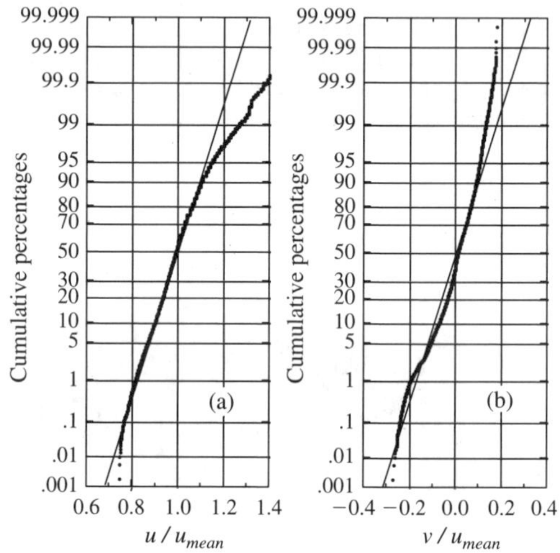

Figure 24. Statistical distributions of u and v.

the data in a range of $x > 5$ mm are plotted. It is clear that the flow rates u and v are at the same deviation. This is considered to be rational from the principle of a two-dimensional Darcy flow.

8 CONCLUDING REMARKS

Tracer Density Time-Integration Method (TDTIM) was proposed as a new scheme of the tracer-aided X-ray CT to visualize the steady water flow in porous rock and to analyze the distribution of flow rate in a fully saturated state.

The two-dimensional theory for the water flow analysis was presented, and it was clarified how the pore-water pressure and the flow rate in rock can be determined by analyzing the transport diffusion process of a tracer with water current in rock, and how the conservation law of the tracer mass and the CT images subtraction technique can be utilized to complete the simultaneous linear equation for the pore-water pressure. Subsequently it was clarified that the coefficients of the simultaneous linear equation can be given by the time-integration of the tracer density for a long period.

A successful case example using a tracer mainly composed of the potassium iodide was presented to make clear the data processing procedure for the determination of the time-integrated tracer density from a time series of the CT images, along with the necessary experimental procedures.

The case example clarified that the TDTIM is a promising tool available for the evaluation of the ununiformity and fluctuations of water flow rate, which is closely associated with the geological discontinuities and heterogeneities in rock.

This is a study followed the paper (Sugawara et al. 2003) on the wetting process analysis to determine the coefficient of permeability of rock, which is deeply dependent upon the effective confining pressure and the matric suction.

REFERENCES

Hounsfield, G.N. 1972. A method of and apparatus for examination of a body by radiation such as X- or Gamma-Radiation: London, British Patent No. 1283915.

International Society of Rock Mechanics. 1979. Suggested methods for determining water content, porosity, density, absorption and related properties and swelling and slake durability index properties, *Int. J. Rock Mech. & Min. Sci.*, 16, 141–156.

Kak, A.C. and Slaney, M. 1988. Principles of Computerized Tomographic Imaging, IEEE Press 1988, New York, USA.

Sugawara, K., Obara, Y., Kaneko, K., Koike, K, Ohmi, M. and Aoi, T. 1997. Visualization of three-dimensional structure of rocks using X-ray CT method, *Proc. of 1st ARMS*, Seoul, Korea, Vol.2, pp.769–774.

Sugawara, K., Kojima, R., Obara, Y., Sato, A. and Shimada, H. 1998a. Crack opening analysis by means of the X-ray CT. J. MMIJ, 114(12), 881–887. (in Japanese).

Sugawara, K., Reid, T.R., Yanagisaki, M. and Kawaguchi, T. 1998b. Measuring the coefficient of permeability of rock by X-ray computed tomography, Memorial Report 1998-5 of Rock Mechanics Laboratory, Graduate School of Science & Technology, Kumamoto University.

Sugawara, K., Sato, A. and Obara, Y. 1999. Crack opening analysis using X-rays CT data, Proc. of 9th Int. Congress on Rock Mechanics, ISRM, Paris, France, pp.1019–1022.

Sugawara, K., Fukahori, D., Iwatani, T., Ikutake, T. and Kubota, S. 2003. Analysis of wetting process of porous dry rock by means of X-ray CT, Proc. of Geo-X, Kumamoto, in press.

Takagi, M. and Shimoda, H. 1991. Handbook of Image Analysis. Tokyo University Publication.

X-ray CT for Geomaterials; Soils, Concrete, Rocks – Otani & Obara (eds.)
© 2004 Swets & Zeitlinger. Lisse, ISBN 90 5809 666 1

Observation of natural gas hydrate dissociation with X-ray CT

Toshiharu Okui
Japan National Oil Corporation, Chiba, Japan

Takashi Uchida
Japan Petroleum Exploration Co. Ltd., Chiba, Japan

Yoshihiro Masuda
University of Tokyo, Tokyo, Japan

ABSTRACT: Dissociation of gas hydrate, which has drawn much attention as an unconventional energy resource, in natural core samples from permafrost was observed with an X-ray CT scanner. Both depressurizing and heating processes, which are considered as typical potential production processes, were simulated in laboratory scale for the field gas production tests from gas hydrate. Dissociation of the gas hydrate was clearly observed as difference of CT values. The difference was mainly caused by gas phase formation. Obtained three-dimensional CT data of inside of the cores were processed to visualize dissociation behavior. Consequently it was observed that dissociation behavior depended on quantity and distribution of hydrates. These results suggested that X-ray CT scanning was suitable for observation of natural gas hydrate dissociation in sediments and useful for evaluation of gas hydrate as an unconventional energy in future.

1 INTRODUCTION

The objective of this study is to evaluate the potential of X-ray CT scanning technique for observation of dissociation behavior of gas hydrate in sediments. This study was conducted as a part of the Mallik project, a research project for gas production from natural methane hydrate under permafrost.

Gas hydrate is a crystalline substance composed of water and natural gas, in which a solid water lattice accommodates guest gas molecules in clathrate cages. While hydrocarbon gases like methane, ethane and propane, and other gases can be occupied in the clathrate structure, the volume of methane hydrate is the most common and enormous in nature. Gas hydrate is widespread in several Arctic sedimentary basins associated with deep permafrost as well as in many deep marine environments along continental margins worldwide.

When considering gas production tests from natural gas hydrate, the results might be influenced by complicated unknown factors in natural environments (Uchida et al. 1999) and condition control is difficult. Therefore, dissociation experiments were planned to collect basic dissociation data of gas hydrate in the real core samples under simply controlled conditions. Simple experimental dissociation data are helpful to understand the gas production from gas hydrate in sediments. Among the laboratory tests, direct observation with X-ray CT were expected to give us much visual information on dissociation behavior of gas hydrate in sediments. Both depressurization and heating methods in the production tests were simulated in the laboratory.

2 EXPERIMENTAL PROCEDURE

2.1 *Apparatus*

2.1.1 *X-ray CT scanner*

The X-ray CT scanner "Toshiba X-force (of scanner TCT series)", which was originally designed for medical use for a cross-sectional image of a human body, has been modified at our laboratory to observe fluid flow in rock core samples (Oshita et al. 2000). This facility was used for the observation of gas hydrate dissociation in sediments this time. Conditions for the measurement are as follows. Diameter of observation area is 180 mm, thickness of a slice is 2 mm, voltage of X-ray source is 130 kV, and current of X-ray source

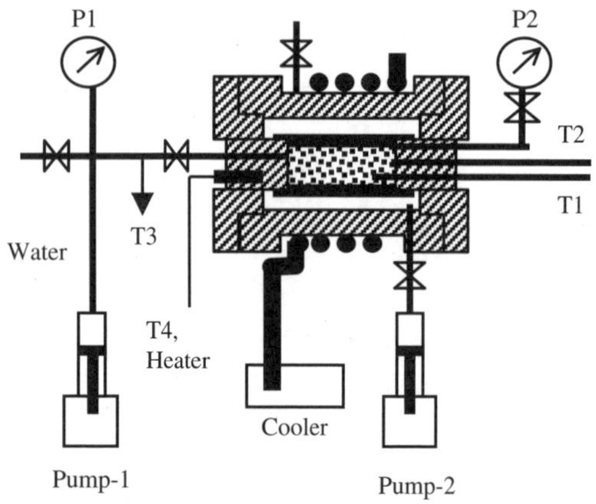

Figure 1. Core holder and condition control system. The pump-1 is for pore pressure and the pump-2 is for confining pressure control.

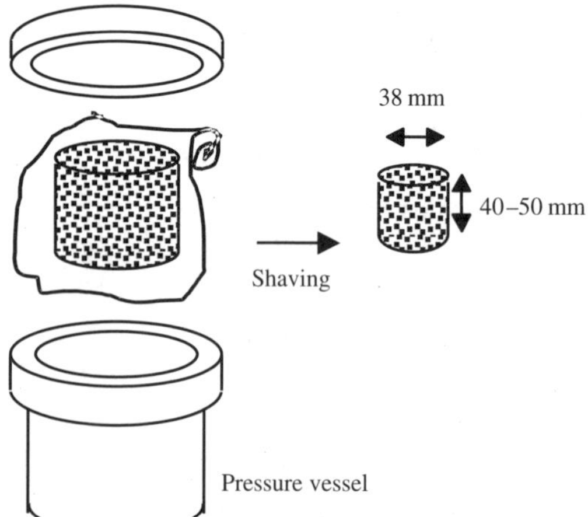

Figure 2. Preparation of the specimen including gas hydrate.

is 150 mA. Resolution of CT image is 0.35 mm in a pixel size. The thickness of a slice was determined as 2 mm from the balance of scanning speed and resolution. The data are accumulated as a set of three-dimensional CT value of each pixel in the core at each moment. CT change in an image is emphasized by subtracting the data between before and after dissociation.

2.1.2 *Core holder*

A diagram of a core holder is shown in Figure 1. Pore pressure and confining pressure are controllable independently. The rubber sleeve equipped in the core holder tightly binds the side surface of a cylindrical core and the core can be pressurized by water from outside of the sleeve. Inner pore pressure is directly controlled by another water pump. Confining pressure is always kept 3.5 MPa higher than inner pressure. Although typical pore pressure is set up to 10 MPa as the static water pressure at 1000 m deep, the corresponding confining pressure was simply determined from technical experiences to prevent breakage of the sleeve.

2.1.3 *Pump*

Each pressure was controlled and monitored with an automatic water pressure pump made by ISCO. Pressure can be controlled by accuracy of 7 kPa (1 psi) and measurable minimum flux is 0.001 cm^3 per minute.

2.2 *Procedure*

2.2.1 *Sample preparation*

The preparation process of a core sample is shown in Figure 2. The samples were frozen at the well site. They were wrapped in vinyl bags, put into the pressure vessels, pressurized with nitrogen up to 4 MPa, and transferred to Japan at below 0 degree C with dry ice. The samples were picked out in a freezing room at minus 15 degrees C and shaved into cylindrical shape just before each dissociation test to get uniform confining pressure. Diameters of all cores were constantly 38 mm, and lengths varied from 35 mm to 61 mm. At the same time a small piece was subdivided from the same block to measure released gas volume from the sample separately to estimate gas volume from the sample for the CT observation.

The shaved frozen sample was quickly introduced into the rubber sleeve of the core holder. The holder was beforehand chilled to 10 degrees C by circulated cold water. A thin thermocouple was inserted along the side surface of the specimen. The core was bound tightly by the plugs from both ends immediately. The end plugs had holes connected to a pump. The inner pressure was pressurized up to 10 MPa directly with water by the pump. At the same time confining pressure was controlled by another pump from outside of the rubber sleeve to be always 3.5 MPa higher than the inner pressure. After that, the core was held until the temperature and pressure became stable after melting of ice (usually 90 minutes). After that, the original conditions of the underground (pressure, temperature and composition) were reproduced.

2.2.2 *Dissociation and observation*
(a) – Depressurization process

Pressure profile during the depressurization process is shown in Figure 3. At the constant temperature, inner pore pressure was decreased step by step. Confining pressure was decreased correspondingly. Estimated equilibrium pressure of pure methane hydrate at 10 degrees C was about 7.5 MPa; therefore, pressure was decreased carefully after 8 MPa. Under the pressure

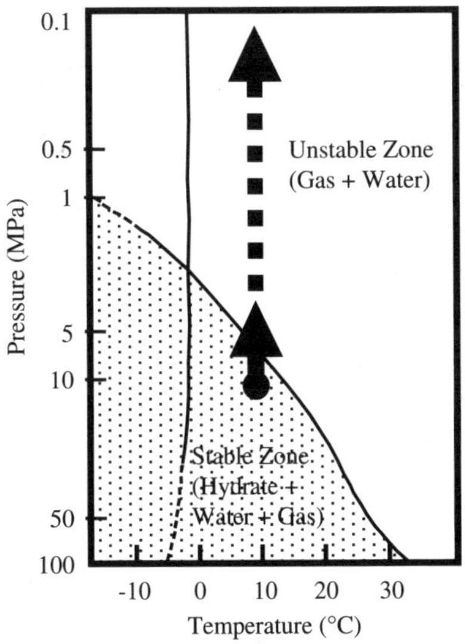

Figure 3. Procedure for depressurization.

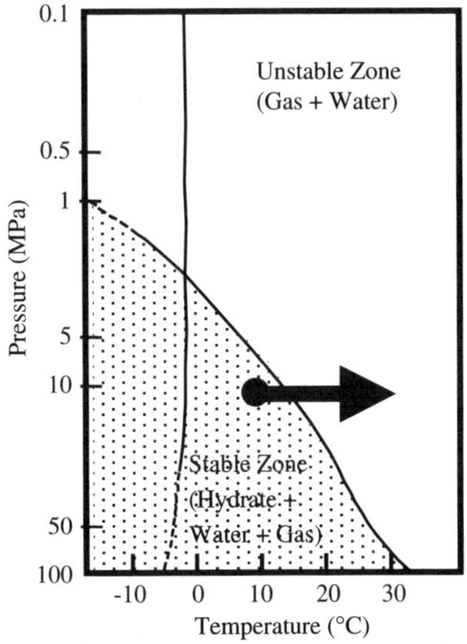

Figure 4. Procedure for heating.

close to the equilibrium pressure, the sample was scanned by X-ray CT just before and after the depressurization. After that, CT scanning intervals were 5 minutes until the gas release finished. Amount and rate of released gas were measured as drawn volume of the syringe of the pump at each constant pressure. After that, pressure was lowered again by 0.5 MPa to begin the next step. Final pressure was 0.1 MPa.

Finally total dissociated gas was measured in an overturned scalpel cylinder in water bath. Gas sample was collected to submit for composition analysis by gas chromatography.

2.2.3 *Dissociation and observation (b) – Heating process*

Temperature profile during the heating process is shown in Figure 4. An electric heater was inserted in an end plug to heat one end of the core. The shaved core sample was bound in the holder and stabilization at 10 degrees C and 10 MPa. First pressure was decreased to 8 MPa to move the condition closer to the equilibrium line, and then the heater was turned on. Heating rate was surveyed in advance with a typical sandstone core so that it would take 15 minutes for the dissociation front to move from one end to the other to scan 3 or 4 times during the dissociation.

The real natural core was scanned before turning on the heater, and was scanned again just after heating began. After that, scanning intervals were 5 minutes. After 20 minutes, temperature rise at the other end was detected and it became constant at 33 degrees C in the next 20 minutes. Since no more volume change of the pump under constant pressure was observed, dissociation was estimated to finish. After that, pressure was carefully decreased to 0.1 MPa again step by step until gas expansion was not detected. Finally total dissociated gas was measured in the underwater overturned scalpel cylinder and gas samples for composition analysis were collected.

3 RESULTS AND DISCUSSION

3.1 *General matters*

Figures 5 & 6 are the results of the X-ray CT observation for gas hydrate in sediments in cores naturally obtained. In both depressurization and heating processes hydrate dissociation was successfully visualized. Each image is of an axially divided quarter block; therefore, the indicated surface is the inside of the sample. The pictures are subtracted images of CT values between each moment and before dissociation. The darkness corresponds to difference of CT values, which basically reflect density of materials. The clear images of subtracted data suggested that sand grains of the samples were bound tightly by confining pressure during the dissociation even though they were unconsolidated.

Dimensional resolution of CT value was bigger than size of both hydrate and sediment grains; therefore, the CT value change was suggested to depend on gas phase generation. As length of one side of one pixel of the CT data was 0.35 mm, the acquired CT value was the average of the data of the material in a cube whose one side is 0.35 mm. Diameter of the

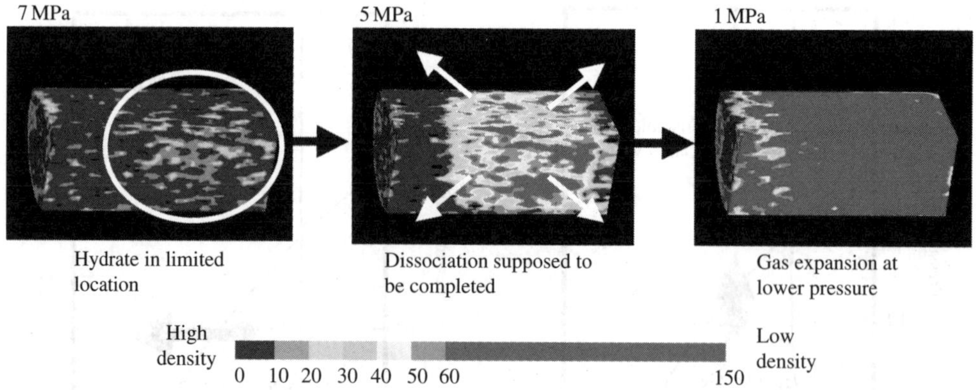

Figure 5. Dissociation behavior of gas hydrate in natural sediments with depressurization (hydrate saturation in pore: 20%).

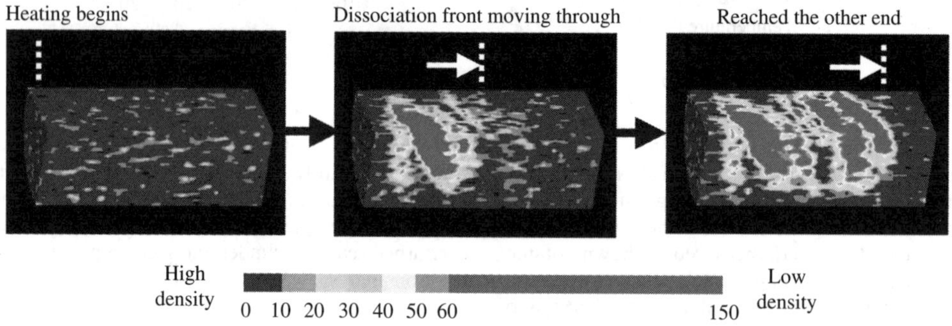

Figure 6. Dissociation behavior of gas hydrate in natural sediments with heating (hydrate saturation in pore: 10%).

sediment grains mainly distributed from 0.125 mm to 0.250 mm and pore size distributed mainly from 5 to 50 microns (Uchida et al., in press). Since the distribution is smaller than the resolution of the CT scanner, CT value is acquired as average of the mixture of sediment (minerals mainly composed of SiO_2), water, gas hydrates and gas filling the residual space.

CT value simply means the density of the observed material. CT value of minerals, hydrate, and water differs but the difference is not so obvious. When those materials are mixed up, only dissociation of hydrate, which is included less than 25% in volume, cannot be detected as a change of the average CT value. Therefore, the visualized hydrate dissociation behavior in this measurement was mainly detected as generation of gas whose density is quite smaller than other solid and liquid materials in this system, especially when it expanded at lower pressure.

As it is indicated in Figures 5 & 6, typical trends of gas hydrate dissociation in the depressurization and heating process were observed. The following discussion is about dissociation behavior of gas hydrate in sediments depending on processes for dissociation and on occurrence of hydrate (Okui et al., in press).

3.2 *Depressurization process*

Images in Figure 5 indicate dissociation behavior of gas hydrate in the core sample composed of medium-grained sand in depressurization process. Gas hydrate saturation calculated from subdivided specimen from the same core sample was about 20%. In this case it was detected that every gas hydrate in the whole core uniformly began to dissociate immediately after the pore pressure was decreased from 7.5 MPa to 7.0 MPa.

Even at relatively high pressure, dissociation might have completed when pressure was decreased to just below the corresponding equilibrium pressure; however, it could not be detected as enough CT value change as long as the released gas was compressed and volume of the gas phase was small. It would be difficult to detect the dissociation at high pressure because CT value change was mainly caused by gas phase appearance and detected value was average of the density of the mixed materials in the space of the minimum resolution, as described above.

After the dissociation, expansion of the released gas at lower pressure was also observed. Finally all area in the image uniformly turned to the color of low density.

The visualized dissociated gas distribution at a little lower pressure (the middle image of Figure 5, for example) indicates the original distribution of gas hydrate. In this case it was indicated that gas hydrate mainly distributed inside of this sample. Dissociation around the surface of the specimen might occur during the sample preparation process.

3.3 *Heating process*

Figure 6 shows the dissociation behavior of the gas hydrate in the core sample composed of coarse-grained sand with heating at constant pressure (8 MPa). In these pictures, the right edge of the sample was heated by an electric heater as indicated in the Figure 1. In those three pictures, it was observed that the dissociation front moved from the right to the left. It took 15 minutes for the dissociation front to pass through from right edge to the left. No further change was observed until the temperature and pressure became stable as far as it was pressurized at 8 MPa.

Gas hydrate saturation calculated from released gas volume from another small piece of the same core block was 10%. Amount of hydrate was not so much but the unique characteristic of this sample was uneven distribution of gas hydrate in the core. There were some layers of dissociated gas, reflecting the original distribution of gas hydrate in sediments.

Additionally, it was observed that dissociated gas had remained at the original position at 8 MPa and expanded with depressurization. Since the equilibrium temperature at 8 MPa is approximately 11 degrees C, dissociation of gas hydrate would have completed after the 20-minute continuous heating at 33 degrees C. This result suggested that the released gas could not come out from the core only on heating. Gas hydrate saturation (10%) was not so much but all the released gas stayed at the original position.

In summary about the CT observation of gas hydrate dissociation, condition control will certainly dissociate the gas hydrate; however, as long as it is pressurized, the dissociated gas would remain at the original position. Further method to enhance gas production, such as additional water injection to wipe out the dissociated gas, might be required for more efficient gas production from gas hydrate in sediments.

4 CONCLUSIONS

Dissociation of gas hydrate in natural sediments in both processes of depressurization and heating could be clearly visualized by X-ray CT scanning. Distribution of gas hydrate was distinguished with the dissociated gas. It was observed that dissociation behavior of gas hydrate in sediments strongly depended on the dissociation process and distribution of the gas hydrate in the core.

In the depressurization process with confining pressure, gas hydrate in the cores with less saturation (10% in pore, for example) dissociated uniformly and quickly. After dissociation, released gas expanded and diffused easily in the core under lower pressure.

In heating processes, it was indicated that heat transfer was fast enough and gas hydrate exposed to the unstable conditions dissociated smoothly. However, some dissociated gas would stay at the original position under high pore pressure even after diffusion. An additional operation, such as wiping out the released gas by water, might be useful to complete gas production from gas hydrate.

ACKNOWLEDGEMENT

This work was the first attempt for us to utilize X-ray CT scanner for gas hydrate research. It was completed by cooperation of a lot of people from various organizations. We are deeply indebted to Messrs. T. Munakata, Y. Tsuchiya and K. Oseto of Japan National Oil Corporation for their special technical supports and useful comments for use of X-ray CT scanner. We are also grateful to Messrs. T. Ueyama and N. Horinouchi of the University of Tokyo, Drs. T. Takayama, A. Waseda, J. Mikami and T. Takahashi of Japan Petroleum Exploration Co., Ltd. for useful discussion with them and their efforts for the setting of facilities and measurement of various parameters in the experiment.

REFERENCES

Oshita, T., Okabe, H. & Namba, T. 2000. Early Water Breakthrough –X ray CT Visualizes How It Happens in Oil-Wet Cores. *The 2000 SPE Asia Pacific Conference on Integrated Modeling for Asset Management; Proc. intern. symp., Yokohama, 25–26 April 2000.* SPE59426. Richardson: the Society of Petroleum Engineering.

Uchida, T., Matsumoto, R., Waseda, A., Okui, T., Yamada, K., Uchida, T., Okada, S. & Takano, O. 1999. Physicochemical properties of natural gas hydrates and associated hydrate-bearing sediments obtained from the JAPEX/JNOC/GSC Mallik 2L-38 research well. In Dallimore, S., Uchida, T. and Collett, T. (eds.), *Scientific Results from JAPEX/JNOC/GSC Mallik 2L-38 Gas Hydrate Research Well, Mackenzie Delta, Northwest Territories, Canada, Geological Survey of Canada Bulletin* 544: 205–228.

X-ray CT for Geomaterials; Soils, Concrete, Rocks – Otani & Obara (eds.)
© 2004 Swets & Zeitlinger. Lisse, ISBN 90 5809 666 1

Characterization of weathering process of rocks by X-ray CT and radiance spectra measurements

K. Koike & T. Yoshinaga
Department of Civil Engineering, Faculty of Engineering, Kumamoto University, Kumamoto, Japan

K. Nishiyama
Faculty of the Integrated Arts and Sciences, University of Tokushima, Japan

ABSTRACT: Changes of inner structures (textures), physical properties, and chemical compositions of rocks with the progress of weathering are significant in the field of engineering geology. Combination of them contributes to understand comprehensively the process of weathering. A nondestructive test is required to visualize inner structures. Rock density is one of the important physical properties. Amount and kind of clay minerals and crystal structure of quartz, the main constituent mineral of rocks, are key factors of chemical compositions related to weathering. To extract these properties, we focused on X-ray CT scan image and radiance spectra of rocks with different degrees of weathering. The reflectance and emissivity spectra in the wavelength ranges of electromagnetic waves, 0.485–2.5 μm and 8–14 μm, respectively were used for the radiance spectra. Three types of rocks, granite, sandstone, and welded tuff, were examined in this study. The weathering features were clearly shown for the samples in the degree of absorption of the reflectance and emissivity spectra at the specific wavelengths such as 1.4, 1.9, 2.5, and 9 μm, which results from the occurrence of clay minerals. In addition, the weathering can be characterized by the large increase of reference in the short-wave infrared region as compared to the reflectance in the visible and near infrared regions, and the flattening of emissivity spectra with the progress of weathering. The CT images clarified the characteristics of changes in the inner structure and density with the weathering and their relation to the changes of mineral compositions inferred from the radiance spectra.

1 INTRODUCTION

Wavelengths of electromagnetic waves from visible to short-wave infrared regions and thermal infrared region are used for the remote sensing by optical sensors, because the transmissions of waves through the atmosphere are high. This phenomenon is known as atmospheric windows. Within the ranges, all materials have the reflectance for the sunlight and the emissivity based on the Planck's law, which are variable with the wavelength. These intrinsic properties are termed radiance spectra composed of reflectance and emissivity spectra.

As for rocks and minerals, reflectance and emissivity spectra differ with the kinds. Due to this property, discriminations of lithologies by combining and processing several band data of the earth-observation satellites have been widely carried out (e.g., Goetz & Rowan, 1981; Kruse et al., 1990). Assemblage of clay minerals such as alunite, sericite, montmorillonite, and kaolinite can be used as a good exploration index of metal deposits, because they are associated with hydrothermal alteration of rocks. Extraction of such assemblage from satellite images, which uses generally the absorption pattern of reflectance of clay minerals, is a typical analysis in satellite remote sensing (e.g., Rowan & Kahle, 1982; Crósta et al., 1998). Absorption of emissivity is also an important phenomenon. Emissivity in thermal infrared bands can be applied to discriminate lithologies (Crowley & Hook, 1996; Watson et al., 1996), and to estimate SiO_2 content (Ninomiya, 1995). As ground-truth data for satellite image interpretations, laboratory experiments for reflectance and emissivity spectra have been accumulated to construct spectral databases (Salisbury et al., 1994)

The main purposes of such conventional geologic remote sensing are identification of rocks and minerals. Due to this, the targets of laboratory spectral experiments have been restricted to standard geological samples. Reflectance and emissivity spectra must be variable with physical properties as well as particle sizes, but there are few researches on this topic. Remote sensing techniques have high potentiality applicable to various fields, not limited to geological identification. In their applications to engineering geology, weathering is one of the most important factors, which controls spatial and temporal changes of physical properties of rock masses. Charactering degree of weathering by remote sensing can contribute extraction of weakened portions of rock masses, estimation of hydraulic properties, and assessment of geologic hazards such as landslide and slope collapse.

For this purpose, we examine the influences of weathering upon reflectance and emissivity spectra of rock samples as a fundamental study. Three geologic types, granite, sandstone, and welded tuff, are used. Weathering indexes are defined using the spectra and then, validness of the indexes is evaluated by correlation analysis between the indexes and physical properties. An X-ray CT scan technique is applied to visualize inner structures of rock samples, and CT values, which are related to density of samples, are used as physical properties for the examination.

2 WEATHERING INDEXES USING REFLECTANCE AND EMISSIVITY SPECTRA

2.1 *Definition of indexes*

Two field spectrometers, FPR-2000 and μFT-IR, were used to obtain reflectance data within 0.485 to 2.5 μm and emissivity data within 8 to 14 μm, respectively, of rock samples. FPR-2000 cannot measure continuous spectra of reflectance, and number of band (wavelength range) is limited to 14. Although the reflectance spectra are discrete, the bands were selected to obtain important characteristics of the spectra. Figure 1 shows the outline of measurement systems.

Ferric ions, Fe^{2+} and Fe^{3+}, cause wide absorption in the ranges 0.4 to 0.6 μm and 0.8 to 1 μm. Clay minerals contain hydroxyl (OH) and water molecule (H_2O). Vibration of OH and bending of H_2O cause the strong absorption of reflectance at 1.4, 1.9, and 2.1 to 2.4 μm. The absorption at 1.4 μm is related to OH only. Accordingly, ferric oxide and clay minerals have specific reflectance spectra in the wavelength range 0.485 to 2.5 μm. There is also a remarkable absorption of emissivity in the range 8 to 14 μm, which is associated with the asymmetric vibration of Si-O-Si at 9 μm, and its symmetric vibration within 12 to 13 μm. These vibrations cause strong and weak absorptions of emissivity, respectively. The depth of absorption and the wavelength at which emissivity minimizes are known to be variable with silica content and crystal structures of silicates (three-dimensional, sheet, chain, and isolated tetrahedral structures).

To express definitely the absorption characteristics of reflectance and emissivity spectra related to weathering by considering the above physical mechanism, we define the four indexes as follows. Figure 2 shows the indexes schematically.

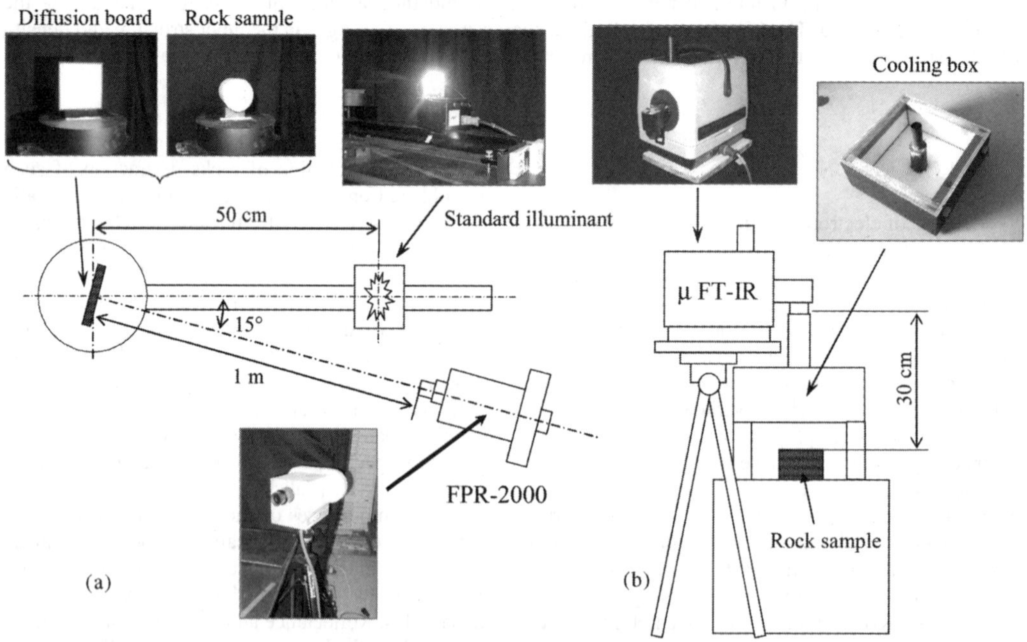

Figure 1. Outline of measurement systems composed of field portable spectrometers for obtaining (a) reflectance spectra and (b) emissivity spectra.

(1) I_{Fe}: an index for absorption depth of reflectance associated with occurrence and abundance of ferric oxide minerals. A line connecting the two reflectance data at 0.485 and 0.98 μm, which are located in the absorption wavelengths of ferric ions, is used as baseline. The difference between the baseline and the local maximum of reflectance at 0.74 or 0.83 μm is used to define I_{Fe}.

(2) I_{clay}: an index for absorption depth of reflectance associated with occurrence and abundance of clay minerals. Two baselines are set by connecting the reflectance data pairs at 1.4 and 1.9 μm, and 1.9 and 2.5 μm. The sum of differences between the baselines and the local maximums of reflectance at 1.64 and 2.06 μm is used to define I_{clay}. These local maximums may be specific to our measurement system as well as I_{Fe}, but the idea for defining the indexes is versatile.

(3) λ_{min}: the wavelength at which the emissivity takes the minimum. Importance of the wavelength is described above.

(4) $\Delta\varepsilon$: the difference between the maximum and minimum values of emissivity spectra. It is difficult to define these values, because the spectra oscillate finely. For this problem, smoothing of the spectra is adopted to obtain the $\Delta\varepsilon$ by fixing the location of λ_{min} (Fig. 2).

2.2 *Validation of the indexes*

To validate the four indexes, reflectance and emissivity spectra of coarse granite samples of the Hiroshima granite type were measured. Their degrees of weathering were evaluated by an X-ray CT scan method using the Toshiba Toscaner-23200 mini. Figure 3 shows the cross-sections of CT images of the samples, which indicates the degree of weathering increases in the order of sample number. In the CT image of No. 4 sample, the portions with small CT values are connected resulting from the leaching of constituent minerals along grain boundaries and cracks.

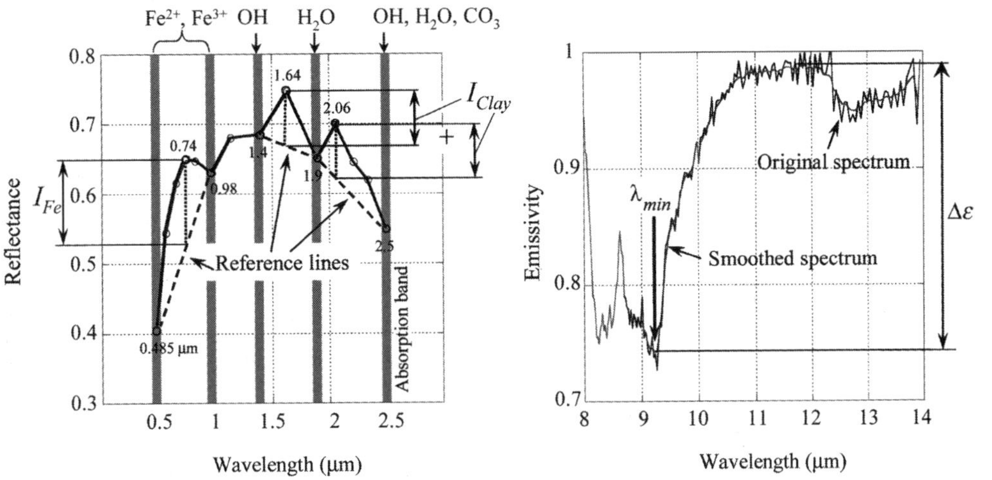

Figure 2. Schematic definitions of four indexes, I_{Fe}, I_{Clay}, λ_{min}, and $\Delta\varepsilon$, based on reflectance spectra and emissivity spectra to estimate weathering degree of rocks. Chemical components related to absorption of reflectance are shown in left figure.

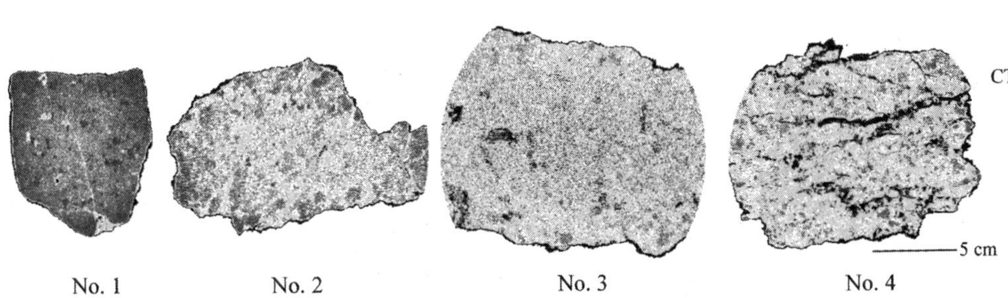

Figure 3. X-ray CT images of four granite samples of Hiroshima type.

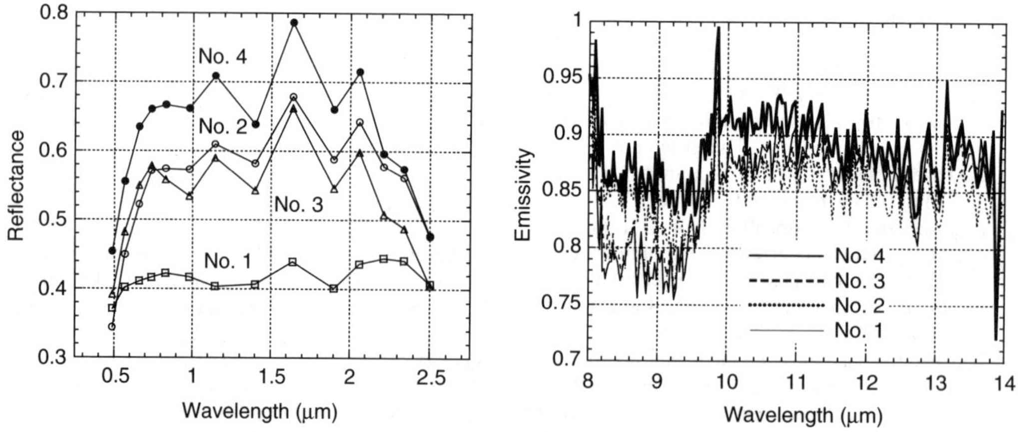

Figure 4. Reflectance and emissivity spectra of granite samples. Weathering degree increases from No.1 to No. 4 samples.

Table 1. Values of two reflectance indexes (I_{Fe} and I_{clay}) and two emissivity indexes (λ_{min} and $\Delta\varepsilon$) of granite samples shown in Figure 3.

Sample No. (weathering degree)	I_{Fe}	I_{clay}	λ_{min} (μm)	$\Delta\varepsilon$
1 (weak)	0.03	0.07	9.2	0.14
2 ↓	0.12	0.19	9.4	0.08
3	0.12	0.21	9.2	0.12
4 (strong)	0.11	0.26	9.6	0.10

Figure 4 shows the reflectance and emissivity spectra of the samples. It is obvious that the shapes of reflectance spectra are similar regardless of the degree of weathering. The absorptions of reflectance at 1.4 μm and 1.9 μm are deeper with increase of the weathering, which is caused by large amount of clay minerals. In fact, remarkable occurrence of montmorillonite and kaolinite were confirmed by the X-ray diffraction analysis. Similar to the reflectance spectra, the emissivity spectra of all the samples have similar shapes.

The four weathering indexes for the samples are summarized in Table 1. Although the difference of I_{Fe} is small except the No. 1 sample, the values of I_{clay}, λ_{min}, and $\Delta\varepsilon$ correspond generally with the degree of weathering. Among them, I_{clay} has high correlation. It can be confirmed, therefore, that the degree of weathering is expressed more or less in the indexes.

3 WEATHERING INDEXES AND PHYSICAL PROPERTIES USING TERRACE GRAVELS

3.1 *Relationship between CT values and geologic ages*

To understand relationship between degree of weathering and radiance spectra, we used terrace gravels in the Miyazaki Plain situated in west Kyushu, southwest Japan. Due to the interaction between the sea-level changes and the tectonic movements, there are several terraces with different geologic ages in the plain. The gravels are suitable to a weathering study, because their ages of emergence were determined by the tephrochronology (Nishiyama et al., 2001). They are classified into two lithologies, wacke sandstone with fine particles and welded tuff of acidic rocks. The sandstone originates from the Shimanto supergroup and consists mainly of quartz with a subordinate amount of plagioclase. For the measurement, samples of 105 sandstones and 31 welded tuffs were collected from the gravel bar of recent river floodplain and the 8 terrace deposits with geologic ages of 20, 40, 70, 90, 110, 120, 250, and 350 ka (1 ka means 1,000 years ago). It can be considered that weathered portions of the gravels were eroded in the process of transportation by waters and then, fresh portions only were remained.

By this mechanism, the age of emergence of terrace is regarded as the start of weathering process. Therefore, the above terrace geologic ages can be converted to the duration of weathering of the gravel samples.

The degrees of weathering of the samples were evaluated by the X-ray CT scan technique. Figure 5 shows representative samples and their CT images at different duration of weathering. A characteristic is detected from the CT images of sandstone samples in that the CT values are almost uniform in each sample. It signifies that the clay minerals, which are the main cementation materials between the particles, have been leached homogenously in the space with the time (Nihiyama et al., 2001). As for the welded tuff samples, the CT images show clearly the formation of weathering rinds in the samples of 90 ka. The rinds may have been associated with the front of chemical reactions such as oxidation.

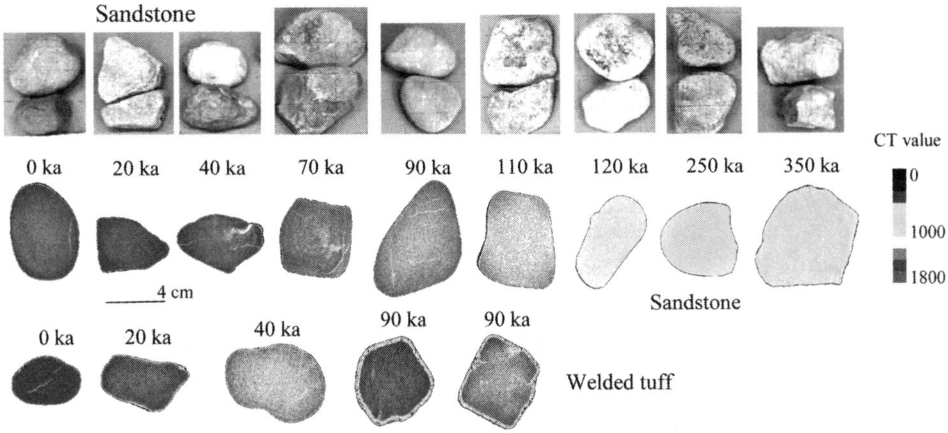

Figure 5. Photographs and X-ray CT images of selected terrace gravels of Shimanto sandstone and welded tuff with different geologic ages. Geologic ages are regarded as duration of weathering.

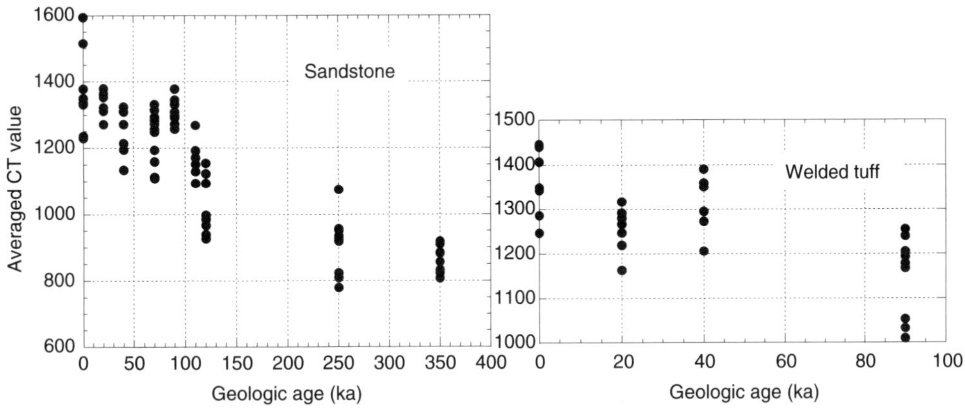

Figure 6. Relationship between averaged CT values and duration of weathering of sandstone and welded tuff samples.

Figure 6 represents the relationship between the duration of weathering and the averaged CT values of each sample. Although the CT values have range 200 to 400 at the same duration of weathering, a trend that the CT values decrease generally with the time is clearly seen. Another interesting feature is detected from the sandstone samples in that the CT values change abruptly between 110 and 120 ka. Based on the oxygen isotope stage, the time of 120 ka corresponds with the highest sea-level period during the last interglacial stage (Marine Oxygen Isotope Stage: MIS 5e). It can be considered that the weathering had proceeded rapidly due to such environment.

3.2 *Characteristics of reflectance spectra*

All the samples were measured for their reflectance spectra. Figure 7 shows the representative data at each duration of weathering.

As for the sandstone samples, the reflectance increases wholly with the time, and the increase of reflectance in the short-wave infrared region is larger than that in the visible to near infrared regions shorter than 1 μm. This corresponds to the characteristic detected from the granite samples (see Fig. 4). Another remarkable point is the deepener of reflectance absorption at 1.9 μm with the time. Absorption at 1.4 μm is not clear, which signifies the small content of the clay minerals with hydroxyl. Based on the X-ray diffraction, spectra of crystalline clay minerals such as montmorillonite and kaolinite were not detected even from the samples of 350 ka. Existence of goethite and hematite was confirmed from the diffraction analysis. These ferric minerals are considered to originate from ferrihydrite, which is amorphous hydration oxide with H_2O molecule (Torrent et al., 1982). Therefore, the absorption at 1.9 μm may be caused by the occurrence of ferrihydrite. Although the generation mechanism of

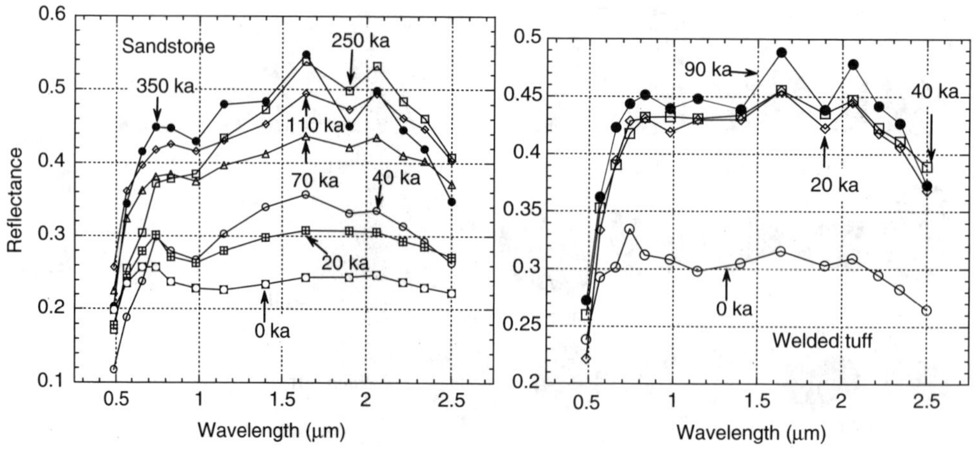

Figure 7. Typical reflectance spectra of sandstone and welded tuff samples with different duration of weathering.

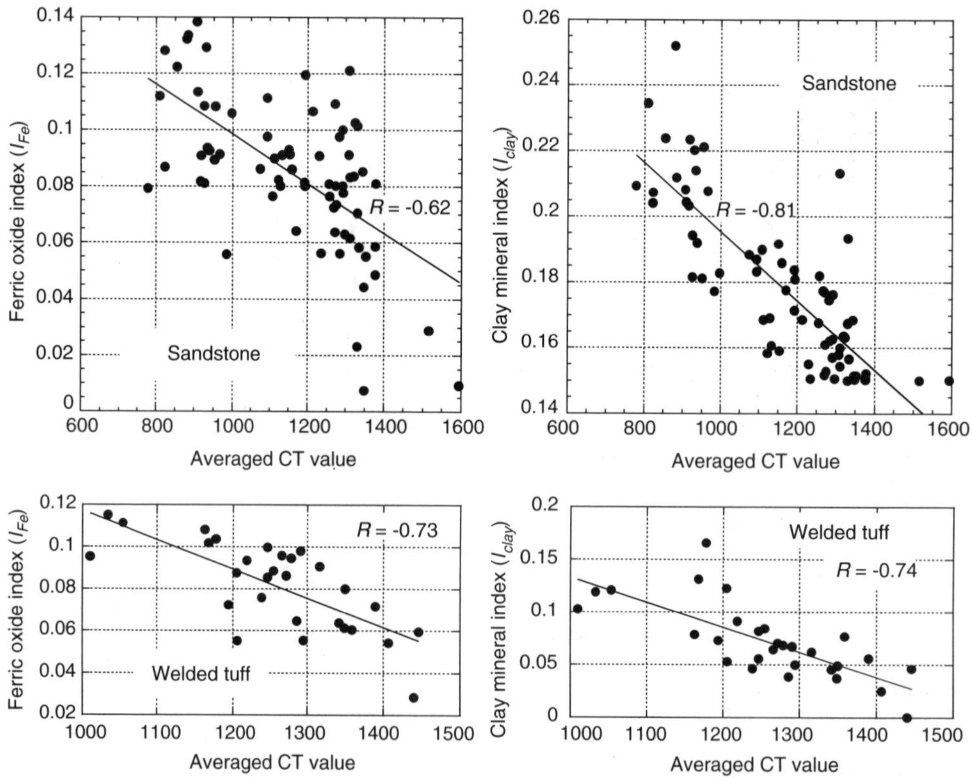

Figure 8. Relationship between averaged CT values and two reflectance indexes, I_{Fe} and I_{Clay}, of all sandstone and welded tuff samples with a regression line. R denotes correlation coefficient.

welded tuff is different from the sandstone, reflectance spectra and their temporal change are similar to those of the sandstone samples. For that reason, similarities of major minerals such as quartz and chemical components can be considered in both the sample types.

Relationships of I_{Fe} and I_{clay} with the averaged CT values are depicted in Figure 8. Both indexes tend to

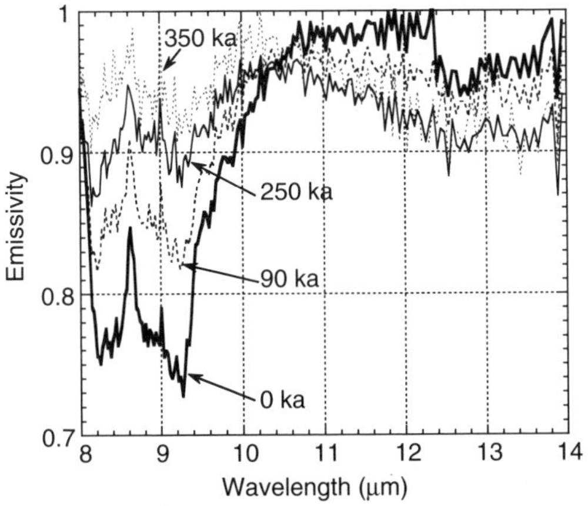

Figure 9. Typical emissivity spectra of sandstone samples with different duration of weathering.

decrease with the increase of the averaged CT values. The correlation is stronger in I_{clay} and the values of I_{Fe} are scattered for the sandstone, while the correlations are almost the same for the welded tuff. The sandstone samples of 350 ka are colored especially by red, which indicates the conspicuous occurrence of hematite. Hematite may cover the sample surfaces only and not be distributed uniformly inside the rocks. It can be inferred from Figure 8 that I_{Fe} is an index related to surface conditions and has weak correlation with physical properties of rocks.

3.3 *Characteristics of emissivity spectra*

The number of emissivity spectra data is smaller than the reflectance data, because some samples are too small to obtain accurate emissivity data. As similar to the reflectance spectra, representative spectra at each duration of weathering are selected from the sandstone samples whose number and duration range are much larger than the welded tuff samples, as shown in Figure 9. The emissivities in the range 8 to 10 μm increase with the progress of weathering, which is similar to the characteristic found by the granite samples (see Fig. 4). Another important feature is that λ_{min} is almost 9.2 μm and not variable with the duration for both the sandstone and welded tuff.

There is a relationship between the averaged CT values and $\Delta\varepsilon$ as indicated by the correlation coefficient 0.52, but such correlation is weak for the welded tuff samples (Fig. 10). The trend of the sandstone samples is similar to the graph (Fig. 11) which shows the relationship between $\Delta\varepsilon$ and the duration of weathering. The values of $\Delta\varepsilon$ decrease gradually with the time and have no discontinuous change around 120 ka. It is noted that the gradients of regression curve in the graph become larger with the decrease of duration.

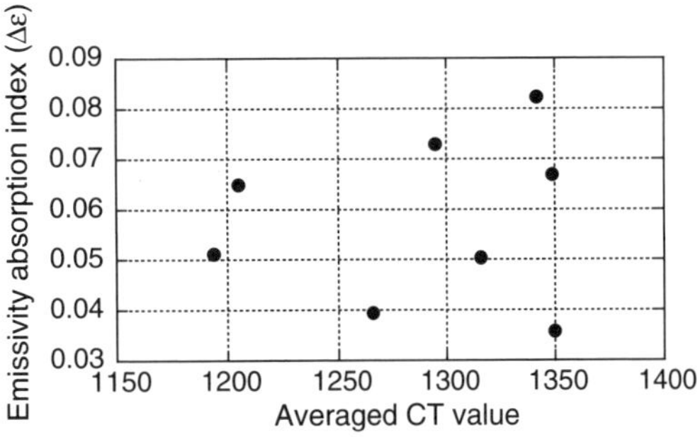

Figure 10. Relationship between emissivity absorption index, $\Delta\varepsilon$, and averaged CT values of the welded tuff samples.

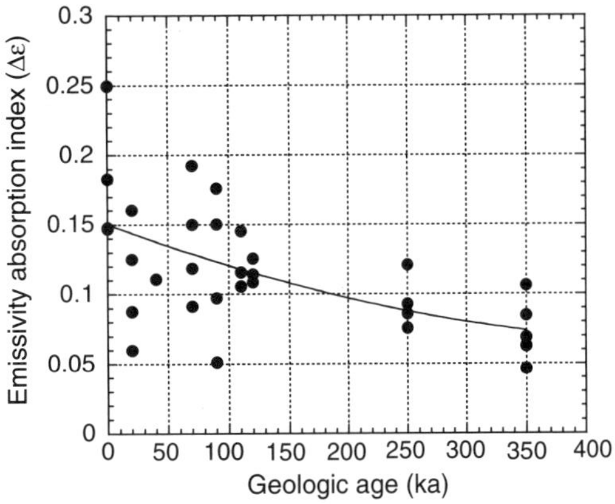

Figure 11. Relationship between emissivity absorption index, $\Delta\varepsilon$, and duration of weathering of sandstone samples.

Accordingly, the generation velocity of clay minerals is interpreted to have been large at the early stages of weathering and become gentle with the time.

4 DISCUSSIONS

An important characteristic was found by this study that the reflectance spectra increase with the progress of weathering, but the shapes of spectra do not change. One plausible reason is the increase of Rayleigh scattering intensity for electromagnetic waves. Enlargement of roughness of sample surface, which is associated with leaching of constituent minerals, can cause the increase of intensity. It has been well known that the reflectance increases with the decrease of mineral particle sizes (Crowley, 1986). Because such decrease makes the surface roughness larger, the above estimation is reasonable.

With progress of weathering, the existence of clay minerals is conspicuous in the reflectance spectra.

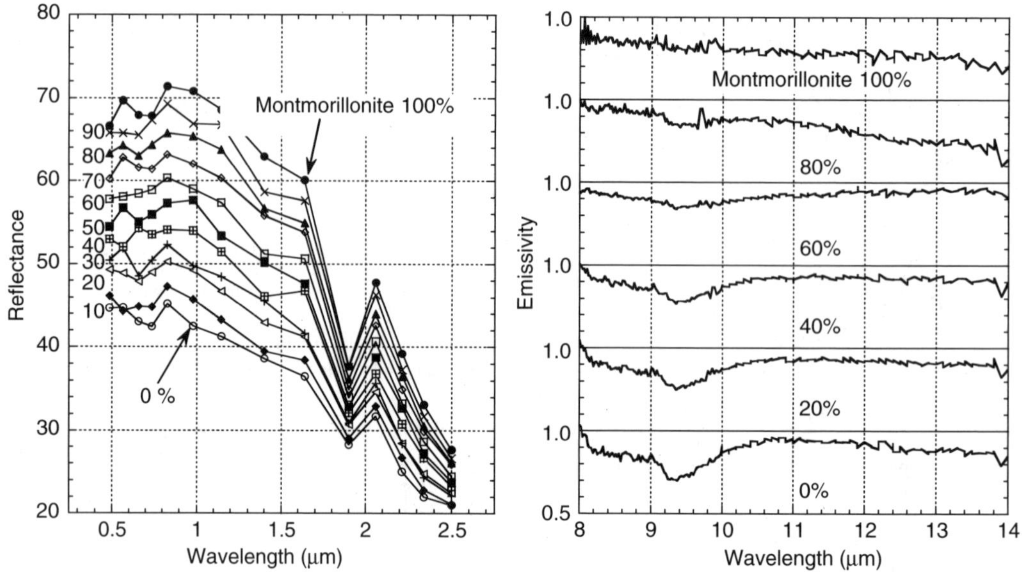

Figure 12. Changes of reflectance and emissivity spectra with different area ratio between granodiorite and montmorillonite.

Figure 12 represents change of reflectance spectra with mixture ratio of granodiorite and montmorillonite, which demonstrates that the absorption of reflectance at 1.9 μm becomes large with the increase of montmorillonite. This figure also indicates that the reflectance spectra are related to the conditions of sample surfaces. However, the CT values are volumetric physical quantities. A factor is required to connect surface and volume conditions and explain why I_{clay} has better correlation with physical properties than I_{Fe}.

Difference in spatial distributions between clay minerals and ferric oxide minerals can be one of the factors. Although clay minerals must be locally biased related to the distribution of initial minerals, the bias is small from a wide viewpoint and then distributions can be regarded to be uniform. Contrary to it, the distributions of ferric oxide minerals are limited to be near surfaces, because they originate from the reaching of Fe, which is contained in biotite and chlorite with small quantities, and precipitation and crystallization of Fe. The generation is controlled by oxidation-reduction potential. Therefore, the minerals may not be distributed uniformly in the volume.

Although the correlation with physical property is weak as compared to I_{clay}, $\Delta\varepsilon$ can also be used as an index for estimating degree of weathering. Figure 12 also shows change of emissivity spectra with mixture ratio. Because $\Delta\varepsilon$ decreases with increasing mixture ratio of montmorillonite, $\Delta\varepsilon$ is considered to be associated with content of clay minerals. This mechanism is the same as I_{clay}.

As for λ_{min}, distinct relationship between it and CT values was not found for the granite, sandstone, and welded tuff samples. A plausible reason is that these samples are composed mainly of quartz. Quartz is the mineral that has the strongest resistance against weathering. However, there is a special case in that λ_{min} is correlated well with physical properties as noted by Koike et al. (submitted). In the case where the connection strength of Si-O is decreased and crystallinity of quartz is weakened with progress of weathering, that correlation may occur.

5 CONCLUSION

As a fundamental step for application of remote sensing technique to engineering geology, we focused on the weathering that is one the most important phenomenon in this field, and examined the physical properties of rock samples and their radiance spectra. X-ray CT values were used for the physical properties. The main results obtained are as follows.

(1) CT images are useful to visualize inner structures of rocks associated with weathering and determine degree of weathering. For the lithologies of this study, the weathered granite samples showed channeling patterns that consist of small CT values; uniform distributions of CT values were observed in the sandstone samples; and the formations of weathering rinds were observed in the welded tuff samples. These differences originate from

constituent minerals, chemical compositions, and textures.

(2) The shapes of reflectance and emissivity spectra are similar regardless of the degrees of weathering of the samples. The reflectance spectra increase with the progress of weathering, which may result from the increase of Rayleigh scattering intensity associated with enlargement of roughness of sample surface.

(3) A reflectance index, I_{clay}, had the highest correlation with the physical properties among the four weathering indexes. Relatively uniform spatial distributions of clay minerals can be a reason for that. The distributions of ferric oxide minerals may be limited to be near surfaces due to the chemical properties of ferric ions. An emissivity index, $\Delta\varepsilon$, is also useful for estimating degree of weathering, because it is associated with content of clay minerals. Another emissivity index, λ_{min}, can be used only in the case where the connection strength of Si-O is decreased and crystallinity of quartz is weakened with progress of weathering.

REFERENCES

Crósta, A.P., Sabine, C. & Taranik, J.V. 1998. Hydrothermal alteration mapping at Bodie, California using AVIRIS hyperspectral data. *Remote Sensing Environ.* 65: 309–319.

Crowley, J.K. 1986. Visible and near-infrared spectra of carbonate rocks: reflectance variations related to petrographic texture and impurities. *J. Geophys. Res.* 91: 5001–5012.

Crowley, J.K. & Hook, S.J. 1996. Mapping playa evaporite minerals and associated sediments in Death Valley, California, with multispectral thermal images. *J. Geophys. Res.* 101: 643–660.

Goetz, A.F.H. & Rowan, L.C. 1981. Geologic remote sensing. *Science* 211: 781–791.

Koike, K., Yoshinaga, T., Mizukami, Y. & Nishiyama, K.; Weathering indexes of rock physical properties using reflectance and emissivity spectra. *J. Remote Sensing Society of Japan* (submitted).

Kruse, F.A., Kierein-Young, K.S. & Boardman, J.W. 1990. Mineral mapping at Cuprite, Nevada with a 63 channel imaging spectrometer. *Photogramm. Eng. Remote Sensing* 56: 83–92.

Ninomiya, Y. 1995. Quantitative estimation of SiO_2 content in igneous rocks using thermal infrared spectra with a neural network. *IEEE Trans. Geosci. Remote Sensing* 33: 684–691.

Nishiyama, K., Mizukami, Y., Koike, K. & Matsukura, Y. 2001. Temporal changes in pore structure of sandstone gravel due to weathering. *J. Japan Soc. Eng. Geol.* 42: 2–14.

Salisbury, J.W., Wald, A. & D'Aria, D.M. 1994. Thermal infrared remote sensing and Kirchhoff's law: I. Laboratory measurements. *J. Geophys. Res.* 99: 11897–11911.

Rowan, L.C. & Kahle, A.B. 1982. Evaluation of 0.46–2.36 μm multispectral scanner image of the East Tintic mining district, Utah for mapping hydrothermally altered rocks. *Econ. Geol.* 77: 441–452.

Torrent, J., Guzman, R. & Parra, M. 1982. Influence of relative humidity on the crystallization of Fe (III) oxides from ferrihydrite. *Clays and Clay Minerals*, 30: 337–340.

Watson, K., Rowan, L.C., Bowers, T.L., Anton-Pacheco, C., Gumiel, P. & Miller, S.H. 1996. Lithologic analysis from multispectral thermal infrared data of the alkalic rock complex at Iron Hill, Colorado. *Geophysics*, 61: 706–721.

X-ray CT for Geomaterials; Soils, Concrete, Rocks – Otani & Obara (eds.)
© 2004 Swets & Zeitlinger. Lisse, ISBN 90 5809 666 1

Preliminary results of X-ray micro-tomography applied in conservation and restoration of natural building stones

V. Cnudde & P. Jacobs
Department of Geology and Soil Science, Ghent University, Ghent, Belgium

ABSTRACT: X-ray micro-tomography (μCT) is a promising non-destructive imaging technique based on measurements of X-ray attenuation by opaque objects. This technique provides information on the internal structure of small samples with to date a maximum resolution of 10 μm for commercial systems (Skyscan 1072). Because μCT can be used to determine total porosity and pore-size distributions inside rock samples, it can be applied in the study of weathering and restoration phenomena occurring in natural building stones. In this first phase of investigation, μCT was tested out (i) to non-destructively determine porosity based on 3D-images, (ii) to visualise the presence of water repellents and consolidation products inside stone samples, (iii) to monitor the protective effects of these products during weathering in order to understand the underlying weathering mechanisms and (iv) to provide advise on the suitability of products for the treatment of a particular rock type. Maastricht limestone and Bray sandstone have been selected for this study because of their high porosity and their very pure mineralogical composition. Measurement results of treatments with consolidants and water repellents (with and without bromine doping) are demonstrated. Home-made software for image analysis of the 3D-reconstruction of the spatial distribution of these treatment products is presented.

1 INTRODUCTION

Every type of natural building stone has to deal with deterioration. Because of the increasing interest in preserving historic structures, a wide variety of water repellents and consolidants were developed in an attempt to minimise the rate of stone decay and to strengthen decayed stone. For the moment no single method has been found to be successful on all stone types and the knowledge of the medium and long-term performance of consolidants and water repellents is minimal, Young et al. (2003). The penetration depth of a treatment and the changes in porosity are two factors which can be involved in assessing the performance of any consolidant or water repellent treatment, Young et al. (2003).

During conservation and restoration procedures, porosity influences to a large extend the action of water repellents and consolidating products. Because pore size controls capillary action, water and other liquids can be differently absorbed on different stone types with different pore size distributions. The surface tension of a liquid, its viscosity and the pore size determine the weathering rate and the penetration depth inside a stone. The most important characteristics, that have an influence on liquid transport in a porous medium are porosity, numeric density, pore shape (size, length, volume, hydraulic radius and tortuosity) and pore connectivity, together called the "genus per unit volume", Perret et al. (1999).

The ability of stone consolidants to penetrate weathered stone is one of the main factors controlling their performance, Clifton (1980). When a consolidant penetrates the stone superficially, it tends to fill only the pores of the surface layers, thereby reducing its permeability. This might result in the accumulation of salt and moisture behind the treated layers, which could provoke extra tension inside the stone, thereby enhancing further decay. A good consolidant should penetrate the weathered stone to a depth to which all incoherent material is solidified and attached to the sound core of the stone, Torraca (1975). Determining the penetration depth of restoration products used to consolidate or to protect natural building stones from weathering is therefore crucial if the application of conservation products is planned. Existing test methods for measuring penetration depth are water droplet absorption time (only for water repellent treatments), visual observation of colour changes on wetting and drying (mainly for water repellent treatments), water vapour permeability and strength tests, Young et al. (2003). However, all these tests are very superficial and operate at another magnification level than X-ray micro-tomography (μCT). To assess this penetration depth and the effectiveness of a certain restoration product, μCT technology can be applied thanks to its non-destructive character.

Every type of natural building stone has its own petrophysical characteristics and each rock type reacts differently on the various restoration products available on the market. Porosity, a basic feature of a rock, is a measure for pore space and two types can be defined. Absolute porosity refers to the total void space, but as part of the porosity will reside within grains, effective porosity is more important, WTCB (1997). This effective porosity characterises the reservoir properties of a rock and together with permeability it also determines the ability of a stone to transmit fluids.

The porosity and pore size distribution of a stone can have a major effect on its durability, Clifton (1980). Therefore it can be harmful if a stone consolidant reduces the size of large pores, but does not completely close them.

Several methods exist to determine porosity. Each method like water absorption, mercury porosimetry, N_2-absorption and image analysis of microscopical thin sections, presents certain limits and disadvantages. By using water absorption, the total open porosity can be determined but no information is generated about the pore size distribution. Mercury porosimetry provides information about the total open porosity and gives an estimation of the pore size distribution, but due to the "ink-bottle-effect" it can overestimate the smallest pores and underestimates the bigger ones, Diamond (2000). Image analysis on thin sections adequately describes the pores in 2D, but necessitates stereology to calculate their position in 3D, DeHoff (2002), Wojnar (2002). When analysing thin sections, it has to be taken into account that the pore size distribution results determined in 2D should be handled with care. Because only 3D analysis is capable of producing precise information about internal structures of objects, μCT was used in this study.

2 EXPERIMENTS

2.1 *Materials*

2.1.1 *Stone*

For this study, porous local Belgian natural building stones with a pure (mono-)mineralogical composition have been selected. The sandstone of Bray, a quartz arenite of Upper-Landenian age (Palaeocene, Tertiary), was used for the construction of different important monuments in Binche, Bray, Aulne and Mons (Belgium). This sedimentary detrital stone is a continental deposit mainly consisting of quartz grains consolidated with siliceous cement, De Geyter & Nijs (1982). The Bray stones differ from other natural building stones from the Belgian Tertiary formations due to their higher hardness and SiO_2 content, their preponderant quartzitic texture and the absence of glauconite (Fig. 1).

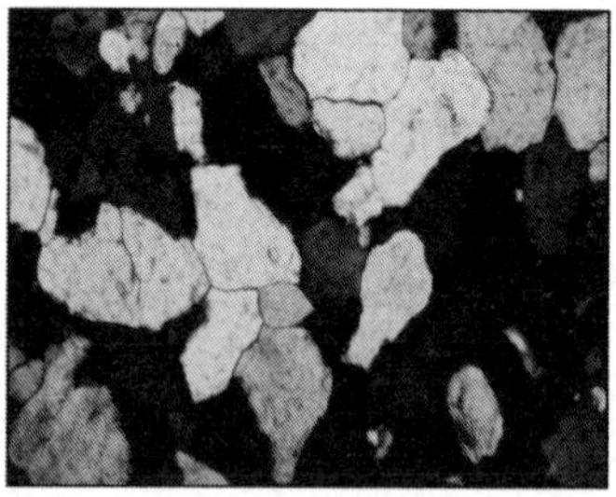

Figure 1. Sandstone of Bray (magnification 100×).

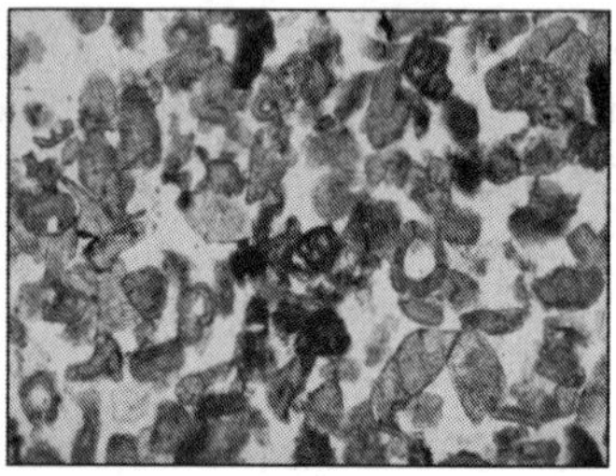

Figure 2. Limestone of Maastricht (magnification 100×).

The limestone of Maastricht is a yellow highly porous bioclastic limestone that can be found in Southern Limbourg (Belgium) and in the region of Maastricht (the Netherlands). In Sibbe (the Netherlands) the famous "Sibberstone" (Maastrichtian, Upper Cretaceous) is still excavated for use as a building material, Carchon (1986). Very characteristic for this soft and porous stone is the formation of a "calcin" which is a thin superficial greyish layer of recrystallised calcite and effectively protects the limestone against weathering, Nijs (1985). The limestone contains at least 90 to 98% of calcite and is mainly built up of microfossils. Unlike typical chalk, it lacks a real matrix, (Fig. 2). Because of the numerous sand-sized fossil fragments it displays a "sandy" touch.

2.1.2 *Water repellents and consolidants*

Because at present more than 90% of the water repellents consist of siloxane, WTCB (2002), a water repellent based on methylethoxypolysiloxane was used. Ethylsilicates were applied as consolidant, because it was reported that it guarantees the best results in consolidation, De Clercq et al. (1999), De Witte (1990) and WTCB (1981).

2.2 *Methods*

2.2.1 *X-ray micro-tomography (μCT)*

X-ray computer tomography (CT) has experienced spectacular developments in recent years, Jacobs et al. (1995). This technique revolutionised medical radiology by producing images of high accuracy and clinical detail. The X-ray micro-tomography (μCT) analysis are based on measurements of the attenuation of X-rays for different positions of an object, depending on the atomic number and the density of the object. It provides information about the internal structure and petrophysical properties of materials, with a maximum resolution of 10 μm for commercial systems (e.g. Skyscan 1072). Because μCT allows visualisation and measurement of complete 3D structures, it was tested on natural building stones in order to obtain more information on the properties of the stone's interior. This study was based on the determination of porosity and pore size distribution inside rock samples and on the visualisation of water repellents and consolidates applied on natural building stones.

For our measurements a "Skyscan 1072" micro-tomograph was used. This is a compact desktop system for X-ray microscopy and micro-tomography. In principle, it consists of the combination of an X-ray shadow microscopic system and a computer with tomographic reconstruction software. In order to obtain high-resolution images, small samples are preferred (cores of 8 mm diameter). X-ray source and detector are fixed while the sample rotates around a stable vertical axis. Samples were scanned at a voltage of 130 kV and current at 76 μA. A random movement of 10 with a 4-frame averaging was chosen to minimise noise. The X, Y spatial resolution was 10 μm with the same resolution on the Z axis. During acquisition, X-ray radiographs are recorded at different angles during step-wise rotation between 0° and 180° around the vertical axis.

The basic physical parameter quantified in each pixel of a CT-image is the linear attenuation coefficient μ. Beer's law relates the intensity (I) of X-ray photons passing through the object with thickness h, with the incoming intensity (I_o) and the attenuation coefficient (μ) of the object:

$$I/Io = e^{(-\mu h)} \qquad (1)$$

If several absorbing materials are presented, this relationship is summarised by:

$$I/Io = e^{-(\Sigma \mu_i h_i)} \qquad (2)$$

with index i referring to every type of material occurring in the X-ray beam. The linear attenuation coefficient μ depends on both electron density and atomic number Z:

$$\mu = \rho\,(a + bZ^{3,8}/E^{3,2}) \qquad (3)$$

where a represents the nearly energy-independent Klein-Nishina coefficient and b is a constant. The first term stands for the Compton scattering, predominant at X-ray energies above 100 kV (where the Skyscan 1072 frequently operates), while the second accounts for the photoelectric absorption, which is more important at energies below 100 kV, Jacobs et al. (1995).

2.2.2 *3D-software*

μCT images always contain a certain amount of noise. This noise can be reduced in two ways. The first one is to take care of all parameters that are responsible for the production of noise. Therefore random movement and frame averaging are applied during acquisition of data. The μCT operation procedure was optimised to produce the best images by reducing artefacts like beam hardening, ring, star and line artefacts as much as possible.

Beam hardening is the most frequently encountered artefact and causes the edges of an object to appear darker (thus denser) than the centre. This artefact is the result of the preferential attenuation of the lower-energy X-rays than higher-energy ones by the object. Because the μCT uses a polychromatic beam, the lower energy parts of the X-ray spectrum are preferentially attenuated when passing through an object, Ketcham & Carlson (2001). To reduce this artefact, an Al-filter is placed between the X-ray source and the object to absorb the low photon-energies before they reach the object.

Line artefacts are bright lines due to abnormally bright pixels in the sinogram. They are caused by cosmic rays or high energy X-rays that directly hit the detector, Van Geet (2001).

Very dense inclusions can create a secondary radiation resulting in star artefacts. Because this secondary radiation especially consists of low X-ray energies, the Al-filter also reduces these star artefacts.

Ring artefacts, which appear as circles centred on the rotation axis, are caused by detector inaccuracies. If a pixel continuously registers corrupt information, this will result in ring artefacts after reconstruction of the image. To minimise these, flat field corrections and a random movement is applied on the object, together with its active area on the detector, Van Geet (2001).

After acquisition, the images can be corrected by selecting tools in the reconstruction software specially designed to reduce beam hardening and ring artefacts.

The second way to reduce noise is to post-filter the image. The TELIN group (Image Processing) of the

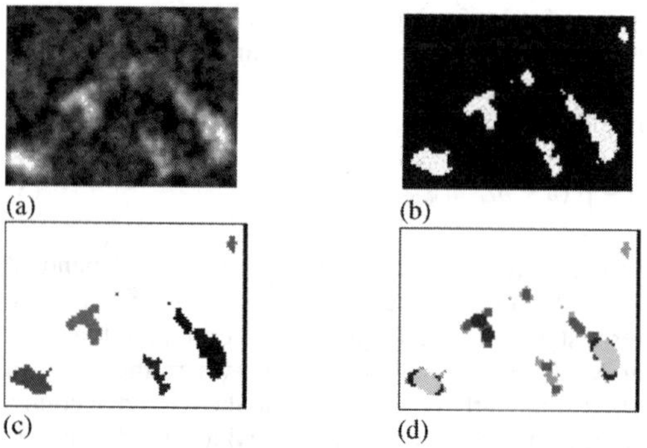

Figure 3. (a) Selected area inside an original image (1 pixel = 9 μm); (b) Segmented image by region growing; (c) Labelling of the different objects; (d) Maximum opening applied on the segmented image.

Ghent University (Faculty of Applied Sciences) developed filter techniques to reduce noise. As Poisson and Gaussian filter techniques produced rather limited results and filters based on Markov Random Fields and steerable filters ameliorated the image reconstruction results but without fundamentally influencing the histogram, it was therefore decided to focus on a performant segmentation technique that adequately deals with noise. Various segmentation methods exist to divide the image into material and pores. Image segmentation is the key to quantitative interpretation of image data, Soille (1999). Different thresholding methods can be used, like pre-selected values from a histogram and edge-based or region growing segmentations. Because the histogram of the μCT images never showed a bimodal distribution, a more complex segmentation technique was needed. As most image analysis programs operate in 2D, new software had to be developed to perform thresholding in 3D. With the help of 3D region growing, the grey-value images were converted into binary ones (Fig. 3a–b). The different objects were labelled, after which the 3D images were quantitatively interpreted. This enabled quantification of properties like maximum opening, pore volumes, neck determination and pore-size distribution (Fig. 3c). To determine the pore-size distribution, a morphological opening operator was used, Soille (1999). This mathematical morphological filtering is function of its structuring element's shape and recovers most structures lost by erosion (Fig. 3d). The principle consists in dilating the image that previously has been eroded using the same structuring element (SE). In theory, an isotropic SE must be used to ensure that measurements are equivalent in every direction of the 3D space, Pierret et al. (2002). In the home-made software a volume that approximates the shape of a sphere was thus used as SE to define a really isotropic filter. The opening of a network is a

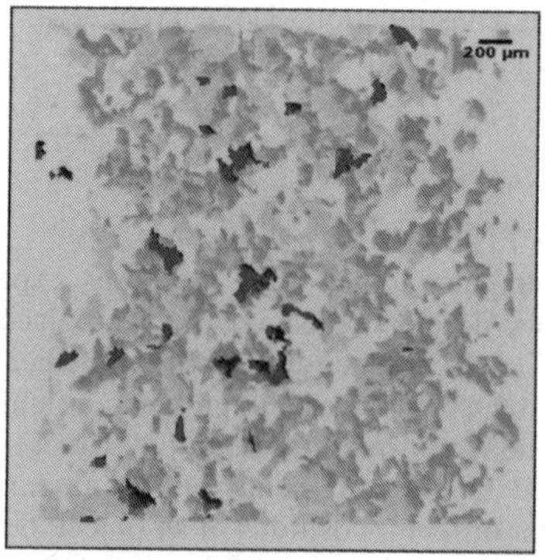

Figure 4. Selected volume inside sandstone sample B221, where the darkest grey stands for pores with maximum opening smaller or equal to 44 μm, medium grey for pores with a maximum opening between 62 μm and 80 μm and the lightest grey for pores with a maximum opening equal or larger than 98 μm.

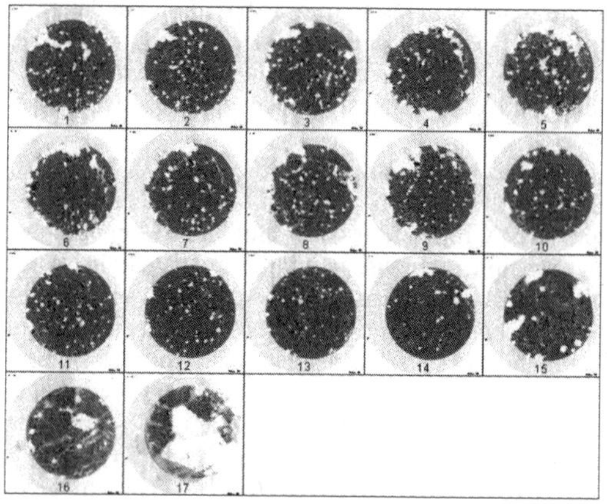

Figure 5. Cross-sections through consolidated crushed limestone.

relevant parameter for water absorption because it provides information about the maximum opening, which represents the largest "sphere" that can be included into a network. All selected objects are relabelled after determination of all their properties. This enables to select objects in 3D based on certain properties like maximum opening (Fig. 4).

2.2.3 *Visualisation of water repellents and consolidants*

On μCT images water repellents and consolidants tend to produce grey values similar to the stone's. Cross-sections of a consolidated crushed limestone image that the consolidant is very hard to localise inside the stone (Fig. 5). Only in cross-section 17 the consolidant is visible because of its high concentration. From the moment the consolidant envelopes the grains with a thin film, the consolidant is very difficult to separate from the grain itself. Because water repellents intend to form even thinner films than consolidants, doping will be necessary for their visualisation inside a stone sample.

3 RESULTS AND DISCUSSION

3.1 *Testing the software*

One of the major problems in this kind of research is reliability and validity of the results. Natural building stones can be very heterogeneous. It is therefore irrelevant to discuss the representativity of the pore research results obtained on such small samples. However, it is crucial to assure that pore measurement results reflect as close as possible reality, even in case of small samples. The newly developed software was therefore first tested on glass spheres and cylinders with a known diameter. Secondly small cylinders of stone samples that already underwent water absorption and mercury porosimetry were scanned.

Several glass spheres with different diameters ranging from 1000 μm to 75 μm were scanned. The glass spheres with diameters smaller than 150 μm showed more artefacts in the reconstructed images due to software limitations. Under the microscope as well as on the μCT images, it was clear that the small spheres were not perfectly spherical (Fig. 6).

The imperfect spherical shape renders a difference between the results of the maximum opening and the sieving results. Figure 7 illustrates the 3D image of glass spheres with a sieving diameter between 500 and 595 μm. The software determined a maximum opening of 460 μm for these glass spheres due to their imperfect spherical shape. This diameter is smaller than sieving results would suggest, but it can nevertheless be accepted as it is larger than the smallest sieve diameter of 420 μm. For the spheres between 149 μm and 177 μm, the software indicated a maximum diameter of 168 μm, Table 1.

For control, glass cylinders were scanned because of their more regular shapes (Fig. 8). The diameters of the tubes, 0,9 mm and 1,2 mm, were easily determined by the software.

The problem with the glass spheres and tubes is their regular shape and size, which do not correspond with the shape and size of the pores. The fact that glass spheres and tubes are composed of two phases, glass and air, makes thresholding of their images a lot

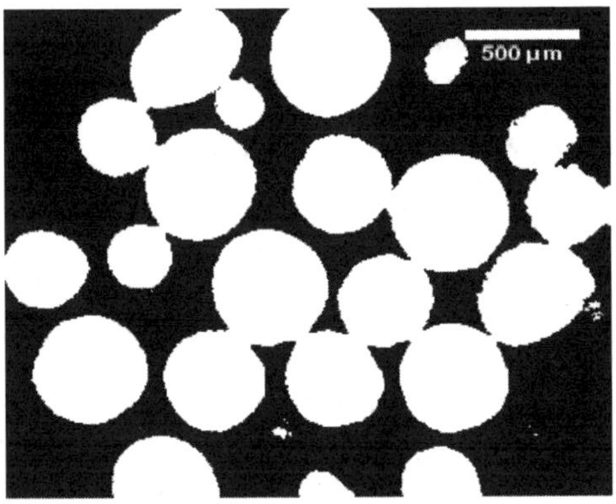

Figure 6. Thresholded cross-section of scanned glass spheres.

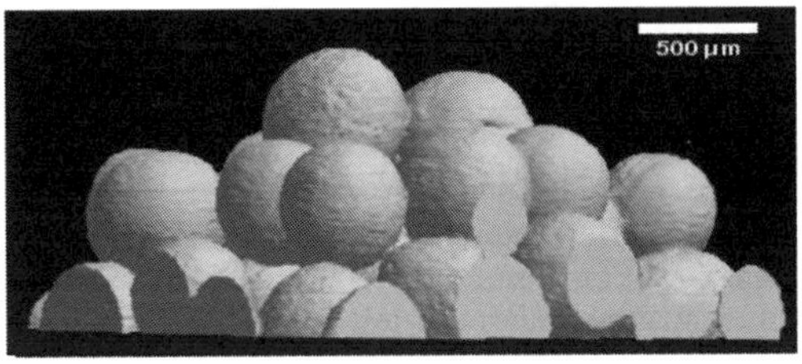

Figure 7. 3D image of scanned glass spheres (pixel size: 7.33 μm).

Table 1. Software results of sieved spheres.

Phi	mm	μm	Software (μm)
2.75	0.149	149	168
2.5	0.177	177	
2.25	0.21	210	
2	0.25	250	
1.75	0.297	297	
1.5	0.354	354	
1.25	0.42	420	
1	0.5	500	462
0.75	0.595	595	
0.5	0.707	707	
0.25	0.841	840	
0	1	1000	

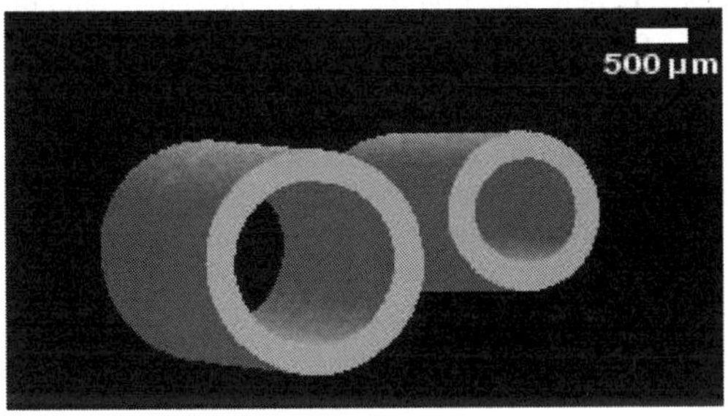

Figure 8. 3D image of scanned glass cylinders.

Table 2. Total porosity results of samples M285 and B6.

M285:
Total porosity determined by water absorption: 51.7%
Total porosity determined with mercury porosimetry: 50.71%

B6:
Total porosity determined by water absorption: 12.3%
Total porosity determined with mercury porosimetry: 11.2%

Total porosity determined on the μCT images with the newly developed software

Subsample M285	55%	B6a	14%
Subsample M285a	50%	B6b	20%
Subsample M285b	46%	B6c	17%
Subsample M285c	53%	B6d	16%
Subsample M285f	50%		
Average M285	51%	Average B6	17%

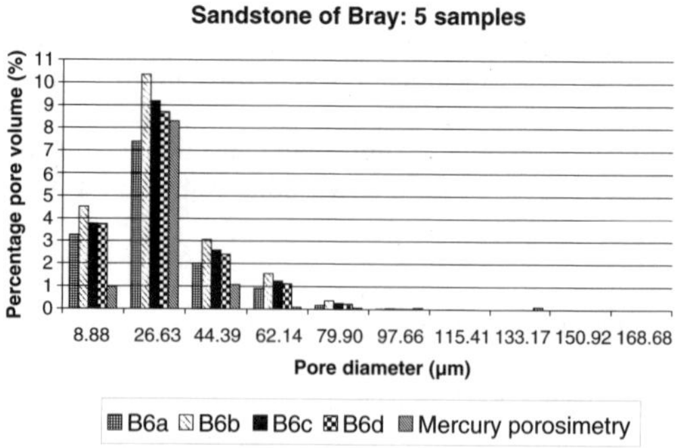

Figure 9. Results of pore-size distribution determined with mercury porosimetry on 1 sample and μCT image analysis on 4 subsamples all cut from the same large sample.

easier than for natural building stones, where the material is composed of several minerals generating different grey values. To test the software in more realistic conditions, sandstone and limestone samples were used. Samples were taken from a larger sample that first underwent water absorption and mercury porosimetry (part of the samples). Table 2 represents the measurement results for limestone sample M285 and for sandstone sample B6. Total porosity results determined through the different techniques showed to be very similar. Everything will depend on the way the μCT images are thresholded. For limestone, parameters for thresholding apparently provide similar results for porosity, but in the case of the sandstone samples the discrepancy between both porosity amounts is hereby a result of the choice of the thresholding parameters than anything else.

Because μCT does detect pores smaller than 10 μm, these results represent more an indication than an absolute correct value. Differences in results between water absorption, mercury porosimetry and μCT also depend on the different sizes of the examined samples. Because natural building stones can be very heterogeneous, they can show different results in porosity depending on the size of the sample and on the location where it was taken. Mercury porosimetry and analysis of μCT images generate different results for the pore size distribution (Fig. 9). This is logic as both techniques were applied on samples of different sizes and determine pore size in a completely different way based on different physical principles.

Mercury porosimetry bases its results on the fact that it considers the pores to be capillaries. Pore diameter is therefore calculated on basis of cylinders, while the software for the μCT images calculates the diameter based on spheres. To compare the accuracy of the results obtained by the different measurement techniques, the same sample should be investigated. Because mercury porosimetry and software operate on a completely different physical basis, results will be difficult to compare.

Both techniques have their own specific limitations. X-ray micro-tomography has its limits in resolution (actually around 10 μm) and μCT images will always contain a certain amount of noise. Mercury porosimetry deals only with the effective porosity. Moreover, the high pressure applied during measurement can create additional small pores. Due to the "ink-bottle-effect" it overestimates small pores and underestimates large pores, Diamond (2000) and Roels et al. (2000).

Another possibility to compare the software results is by microscopical thin section analysis. Even if a performant image analysis technique for thin sections could be applied, results will always be in 2D while μCT results are always in 3D. Stereological corrections could rectify the 2D results, but will remain an estimation. If several thin sections could be made consecutively, a stack of 2D images could create a 3D view. However it seems to be almost impossible and very time-consuming to produce a stack of 2D images obtained from equidistant thin sections. The only real solution would possibly consist in scanning reference material with known pore parameters.

3.2 *Visualisation of water repellents*

For the visualisation of the water repellents a bromosilane was mixed with a methylethoxypolysiloxane in a 1/2 ratio and applied on Bray sandstone with 14% porosity. The doped water repellent acts in the same way as the non-doped and was specially chosen to avoid chromatic separation. Because bromine has a higher atomic number, incident X-rays are better attenuated and make the hydrofuge more visible. By doping the water repellents, better attenuation was achieved and

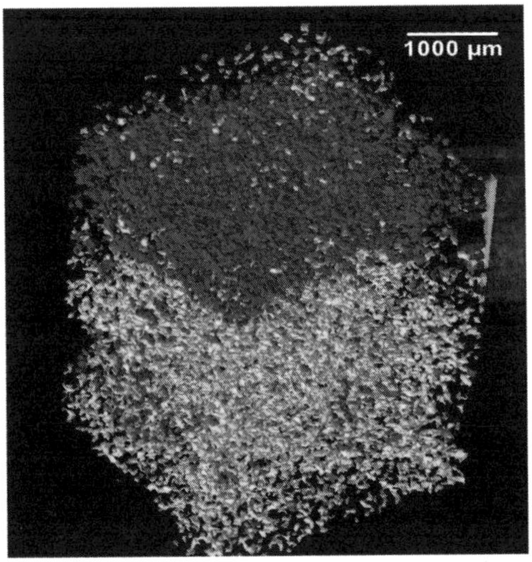

Figure 10. Visualisation of a water repellent (dark) in the sandstone of Bray.

a clear visualisation of the location of the products could be obtained (Fig. 10).

Cross-sections 1 to 12 (Fig. 11) of the Bray sandstone treated with a doped hydrofuge show the presence of the hydrofuge as a dark colour. With this method it is possible to determine the impregnation depth of the hydrofuge and its exact localisation. Scanning the sample with the doped product showed that the siloxane did not penetrate into the lower parts, while it was obviously present in the upper sample parts. Figure 12a shows a cross-section of the lower part of the sample, while Figure 12b displays a cross-section in the upper part. In both images black represents pores while white stands for doped product. In this case the product completely filled parts of the pore network. These results indicate that it is possible with μCT to verify if a water repellent or similar product could block pores or not. These results were confirmed by microscopical research, which indicated that certain pores where indeed completely filled with the hydrofuge.

A 3D reconstruction clearly visualises the presence of the doped product inside the natural building stone (Fig. 12).

When doped hydrofuge was applied on the Maastricht limestone, which has a much higher porosity, the hydrofuge seemed to be absorbed by the whole sample rendering it in general darker on the cross-sections. Another way of solving the visualisation problem is increasing the object thickness h (Beer's law). But due to size limitations for the object within the X-ray tomograph chamber, this second method could not be used.

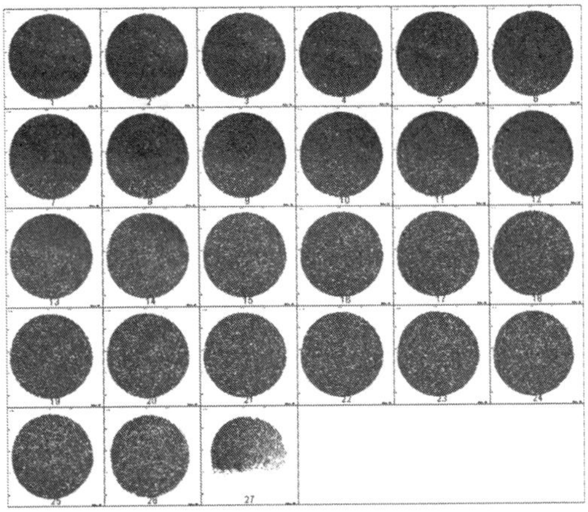

Figure 11. Cross-sections of Bray sandstone treated with doped hydrofuge.

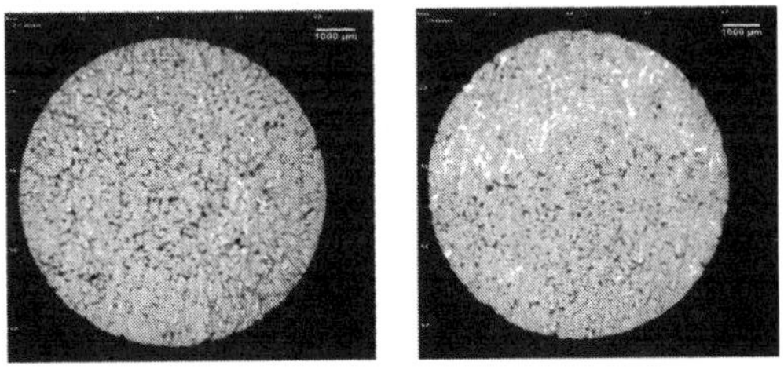

(a) (b)

Figure 12. (a) Cross-section of the lower part inside a Bray sandstone sample where no product occurs (b) Cross-section of the upper part inside the same sandstone sample where water repellent does occur (white colouring).

3.3 *Changes in porosity due to consolidation*

For the visualisation of the consolidant (a tetraethylsilicate), a bromo-silane was mixed with the methyl-ethoxypolysiloxane in a 1/4 ratio and applied on very porous Maastricht limestone. The limestone was scanned before and after treatment. Because the consolidant could spread over the whole sample in a thin film, in general cross-sections coloured darker. The software detected changes in total porosity and partial porosity due to consolidation. μCT scanning indicated a total porosity of 39.6% after consolidation, which was 6.4% lower than initially. The results of the partial porosimetry indicate that the upper part of the sample (Fig. 13, volume No. 0–100) had an average porosity of 47% before treatment while the bottom showed an average porosity of 42%, which is 5% lower. After applying the consolidant on top of the sample, the porosity in the top dropped down to 39%. The average porosity of the bottom was 37%, so only 2% lower than the upper part. These results suggest that the consolidant had an influence on the porosity

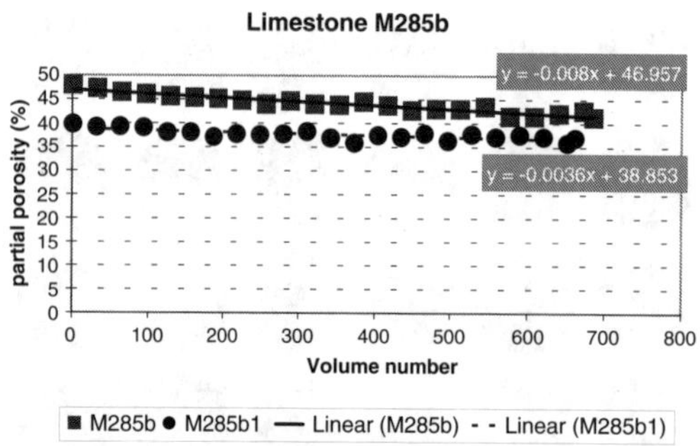

Figure 13. Partial porosity results of a Maastricht limestone sample before and after treatment with consolidant.

of the whole sample, which was not higher than 2 cm. This was confirmed in the research of De Clercq et al. (1998), where ethyl-silicate showed to have a large impregnation depth and tends to spread more equally over the sample instead of concentrating at the top. In the region where the consolidant was applied, porosity values were more reduced than in other areas of the sample.

These results also indicate that the consolidant did not just concentrate on the upper part of the sample, which could be harmful during further weathering. For other samples similar results were obtained. Future research will be carried out to determine the influence of several consolidation treatments on porosity.

4 CONCLUSION

Due to its non-destructive character and its resolution down to porosity scale, the technology of μCT offers a large potential of application. Further studies need to be carried out, but the first results show a promising future for the μCT-technique. Its 3D visualisation capacity offers the big advantage that further non-destructive profound investigation can be accomplished, which could provide new insights to optimize conservation and restoration techniques of building materials.

μCT in combination with our new developed 3D-software makes it possible to determine porosity and pore-size changes due to external factors like consolidation or weathering. The impregnation depth of different types of consolidants into different types of natural building stones can be studied. Questions whether it is better to apply a consolidant several times or one application is sufficient, will most probably be answered. More tests will be carried out in order to monitor the influences of water repellents and consolidants on stones when submitted to all kinds of weathering forms.

REFERENCES

Carchon, P. 1986. Petrografie van de kalkstenen van het Krijt van Maastricht. Unpublished licentiate thesis UGent, Faculty of Sciences.

Clifton, J.R. 1980. Stone Consolidating Materials – A Status Report. Center for Building Technology, National Engineering Laboratory, National Bureau of Standards, NBS technical note 1118. Washington: Dept. of Commerce, National Bureau of Standards.

De Clercq, H., De Witte, E., De Bruyn, R. & Pien, A. 1998. Restauratie van buitenmuren. WTCB-Tijdschrift, herfst 1998.

De Clercq, H., De Witte, E., De Bruyn, R. & Pien, A. 1999. Restauratie van buitenmuren, steenversteviging. WTCB-tijdschrift, herfst 1999: 3–10.

De Geyter, G. & Nijs, R. 1982. Petrografisch onderzoek van natuurlijke bouwstenen uit Belgische Tertiaire formaties. Het kwartsiet van Tienen (Formatie van Landen). Natuurwetenschappelijk Tijdschrift 64: 41–59. Gent, 1982.

De Witte, E. 1990. Natuursteen in de monumentenzorg: vervangen of conserveren? Bulletin de la Société belge de Géologie, 99-2: 197–205, Brussel.

DeHoff, R.T. 2000. Probes, population, samples, measurements and relations in stereology. Images Analysis and Stereology 19: 1–8.

Diamond, S. 2000. Mercury porosimetry – An inappropriate method for the measurement of pore size distributions in cement-based materials. Cement and Concrete Research, 30: 1517–1525.

Jacobs, P., Sevens, E. & Kunnen, M. 1995. Principles of computerised X-ray tomography and applications to building materials. The Science of the Total Environment 167: 161–170.

Ketcham, R.A. & Carlson, W.D. 2001. Acquisition, optimization and interpretation of X-ray computed tomographic imagery: applications to the geoscience. Computers & Geosciences, Vol. 27 (4): 381–400. Elsevier Science Ltd.

Ministerie van het Waalse Gewest 1996. Pierres à bâtir traditionnelles de la Wallonie. Manuel de terrain.

Nijs, R. 1985. Petrographical characterization of calcareous building stones in Northern Belgium. Vth International Congress on Deterioration and Conservation of Stone, Lausanne, 25-27.9.1985: 13–21.

Perret, J., Prasher, S.O., Kantzas, A. & Langford, C. 1999. Three-dimensional quantification of macropore networks in undisturbed soil cores. Soil Science Society of America Journal 63: 1530–1543.

Pierret, A., Capowiez, Y., Belzunces, L. & Moran, C.J. 2002. 3D reconstruction and quantification of macropores using X-ray computed tomography and image analysis. Geoderma, 106, 3–4: 247–271.

Price, C. 1996. Stone Conservation. An Overview of Current Research. The Getty Conservation Institute, Los Angeles, 73 pp.

Roels, S., Elsen, J., Carmeliet, J. & Hens, H. 2000. Characterisation of pore structure by combining mercury porosimetry and micrography. Materials and Structures 34: 76–82.

Soille, P. 1999. Morphological image analysis. Principals and applications. Berlin, Heidelberg: Springer-Verlag.

Torraca, G. 1976. Brick, Adobe, Stone and Architectural Ceramics: Deterioration Processes and Conservation Practices. In: Preservation and Conservation: Principles and Practices: 95–97. The Preservation Press, Washington, D.C.

Van Geet, M. 2001. Optimisation of microfocus X-ray computer tomography for geological research with special emphasis on coal components (macerals) and fractures (cleats) characterisation. Unpublished PhD, KULeuven.

Wojnar, L. 2002. Stereology from one of all the possible angles. Images Analysis and Stereology 21: 1–11.

WTCB Technische Voorlichting 138: De siliciumsamenstellingen. Vochtwerende produkten in de massa en op de oppervlakte. Konsolidatiemiddelen. Kitten. September 1981.

WTCB Technische Voorlichting 205: Natuursteen. September 1997.

WTCB Technische Voorlichting 224: Waterwerende oppervlaktebehandeling. June 2002.

Young, M.E., Cordiner, P., Murray, M. 2003. Chemical consolidants and water repellents for sandstones in Scotland. Historic Scotland Research Report pp. 266, ISBN 1-903570-20-4.

X-ray CT for Geomaterials; Soils, Concrete, Rocks – Otani & Obara (eds.)
© 2004 Swets & Zeitlinger. Lisse, ISBN 90 5809 666 1

Characterization of asphalt concrete using X-ray tomography

L. Wang
Louisiana State University/Southern University, Baton Rouge, USA

ABSTRACT: X-ray computerized tomography (XCT) has been widely used in the characterization of asphalt concrete in the last five years. This paper reviews the state-of-the-art development using XCT in the characterization, modeling and simulation of asphalt concrete.

1 INTRODUCTION

X-ray Computerized Tomography (XCT) is a powerful tool for nondestructive evaluation of the microstructure of materials. It was invented for use in medical diagnosis. Since the very beginning of its invention, researchers in civil engineering started applying it in the characterization of soil-water systems, rock, and cement concrete. However, only in the last five years, has it been widely used in the characterization of asphalt concrete. This paper reviews the applications of XCT in the characterization, modeling and simulation of asphalt concrete.

Use of XCT in characterizing aggregates and asphalt mixture started about five years ago [Shashidhar, 1999]. XCT systems used in these applications usually have a large penetrating capability, and high resolution up to 5–10 micrometers. It has many advantages over optical imaging. Although it is still quite expensive at present stage, there are three systems in the United States that are mainly dedicated to the study of aggregates, asphalt concrete, cement concrete and soils. Compared with other methods to image the microstructure of asphalt concrete, XCT has quite a few advantages including the ability to acquire 3D data set, no need for sample preparation, and non-destruction to suit unique requirements of asphalt core analysis. The review will focus on how XCT is applied to the characterization of aggregates, the internal structure of asphalt concrete, and computational simulation of mixture properties using the microstructures characterized from XCT.

2 APPLICATIONS IN CHARACTERIZATION

2.1 *Aggregate characterization*

The characterization of shape, angularity and texture of aggregates is an important research area. By using XCT, true 3D characteristics can be quantified. Using XCT and digital image analysis, the X,Y and Z coordinates of the surface points on an aggregate particle can be abstracted and represented. With this information, the lengths in different orientations can be computed to perform multiple ratio analysis; the surface area can be accurately calculated [Wang, 1998; Wang and Frost, 2003d]; the mass momentums can be also computed for performing DEM simulation [Wang et al, 2003f]; and the volume and surface area can be used to define shape factors [Wang et al, 2002a; Garboczi, 2002]. In addition, the quantities obtained from the 3D dataset can also be used to correlate and verify quantities obtained through 2D datasets [Wang et al, 2002a]. Surface coordinates represent the surface irregularity and can be used to quantify roughness and texture using either Fourier analysis [Wang et al, 1997; Garboczi, 2002; Wang et al, 2003g] or wavelet analysis [Kim et al, 2002]. XCT can also be used for evaluating gradation effects of aggregates on such as Volume in Mineral Aggregates (VMA) and particle orientation distribution etc.

2.2 *Mixture characterization*

The property of asphalt concrete is very complicated: binder is much stiffer at lower temperature than at higher temperature. Thereby, asphalt concrete demonstrates a duality in properties: loads are mainly transmitted through the particle skeleton at higher temperature to demonstrate its granular behavior but transmitted through both particle contacts and binder at lower temperature to demonstrate its continuum behavior. By the skeleton view, the average number of contacts for coarse aggregates, the contact normal distribution, the branch vector distribution, and the particle orientation distribution are relevant. By the continuum view, mean solid path, the air void surface area, the damage tensor, and the local void volume fraction and its gradient are relevant. The quantification of the parameters in the skeleton view usually requires block 3D datasets. The quantification of the parameters in the continuum scheme can make use of the stereology methods [Kanatani, 1984a, 1984b, 1985] by using few sectional dataset.

2.2.1 *Void area fraction and damage tensor*

Voids do not transfer load and can be considered as inherent damage although a certain amount of voids is needed to avoid bleeding. Its effect on mechanical properties can be illustrated by the effective stress concept. Equations (1) and (2) represent the definitions of nominal stress and effective stress.

$$\sigma_n = \frac{F}{A} \tag{1}$$

$$\sigma_e = \frac{F}{A - A_v} = \frac{F}{A}\frac{1}{1-\varphi} = \sigma_n \frac{1}{1-\varphi} \tag{2}$$

Where F is the total force applied normal to a cross-section, A is the cross-section area, A_v is the area of air voids contained in A, σ_n is the nominal normal stress, σ_e is the effective stress and φ is the areal fraction of voids ($\varphi = A_v/A$, in continuum damage mechanics, this parameter is named as damage scalar and the effective stress dominates the deformation). The area fraction usually varies with orientations and can be represented by a second order fabric tensor.

By stereology principles [DeHoff and Rhines, 1968; Underwood, 1970], the average of the areal fractions of voids in different orientations is equal to the void volume fraction or air void content. However, engineering practice indicates that the distribution of the void is also important. X-ray tomography imaging can be used to determine not only the total air void content but also the void content inhomogeneity and anisotropic distribution. Using stereology and virtual cutting techniques, Wang et al [Wang et al, 2002b] quantified the damage scalar and damage tensor and the effective damage defined in [Murakami, 1988; Voyiadjis and Katta, 1999] and related these quantities to mixture performance for the mixes of the WesTrack project [Epps et al, 1997]. They have demonstrated that these parameters have good correlation with performance.

In addition to the total air void content, the shape, the size distribution, the void connectivity, and the spacing among voids are also important to mixture properties according to mechanics principles. Interested readers are refered to the cited reference in this section and [Wang et al, 2001a; Wang et al, 2003e]. The following addresses these parameters separately.

2.2.2 *Specific void surface area (damaged surface area) and aggregate surface area*

The specific void surface area and/or damaged surface area (area per unit volume) is an overall evaluation of the severity of the damaged continuum (i.e. the level of fracture, fatigue cracking etc.). Generally speaking, the distribution of the void/damaged surface areas around the orientations is not uniform. If the distribution can be approximated by a second order fabric tensor, the distribution may be represented as:

$$S(n) = \frac{S_v}{4\pi}(1 + S_{ij}n_i n_j) \tag{3}$$

where $S(n)$ is the distribution density function of the specific void or damaged surface area, n is the unit normal to a unit sphere, and n_i and n_j are the directional cosines. S_v is the specific damaged surface area. S_{ij} is the second order fabric tensor representing the orientational variation of the distribution.

In brief, the distribution function has two parameters: the specific damaged surface area S_v and its anisotropic characteristics represented as the fabric tensor S_{ij} [Wang et al, 2001a; Wang et al, 2002b]. If aggregate surfaces are used, the method can also quantify the total surface areas of the aggregates and its orientational distribution, which is related to the concept of surface energy [Cheng et al, 2002].

2.2.3 *Average size and the shape tensor of the defects*

If an elliptical void is embedded in a continuum subjected to far field uniform tension (in 2D), the stress at the void edge varies with orientations. The ratio between the largest stress and the far field stress is named Stress Concentration Factor (S_c see Equation (4)).

$$S_c = (1 + 2\frac{b}{a}) \tag{4}$$

Where a and b are the lengths of the semi-axis of the ellipsis.

Equation (4) indicates that the stress concentration factor is related to the shape and orientation of the ellipsis. Wang et al [2002b] defined the overall shape of many voids in a tensorial format in Equation (5).

$$\delta(n) = \delta(1 + \delta_{ij}n_i n_j) \tag{5}$$

Where $\delta(n)$ represents the average length of the intersecting lines over all the voids/defects in orientation n; δ_{ij} is the shape tensor and δ is the average size of all the voids/defects over all the orientations. The average size is also important factor: a large void will more likely induce larger localization of strains and may cause local instability, which may propagate.

2.2.4 *Mean solid path*

When two cavities are far away, their interaction is negligible. However, when two cavities are close they will interact with each other to further weaken the material. The spacing among the two voids is an indication of the strength of interaction and is an important parameter [Lacy et al, 1997; Lacy et al, 1999]. As the distribution of the average spacing among the voids and/or damaged surfaces is usually not isotropic, tensors are needed to represent these distributions. Equation (6) represents the case where the anisotropy of the distribution can be represented by a second order fabric tensor.

$$\lambda(n) = \lambda(1 + \lambda_{ij} n_i n_j) \tag{6}$$

where $\lambda(n)$ is a function representing the orientational variations of the mean solid path among the damaged surfaces; n is the unit normal to a unit sphere; and n_i and n_j are the directional cosines. λ is the mean solid path in all orientations among the voids/damaged surfaces. It can be obtained by placing test lines in different orientations and measuring the spacing among the cracked surfaces in different orientations and averaging them [Kuo et al, 1998]. λ_{ij} is the second order mean solid path tensor representing the orientational variations of the mean solid path. An example application to the WesTrack project indicates that ranking by this perimeter (λ) is consistent with the field performance of the three mixes of the project.

2.2.5 *Spacing-size ratio*

The spacing between voids/defects and the size of the voids/defects are important variables in non-local damage theories. Chudnovsky et al [1987a, 1987b] developed a simple model addressing the interaction of two cracks, in which the two important model parameters are the spacing between the two crack tips and the sizes of the cracks. Based on this theory, Wang et al [2002b] quantified the ratio of λ/δ for the three mixes of the WesTrack project and obtained a good correlation between λ/δ and the mixture performance.

2.2.6 *Local void volume fraction and its gradient*

In addition to the quantities reviewed in the previous sections, the spatial distribution of voids may be characterized by the local volume fraction of voids/defects (γ) and its spatial gradients ($grad\phi$). There are several theories including continuum mixture theory [Green and Naghdi, 1967; Goodman and Cowin, 1972; Arduino, 1996; Krishnan and Rao, 2000; Krishnan and Rao, 2001], material force mechanics [Maugin, 1993], and micro-mechanics [Nemat-Nasser, 1999] that relate the local volume fractions of the constituents and the mechanical properties of the mixture.

Wang et al [2003a] developed a method to quantify the local void volume fraction and its gradient and related them to stress analysis in the mixture theory scheme [Wang et al, 2003b]. This study indicated that local void volume fraction and its gradient may serve as a performance related internal variable in mixture constitutive modeling.

2.2.7 *Skeleton view of the mixture*

In the skeleton view of the mixture, the average number of contacts per particle of coarse aggregates, the contact normal distribution (number of contacts in different orientations), the branch vector distribution (number of branch vectors in different orientations), and the particle orientation distribution (number of particles with their particle orientations in certain range) are important parameters. These parameters have been shown to be related to the strength and deformation of granular materials. They have been used in micromechanics [Chrisoffersen et al, 1981; Chang and Ma, 1991; Rothenburg and Bathurst, 1992], doublet mechanics [Granik and Ferrari, 1993; Ferrari et al, 1997], and Distinct Element Method (DEM) [Cundall and Strack, 1979].

Wang et al [2001b] used branch vector distribution to approach the contact normal distribution using three-subspace sampling. Recently, Wang et al [2003c], by reconstructing each individual particle, and detecting the contacts between the particles, came up with an accurate quantification method. The distribution is represented as a fabric tensor through minimizing the differences between the tensorial evaluations and the actually observed data [Wang, 2003e].

3 APPLICATIONS IN COMPUTATIONAL SIMULATION

Three typical computational simulation techniques include the Finite Element Method (FEM), the Distinct Element Method (DEM) and the Boundary Element Method (BEM). These three methods have been all applied to simulate the properties of asphalt concrete. Chang and Meegoda [1999] developed a DEM program to incorporate viscoelastic contacts; Buttlar and You [2001] applied DEM and imaging techniques to model also the irregular shape of the aggregates but on a 2D structure. Most recently, Fu and Wang [2003] developed a new method to use X-ray tomography imaging and a clump technique to represent the true 3D particle shape for DEM simulation. It is anticipated that DEM will find more and realistical applications when better contact models and real particle shapes and roughness can be incorporated.

3D FEM simulation of asphalt concrete properties using X-ray tomography imaging was achieved by Wang et al [1999]. Masad et al [2001] have used FEM and 2D images to evaluate the strains and the properties of asphalt concrete. Papagiannakis et al [2002] also incorporates the viscoelastic properties of the binder into the simulation for a 2D and two-phase case. Sadd et al [2003] developed a method to approximate aggregates as ellipsis and developed a contact model to simulate indirect tensile test for asphalt concrete. More recently, Wang et al [Wang, 2003h; Wang et al, 2003i] incorporates the randomly distributed voids of real asphalt concrete specimens and used the Stress Concentration Factor as a performance indicator. Results indicated that the stress concentration factor may serve as a good candidate for mixture performance. Currently FEM is more matured than the DEM approach. It is anticipated that this method will become widely accepted in the near future when realistic constitutive models on mastics and binder can be developed.

BEM application has recently been developed by Birgisson and his colleagues [Birgisson et al, 2002]. This approach has its unique features in reducing the simulation time because only the elements at the boundaries of interest are needed.

4 OTHER APPLICATIONS

There are many other applications including using XCT for cracking detection [Braz et al, 1999; Read, 2000; Offrel and Magnusso, 2002], forensic study, evaluation of the internal structure evolution during compaction [Jonsson et al, 2002; Masad et al, 2002; Tashman et al, 2002] and permeability study. It is believed that XCT would find more applications in the characterization of aggregates and asphalt concrete in the near future with overall improvements in detector technology, image processing and analysis, and computational software development.

5 SUMMARY AND CONCLUSIONS

X-ray Computerized Tomography has been successfully used in the characterization of aggregates and asphalt concrete in many aspects. Its unique capability to obtain the 3D microstructure of these materials nondestructively allows the fundamental mechanism of strength, deformation and permeability of asphalt concrete be better understood. The microstructural quantifies will also enhance the modeling of these materials. It is anticipated that XCT in conjunction with modeling and computational techniques will make the digital specimen and multiple functional digital tester techniques realistic in the near future to improve the understanding of the behavior of asphalt concrete and to enhance mix design and performance predictions.

REFERENCES

Arduino, P. (1996). Multiphase Description of Deforming Porous Media by the Finite Element Method. Ph.D. Dissertation, Georgia Institute of Technology, Atlanta.

Buttlar, W.G. and You, Z. (2001). Discrete Element Modeling of Asphalt Concrete: Microfabric Approach. Transportation Research Record, No. 1757, pp. 111–118.

Birgisson, B., Sangpetngam, B. and Roque, R. (2002). Predicting Viscoelastic Response and Crack Growth in Asphalt Mixtures with the Boundary Element Method. Transportation Research Record, No. 1789, pp. 129–135.

Braz, D., Da Motta, L.M.G. and Lopes, R.T. (1999). Computed tomography in the fatigue test analysis of an asphaltic mixture. Applied Radiation and Isotopes, *Appl Radiat Isot*, Vol. 50, No. 4, pp. 661–671.

Chang, C.S. and Ma, L. (1991). A Micromechanical-Based Micropolar Theory for Deformation of Granular Solids. *Int. J. Solids Structures*, Vol.28, No.1, pp. 67–86.

Chang, G.K. and Meegoda, J.N. (1999). Micromechanical Model for Temperature Effects Of Hot-Mix Asphalt Concrete Transportation Research Record, No. 1687, pp. 95–103.

Cheng, D., Little, D.N., Lytton, R.L. and Holste, J.C. (2002). Surface Energy Measurement of Asphalt and its Application to Predicting Fatigue and Healing in Asphalt Mixtures. Transportation Research Record, No. 1810, pp. 44–53.

Christoffersen, J., Mehrabadi, M.M. and Nemat-Nasser, S. (1981). A Micromechanical Description of Granular Material Behavior. *Journal of Applied Mechanics*, Vol. 48, pp. 339–344.

Chudnovsky, A., Dolgopolsky, A. and Kachanov, M. (1987a). Elastic Interaction of a Crack with a Microcrack Array-I. Formulation of the Problem and General Form of the Solution. *Int. J. Solids and Structures*, Vol. 23, No. 1, pp. 1–10.

Chudnovsky, A., Dolgopolsky, A. and Kachanov, M. (1987b). Elastic Interaction of a Crack with a Microcrack Array-II. Elastic Solution for Two Crack Configurations (Piecewise Constant and Linear Approximations). *Int. J. Solids and Structures*, Vol.23, No.1, pp. 11–21.

Cundall, P.A. and Strack, O.D.L. (1979). A distinct element model for granular assemblies. *Geotechnique*, Vol. 29, pp. 47–65.

DeHoff, R.T. and Rhines, F.R. (1968). Quantitative microscopy. McGraw-Hill, New York.

Epps, J., Monismith, C.L., Alavi, S.H., and Mitchell, T.M. (1997). WesTrack Full-Scale Test Track: Interim Findings. http://www.westrack.com/wt_04.htm

Ferrari, M., Vladimir, T., Granik, A.L., Nadeau, J.C. (Eds.) (1997). Advances in Doublet Mechanics, Springer.

Fu, Yanrong and Linbing Wang (2003). A Practical Method to Represent Particles of Irregular Shape in DEM Simulation. In Submission to ASCE EM 17 2004.

Garboczi, E.J. (2002). Three-dimensional Mathematical Analysis of Particle Shape Using X-ray Tomography and Spherical Harmonics: Application to Aggregates Used in Concrete. Cement and Concrete Research, Vol. 32, No. 10, pp. 1621–1638.

Green, A.E. and Naghdi, P.M. (1967). A Theory of Mixtures. *Arch. Rat. Mech. Anal.*, Vol. 24, pp. 243–263.

Granik, V.T. and Ferrari, M. (1993). Microstructural Mechanics of Granular Media. Mechanics of Materials, Vol.15, pp. 301–322.

Goodman, M.A. and Cowin, S.C. (1972). A Continuum Theory for Granular Materials. Arch. Rational Mechanics Analysis. Vol.44, pp. 248–266.

Jonsson, M., Partl, M.N. and Flisch, A. (2002). Comparison of Different Compaction Methods Using X-ray Computer Tomography. EMPA Report.

Kanatani, K.I. (1984a). Stereological determination of structural anisotropy. *Int. Engng. Sci.* Vol.22, No.5, pp 531–546.

Kanatani, K.I. (1984b). Distribution of Directional Data and Fabric Tensors. *Int. J. Engng. Sci.* Vol.22, No.2, pp. 149–164.

Kanatani, K.I. (1985). Procedures for stereological estimation of structural anisotropy. *Int. Engng. Sci.* Vol.23, No.5, pp. 587–598.

Kim, H., Haas, CT., Rauch, AF., and Browne, C. (2002). Wavelet-Based Three-Dimensional Descriptors of Aggregate Particles. Transportation Research Record, No.1787, pp. 109–116.

Krishnan, J.M. and Rao, C.L. (2000). Mechanics of Air Voids Reduction of Asphalt Concrete Using Mixture Theory. *International Journal of Engineering Science*, Vol.38, pp. 1331–1354.

Krishnan, J.M. and Rao, C.L. (2001). Permeability and Bleeding of Asphalt Concrete Using Mixture Theory. *International Journal of Engineering Science*, Vol.39, pp. 611–627.

Kuo, C.Y., Frost, J.D. and Chameau, J.L. (1998), "Image Analysis Determination of Stereology Based Fabric Tensors", *Geotechnique*, Vol.48, No. 4, pp. 515–525.

Lacy, T.E., McDowell, D.L., Willice, P.A. and Talreja, R. (1997). On Representation of Damage Evolution in Continuum Damage Mechanics. *International Journal of Damage Mechanics*, Vol.6, pp. 62–95.

Lacy, T.E., McDowell, D.L., Willice, P.A. and Talreja, R. (1999). Gradient Concept for Evolution of Damage. Mechanics of Materials, Vol.31, pp. 831–860.

Masad, E., Somadevan, N., Bahia, H.U. and Kose, S. (2001). Modeling And Experimental Measurements of Strain Distribution in Asphalt Mixes. *Journal of Transportation Engineering*, Vol.127, No.6, pp. 477–485.

Masad, E., Jandhyala, V.K., Dasgupta, N., Somadevan, N. and Shashidhar, N. (2002). Characterization of Air Void Distribution in Asphalt Mixes Using X-Ray Computed Tomography. *Journal of Materials in Civil Engineering.* Vol.14, No.2, pp. 122–129.

Maugin, G.A. (1993). Momentum and Pseudomomentum in Matter (Newtonian versus Eshelby Mechanics), Proc. Roy. Soc. London., A.

Murakami, S. (1988). Mechanical modeling of material damage. *J. Appl. Mech.*, Vol.55, pp. 280–286.

Nemat-Nasser, S. and Hori, M. (1999). Micromechanics: Overall Properties of Heterogeneous Materials. North Holland.

Offrel, P. and Magnusson, R. (2002). Computerized Tomography as a Tool for Crack Analysis in Asphalt Layers. *International Journal of Road Materials and Pavement Design*. Vol.3, No.1, pp. 49–72.

Papagiannakis, A.T., Abbas, A. and Masad, E. (2002). Micromechanical Analysis of Viscoelastic Properties of Asphalt Concretes. Transportation Research Record, No.1789, pp. 113–120.

Read, J.M. (2000). New Method for Measuring Crack Propagation in Asphalts. *International Journal of Pavement Engineering*. Vol.1, No.1, pp.15–34.

Rothenburg, L. and Bathurst, R.J. (1992). Micromechanical Features of Granular Assemblies with Planar Elliptical Particles. *Geotechnique*, Vol.42, No.1, pp. 79–95.

Sadd, M.H., Dai, Q.L., Parameswaran, V. and Shukla, A. (2003). Simulation of Asphalt Materials Using Finite Element and Micromechanical Model with Damage Mechanics. TRB 2003.

Shashidhar, N. (1999). X-ray tomography of asphalt concrete. Transportation Research Record, No.1681, pp. 186–192.

Tashman, L., Masad, E., D'Angelo, J., Bukowski, J., and Harman, T. (2002). X-Ray Tomography to Characterize Air Void Distribution in Superpave Gyratory Compacted Specimens. *International Journal of Pavement Engineering*. Vol.3, No.1, pp. 19–28

Underwoood, E.E. (1970). Quantitative Stereology, Addison-Wesley, Reading.

Voyiadjis, G.Z. and Kattan, P. (1999). Advances in Damage Mechanics: Metals and Metal Matrix Composites, 542 p., Elsevier, Oxford, ISBN 0-08-043601-3.

Wang, L.B., Lai, J.S. and Frost, J.D. (1997). Fourier Morphological Descriptors of Aggregate Profiles. 2nd international Conference on Image Technology Applications in Civil Engineering, Sweden.

Wang, L.B. (1998). An Evaluation of the Microstructures and the Macro-Behavior of Unbonded and Bonded Granular Materials, Ph.D. Thesis, School of Civil and Environmental Engineering, Georgia Institute of Technology.

Wang, L.B. (1999). 3D FEM Simulation for WesTrack Mixes from X-ray Tomography Images. Research Report, School of Civil and Environmental Engineering, Georgia Institute of Technology.

Wang, L.B., Frost, J.D. and Shashidhar, N. (2001a). Microstructure Study of Westrack Mixes from X-ray Tomography Images. TRR No.1767, pp. 85–94.

Wang, L.B., Frost, J.D. and Lai, J.S. (2001b). "*Quantify the Doublet Distribution of Granular Materials*". Submitted to the special issue on microstructure characterization and modeling of ASCE, *Journal of Engineering Mechanics*, Vol. 127, No.7, pp. 720–729.

Wang, L.B., Frost, J.D. and Mohammad, L. (2002a). Three-Dimensional Aggregate Evaluation Using X-ray Tomography Imaging, TRB 2002.

Wang, L.B., Frost, J.D., Voyiadjis, G. and Harman, T.P. (2002b). Quantification of Damage Parameters Using X-ray Tomography Images. *Journal of Mechanics of Materials*, Vol.35, pp. 777–790.

Wang, L.B., Wang, Y.P., Mohammad, L. and Harman, T. (2003a). Voids Distribution and Performance of Asphalt Concrete. *International Journal of Pavement*, Vol.1, No.3.

Wang, L.B., Wang, X., Mohammad, L.M. and Wang, Y.P. (2003b). Evaluation of the mechanical properties of asphalt concrete using mixture theory. ASCE, *Journal of Materials in Civil Engineering*.

Wang, L.B., Park, J.Y., Frost, J.D. and Harman, T. (2003c). Quantification of the Contact Normal, Branch Vector and Particle Orientation Distribution Using X-ray Tomography Imaging. In Submission to ASCE, *Journal of International Geomechanics*.

Wang, L.B. and Frost, J.D. (2003d). Quantification of Aggregate Specific Surface Area Using X-ray Tomography Imaging. ASCE Geotechnical Special Publication, In Press.

Wang, L.B. (2003e). Enhancing Rutting Performance of Flexible Pavements (Characterization of Asphalt Concrete Using X-ray Computerized Tomography). FHWA MIHE Research Report.

Wang, L.B., Frost, J.D. and Lai, J.S. (2003f). 3D Digital Representation of the Microstructure of Granular Materials. *Journal of Civil Engineering Computing*, In Press.

Wang, L.B. Jin-Young Park and Louay Mohammad (2003g). Quantification of Morphology Characteristics of Aggregate from Profile Images. 2003 TRB.

Wang, L.B. (2003h). Stress Concentration Factor of Poroelastic Material by FEM Simulation and X-ray Tomography Imaging. ASCE Engineering Mechanics Conference, Seattle, WA.

Wang, L.B., Wang, Y.P., Mohammad, L. and Chris Abadie (2003i). Stress Concentration Factor as a Performance Indicator. In Submission to 2004 TRB.

X-ray CT for Geomaterials; Soils, Concrete, Rocks – Otani & Obara (eds.)
© 2004 Swets & Zeitlinger. Lisse, ISBN 90 5809 666 1

Author Index